The American Handbook of Psychiatric Nursing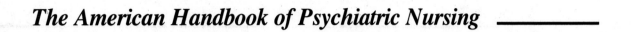

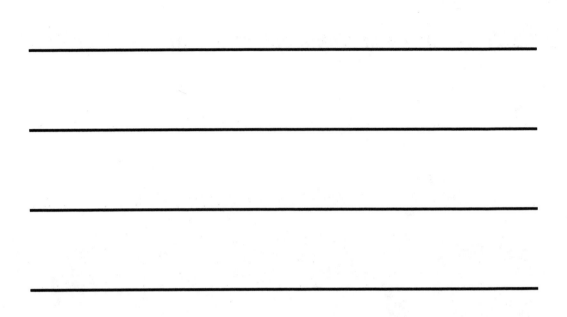

 J. B. Lippincott Company

Philadelphia

New York

St. Louis

Mexico City

London

São Paulo

Sydney

The American Handbook of Psychiatric Nursing

Suzanne Lego, RN, PhD, CS, Editor

Private Practice, New York City

and Demarest, New Jersey

45 Contributors

Sponsoring Editor: William Burgower
Manuscript Editor: Helen Ewan
Indexer: Sandra King
Art Director: Tracy Baldwin
Designer: Arlene Putterman
Production Supervisor: Kathleen P. Dunn
Production Coordinator: Charles W. Field
Compositor: Hampton Graphics
Printer/Binder: Murray Printing Company

6 5 4 3

Library of Congress Cataloging in Publication Data
Main entry under title:

The American handbook of psychiatric nursing.

  Bibliography: p.
  Includes index.
  1. Psychiatric nursing—Handbooks, manuals, etc.
2. Psychotherapy—Handbooks, manuals, etc. I. Lego,
Suzanne. [DNLM: 1. Psychiatric nursing. 2. Mental
disorders—Nursing. WY 160 A5118]
RC440.A55 1984   610.73′68   83-24882
ISBN 0-397-54370-0

The authors and publisher have exerted every effort to ensure
that drug selection and dosage set forth in this text are in
accord with current recommendations and practice at the time
of publication. However, in view of ongoing research,
changes in government regulations, and the constant flow of
information relating to drug therapy and drug reactions, the
reader is urged to check the package insert for each drug for
any change in indications and dosage and for added warnings
and precautions. This is particularly important when the
recommended agent is a new or infrequently employed drug.

To Dick and Rich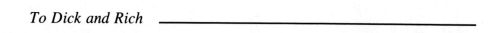

Contributors

LINDA BARILE, RN, MN
Assistant Professor, Quinnipiac College, Hamden, Connecticut

LINDA S. BEEBER, RN, MA
Assistant Professor, Psychiatric–Mental Health Nursing, Syracuse University, College of Nursing, Syracuse, New York

JANET CRAIG, RN, MSN
Clinical Director of Nursing, Marshall Pickens Hospital, Greenville, South Carolina

JOAN CUNNINGHAM, RN, MA
Assistant Professor of Nursing, County College of Morris, Randolph Township, New Jersey

CANDY DATO, RN, MS
Clinical Specialist, St. Luke's–Roosevelt Hospital, New York, New York

THERESA S. FOLEY, RN, PhD, CS
Assistant Professor, School of Nursing, University of Michigan, Ann Arbor, Michigan

JOYCE J. FITZPATRICK, RN, PhD, FAAN
Dean, School of Nursing, Case Western Reserve University, Cleveland, Ohio

KAREN DAVIS FRANK, RN, MA
Psychiatric Coordinator, Englewood Hospital, Englewood, New Jersey

ELEANOR RODIO FURLONG, RN, MA
Director of Nursing, Ancora Psychiatric Hospital, Hammonton, New Jersey

SHIRLEY TeMAAT HOLLINGSWORTH, RN, MPH
Assistant Professor, Widener University, School of Nursing, Chester, Pennsylvania

SUSAN L. JONES, RN, PhD
Associate Professor of Nursing, Kent State University, Kent, Ohio

MAUREEN SHAWN KENNEDY, RN, MA
Director of Education, Medical Media Associates, Livingston, New Jersey

NORINE J. KERR, RN, MN
Clinical Nurse Consultant, Western Missouri MHC, Kansas City, Missouri

TERRIE KIRKPATRICK, RN, MS
Staff Development Instructor, Marshall Pickens Hospital, Greenville, South Carolina

KATHLEEN O'BRIEN KOBBERGER, RN, MS
Clinical Specialist, Fair Oaks Hospital, Summit, New Jersey

SUZANNE LEGO, RN, PhD, CS
Private Practice, New York City and Demarest, New Jersey

NADA LIGHT, RN, MA
Formerly Instructor, Graduate Program in Child Psychiatric Nursing, College of Physicians and Surgeons, Columbia University, New York, New York

MAXINE E. LOOMIS, RN, PhD, CS, FAAN
Director, Doctoral Program, College of Nursing, University of Illinois at the Medical Center, Chicago, Illinois

KEM BETTY LOUIE, RN, PhD
Assistant Professor, Villanova University, Villanova, Pennsylvania

MARIE McGILLICUDDY, RN, PhD
Associate Professor, Herbert H. Lehman College, City University of New York, Bronx, New York

KATHLEEN MCQUADE, RN, MA
Clinical Nurse Specialist in Human Relations, St. Vincents Hospital, New York, New York

SHARON WARD MILLER, RN, MA
Instructor, Staff Development, New York Hospital–Cornell Medical Center, Westchester Division, White Plains, New York

JEAN MOORE, RN, MS
Regional Training Coordinator, N.Y.S. Office of Mental Health, Albany, New York

VIOLA MOROFKA, RN, PhD
Associate Professor of Nursing, Kent State University, Kent, Ohio

TERRY MORTON, RN, MS
Director of Nursing, Bangor Mental Health Institute, Bangor, Maine

THOMAS F. NOLAN, RN, PhD
Professor of Nursing, Sonoma State University, Rohnert Park, California

ANITA WERNER O'TOOLE, RN, PhD
Professor of Nursing, Kent State University, Kent, Ohio

RACHEL PARIOS, RN, MSN
Psychiatric Nurse Administrator, Beth Israel Medical Center, Newark, New Jersey

KATHLEEN REKASIS, RN, MSN
Nurse Coordinator, Chicago Lakeshore Hospital, Chicago, Illinois

LISA ROBINSON, RN, PhD
Professor, Psychiatric Nursing, University of Maryland, Baltimore, Maryland

JOHN ROSATO, RN, MS
Nurse Administrator, Austin State Hospital, Austin, Texas

LINDA ST. GERMAIN, RN, MSN
Nurse Coordinator, Chicago Lakeshore Hospital, Chicago, Illinois

NANCY SARGENT, RN, MSN
Associate Director of Nursing, Friends Hospital, Philadelphia, Pennsylvania

THOMAS A. SHERWOOD, RN, MA, MPH, MEd
Chief, Nursing Services, Veterans Administration Medical Center, Coatesville, Pennsylvania

MARIE C. SMITH, RN, MA, CS
Instructor, Herbert H. Lehman College, City University of New York, Bronx, New York

MARIE E. SNYDER, RN, MS, JD, CS
Snyder and Sweeney, Attorneys-At-Law, Boston, Massachusetts

ARDIS R. SWANSON, RN, PhD
Associate Professor, Graduate Programs, SEHNAP, New York University, New York, New York

CYNTHIA M. TAYLOR, RN, MSN, CS
Private Practice, Chicago, Illinois

MARTHA MERRITT TOUSLEY, RN, MS
Director of Staff Development, Fair Oaks Hospital, Summit, New Jersey

ELIZABETH MERRILL VARCAROLIS, RN, MA
Associate Professor of Nursing, Manhattan Community College, City University of New York, New York, New York

MARY WEBSTER, RN, MS
Psychotherapist, Elizabeth General Medical Center, Elizabeth, New Jersey

SHEILA RAFTER WEBSTER, RN, MA
Former Director, Outpatient Clinic, South Beach Psychiatric Center, Brooklyn, New York

SHEILA ROUSLIN WELT, RN, MS
Private Practice, New York City, Ridgewood, and Morristown, New Jersey

JOAN SMITH WINTER, RN, MA, CS
Coordinator, Mobile Outreach Team, St. Luke's–Roosevelt Hospital, New York, New York

MARY ANN ZILLMAN, RN, MSN
Nursing Care Coordinator, Mt. Sinai Hospital Medical Center of Chicago, Chicago, Illinois

Foreword

When I became an RN, more than a half-century ago, there were exceedingly few textbooks on psychiatric nursing. There was, of course, the first text, written in 1920 by a nurse, Harriet Bailey. Slowly, other publications by psychiatric nurses began to appear. In the last decade, there has been a proliferation of psychiatric nursing texts. This is a positive development. It suggests not only that there are more experts in this clinical area of nursing but greater interest in clarifying the many dimensions of psychiatric nursing from different standpoints. Yet there is a noticeable gap in psychiatric nursing literature, which *The American Handbook of Psychiatric Nursing* fills.

In the last few decades, two major developments have made it more difficult for psychiatric nurses to keep up with new knowledge and practical know-how. There has been a veritable explosion of knowledge, particularly in the behavioral sciences and in the field of psychiatric–mental health care. And there is exciting progress in the development of theory and theory application related to nursing practice. Each new nursing textbook helps nurses to keep in touch with aspects of these two evolving trends.

The merit of *The American Handbook of Psychiatric Nursing* is that it is a comprehensive reference manual. It covers a broad range of theoretical and practical knowledge on clinical problems. It also addresses forms of service other than direct clinical practice in which psychiatric nurses are engaged, as well as contemporary issues that impinge upon and influence the environment in which nurses work. It is written in clear, succinct form—some of it outlined—and is arranged for ease of use. The work is in a sense both a textbook and desk manual, a book to be studied in depth or to be consulted briefly at the point of need for specific information. This work, then, summarizes a great deal of current information relevant to the broad and complex workrole of psychiatric nurses. It fills a gap by providing in one publication a readily available way to keep up with what is new in the field of psychiatric–mental health nursing.

Hildegard E. Peplau
Professor Emerita, Rutgers University

Preface

Psychiatric–mental health nurses are called upon today to function in many varied ways. Broadly speaking, we are administrators, teachers, supervisors, clinical specialists, and, although "bedside" hardly seems applicable, we are "client-side" practitioners.

The American Handbook of Psychiatric Nursing is designed to help psychiatric nurses keep up with the myriad of roles, therapies, practices, and procedures that our field now comprises. Tables, lists, outlines, and charts are provided to make information easily accessible. At the same time, theory is integrated throughout the manual so that the reader can appreciate the rationale for nursing actions.

The first nursing action is assessment. Part I is written to help the nurse to gather data about the client, to apply these data to diagnostic categories, and to formulate a treatment plan based on all the data.

Psychiatric–mental health nurses are called upon today to design structures that provide specific mental health services. If we do not design them ourselves, we should be familiar with ideal conditions for these structures. The chapters in Part II are written by nurses who have learned what works and what does not.

Next we must choose a therapeutic modality for each client. Part III provides twenty different therapeutic modalities commonly practiced by psychiatric–mental health nurses.

Specific clients have specific needs, whatever mode is chosen. The nurse who works side by side with clients in hospitals, day treatment programs, and so forth must know how to help these clients daily over time. Part IV presents fifteen kinds of specific clients whom nurses encounter in these settings.

Part V includes procedures used in inpatient settings. These are brief chapters, since the essence of psychiatric–mental health nursing is communication.

The final parts of the manual describe broad areas of psychiatric–mental health nursing that deserve to be examined separately. These include psychopharmacology and legal, women's, and cultural issues.

My choice of the word "client" over "patient" deserves a brief explanation. William Safire wrote, "Lawyers have clients, doctors have patients." Where does this leave nurses? While I have often thought of the word "client" as a euphemism, after careful consideration, I concluded that "client" could be used in any situation, but "patient" would be inappropriate in some chapters, particularly those involving holistic approaches such as relaxation. However, our language does not allow for a total conversion, and the familiar terms, "inpatient," "outpatient," patient government, and a few others, remain.

In the tradition of the *Lippincott Manual of Nursing Practice,* this book is written in simple, practical terms designed to make the material immediately usable. It is written for the practitioner, the student, the instructor, and the administrator. Because of its broad scope within the field of psychiatric–mental health nursing, it should be helpful to beginners as well as to experienced clinicians.

Suzanne Lego, RN, PhD, CS

Acknowledgments

I would like to thank the 44 contributors without whom this book would not have been possible. Each chapter was reviewed by two or more reviewers, usually experts in the area of practice being described. I want to thank the reviewers who reviewed large sections of the book, including Linda Barile, Anita Werner O'Toole, Marie Smith, Cynthia Taylor, and Sheila Rouslin Welt. Reviewers who lent their much appreciated expertise in specific areas were Virginia Trotter Betts, Steve Lipton, Mary McAndrew, Virginia Moore, Shirley Smoyak, Katherine VanSavage-Fink, and Rory Zahourek.

My mentor, Hildegard E. Peplau, was kind enough to write the Foreword and to review a part of the book; she has been a constant source of help and encouragement throughout my career. I want to thank Earl Shepherd, who got the project going and offered many helpful suggestions, and my editor, Bill Burgower, who has been deeply involved in the project from start to finish, even after a change of positions at J. B. Lippincott Company.

I appreciate the efforts of Joyce Logan, who typed the first draft, and Mary Loch and Carol Lee Shanley, who worked long and obsessionally on the final draft, typing and proofreading.

On a personal note, I would like to thank my husband and friend, Dick, who stood in line at the South Hackensack post office approximately 198 times to mail manuscripts to authors and reviewers and who, without a word, took over the running of our household during the last month of manuscript preparation. And a thank-you to my son, Rich, who faithfully asked every evening, "How many more chapters?"

Contents

Part IV   Counseling Specific Clients

Part V *Psychiatric Nursing Procedures*

Part I

Assessment and Planning

1

Psychiatric Nursing Assessment

Mary Webster

OVERVIEW

Description
Role of the Nurse
Goals
The Psychiatric Interview
The Psychosocial History
Assessment of Current Status
Mini-mental State Examination

Description* The psychiatric nursing assessment provides an opportunity for the nurse to gather data to be used in treatment of the client. Specific information about the client's thoughts, feelings, and behaviors is obtained. In addition, the environmental stimuli that affect these thoughts, feelings, and behaviors are investigated.

There are three basic elements of a psychiatric nursing assessment:

1. Psychosocial history
2. Determination of current status
3. Mental status examination

The most widely used assessment *tool* is the psychiatric interview. The assessment may be completed in a single, initial interview or in several interviews of shorter duration, when the assessment is part of the total evaluation of a client whose primary problem is physical illness.

The assessment interview may take place in a variety of clinical settings. These include

1. Emergency rooms
2. Medical–surgical units
3. Intensive care units or cardiac care units
4. Psychiatric inpatient units
5. Crisis units
6. Community mental health centers
7. Private practice

Role of the Nurse The role assumed by the nurse in the psychiatric nursing assessment will depend on the level of nursing preparation and the practice setting. The psychiatric nurse in a psychiatric or medical setting offers direct care through the nurse–client relationship. Assessment is used to elicit sufficient information to identify problems and to formulate beginning plans for intervention. This formulation, or nursing diagnosis, should be an accurate, concisely worded statement that[8]

1. Describes the client's condition and circumstances affecting his response
2. Points to primary or contributory causes
3. Points by implication to the nursing actions needed to prevent, minimize, or alleviate the problem

   Ex: "Anxiety and depression related to fear of impending surgery for possible carcinoma of the breast."

   Ex: "Severe anxiety and depression related to the recent death of husband, leading to inability to fulfill usual daily activities."

Goals The clinical specialist in psychiatric nursing is often responsible for the initial assessment and diagnosis of the client. The goals of the clinical specialist are to

A. **IDENTIFY PSYCHIATRIC EMERGENCIES**

Emergencies such as acute drug reactions, alcoholic coma, and suicidal and assaultive impulses and behaviors may necessitate immediate intervention.

B. **ASSESS THE NEED FOR CONSULTATION**

Other mental health professionals may be needed to aid in assessment and treatment recommendations. These may include

1. Physician to provide a medical examination

---

*For simplicity, the nurse will be referred to as "she," and the client as "he."

2. Psychiatrist to perform a psychiatric evaluation, medication assessment, or involuntary commitment
3. Psychologist to administer psychological tests to assess the extent of thought disorder or level of intellectual functioning
4. Neurologist to rule out organicity, seizure disorder, or brain lesion
5. Psychiatric social worker to assess family and community support systems, referrals to other agencies, or need for emergency housing

C. **FORMULATE AN UNDERSTANDING OF THE CLIENT'S PREMORBID LEVEL OF FUNCTIONING**
This would include ego strengths and deficits.

D. **FORMULATE AN UNDERSTANDING OF THE CLIENT'S PSYCHOPATHOLOGY**
This will enable the clinical specialist to fulfill the multiaxial diagnostic classification system of the DSM III (see Appendix B).

E. **ESTABLISH TREATMENT RECOMMENDATIONS**
Recommendations should be acceptable to the client and his family.

F. **FORMULATE A PROGNOSIS**

The Psychiatric Interview

1. The psychiatric interview is a goal-directed communication between the nurse and the client. It provides an opportunity for the nurse to experience who the client is and to understand how he has developed through the course of his life events.[2]
2. The purpose of the interview is to establish rapport with the client and to gain knowledge of his usual activities and how he perceives himself and those in his environment.
3. The interview provides factual information about the client and affords the nurse the opportunity to observe such personal characteristics of the client as appearance, speech, and nonverbal communications.
4. Interviews with informants other than the client provide independent information that may corroborate the client's perceptions of his situation or point to important inconsistencies. This source of information is particularly important when the client is inaccessible (severely delusional, confused, catatonic) or uncooperative. Chart 1–1 shows nursing actions and their theoretical rationale when interviewing.

The Psychosocial History[1,11]

The psychosocial history is better understood if it is organized into identifying data, chief complaint, present problem, and past personal history.

Identifying Data

1. Age
2. Sex
3. Race and ethnic affiliation
4. Marital status
5. Number and ages of children/siblings
6. Spouse/parents' ages (still living)
7. Living arrangements
8. Occupation
9. Education
10. Religion—degree of commitment

Chart 1–1
NURSING ACTIONS AND THEORETICAL RATIONALE WHEN INTERVIEWING

Nursing Action	*Theoretical Rationale*
The nurse introduces herself by name, title, and role. The nurse addresses the client by name and asks how he prefers to be addressed.	Addressing the client by name and introducing herself by name and title is a way for the nurse to convey respect for the client.
The nurse provides an interview room that is private and quiet, and does not contain distracting objects. When a room is unavailable, as in the CCU, some measure of privacy is provided by using curtains and screens. Interruptions and interference by other staff members are kept to a minimum.	Privacy encourages the reticent, embarrassed client to disclose his personal problems and feelings. It also eliminates some of the client's concerns about confidentiality. Distracting objects may prove disturbing to a confused, disoriented, or psychotic client. The psychiatric interview is demanding of both the client and the nurse and requires concentration.
The nurse provides two chairs of equal size and comfort and a choice of seating. Additional seating should be available for family interviews and consultations.	The choice of where he sits provides clues to the client's need for personal space, fears of interpersonal closeness, and possible suspiciousness.
The nurse makes prior arrangements and establishes a protocol to provide for safety and security for the client and herself. This is particularly important in the emergency room or other medical treatment settings.	Medical paraphernalia is potentially dangerous and may also frighten the client. Help is sometimes needed to manage the confused, assaultive, or suicidal client. Prior arrangement for this help will allay the nurse's anxiety. Limit setting is also reassuring to the disturbed or impulsive client.
The nurse begins with an open-ended question (a question that indicates a general inquiry, defines an area of interest, but leaves a wide range of interpretation possible). Ex: "What brought you here today?" The nurse uses the kind of response, verbal or nonverbal, that encourages the client to say more. The response may be anything from an expectant look to a request to "tell me more about that."	The open-ended question is broad and allows the client to verbalize his views, thoughts, and feelings. The closed question tends to elicit facts only. Direct, more specific questions are asked (to get additional information) after the client has told his story. This response is nonrestrictive and does not sharply define the answer for the client, but rather elicits spontaneous and individualistic responses that describe how he sees his problem.
The nurse communicates with the client by the use of silences. Silences, on the part of both the client and the nurse, are accompanied by facial and bodily expression, gestures, or postures that convey meaning. If, for example, the client transmits a feeling of anger, the nurse might state something about the anger and ask the client to put it into words.	The nurse's silence can convey concern and interest, and can facilitate continued communication. The nurse can determine the possible meaning of the client's silences by observing his nonverbal communication and by examining her empathic response.
The nurse uses responses that convey support, empathy, and understanding. Ex: "You seem to feel guilty about being unable to work."	This type of response affirms that the nurse accepts the feelings and information the client has offered with concern but without criticism.
The nurse uses confrontation and interpretation to make explicit a connection between a feeling or symptom and the client's interpersonal or intrapsychic life. Ex: "You seem to have these headaches at times when you are most angry."	This encourages the client to make his own additional connections and to explore matters further.
The nurse pays attention to the interview content (words spoken), as well as to the process (what is happening) between the client and the nurse. Ex: The client states that he feels relaxed but fidgets in his chair and cannot make eye contact.	By attending to the two levels of a message, the content and the process, the nurse may more accurately assess the client, what is occurring in the interview, and what may be occurring in his life.

Chief Complaint   The chief complaint is the presenting problem for which the client is seeking professional help. The chief complaint should be stated in the client's own words.

History of the Present
Problem

1. When did the problem begin?
2. How does the client describe his symptoms?
3. What has happened recently to upset the client? The amount of stress the client has been recently experiencing can be estimated by using the Holmes and Rahe Social Readjustment Rating Scale (see Table 1–1.)[6] An accumulation of 200 or more life change units in 1 year can trigger a physical or psychiatric problem.
4. Has there been a change in somatic functioning—sleep disturbance, appetite or weight change, or change in sexual interest or performance?
5. Has there been a change in the client's mental status—feelings of anxiety or depression?

Past Personal History

A. **INFANCY**
   1. Did the client's mother experience prenatal difficulties or problems during labor and delivery?
   2. Was the client breast fed or bottle fed?
   3. Are there memories of toilet training, motor development, or early or delayed use of language?

B. **CHILDHOOD**
   1. What childhood diseases or hospitalizations occurred?
   2. How would he describe his relationship with each of his parents?
   3. Were there nightmares, enuresis, or phobias?
   4. How did he adjust to school and peers?
   5. Was there any child abuse or sexual abuse?
   6. Did his parents drink? How much?

C. **ADOLESCENCE**
   1. How did the client react to the onset of puberty?
   2. How did the parents react?
   3. Did he feel adequately prepared for the maturational changes?
   4. How did he relate to his family?
   5. Was he overcompliant or aggressively rebellious?
   6. How did he relate to his peers?
   7. Did he feel part of the "in-group" or isolated and different?
   8. How did he react to any sexual experimentation?
   9. Was there acting-out behavior involving drugs, sex, or truancy, or difficulties with breaking the law?

D. **ADULTHOOD**
   1. What level of education did the client achieve?
   2. Does he feel that he accomplished his educational objectives?
   3. What is his work history?
   4. Does he feel satisfied with his work?
   5. Was there interruption of education or work owing to physical or psychological difficulties?
   6. What is his sexual orientation or preference?
   7. Does he feel comfortable with his sexual/marital relationships?

Table 1–1
HOLMES AND RAHE SOCIAL READJUSTMENT RATING SCALE

Rank	Life Event	Life Change Units
1.	Death of spouse	100
2.	Divorce	73
3.	Marital separation	65
4.	Jail term	63
5.	Death of close family member	63
6.	Personal injury or illness	53
7.	Marriage	50
8.	Fired at work	47
9.	Marital reconciliation	45
10.	Retirement	45
11.	Change in health of family member	44
12.	Pregnancy	40
13.	Sex difficulties	39
14.	Gain of new family member	39
15.	Business readjustment	39
16.	Change in financial state	38
17.	Death of close friend	37
18.	Change to different line of work	36
19.	Change in number of arguments with spouse	35
20.	Mortgage over $10,000	31
21.	Foreclosure of mortgage or loan	30
22.	Change in responsibilities at work	29
23.	Son or daughter leaving home	29
24.	Trouble with in-laws	29
25.	Outstanding personal achievement	28
26.	Wife begin or stop work	26
27.	Begin or end school	25
28.	Change in living conditions	25
29.	Revision of personal habits	24
30.	Trouble with boss	23
31.	Change in work hours or conditions	20
32.	Change in residence	20
33.	Change in schools	20
34.	Change in recreation	19
35.	Change in church activities	19
36.	Change in social activities	18
37.	Mortgage or loan less than $10,000	17
38.	Change in sleeping habits	16
39.	Change in number of family get-togethers	15
40.	Change in eating habits	15
41.	Vacation	13
42.	Christmas	12
43.	Minor violations of the law	11

(Reprinted with permission from Holmes T, Rahe R: The Social Readjustment Rating Scale. J Psychosom Res 11:216, © 1967, Pergamon Press, Ltd.)

8. Is there any sexual dysfunction?
9. If client is female, has there been any difficulty conceiving, pregnancies, or abortions?
10. Does the client drink or use drugs? How much?

E. **MEDICAL HISTORY**
1. Has the client experienced any significant illness, injury, or surgery?
2. Did he require hospitalization?
3. How did he react to the illness or hospitalization?
4. Is he taking any prescribed or illicit drug?
5. Does he have any allergies?
6. Has he experienced any significant side effect of psychotropic medication?

F. **FAMILY HISTORY**
1. Who constitutes the client's nuclear family, extended family, and family of origin?
2. Was he an only child, the youngest, or oldest child?
3. Were there breakdowns in the family unit due to separation, divorce, or death?
4. Is there a history of physical or psychiatric illness in family members?
5. Is there a history of suicide attempts or completed suicide, alcoholism, or child abuse?

G. **PAST PSYCHIATRIC HISTORY**
1. Has the client received any psychiatric treatment in the past?
2. Has he been hospitalized for this treatment?
3. What medications were prescribed?
4. Did he receive electroconvulsive therapy?
5. What were the results of any treatment modality?

Assessment of Current Status

Physical Characteristics   Describe apparent age, manner of dress, personal hygiene, attitude toward the interviewer, posture, gait, gestures, facial expressions, and mannerisms. Is the client's attitude toward the interviewer cooperative, fearful, suspicious, or manipulative? Describe any indication of the client's identification with a subculture (for example, males with earrings, dyed hair, track marks).

Speech   Is it soft or loud, hesitant, slurred, pressured, rapid, mumbled, or whispered? Do his style and vocabulary convey archness, coyness, suspiciousness, arrogance, secretiveness, superiority, humor, or pretentiousness? Does he use loud expletives? Does he use speech to plead, frighten, command, seduce, shock, intimidate, or distract the nurse?[10]

Psychomotor Activity   Does the client display tics, agitation, twitches, psychomotor retardation, or hyperactivity? Does he touch the examiner, become combative, or display waxy flexibility? Is his body limp, rigid, agile, or clumsy?[7]

Mood   Mood is a pervasive and sustained emotion that colors the person's perception of the world.[7] How does the client say he feels? Describe depth, intensity, duration, and fluctuations of mood. Is client depressed, despairing, irritable, anxious, terrified, angry, expansive, euphoric, empty, or guilty?

Affect Affect is a person's emotional feeling tone and its outward manifestations.[5] Is affect depressed, blunted or flat, fearful, or angry? What is the range of affective expression? Is it consistent, labile, anhedonic, or appropriate to the situation and feelings verbalized?

Perception Perception is the awareness and intended integration of sensory impressions of the environment and their interpretation in light of experience.[9] Are there distortions in the client's perception of reality, including illusions, hallucinations, derealization, or depersonalization?

Orientation (See mini-mental state examination)
1. Does the client identify the date correctly? Can he estimate the time of day? The month and year?
2. Does the client know where he is?
3. Does the client know who the examiner is? Is he aware of the roles or names of the people with whom he is in contact?

Thought Processes Are there illogical stream of thought, lack of productivity, overabundance or paucity of ideas, flight of ideas, blocking, looseness of associations, tangentiality, circumstantiality, evasiveness, rambling, clanging, or use of neologisms?

Content of Thought
1. Is there preoccupation with illnesses, compulsions, phobias, homicidal or suicidal ideation, or specific antisocial urges?
2. Are there thought disturbances (delusions, ideas of reference and influence)? What meaning does the client attribute to these?
3. What is the client's capacity for abstract thinking? This can be assessed by the use of proverbs. The ability to interpret proverbs shows that the client has an intact fund of general information, the ability to apply this knowledge to unfamiliar situations, and the ability to think in the abstract. Client interpretations may be concrete, semiabstract, or abstract.[12] Tell the client, "I am going to tell you a saying which you may or may not have heard before. Explain in your own words what the saying means."
   Example: "Rome wasn't built in a day."
   • Concrete—"It took a long time to build Rome." "You can't build cities overnight."
   • Semiabstract—"Don't do things too fast."
   • Abstract—"Great things take time to achieve." "If something is worth doing, it is worth doing carefully."
4. Information and Intelligence—Is general grasp of information congruent with educational level achieved and intelligence?
5. Concentration—Is the client able to sustain attention over an extended period of time? Assess ability to concentrate by asking the client if he has had difficulty concentrating on tasks at home or at work. Ask the client to, "Count backwards from 100 by 7s (serial sevens—100, 93, 86, 79, 72)." If client cannot subtract 7s, can he do easier tasks—4×5, 7×3? Does anxiety, depression, or level of consciousness appear responsible for any difficulty?

Memory Memory is a general term for a mental process that allows the individual to store experiences and perceptions for recall at a later time.[12] Assess the client for
1. Remote memory—childhood data, events occurring when client was free of current problem

2. Recent past memory—the past few months
3. Recent memory—the past few days

Judgment   Judgment is the client's ability to form an opinion by discerning and comparing.[13] Is the client aware of the probable consequences of his social behaviors? Test judgment by asking the client what he would do in an imaginary situation, for example, if he found a stamped, addressed envelope in the street. Repeat questions and watch for a pattern of response that is not random in order not to misinterpret or overestimate the client's judgment.

Insight   Does the client understand and realize the significance of his symptoms and of the situation in which he finds himself?

Ego Strengths   Table 1–2 lists ego functions and their component factors, sample interviewing questions for assessing these factors, and some possible disturbances.[3]

(Text continues on page 15)

Table 1–2
EGO FUNCTIONS AND COMPONENT FACTORS, INTERVIEW QUESTIONS, POSSIBLE DISTURBANCE

Ego Function and Component Factors	Interview Questions	Possible Disturbance
1. Sense of Reality of the World and of the Self		
a. The experience of external events as real and as embedded in a familiar context	Do people and things around you sometimes feel unreal to you, foggy, or seen through a haze?	Alienation, emotional isolation; depersonalization; derealization; dreamlike states; fugues; major dissociations; identity diffusion
b. The experience of one's body (or parts of it) and its functioning and one's behavior as familiar and unobstructive, and as belonging to oneself	Have people or things ever looked closer or farther away, larger or smaller than you know they actually are?	
c. The degree of development of individuality, uniqueness, sense of self, and self-esteem	Have you ever had strange feelings in various parts of your body that could not be explained by something physical?	
d. The degree of separation of one's self-representations from one's object representations (*i.e.,* clarity of ego boundaries)	Have you ever had trouble feeling physically separate from and independent of others?	
	Do you ever feel that you can read someone's mind, or they yours?	
	Do you spend time wondering, ''Who am I?''	
2. Regulation and Control of Drive, Affect, and Impulse		
a. The directness of impulse expression, ranging from primitive acting out, through the activity of the impulse-ridden character, through neurotic acting out, to relatively indirect forms of behavioral expression	Do you have a lot of drive to be physically active or do you ever find it difficult to ''get going?'' Do you tend to be excitable and emotional about things? Do you consider yourself to be an overcontrolled or undercontrolled person?	Temper outbursts; habit and conduct disorders; low frustration tolerance; acting out; homicidal or suicidal tendencies; impulsiveness; drive-dominated behavior; chronic irritability and rage; excessive control of impulse

(continued)

Table 1–2
(continued)

Ego Function and Component Factors	Interview Questions	Possible Disturbance
b. The effectiveness of delay and control mechanisms; the degree of frustration tolerance	Do you ever have rapid changes in your mood? Are you a patient or impatient person? Are you easily frustrated? How well do you think you tolerate anxiety?	
3. Object Relations a. The degree and kind of relatedness to others (taking into account narcissism, symbiosis, separation–individuation, withdrawal trends, narcissistic object choice or extent of mutuality); degree of choice in maintaining object relations b. Primitivity–maturity of object relations—the extent to which present relationships are adaptively or maladaptively based upon older ones c. The extent to which the person perceives and responds to others as independent entities other than as extensions of himself	What were your father and mother like? How was your home life? How do you get along with your girlfriend/spouse/boss? Do you keep getting involved with the same kind of person? Do you prefer to get close to people or keep your distance? How easily are your feelings hurt? Are you sensitive to criticism? How well do you understand others? How well do they understand you? How do you get what you want from others? Who handles what in your household—like making major decisions? Who initiates sexual activity, you or your girlfriend/spouse?	Defensive social overactivity; withdrawal; detachment; symbiotic–dependent attachments; difficulty in perceiving others as separate
4. Thought Processes a. Degree of adaptiveness in memory, concentration, and attention b. The ability to conceptualize—the extent to which abstract and concrete thinking are appropriate to the situation c. The extent to which language and communication reflect primary or secondary process thinking	Do you have trouble concentrating—do you find your mind wandering when you read? What was the most significant thing you remember about your childhood? Do you have thoughts that stick in your mind so you can't get rid of them? How do you think they got there? Do you ever have thoughts that you feel others wouldn't understand?	Magical thinking; autistic logic, attention lapses; inability to concentrate; memory disturbances; concreteness; primitive thought functioning
5. Adaptive Regression in the Service of the Ego (ARISE) a. First phase of an oscillating process—degree of relaxation of perceptual and conceptual acuity with corresponding increase in ego awareness of previously preconscious and unconscious contents and the extent to which these "regressions" disrupt adaptation or are uncontrolled	What do you do when you're alone and you have nothing to do? Do you daydream—what about? Describe one of the most creative ideas you've ever had. Are you ever able to let go and think "crazy" thoughts without being upset or frightened? Do you ever get so carried away with your ideas that you find it difficult to come back down to earth?	Extreme rigidity in character structure and thinking, where fantasy and play are difficult or impossible; regression of any ego function produces anxiety and disruption of creativity; stereotyped thinking; intolerance of ambiguity

Table 1–2
(continued)

Ego Function and Component Factors	Interview Questions	Possible Disturbance
b. Second phase of the oscillating process—extent of controlled use of primary process thinking in allowing new configurations to emerge	What does it feel like when you listen to music you enjoy? Are you an inventive cook or do you prefer to follow recipes?	
6. Defensive Functioning a. Extent to which defense mechanisms, character defenses, and other defensive functioning have affected ideation, behavior, and the adaptive level of other ego functions b. Extent to which defenses have symptomatically succeeded or failed (*i.e.*, degree of emergence of anxiety, depression, and other dysphoric affects) c. Defensive functioning can be pathological or adaptive, depending on whether the defense leads to symptom formation or to healthy social adaptation.	Do things easily upset you? Do you feel you have ways to protect yourself from too many worries and anxiety? Do you have any fears like claustrophobia, fear of travel, or fear of crowds? Do you ever have strange thoughts or nightmares? When things throw you, how well are you able to pull yourself together? Are you concerned about what other people are saying about you?	Emergence of unconscious contents triggering extreme anxiety and panic, which then affect concentration and memory; pervasive feelings of vulnerability; fear of cracking up and falling apart; massive withdrawal from others in an attempt to prevent uncontrolled drive expression
7. Stimulus Barrier a. Sensitivity to external and internal stimuli and degree of adaptation b. Organization and integration of responses to various levels of sensory stimulation (*i.e.*, the effectiveness of management of excessive stimulus input)	Are you very sensitive to light, sound, or temperature? Are you irritable or jumpy when there's too much noise around you? Do you get bored when things are not exciting enough, or does excitement rattle you?	Oversensitivity to bright lights, loud sounds, temperature extremes, and pain, resulting in withdrawal, physical symptoms, or irritability; thresholds too high, which causes inability to perceive social cues and nuances; underresponsiveness to environmental stimuli
8. Autonomous Functioning a. Degree of freedom from impairment of apparatuses of primary autonomy–attention, concentration, memory, learning, perception, motor function b. Degree of freedom from impairment of secondary autonomy—disturbances in habit patterns, learned complex skills, work routines, hobbies and interests	Does reading ever make you tense? Have you ever had trouble with hearing or vision that was not due to a physical illness or defect? Have you had trouble with routine things like getting dressed, walking down stairs, or carrying out your usual work routine? How is your energy level? When you have free time, do you get things done or do you procrastinate?	Functional blindness or deafness; catatonic postures; inability to feed, dress, or care for one's self; disturbances of will, skills, habits; expenditure of great effort to carry out routine tasks

(continued)

Table 1–2
(continued)

Ego Function and Component Factors	Interview Questions	Possible Disturbance
9. Synthetic–Integrative Functioning a. Degree of reconciliation or integration of potentially contradictory attitudes, values, behavior, affects, and self-representations (*i.e.,* role conflicts) b. Degree of active integrating of both intrapsychic and behavioral events, whether contradictory or not	Can you adapt easily to change or does it upset you? Can you pay attention to two things at once? Do you think it possible to do more than one thing well, for instance, can a person be both a leader and a follower or both a teacher and a student? How well organized are you—what sort of things disorganize you? Do you find yourself doing or saying things that seem unlike you? Do you live from day to day or do you plan ahead?	Disorganized behavior, incongruity between thoughts, feelings, and actions, absence of consistent life goals; poor planning; little effort to relate different areas of experience; fluctuating emotional states without appropriate awareness of the change, as in hysterics; minor and major forms of dissociation—from fugues to multiple personalities; many other ego functions affected because this function is such a basic one
10. Mastery–Competence a. Competence, or how well the person actually performs in relation to his existing capacity to interact with and actively master and affect his environment b. The person's subjective feeling of competence with respect to mastering and affecting his environment; person's expectations of success on actual performance (how he feels about how he does and what he can do) c. The degree of discrepancy between actual competence and sense of competence. It may be negative—in which case actual competence exceeds sense of competence. It may be equal—in which case actual competence and sense of competence are congruent. It may be positive—in which case sense of competence exceeds actual competence.	Do you function as well as you believe you are capable of functioning? Do you feel that you generally stay on top of things? Do you like to be in charge of things? Do you live up to your own expectations of yourself? Do you ever feel you are missing out on life? Why? Do you feel very much at the mercy of events, or do you feel that you are the master of your own fate? Do you believe that you could effectively alter your life or influence the people around you to get what you need and want?	The person does almost nothing to alter, affect or interact with his environment, because he is largely unable to use abilities and capacities in relation to reality. What he does can be seen as a passive reaction rather than an active coping. The sense of power is almost nil; the person feels powerless to act effectively, regardless of actual performance.

(Adapted from Bellak L et al: Ego Functions in Schizophrenics, Neurotics and Normals. New York, © John Wiley & Sons, 1973. Reprinted by permission of John Wiley & Sons, Inc.)

The Mini-mental State Examination[4]

Definition The mini-mental state examination (MMS) is a screening instrument for cognitive disorders; it should be used only when the nurse believes the client is disoriented.

Use The MMS is useful in quantitatively estimating the severity of cognitive impairment, and for serially documenting cognitive change.

Description It includes 11 questions and requires only 5 to 10 minutes to administer; this is valuable for use with the elderly client whose cognitive impairment allows him to cooperate for only a short period of time.

Components It is divided into two parts. The first requires vocal responses only, and the maximum score is 21. The second part involves reading and writing, and the maximum score is 9. Adjust for those clients with impaired vision by writing directions in large print and allow for the difficulty in scoring.

Scoring The maximum score is 30. The test is not timed but is scored immediately. Directions for administering the MMS are given in Chart 1–2. Clients scoring 24 or less are

---

Chart 1–2

INSTRUCTIONS FOR ADMINISTERING MINI-MENTAL STATE EXAMINATION

Orientation

1. Ask for the date. Then ask specifically for parts omitted (*e.g.,* "Can you also tell me what season it is?") One point for each correct.
2. Ask in turn "Can you tell me the name of this hospital (town, county, etc)?" One point for each correct answer.

Registration

Ask the patient if you may test his memory. Then say the names of 3 unrelated objects, (for example, car, house, book) clearly and slowly, about 1 second for each. After you have said all 3, ask him to repeat them. This first repetition determines his score (0–3), but keep saying them until he can repeat all 3, up to 6 trials. If he does not eventually learn all 3, recall cannot be meaningfully tested.

Attention and Calculation

Ask the patient to begin with 100 and count backwards by 7s. Stop after 5 subtractions (93, 86, 79, 72, 65). Score the total number of correct answers.

If the patient cannot or will not perform this task, ask him to spell "world" backwards. The score is the number of letters in correct order (*e.g.,* dlrow = 5, dlorw = 3).

Recall

Ask the patient if he can recall the 3 words you previously asked him to remember. Score 0–3.

Language

Naming—Show the patient a wristwatch and ask him what it is. Repeat for pencil. Score 0–2.

Repetition—Ask the patient to repeat the sentence after you. Allow only one trial. Score 0–1.

3-Stage command—Give the patient a piece of plain, blank paper and repeat the command. Score 1 point for each part correctly executed.

Reading—On a blank piece of paper print the sentence "Close your eyes" in letters large enough for the patient to see clearly. Ask him to read it and do what it says. Score 1 point only if he actually closes his eyes.

Writing—Give the patient a blank piece of paper and ask him to write a sentence for you. Do not dictate a sentence; it is to be written spontaneously. It must contain a subject and verb and be sensible. Correct grammar and punctuation are not necessary.

Copying—On a clean piece of paper, draw intersecting pentagons, each side about 1 in, and ask him to copy it exactly as it is. All 10 angles must be present and 2 must intersect to score 1 point. Tremor and rotation are ignored.

Estimate the patient's level of sensorium along a continuum, from alert on the left to coma on the right.

(Adapted from Folstein M et al: Mini-mental state: A method for grading the cognitive state of patients for clinicians. J Psychiatr Res 12:189, © 1975, Pergamon Press, Ltd. Reprinted with permission.)

considered positive for the presence of cognitive disorders. A score of 20 or less is found essentially in clients with dementia, delirium, schizophrenia, or affective disorder, and not in normal elderly people or in clients with a primary diagnosis of neurosis or personality disorder. Chart 1–3 shows the score sheet.

Chart 1–3
SCORE SHEET—MINI–MENTAL STATE

Name _____   Unit _____

Date _____

Maximum Score	Score	
		Orientation
5	( )	What is the year (season, date, day, month)?
5	( )	Where are we: (state, county, town, hospital, floor)?
		Registration
3	( )	Name 3 objects: 1 second to say each. Then ask the patient all 3 after you have said them. Give 1 point for each correct answer. Then repeat them until he learns all 3. Count trials and record. Trials:
		Attention and Calculation
5	( )	Serial 7's. 1 point for each correct. Stop after 5 answers. Alternatively spell "world" backwards.
		Recall
3	( )	Ask for the 3 objects repeated above. Give 1 point for each correct.
		Language
9	( )	Name a pencil, and a watch (2 points). Repeat the following: "No ifs, ands, or buts" (1 point).

Follow a 3-stage command:
    "Take a paper in your right hand, fold it in half, and put it on the floor" (3 points).
Read and obey the following:
    CLOSE YOUR EYES (1 point).
Write a sentence (1 point).
Copy design (1 point).
Total score
ASSESS level of consciousness along a continuum.

_____
Alert   Drowsy   Stupor   Coma

Examiner _____

(Adapted from Folstein M et al: Mini-Mental State: A method for grading the cognitive state of patients for clinicians. J Psychiatr Res 12:189, © 1975, Pergamon Press, Ltd. Reprinted with permission.)

References

1. Backer B et al (eds): Psychiatric Mental Health Nursing: Contemporary Readings. New York, D Van Nostrand, 1978
2. Batzer S: Psychiatric Evaluation. In Stuart G, Sundeen S (eds): Principles and Practice of Psychiatric Nursing, St Louis, CV Mosby, 1979
3. Bellak L et al: Ego Functions in Schizophrenics, Neurotics and Normals. New York, John Wiley & Sons, 1973
4. Folstein M, Folstein S, McHugh P: Mini-Mental State: A method for grading the cognitive state of patients for clinicians. J Psychiatr Res 12:189, 1975
5. Fracier S et al: A Psychiatric Glossary. Washington, DC, American Psychiatric Association Publications Office, 1975
6. Holmes T, Rahe R: The social readjustment rating scale. J Psychosom Res 11:216, 1967
7. Kaplan H, Sadock B: Psychiatric report. In Friedman A et al (eds): Contemporary Textbook of Psychiatry, III, Vol 1. Baltimore, Williams & Wilkins, 1980
8. Reynolds J, Logsdon J: Assessing your patient's mental status. Nursing '79, 9:33, 1979
9. Rowe C: An Outline of Psychiatry. Dubuque, Iowa, William C Brown, 1980
10. Simon N: Psychological assessment: Gathering data. In Simon N (ed): Psychological Aspects of Intensive Care Nursing. Bowie, Maryland, Robert J Brady, 1980
11. Slaby AE, et al: Handbook of Psychiatric Emergencies. New York, Medical Examinations Publishing Co, 1975
12. Strub R, Black FW: The Mental Status Examination in Neurology. Philadelphia, FA Davis, 1977
13. The New Merriam Webster Pocket Dictionary. New York, Pocket Books, 1971

Bibliography

Fauman B, Fauman M: Emergency Psychiatry for the House Officer. Baltimore, Williams & Wilkins, 1981
Taylor MA: The Neuropsychiatric Mental Status Examination. New York, SP Medical and Scientific Books, 1981

2

Differential

Diagnosis

Mary Webster

Introduction	Once the nurse has done a thorough assessment, using the psychiatric interview to obtain the psychosocial history, assessment of current status, and, if needed, a mental status examination, data are then available for a provisional diagnosis. The masters prepared psychiatric nurse may be asked to carry out this function. This chapter lists common presenting symptoms, possible diagnoses, and factors to aid in differential diagnosis.
Depression	Depression has been defined psychiatrically as a morbid state of deep sadness and dejection. Table 2–1 shows possible diagnoses and differential factors when the client is depressed.

Table 2–1
DEPRESSION—POSSIBLE DIAGNOSES AND DIFFERENTIAL FACTORS[1-3]

Possible Diagnosis	*Differential Factors*
1. Major depressive episode	Onset—develops over a period of days to weeks, sometimes occurs suddenly following stress. No precipitating event is necessary.[1] Age—may occur at any age; age of onset evenly distributed throughout adult life[1] Sex—is more common in females. Appetite and sleep disturbance, psychomotor agitation or retardation, anhedonia, impaired concentration, and suicidal ideation may occur.[1] Diurnal variations found—clients feel better in the afternoon than in the morning.[1]
2. Dysthymic disorder (depressive neurosis)	Onset—variable, usually few days to weeks or months[1] Age—may occur at any age, but often begins in early adulthood[1] Mild intermittent or sustained depression of at least 2 years' duration[1] may occur. Insomnia or hypersomnia may occur. May occur as a reaction to stress superimposed on a characterological disorder[1] No diurnal variation is seen.
3. Bipolar disorder depressed	Onset—sudden[1] Sex—common in both sexes[1] Has had one or more manic episodes[1] Genetic factors—often there is a history of affective disorder in family.[1]
4. Organic affective syndrome with depression	Depressed mood, but consciousness is clear[1] An organic cause such as reserpine intoxication or hypothyroidism can be identified.[1]
5. Organic brain syndrome (delirium, dementia, etc)	Depression is found as a reaction to the cognitive impairment, such as memory disturbance, caused by illness with an organic factor.[1] In early mild dementia, the client may be unconsciously aware of impairment and responds with depression before becoming consciously aware of deficits.[1] Depression is a common early symptom of temporal and frontal tumors and of hydrocephalus.[1]
6. Schizophrenia	Onset—adolescence or early adulthood[1] Sex—common in both sexes[1] Depression is often superimposed on psychotic symptoms.[1] The depressive symptoms are brief in duration compared to the psychotic symptoms.[1] Familial pattern can be identified.[1]

Euphoria	The client who is euphoric displays an exaggerated feeling of physical and emotional well-being. This behavior is not congruent with objective events in the client's life. Table 2–2 shows possible diagnoses and differentiating factors.
Hallucinations	The client who is hallucinating has a sensory experience that may be auditory, visual, tactile, or olfactory and that has no external stimuli. This occurs in the waking state. Table 2–3 shows possible diagnoses and differential factors when the client is hallucinating.
Disorientation	The client who is disoriented has lost a sense of the time, the place, and even personal identity. Table 2–4 shows possible diagnoses and differential factors.
Depersonalization	The client who is depersonalizing has a feeling of strangeness about the self and the surroundings. Table 2–5 shows possible diagnoses and differential factors when this symptom is presented.

(Text continues on page 24)

Table 2–2
EUPHORIA—POSSIBLE DIAGNOSES AND DIFFERENTIAL FACTORS[1-3]

Possible Diagnosis	*Differential Factors*
1. Bipolar disorder, manic	Onset—begins suddenly with rapid escalation of symptoms over a few days[1] Age—before age 30[1] Duration—a week or more of hyperactivity, loquaciousness, flight of ideas, grandiosity, decreased need for sleep, buying sprees, reckless driving, and impaired judgment[1] often occur. Family history of affective disorder often found[1]
2. Organic mental disorders a. Phencyclidine-induced intoxication (street names—PCP, THC, angel dust, crystal, and Peace Pill)	Effect such as euphoria is associated with mode of use and dosage; a mild "floaty" euphoria can result 5 minutes after smoked, sniffed, or taken intravenously[1] Symptoms appear about 1 hour after substance is ingested.[1] Euphoria is associated with use of less than 5 mg of PCP.[1] Age—peak use between 18 and 25 years, less common under 18[1] Acute ingestion is often misdiagnosed as schizophrenia, paranoid type.[1] Most users are unaware of PCP and believe that they are using marijuana.
b. Cocaine intoxication	"Rush," or elation (marked euphoria accompanied by increased motor activity),[3] may occur within a few minutes of smoking cocaine "base," sniffing the crystalline flakes or powder, or intravenous use.[1]
c. Opioid intoxication (natural opioids, such as heroin and morphine, and synthetics with morphinelike action, such as meperidine and methadone)	A single dose of morphine taken intravenously reaches its peak "high" in 5 minutes or less.[1] Used orally, intravenously, intranasally, or subcutaneously (skin-popping).[1] Pupillary constriction is usually present, with dilated pupils seen in severe overdose. Drowsiness, slurred speech, and impaired attention and memory occur.[1]
3. Bilateral frontal lobe syndrome	Euphoria, with a tendency toward jocularity, short-lived irritability, and social inappropriateness can be seen before dramatic cognitive deficits are found in formal mental status testing.[1] Emotional disinhibition and euphoria do not result in constructive activity, although on first impression the client seems productive and interested in the environment.[1] Subtle alterations in cognition occur without disorientation or memory disturbance.[1]

Table 2–3
HALLUCINATIONS—POSSIBLE DIAGNOSES AND DIFFERENTIAL FACTORS[1-3]

Type	Possible Diagnosis	Differential Factors
Auditory hallucinations	1. Schizophrenia	The content may be pleasant; more often it is abusive. "Voices" are usually continuous.[2] "Command" auditory hallucinations give "orders" to the client.[1] Associated with other psychotic symptoms
	2. Amphetamine intoxication	Often misdiagnosed as schizophrenia, paranoid type[1] There is a history of repeated paranoid episodes with good recovery.[1] May have tactile or olfactory hallucinations as well[1] Urine screening for amphetamine is positive. History may reveal use of sedatives for sleep and amphetamines for staying awake.
	3. Temporal lobe epilepsy	Transient auditory hallucinations or visual hallucinations prior to seizure (aura) or during seizure itself (ictal phenomena) occur.[2] Often associated with deja vu experiences (the sensation that an experience happening for the first time has occurred previously)[3] Associated with feelings of depersonalization, illusions, delusions, sexual feelings, paranoia, fear, and anger Amnesia for behavior during the seizure occurs.[1] Sometimes associated with violent behavior, confused state postseizure (postictal)
Visual hallucinations	1. Delirium due to infectious disease (influenza encephalitis)	Colorful or vivid visual hallucinations in combination with fever, clouded consciousness occur.[1] Neck rigidity is seen. Fluctuation in levels of consciousness with exacerbation of symptoms during sleepless nights or in the dark occur.[1] Lucid intervals may occur at any time, but most commonly in the morning.[1]
	2. Hallucinogen hallucinosis	Onset—usually within 1 hour of ingestion[1] Duration—LSD, most common hallucinogen, lasts about 6 hours; with other hallucinogens duration may be under an hour to a day or two.[1] History of recent ingestion of a hallucinogen such as LSD, mescaline, "peyote", psilocybin, dimethyltryptamine (DMT), dimethoxymethylamphetamine (STP; "serenity", "tranquility"), or morning glory seeds[3] Perceptual changes occur without a disturbance in consciousness, intellectual abilities, or mood, or without delusions.[1] Visual hallucinations are often of geometric forms and figures and sometimes of persons and objects.[1] Associated physical symptoms are pupillary dilation, tachycardia, sweating, palpitations, tremors, blurring of vision, and incoordination.[1] Hallucinations are associated with depersonalization, derealization, illusions, and synesthesias (seeing colors when a loud sound occurs).[1]

(continued)

Table 2–3
(continued)

Type	Possible Diagnosis	Differential Factors
	3. Alcohol withdrawal delirium (delirium tremens)	Onset—usually on the second or third day after the cessation or reduction of alcohol. Rarely appears more than a week after abstinence.[1] Age—usually after 5–15 years of heavy episodic alcohol abuse[1] Sex—four times more prevalent in males[1] Anxiety, tremors of the hands, tongue, and eyelids (most obvious is the hands), restlessness, and hypersensitivity to noise and light occur.[1] Nausea is common, especially in the morning, associated with anorexia. Isolated, visual hallucinations occur, when it is dark and client is alone.[3] Psychotic behavior occurs within a week after cessation or reduction of heavy alcohol intake.[3] Hallucinations—small animals such as mice, beetles, and snakes are seen, and "felt" crawling on the body, producing anxiety and intense terror.[2] Tachycardia, sweating, redness of face, insomnia, elevated blood pressure, and dilated pupils occur.[1] Delusions are in keeping with the hallucinations.[3] Seizures may occur.[1]
Olfactory hallucinations	1. Schizophrenia	Smell of poisonous gas or dead bodies is reported.[2] Delusion that the body emits a foul odor that they themselves cannot smell occurs[2]
	2. Temporal lobe epilepsy	Often ushered in by the odor of burning paint or rubber[2]
Tactile hallucinations (invariably this symptom is associated with a delusional interpretation of the sensation)[2]	1. Cocaine intoxication	Formication, the sensation of something crawling or creeping on or under the skin ("cocaine bug") occurs.[3]
	2. Delirium tremens	Sensation of insects crawling over the body is reported. There is a history of alcohol abuse. Other alcohol withdrawal symptoms are present.
	3. Schizophrenia	Sexual hallucinations are present in which the male feels that erections and orgasms are forced on him.[2] Females complain of rape and a sensation of a penis in the vagina.[2]
Somatic hallucinations (hallucinations involving the perception of a physical experience localized within the body)[1]	1. Schizophrenia	Must be distinguished from hypochondriacal preoccupation and tactile hallucination Example—feeling of electricity running through the body[2]
Kinesthetic hallucinations	1. "Phantom limb"	Experience of feeling the limb, or other part of the body that has been surgically removed, as if it were still present occurs.[2] The experience of "phantom limb" may be very painful but usually diminishes over time.

Table 2–4
DISORIENTATION—POSSIBLE DIAGNOSES AND DIFFERENTIAL FACTORS[1-3]

Possible Diagnosis	Differential Factors
1. Organic mental disorder (for example, metabolic disorder or drug or alcohol intoxication)	Time sense is the first to be lost, followed by loss of sense of place and then person.[1] In acute organic states, it is combined with clouding of consciousness, and in chronic organic states, with memory disorders.[1] Disorientation is usually reversible in deliria, but usually irreversible in chronic disorders such as senile and presenile dementia.[3]
2. Epilepsy	Associated with confusion after a grand mal seizure or following sleep. History of seizures is present. May also occur as an ictal twilight state—associated with a disturbance of consciousness. Early symptoms include searching movements of the head and eyes, lip smacking, masticatory movements, and swallowing.[5]

Table 2–5
DEPERSONALIZATION—POSSIBLE DIAGNOSES AND DIFFERENTIAL FACTORS[1-3]

Possible Diagnoses	Differential Factors
1. Depersonalization disorder	Onset—rapid[1] Age—usually begins in adolescence, rarely over 40[1] Mild depersonalization, without social or occupational impairment, is estimated to occur at some time in 30%–70% of young adults.[1]
2. Schizophrenia	Associated with other psychotic symptoms
3. Affective disorders	History of same occurs.
4. Organic mental disorders	Client is of advanced age.
5. Anxiety disorders	Absence of major psychiatric illness; is accompanied by pounding heart, perspiration, increased blood pressure, hyperventilation
6. Personality disorders	History of maladaptive stress-coping devices is present.
7. Epilepsy	History of same, familial history, and EEG changes, are usually present but not always.

Clients often use speech in a private, idiosyncratic way. Some of these patterns of speech have been categorized and described. Table 2–6 shows presenting symptoms, possible diagnoses, and differential factors.

Table 2–6
SPEECH AND VERBAL SYMPTOMS—POSSIBLE DIAGNOSES AND DIFFERENTIAL FACTORS[1-3,5]

Presenting Symptom	Possible Diagnosis	Differential Factors
Mutism	1. Stupor (organic—caused by CVA, diabetic coma, drug and alcohol intoxication)	Occurs in all stuporous states (profound unconsciousness) Incontinence of urine and feces occurs.
	2. Schizophrenia, catatonic type	Psychological pillow (head and neck elevated as if resting on a pillow) may occur.[5] Incontinence occurs, unless client is assisted to toilet.
	3. Severe depressive disorders	No incontinence occurs. Associated with other depressive symptoms such as psychomotor retardation Sadness of the face is present but without the entirely expressionless look of a catatonic stupor.[2]
	4. Conversion disorders (hysteria)	No organic cause can be identified. Can occur as an isolated symptom in hysteria; not as common as in hysterical aphonia (inability to produce normal speech)[1] No incontinence occurs.
Perseveration (a thought that was relevant to a discussion is repeated several times)[2]	1. Organic states	Most commonly seen in dementias (organic brain syndrome characterized by decreased intellectual ability, which impairs social or occupational functioning)[1]
	2. Schizophrenia, catatonic type	Associated with other schizophrenic symptoms, but not seen frequently
Echolalia (pathologic repetition of the words or phrases of another person)[3]	1. Organic disorders (dementias)	Associated with impaired cognitive functioning Often seen with echopraxia
	2. Schizophrenic disorders	Associated with other psychotic symptoms, including echopraxia
	3. Mental retardation (IQ below 70)	Onset—before age 18[1] Sex—twice as common in males[1] There is impairment in adaptive functioning.
Logorrhea (uncontrollable, rapid, excessive talking)[2]	1. Bipolar disorder, manic	May progress into flight of ideas Associated with other symptoms of bipolar disorder, manic
Blocking (difficulty in recalling or interpreting a stream of speech or thought because of emotional forces, usually conscious)[3]	1. Schizophrenia	May be associated with preoccupation, auditory hallucinations, or suspiciousness in paranoid states There is overproductivity of thoughts, which become jumbled and interfere with logic. ''Empty thoughts'' or paucity of thought may be reported.
	2. Depressive disorders	Associated with psychomotor retardation, short attention span, and poor concentration[1]

Disturbance of Motor Behavior	Psychiatric clients sometimes display motor behavior that is unusual or out of the ordinary. Table 2–7 shows presenting symptoms, possible diagnoses, and differential factors.
Memory Disturbance	Clients are sometimes unable to remember recent events or past events, or can remember one and not the other. Table 2–8 shows presenting symptoms, possible diagnoses, and differential factors.

Table 2–7

DISTURBANCE OF MOTOR BEHAVIOR—POSSIBLE DIAGNOSES AND DIFFERENTIAL FACTORS[1-5]

Presenting Symptom	Possible Diagnosis	Differential Factors
Variations of usual motor behavior	1. Bipolar disorder, manic	Excess of expressive movements involving hands and upper trunk occurs. There is absence of hallucinations.
	2. Depressive disorders	Slow, tired, constricted movements occur. Sad facial expression is observed. Morbid topics are presented. Angulation of the inner end of the fold of skin in the upper eyelid (Veraguth's sign) is sometimes observed.[5] Furrowing between the eyebrows is sometimes seen (Omega sign, Ω).[5]
	3. Schizophrenia	Expressive movements are often severely restricted.[1]
	4. Schizophrenia, catatonic type	Facial movement is stiff, although the eyes may show some aliveness. Face usually appears flat and expressionless, without eye blinking. Excessive grimacing and facial contortions may occur. Sometimes nose is wrinkled with excessively pouted lips, giving the appearance of an animal's snout.[2] Excitement with hyperactivity for a short duration alternating with stupor is sometimes seen. Assaultive behavior occurs.[3] Mild excited states, manifested by restless wandering or senseless moaning, may continue for long periods. Automatic movement to adjust to stimuli is lost in catatonia before voluntary movements are affected.
	5. Acute PCP intoxication	May become violent and assaultive
	6. Temporal lobe epilepsy	May become violent and assaultive after a seizure
	7. Anxiety states	Rapid, excessive, and tremulous active movements may be observed.
Echopraxia (pathologic imitation of movements client is observing)[3]	1. Schizophrenia, catatonic type	Associated with other catatonic symptoms Often is seen with echolalia
	2. Dementias	Seen in older clients with impairment in cognitive functioning
Catalepsy (sudden, transient attack of muscular weakness, with or without loss of consciousness)[3]	1. Narcolepsy	Age—begins in youth or early adulthood Sex—more common in males Sleep attacks may be sudden or may be preceded by an irresistible urge to sleep.

(continued)

Table 2–7
(continued)

Presenting Symptom	Possible Diagnosis	Differential Factors
Catalepsy (continued)		Attacks vary in duration from several minutes to an hour or more.
		Attacks are precipitated by strong emotions, surprise, or anger.
		Obesity is often present.
		EEG is normal in waking state.
		There is rapid entrance into REM sleep.
	2. Schizophrenia, catatonic type	Waxy flexibility (client offers slight resistance when limb is placed in awkward position; position is maintained although uncomfortable) can occur associated with other symptoms of catatonia.[1]
Catatonic state (a state characterized by immobility with muscular rigidity, inflexibility, or excitability)[3]	1. Schizophrenia, catatonic type	Marked psychomotor disturbance associated with stupor, negativism, rigidity, excitement, or posturing. Rapid alteration between the extreme of excitement or stupor sometimes occur. Mutism is often seen. Associated with stereotypy, mannerisms, and waxy flexibility. Incontinence of urine and feces sometimes occur.[1,3]
	2. Major affective disorder	Associated with symptoms of serious depression
	3. Central nervous system conditions[4] (viral encephalitis, frontal lobe tumors)	Evidence of organic mental syndrome occurs. Associated physical findings of specific illness occur. Confirmatory tests and examinations must be done.
	4. Metabolic condition[4] (diabetic ketoacidosis, hypercalcemia, pellagra)	Evidence of organic mental syndrome occurs. Associated physical findings of specific illness occur. Confirmatory tests and examinations must be done.
	5. Toxic agents[4] (mescaline, ethanol, PCP, neuroleptics)	Evidence of organic mental syndrome occurs. Associated physical findings of specific illness occur. Confirmatory tests and examinations must be done.
Perseveration (repeated, useless repetition of a goal-directed act)[2]	1. Schizophrenia, catatonic type	Associated with other symptoms of schizophrenia
	2. Delirium	Age—any age, more common in children and after age 60[1]
		Associated with disorientation, memory impairment[1]
		Psychomotor activity may shift from perseveration to sluggishness and certain features resembling catatonic stupor.[1]
		Abnormal neurologic signs are uncommon.
	3. Mental retardation	Significantly below-average intellectual functioning associated with impairment in adaptive functioning occurs.[1]

Table 2–8
MEMORY DISTURBANCE—POSSIBLE DIAGNOSIS AND DIFFERENTIAL FACTORS[1,3]

Presenting Symptom	Possible Diagnosis	Differential Factors
Amnesia	1. Organic etiology (head injuries, epileptic seizures, metabolic disorder or drug intoxications, brain tumors)	There is disorientation for time and place, the loss of registration of new memories, and some degree of retrograde amnesia (extending backwards over a period of time).[1] Sometimes confabulation and euphoria occur.
	2. Psychogenic amnesia	Onset—sudden with brief duration[3] May be triggered by severe anxiety; often a response to feelings of terror, anger, or guilt[1] Memory for period of time (and often for personal identity) is more or less consciously repressed.[3] There is absence of history of trauma. There are negative neurologic and laboratory findings.
Fugue state (dissociation, flight from the immediate environment characterized by inability to remember what is happening)[3]	1. Dissociative disorders, psychogenic fugue	Sudden, unexpected travel away from home or work occurs.[3] There is assumption of a new identity with an inability to recall prior identity[1] No underlying organic mental disorder is present.[1] Clients appear normal to observers.[3] Amnesia may follow termination of the fugue.[3] Incidence is rare, except in wartime, or in times of natural disasters.[3] May be associated with alcohol abuse[3] Histrionic underlying personality disorder often is present.
Confabulation (falsification of memory in which gaps of memory are filled in by imaginary experiences that seem plausible and are recounted in detail)[3]	1. Amnestic syndrome	Impairment in short- and long-term memory in a state of normal consciousness occurs.[1] Organic factor is present.[1] There is lack of insight into memory deficit. If clients acknowledge problem, they appear unconcerned about it.[1] Apathy, lack of initiative, and emotional blandness are common.[1] Most common form of amnestic syndrome is caused by thiamine deficiency associated with prolonged use of alcohol (Korsakoff's disease).

References

1. Diagnostic and Statistical Manual of Mental Disorders, 3rd ed. Washington, DC, American Psychiatric Association, 1980
2. Hamilton M (ed): Fish's Outline of Psychiatry. England, John Wright and Sons, 1978
3. Rowe C: An Outline of Psychiatry. Dubuque, Iowa, William C Brown, 1980
4. Stoudemire A: The differential diagnosis of catatonic states. Psychosomatics 23:28, 1982
5. Taylor MA: The Neuropsychiatric Mental Status Examination. New York, Medical and Scientific Books, 1981

3

Assessing
Suicide Potential

Mary Webster

OVERVIEW   *Introduction*
Definition
Phenomena Associated with the Suicidal State
Assessment
Emergency Evaluation

Introduction The psychiatric/mental health nurse encounters the potentially suicidal client in a variety of clinical settings, including outpatient departments, inpatient units, emergency rooms, crisis centers, and the general hospital. The threat of suicide is the most common emergency in psychiatric nursing practice. The responsibility for assessing the potential for suicide is an anxiety-provoking experience for the nurse. Therefore, it is essential for the nurse to have an understanding of the suicidal state itself, a conceptual framework for assessing self-destructive behavior, and a willingness to examine personal reactions (countertransference) to the suicidal client.

Definition[5] Suicide is at the extreme end of a continuum of self-destructive behavior that, without intervention, would result in death. The continuum ranges from habitual self-inflicted life-threatening behaviors to isolated highly lethal acts that result in instant death. The suicidal client is one who
1. Is thinking about committing a self-destructive act
2. Is expressing the intent to commit a self-destructive act
3. Has recently attempted or committed a self-destructive act

Phenomena Associated with the Suicidal State[2] It is useful to look upon any suicidal thought or act as an effort by an individual to stop unbearable anguish or intolerable pain by "doing something." The pain results from the following experiences:

A. **DEPRESSION** (See also Chap. 43)
   Depression is a complex feeling ranging from unhappiness to deep dejection and hopelessness, accompanied by feelings of guilt, failure, and worthlessness. The physical concomitants of depression are disturbances in sleeping patterns, changes in appetite, and slowing down of physiologic processes. Depression can be viewed as communication of a self-inflicted state of deprivation, and communication to those in the environment to "do something to help me."

B. **ISOLATION AND WITHDRAWAL**
   The suicidal client may overtly display isolative or withdrawing behaviors, or may attempt to mask them by frantic activity. When clients are asked about the increased activities, they often describe themselves as "going through the motions" and "feeling cut off from others."

C. **HOPELESSNESS AND HELPLESSNESS**
   Feelings of hopelessness and helplessness are very accessible to the client's consciousness and are an accurate indicator of the seriousness of the suicidal state.

D. **HOSTILITY**
   High levels of hostility have been found by some investigators in suicide attempters.[2] Frequently, the suicide attempters' message to significant others is "you should have cared more."

E. **AMBIVALENCE**
   Persons with suicidal ideation often express ambivalence about living or dying. The nurse's interventions are allied with that part of the ambivalence leading to continued life.

F. **"TUNNEL VISION"**
   Suicidal persons are frequently unable to see choices or alternatives that might

improve their situation. The nurse aids the client by exploring and clarifying alternatives other than suicide.

Assessment   Sources of data include
1. Client
2. Significant others, including family and friends
3. Police report
4. Staff in the clinical setting
5. Current therapist, if applicable

Table 3–1 identifies factors influencing suicide potential.

Table 3–1
FACTORS INFLUENCING SUICIDE POTENTIAL[3-5]

Factor	Increased Potential	Decreased Potential
Age	Rises steadily in men over 45 Increasing among adolescents, particularly college students	Young females have low rate Rare among children, but rises rapidly in latency, early adolescence through the early 20s
Sex	Men are three times as likely to *succeed* at suicide. Women succeed more often after age 55	Women are three times as likely to *attempt* suicide. Women over 70 have lower risk.
Race	Caucasians, American Indians, and Eskimos	Blacks have rates ⅓ those of Caucasians, except in urban areas where rates now are approximating those for Caucasians
Marital status	Single persons have twice the rate of married persons. Divorced, separated, and widowed persons living alone have rates 4–5 times higher than those married. In the widowed, risks are greater during the first year of widowhood	Lowest among married persons who have children
Religion	Protestants and those who profess no religious affiliation have highest rates.	Jews and Catholics have lowest rates.
Health history	70% of those who have completed or attempted suicide have one or more active, mostly chronic, illnesses at the time of death. Those who believe they have a serious or chronic illness have high rates.	
Stress	Recent death of a significant person, especially on the anniversary of the death Loss of a significant person through separation or divorce Loss of job, prestige, or status Threat of criminal exposure	

Table 3–1
(continued)

Factor	Increased Potential	Decreased Potential
Life-style	Unstable life-style, which might include a. Inconsistent work history b. Unstable marital and family relationships c. History of previous suicide attempts d. Coping with problems by using drugs or alcohol	
Support systems	Absence of available support system. Support systems might include a. Family b. Friends c. Neighbors d. Clergy and church members e. Physician f. Employer and co-workers g. Social agencies Support systems should be evaluated in terms of their ability to give the *client* support; often family and friends are relying on the client for support.	
Occupation	Higher rates are seen at both socioeconomic extremes. Most significant is a change in status, either higher or lower. Physicians, when adjusted for age and education, have same rates as other groups. Among physicians, psychiatrists rank highest.	
Depression	Depressed mood accompanied by vegetative signs: a. Loss of appetite b. Loss of weight c. Decreased libido d. Difficulty in falling asleep e. Awakening during the night f. Early morning awakening Severe insomnia even in the absence of depression Psychomotor retardation, agitation, and feelings of hopelessness and worthlessness Rates, although higher than usual in the presence of psychomotor retardation, are less ominous than in agitated depression. Rate increases in clients with psychomotor retardation after treatment with antidepressants because client is able to motivate enough energy to activate an attempt.	

(continued)

Table 3–1
(continued)

Factor	Increased Potential	Decreased Potential
Thought disorder	Thought disorder combined with depressed mood and suicidal ideation "Command" hallucinations, voices telling a person to kill himself or join another in the grave Paranoid delusional systems Postpartum psychosis and primary affective disorders	
Family history	Family history of suicide Member of family with unipolar or bipolar depression	
Previous attempts	Almost ¾ of those who ultimately succeed at suicide have had previous attempts.	
Sexual orientation	Confused sexual orientation, particularly when associated with depression, aging, alcohol, or borderline personality disorder[6]	
Lethality of attempt	Men tend to use more lethal methods such as hanging, shooting, or jumping from high distances. When women use a more lethal method (such as those just noted) and survive, they are at high risk for subsequent attempts. Alcohol and tranquilizers, barbiturates, or antidepressants represent a highly lethal combination.	Less lethal methods such as ingestion of moderate amounts of drugs and superficial lacerations of the wrist are often used by women.
Alcohol use	Alcohol abuse figures predominantly in the chronically suicidal person.	

Emergency Evaluation   In situations in which it is not possible to do a complete assessment of the suicidal client (for example, in the emergency room) the mnemonic shown in Chart 3–1 has proved helpful.[1] It is to be used with clients who have just made a suicide attempt but could be modified for use with clients who are threatening suicide.

The nurse should be able to consult with co-workers, supervisors, and other professionals about those clients who are particularly disturbing. In this way, and with additional experience over time, the nurse will gain confidence in assessing the suicidal client.

Chart 3–1
SAD CHILDREN—A SUICIDE POTENTIAL SCALE

S	Support system	Who is at home? How does the client get along with them? Are there others in the environment who can be called upon?
A	Alcohol	Is alcohol abuse involved in the attempt? Is the client a known alcoholic? Is the client sober enough for a final assessment?
D	Depression	How clinically depressed is the client?
C	Communication	Is the client communicating with you? With the family?
H	Hostility	How hostile or angry is the client? Is the anger so strong that the client might commit suicide in order to "punish" significant others?
I	Impulsivity	How impulsive was the suicidal act? Is the client generally impulsive?
L	Lethality	Is the client aware of the lethality of the method? Was the plan well thought out to avoid rescue?
D	Demography	Do demographic variables such as age, sex, and socioeconomic status place the client in a high risk category?
R	Reaction of evaluator	Is your empathic response to the client a feeling of hopelessness or depression? Is there something about the client that makes you feel angry?
E	Events	What events led to the attempt? Has the client had any significant life changes, particularly the loss of a spouse?
N	No hope	Does the client believe there is no hope of things improving? Do you feel hopeless upon hearing about the client's life?

(From DiVasto P et al: A framework for the emergency evaluation of the suicidal patient. J Psychiatr Nurs 17:15, 1979. Reprinted by permission of Journal of Psychosocial Nursing and Mental Health Services, Slack, Incorporated, Medical Publisher)

References

1. DiVasto P et al: A framework for the emergency evaluation of the suicidal patient. J Psychiatr Nurs 17:15, 1979
2. Hatton Y, Valente S, Rork A: Suicide: Assessment and Intervention. New York, Appleton-Century-Crofts, 1977
3. Resnik H: Suicide. In Friedman A et al (eds): Comprehensive Textbook of Psychiatry III. Bowie, Maryland, Williams & Wilkins, 1980
4. Resnik H, Ruben H: Emergency Psychiatric Care. Bowie, Maryland, The Charles Press, 1975
5. Rigdon I, Godbey K: Threats to survival. In Armstrong M et al (eds): McGraw-Hill Handbook of Clinical Nursing. New York, McGraw-Hill, 1979
6. Slaby A, Tancredi L, Lieb J: Clinical Psychiatric Medicine. Philadelphia, Harper & Row, 1981

4

Formulating a Comprehensive Treatment Plan

Martha Merritt Tousley

OVERVIEW

Introduction   The client's treatment plan describes what is to be accomplished during the period of outpatient treatment or during the course of hospitalization. Based on a comprehensive assessment of clients' problems and clinical needs, it is a collaborative effort involving the clients, their families or significant others, and members of the treatment team. Specific problems are identified, goals are set, and methods for achieving them are described. Treatment that is planned and documented can be evaluated more effectively, both internally (by means of the service's quality assurance program) and externally (by accrediting agencies and consumers of health care). To demonstrate the use of the comprehensive treatment plan a case study is presented in Chart 4–1.

Components   A. **PRELIMINARY TREATMENT PLAN**

The preliminary treatment plan is the ''unofficial'' problem list and plan for treatment formulated by the admitting clinician when the client is first admitted to the service or the unit. In a hospital setting, such a plan includes physician's orders and may be based on information from the admissions office.

Chart 4–1
CASE STUDY

Introduction

J.S. is a 20-year-old, part Indian, male student presently working as a stockboy for a local bakery. He came voluntarily to the center because of "problems that are bothering me." He holds a brown belt in judo and describes a growing feeling that he may "lose control" while working out with a partner: "When I'm pinning a guy, I feel like driving him through the mat." He complains of "migraine headaches" which he describes as "continual" (for the last 5 years) and indicated that he had taken "a pain pill" shortly before this initial interview. He says he has petit mal epilepsy, which is controlled with medication. His last hospitalization was 3 months ago, when he was admitted to a general hospital following ingestion of several different pills (Darvon, Dilantin, Phenobarbital, and Talwin). He states that "This was no cry for help—I didn't intend to come back. I was way out on a country road that's seldom plowed, where no one could find me. I was surprised when I woke up in the hospital."

J.S. says that he is a student at a local community college and particularly likes math, although he is not taking any courses this term: "It's hard to concentrate on my studies." He denies any problems at work, yet describes his co-workers as "a bunch of women who bicker among themselves all day." When asked whether he had any friends, he smiled wryly and said, "All the shrinks I've been to ask me that—'How many friends do you have? What's a close friend mean to you?' Then the next question is always 'Do you prefer girls to boys?' Yes I prefer girls." He says he has never found a girl in whom he can confide.

Clinical Data

Client was seen initially at this center 2 years ago, having been referred by the Vocational Rehabilitation Department for psychological testing. Subsequently his case was presented in staff conference, from which emerged a diagnostic impression of "hysterical neurosis, dissociative type, with depressive and schizoid features." J.S. has a history of being in "continuous supportive counseling" since his junior year in high school; he was counseled for 2 months through Vocational Rehabilitation prior to his referral here. After his testing, the choice of whether to return for therapy was left to J.S. He has not returned until today.

Initial Assessment

J.S. was casually dressed but neat and clean. He was soft-spoken and cooperative throughout the session. He displayed some testing behavior at various points, but he was able to verbalize his own feelings of anxiety at these times. The client's affect was generally appropriate to his thought content and somewhat blunted. He seemed rather tense throughout the interview. He was oriented in all three spheres, fully conscious and aware of his surroundings. He seemed fairly bright and was capable of both concrete and abstract thought. His judgment appeared intact, and he was aware that he may be losing control over his aggressive impulses. The diagnostic impression was hysterical neurosis, dissociative type, with depressive and schizoid features; secondary diagnosis was nonpsychotic organic brain syndrome associated with epilepsy.

B. INITIAL TREATMENT PLAN

The initial treatment plan is the plan developed by a designated member of the treatment team within the first 72 hours of the client's hospitalization. It lists presenting problems based on the staff's initial assessment of the client's physical, cognitive, emotional, and behavioral status and specifies immediate treatment recommendations and anticipated period of treatment or length of hospitalization (see Fig. 4–1).

C. ASSESSMENT

The assessment is the accumulated information considered relevant to treatment. It provides the baseline data from which specific needs and problems are identified, and against which progress is measured and includes physical, emotional, spiritual, cognitive, behavioral, socioeconomic, environmental, rehabilitative, or legal aspects.

D. COMPREHENSIVE (MASTER) TREATMENT PLAN

The comprehensive treatment plan is the "official" working plan developed by the multidisciplinary team for the client whose hospitalization exceeds 10 days (see Fig. 4–2).

INITIAL TREATMENT PLAN	(Addressograph)

Admission Date: _____10/1_____ Initial Treatment Planning Date: _____10/1_____

PRESENTING PROBLEMS: List presenting problems based on initial assessment of the client's physical, cognitive, emotional, and behavioral status:

1. Depression
2. Social withdrawal
3. Anxiety
4. Dependency
5. Suspiciousness

IMMEDIATE TREATMENT RECOMMENDATIONS: Specify recommended services, activities, and therapeutic programs. Specify by name and discipline those staff members assigned to implement recommendations:

1. Avoid hospitalization.
2. Supportive short-term outpatient therapy recommended.
3. Client will meet with M. Tousley, M.S., R.N., at Center for one hour per week.
4. Client will enter a No-Suicide Contract with therapist.
5. Progress will be evaluated 8 weeks hence, with client, therapist, and members of treatment team.

ANTICIPATED PERIOD OF HOSPITALIZATION/TREATMENT _____8 weeks_____

SIGNATURE OF INITIATOR _Martha Merritt Tousley, M.S., R.N._

FIG. 4–1 Initial treatment plan. (From Fair Oaks Hospital, Summit, New Jersey. Reprinted with permission)

COMPREHENSIVE TREATMENT PLAN	(Addressograph)

GOAL OF TREATMENT: Specify the outcome that will be observed if the Treatment Plan and activities of the Treatment Team are successful. Identify what it is that the client must accomplish during this hospitalization/period of treatment.

1. J.S. will enter a No-Suicide Contract and behavior will be congruent with that statement.
2. He will open lines of communication with significant other(s) on an adult level.
3. He will recognize signs, symptoms of anxiety & will seek out significant other(s) when he feels anxious.
4. He will return to his studies as a part-time student next term.
5. He will begin evaluating remarks of others, accepting only that criticism that is warranted and/or constructive.

Date First Noticed	PROBLEMS/NEEDS	Date Reviewed	OBJECTIVES/METHODS	Date Achievement Expected	Date Resolved
	List and number significant client PROBLEMS. Specify ways client portrays them. Identify unmet NEED(S) underlying problem(s).		Specify what client must do, step by step, to reach GOAL. Specify MEMBERS and METHODS team will use to facilitate achievement, including FREQUENCY.		
10/1	☐1 DEPRESSION: • Attempted suicide 3 mo. ago; nearly succeeded. • Fears inability to control own aggressive impulses. (NEEDS to feel worthwhile; to have hope for future.)	10/11	J.S. will: • Notify Center when suicidal thoughts occur. • Externalize and verbalize feelings of anger. • Willingly identify and listen to alternatives to suicide. • Recognize and identify own efforts at self-control.	From now on. Within 2 weeks. Within 2 weeks. Within 4 weeks.	
10/1	☐2 SOCIAL WITHDRAWAL: • "No friends at work." • Avoids people: "they hassle me." • Feels "worthless;" fears "being rejected." (NEEDS a sense of belongingness— to feel safe, secure in relationships with others.)		J.S. will: • Visibly relax and converse freely with therapist. • Expose self to developing relationships with others. • Accept comments on strengths, achievements without displaying embarrassment.	By 4th week. By 5th week. By 8th week.	

(continued)

FIG. 4–2 Comprehensive treatment plan. (From Fair Oaks Hospital, Summit, New Jersey. Reprinted with permission)

COMPREHENSIVE TREATMENT PLAN

Date First Noticed	PROBLEMS/NEEDS	Date Reviewed	OBJECTIVES/METHODS	Date Achievement Expected	Date Resolved
10/1	③ *ANXIETY:* • Demonstrates difficulty verbalizing under stress. • Weak tolerance to stress—"clutches" during exams. • Impaired ego function: "can't concentrate on studies." • Loud, nervous laughter when embarrassed. (NEEDS to feel free from overwhelming stress.)	10/11	J.S. will recognize those times when he feels anxious and will: • Share awareness during therapy sessions. • Initiate contact with Significant Other for support. • Explore reality: certain events are inherently stressful. • Identify & explore own successful methods for dealing with stress (e.g. Judo).	By 3rd week. By 3rd week.	
10/1	④ *DEPENDENCY:* • Has been in "supportive counseling" since Jr. year in highschool (6 years). • Sees no way to become financially independent of parents. (NEEDS to trust in himself and in others.)	10/11	J.S. will: • Begin depending on own ability to problem-solve, by making a decision & "owning" the consequences. • Return to studies as a part-time student. • Identify behaviors in therapist & in others that indicate they can be trusted as sincere, dependable.	By 8th week. By Winter Term By 8th week	
10/1	⑤ *SUSPICIOUSNESS:* • Demonstrates hypersensitivity to casual remarks of others. • Places high value on honesty in relationships, yet admits own tendency to deceive others. (NEEDS to deny basic feelings of inadequacy & project onto others.)	10/11	J.S. will: • Spontaneously share current concerns with therapist. • identify behaviors in himself that may lead others to mistrust or misjudge him. • Recognize his own willingness to be more open, honest during sessions.	By 5th week. By 5th week. By 6th week.	

FIG. 4–2 *(continued)*

Terminology   Terms commonly associated with treatment plans are defined in Chart 4–2.

Treatment Plan Review   Problem-oriented multidisciplinary case conferences, with contributions from several team members at one time, are held to review and evaluate progress. The conference includes the various disciplines participating in the care of client, thereby promoting more complete understanding of the client's problems. Figure 4–3 shows a form for documenting the meetings, the Treatment Plan Review Record.

Chart 4–2
TERMINOLOGY

1. *Problem*—Occurs whenever there is an interruption in the client's ability to meet a need. Includes whatever is going on with the client that
   a. Jeopardizes physical or mental health
   b. Causes difficulty for self, family, or those providing care
   c. Is of sufficient importance to require a *plan* for resolution (*e.g.,* further diagnosis, management, observation, education of client or family)
   For purposes of *measurement,* problems are made operational by describing discrete behaviors. When a problem is stated, the nurse lists one or two verbal or nonverbal examples of how she/he has observed the client displaying or acting out that problem.

2. *Problem list*—Identifies which specific problems team members will monitor and use to assess the client's response to treatment. The problem list is
   • *Pertinent*—Information in the assessment is used to generate the list.
   • *Current*—Though not an exhaustive list, it reflects what the client presents *now*. Problems listed are *active* problems.
   • *Dynamic*—As more data are gathered and the client's status changes, problems can be combined, separated, added, redefined, or deleted as resolved. This indicates progress over time. Such changes are dated and further explained in the progress notes.
   • *Identifiable*—Each problem is given its own number. To avoid confusion, the same number is always used to identify the same problem (whether it appears in the nursing care plan, the treatment plan, or the progress notes). Thus, everything done with the client is documented in terms of a specific problem. (When a client has many problems, it is useful to refer to the problem by both its number and its name.)
   • *Clear*—It is stated so clearly and so concisely that it will be meaningful to anyone who reads it.
   • *Precise*—It will point to treatment implications, thereby assisting in planning care and lending direction to the treatment process.
   NOTE: A problem is *not* the same as a diagnosis and should not be stated as such. An official DSM diagnostic label is not useful in planning treatment because, as it stands, it has not been broken down into measurable behaviors. It may be helpful to ask, "What life problems is this diagnosis causing for this person?"

3. *Goal*—Specifies the *outcomes* that will be observed if the treatment plan and activities of the treatment team are successful. Identifies what the client must accomplish during this hospitalization, thereby giving direction to the treatment planning process. The goal is stated clearly, objectively, and in measurable terms, so that any staff member can recognize the desired outcome behavior.

4. *Objective*—Specifies the *process,* that is, what the client must do to reach the goal(s). An objective stated in behavioral terms describes the *behaviors* the client should possess or exhibit if the objective has been met. An objective is
   • *Specific*—It identifies what the client actually should be able to do, step by step, throughout the period of treatment.
   • *Clear*—It communicates clearly to the client what is expected, and it is so precise that any member of the team could apply it to the client's problem.
   • *Reasonable*—It is achievable, given the client's strengths and abilities, and consistent with his/her value system.
   • *Results-oriented*—It is presented in terms of results to be achieved.
   • *Measurable*—It designates the means for measuring progress toward the goal in observable terms.
   • *Pertinent*—It is based on the assessment of the client's needs and is problem related.
   • *Positive*—It states what the client is aiming toward rather than dwelling merely on problems.
   • *Time-limited*—It specifies a deadline.
   • *Identifies a standard*—It implies or states the criteria against which acceptable performance is measured.

5. *Method*—Specifies the methods for achieving the goals. Specifically identifies
   a. Services, activities, or programs prescribed for the client (including referrals outside the agency or hospital)
   b. Which staff members will be assigned to work with the client
   c. Frequency of treatment procedures

TREATMENT PLAN REVIEW RECORD

Note: For *results* of review and evaluation of client's Treatment Plan and progress in attaining goals (including discontinuation, modification or update), see PROGRESS NOTES.

Team Leader: *M. Tousley, M.S., R.N.*

Date of Meetings: initial if present

TREATMENT PLANNING TEAM (Signature)	10/11	10/18	10/25	11/1	11/8	11/15	11/22	12/10
Staff Psychiatrist *R. Taylor, M.D.*	RT		RT	RT				RT
A. Jones, R.N.	AJ	AJ	AJ	AJ		AJ		AJ
Nurse(s)								
S. Smith, M.H.W.	SS			SS	SS		SS	
Mental Health Worker(s)								
R. Brown, A.C.S.W.	RB	RB			RB		RB	RB
Social Worker(s)								
Nurse Clinical Specialist *M. Tousley, M.S., R.N.*	MT	MT	MT	MT	MT	MT	MT	MT
Psychologist *P. Davis, Ph.D.*	PD				PD	PD	PD	PD
Creative Therapist *J. Black, C.T.*	JB							JB
Other								
*Client's Participation in Planning	I	I	I	I	I	I	I	III

*Client's Participation Key:
  I Contributed to Goals or Plans
  II Aware of Plan Content
  III Reviewed Treatment Plan
  IV Refused to Participate
  V Unable to Participate

FIG. 4–3 Treatment plan review record. (From Fair Oaks Hospital, Summit, New Jersey. Reprinted with permission)

A. **PURPOSE**
  1. To *pool* and exchange information so problems are identified and updated.
  2. To *evaluate* client and staff progress in solving problems and reaching goals.
  3. To *modify* approaches as indicated.

B. **FREQUENCY**
  Reviews should occur at least
  1. As frequently as clinically indicated, and as required by survey agencies (for example JCAH)
  2. Following the first 10 days of hospitalization
  3. Within 1 month of the first 10 days
  4. Every 2 months for the first year
  5. Every 3 months after the first year

C. DOCUMENTATION

Treatment planning meetings are documented by recording the results of the review and evaluation of the client's progress in his/her chart. Thus the *product* of the team's effort (that is, the treatment plan) is made accessible and available to all concerned, and continuity of care is provided.

Discharge Summary and Aftercare Plan

This is a summary of the clinical course of treatment with regard to problems as listed in the treatment plan. It includes final assessment of the client's status as well as recommendations and arrangements for further treatment or follow-up care. Figure 4–4 shows a discharge summary and aftercare plan.

FIG. 4–4 Discharge summary and aftercare plan. (From Fair Oaks Hospital, Summit, New Jersey. Reprinted with permission)

DISCHARGE SUMMARY AND AFTERCARE PLAN	(Addressograph) Date: 12-10

DISCHARGE SUMMARY: Summarize clinical course of treatment with regard to problems listed in Treatment Plan. Include final assessment of client's status:

1. *DEPRESSION: J.S. now describes his "only alternative is to reach out to others." On 12/6 he initiated contact with Voc. Rehab. Counselor: "He's someone I can talk to."*
2. *SOCIAL WITHDRAWAL: Is spending evenings with college buddies; accepts invitations "to go out and socialize" 3 times a week ("I'll never meet a girl by sitting home.") Has initiated phone contact with his boss & wife ("a really nice couple").*
3. *ANXIETY: Breaks periods of silence himself by adding comments; speech is more animated; is more relaxed, open and direct in sharing concerns.*
4. *DEPENDENCY: Signed up for 2 courses at college: "to get my grade point up."*
5. *SUSPICIOUSNESS: Acknowledges that he cannot know what another is thinking unless he asks.*

AFTERCARE PLAN: State recommendations and specify whatever arrangements for further treatment (e.g. medication, referral):

J.S. has initiated contact with his counselor from Vocational Rehabilitation office. He can return to the Center whenever he feels a need to do so.

SIGNATURES OF PLANNING PARTICIPANTS:
(Include client and/or significant others when appropriate)

J.S.	*Ann Jones, R.N.*
Martha Tousley, M.S., R.N.	*Rita Brown, A.C.S.W.*
Robert Taylor, M.D.	

Bibliography

Atwood J, Yarnall S (eds): Symposium on the problem-oriented record. Nurs Clin North Am vol 9, 1974

Bower F: The Process of Planning Nursing Care: A Model for Practice, 2nd ed. St Louis, CV Mosby, 1977

Cantor M: Philosophy, purpose, objectives: Why do we have them? J Nurs Adm 3:21, 1973

Cantor M: Achieving Nursing Care Standards: Internal and External. Wakefield, MA, Nursing Resources, 1978

Carnevali D: Nursing Care Planning: Diagnosis and Management, 3rd ed. Philadelphia, JB Lippincott, 1983

Consolidated Standards Manual for Child, Adolescent and Adult Psychiatric, Alcoholism and Drug Abuse Facilities. Chicago, Joint Commission on Accreditation of Hospitals, 1983

Dillman C, Rahmlow H: Writing Instructional Objectives. Belmont, CA, Fearon Publishers, 1972

Gahan D: Using problem-oriented records in psychiatric nursing. In Kneisl C, Wilson H, (eds): Current Perspectives in Psychiatric Nursing: Issues and Trends. St Louis, CV Mosby, 1976

Journal of Nursing Administration Editorial Staff: Planning and Evaluating Nursing Care, 2nd ed. Wakefield, MA, Contemporary Publishing, 1978

Sharp BB, Cox C: Choose Success: How to Set and Achieve All Your Goals. New York, Hawthorne Books, 1970

Wooley FR et al: Problem-Oriented Nursing. New York, Springer-Verlag, 1974

Part II
Designing
Programs

5

Designing a Crisis Center

Kathleen O'Brien Kobberger / Martha Merritt Tousley

Introduction   Setting up a community center for crisis intervention services requires that the nurse be familiar with modern concepts of community mental health as well as with principles of community action.

Process for Developing a Crisis Center

Decision   There is agreement in the community that a crisis center is needed.

Phases[4]   A. GAINING SUPPORT
Certain groups will have vital interest in the project, while others will not. Interest cannot be assumed where there is none; similarly, allies must not be overlooked. History is useful. Learning what mistakes were made in the past can prevent repetition of them.

B. GETTING STARTED
Issues of territoriality may be avoided by involving key members of service agencies already in existence. Supporters already recognized as credible in the community should be enlisted.

C. GETTING APPROVAL
The project is legitimized by obtaining public approval (sponsorship) from influential community members.

D. PLANNING THE STRUCTURE
Preliminary structuring (setting objectives, forming committees) begins, but plans are kept general and flexible.

E. DEVELOPING THE SYSTEM
The planning group establishes itself as a functional system.

F. LAUNCHING THE PROGRAM
This is the most worrisome phase because all the prior work of the planning group is finally put to the test.

G. EVALUATING RESULTS
An ongoing method of evaluating the program should be developed in order to ascertain its effectiveness in reaching stated objectives.

Community Mental   A. STAFFING
Health Principles[4]   Staff includes professional mental health workers as well as volunteer and paid nonprofessionals.

B. CONSULTATION
Professional specialists act not as primary care-givers, but rather as consultants whose role is to provide support and to encourage staff members to be independent.

C. PREVENTION VS. TREATMENT
Efforts are directed at early intervention, eliminating or defusing stressful conditions *before* pathology develops.

D. STRESS VS. PATHOLOGY

Symptoms are related to stressful events in the client's environment, rather than considered to be manifestations of psychiatric disease.

E. NETWORKING

The mental health center works cooperatively with other agencies and is attuned to the needs of the community.

F. ACCOUNTABILITY

Quality assurance requires that the center define its purpose and operationalize its goals so that program and personnel performance can be measured against stated objectives. Documentation is required in order to demonstrate that changes are made according to findings.

Guidelines in Establishing and Maintaining an Effective Crisis Center[1,4]

1. The extent of need in the community is determined by considering the following:
   a. Who decided that such a need exists here?
   b. How was that need determined?
   c. Has the need been documented adequately?
   d. Are anyone's personal motives interfering?
2. The length of time devoted to program planning is less important than the quality of time spent.
3. Having one or two key persons manage the planning process proves more efficient than doing so by committee.
4. Planning continues indefinitely throughout the life of the program.
5. An attitude that values and permits change should be nourished as the program develops.
6. Knowledge of the local power structure keeps the program's goals congruent with changes in the local social, economic, and political climate.
7. Although professional consultations and collaboration are necessary, power and control rightfully belong to the program.
8. The impact of this new crisis service on the operation of existing agencies should be kept in mind.
9. Representatives from other than mental health fields, for example, police, are valuable resources and collaborators.
10. Turnover rate is kept to a minimum by selecting key personnel carefully.
11. Needs of the center's staff members should be recognized and addressed.
12. Alternative plans for permanent funding are included in the earliest planning.
13. Key persons, that is, those from industry, banking, business, are invited to sit on the center's directorial board.
14. Public funding carries a price. It may require surrendering some control or compromising some program goals.
15. The agency acts as though it deserves recognition in the community; it must take up an identifiable space and assume responsibility for a particular type of service.

Affiliation Should the crisis center stand alone, or should it affiliate itself with a local community mental health center (CMHC)?

A. ADVANTAGES OF CMHC AFFILIATION

1. *Funding*—Access to local and federal monies

2. *Acceptance*—Entry into an established community power structure
3. *Quality Assurance*—Quality of mental health service is already being assessed by CMHC.

B. **DISADVANTAGES OF CMHC AFFILIATION**
   1. *Funding*—When local funding is no longer "matched" by federal dollars, certain crisis services may become expendable.
   2. *Control*—Philosophy, purpose, and methods of the crisis center may be inconsistent with those of the CMHC, jeopardizing the crisis center's autonomy.

C. **ALTERNATIVES TO AFFILIATION**
   Alternatives to affiliation with a CMHC might include the following[1]:
   1. Operation by an independent corporation contracting with a number of different agencies to provide service
   2. Conceptualization of the crisis intervention service as a non-mental health program providing its own unique service

Crisis Delivery Systems

A crisis service provides short-term assistance to distressed individuals, families, significant others, or groups. People in crisis can seek such help directly, or they can be referred by others. Comprehensive crisis services can be delivered in the following ways:

Twenty-four-Hour Telephone Counseling

This service is operated predominantly by lay volunteers.[1] It is their responsibility to help with the presenting crisis situation itself and to provide linkage to the other essential crisis services in the community. Crisis center developers should plan ahead for an adequate telephone system because it is difficult to change telephone systems once they have begun operation.[4]

Guidelines for installing a telephone system include the following[1-5]:
1. Install a separate business line in addition to the crisis line.
2. Install rotary connections on the crisis line so that when one crisis line is busy, another will ring automatically.
3. Install a separate telephone instrument for each emergency line. This permits emergency calls during the time that the original incoming call is still on the line, thereby eliminating the need to put a caller on hold.
4. Install an automatic dial telephone with an unlisted number so that outgoing emergency calls can be made.
5. List the center's telephone numbers in all local telephone directories and in adjacent area directories as well.
6. Index both the business and emergency numbers in the white pages section.
7. Index both the business and emergency numbers in the classified section under several eye-catching categories (for example, Crisis Center, Suicide Prevention, and so forth).
8. Include the center's emergency numbers in the emergency listings section located in the front of the telephone directory.
9. Receive calls on a full-time basis in the setting in which the adequate telephone system is in operation. Commercial answering services, for example, carry with them a number of disadvantages:
   a. *Control*—When total responsibility for telephone counseling is not provided by a trained crisis worker, the center's control over the service is diminished considerably.

b. *Ethics*—When a twenty-four-hour service is advertised and something less than that is provided, an ethical question arises as to whether the center is, in fact, providing what it has promised to deliver to the public.

c. *Contact*—When the client's initial contact is not with the crisis worker, the fragile connection with the caller may be broken. Delays in rendering service can result. In addition, callers not wishing to give their names or telephone numbers are prevented from having any access to the crisis worker.

Face-to-Face Counseling Trained crisis workers provide intervention via direct, personal contact in a variety of clinical settings:

A. **WALK-IN SERVICE**

The walk-in service is located in the crisis center itself. A crisis center must have an independent, identifiable base from which its operations are directed and conducted.[4] Consider these questions in planning a base of operations[3,4]:

1. *Location*—Is the proposed center
   - Accessible to the community being served?
   - On a main street?
   - Served by public transportation?
   - Housed in an easily recognized building?
   - Identifiable with a sign?
   - Near adequate parking facilities?
2. *Physical Setting*—Has adequate space been allotted so that
   - Records can be stored?
   - Business can be conducted?
   - Telephone counseling can be provided?
   - Walk-in counseling can be done in separate, private quarters?

B. **MOBILE OR OUTREACH SERVICE**

Deciding whether the center will provide crisis services in the actual crisis setting requires certain considerations:

1. *Criteria*[3]—A mobile service may be indicated when
   - A crisis cannot be assessed adequately over the telephone and the person(s) cannot come to the center
   - Police or rescue squad intervention seems inappropriate, is unavailable, or is refused by the person(s) in crisis
   - The person is a threat to self and cannot or will not come for help
   - The person is a threat to others. In such cases collaboration with police should be considered. Crisis workers are not obliged to put themselves in dangerous situations.
   - Transportation to community resources is urgently needed and no other means of transportation is available
   - A disruption in a family requires resolution
   - It is necessary to remove forcibly a person from the home
2. *Staff*[4]—Usually two crisis workers go to the crisis scene together (too many workers can only add to the confusion).
3. *Equipment*[4]—Certain items prove useful in the operation of a mobile unit:
   - Two-way radio system enables the crisis worker to get to the crisis scene as quickly as possible and facilitates involvement of other community services (for example, police, rescue squad, etc.)

- Maps of the community
- First aid kit
- Flashlights

C. **CRISIS SETTING**

Wherever crisis service is rendered, the rapport between crisis worker and the person(s) in crisis is enhanced when certain conditions exist[5]:

1. *Quiet*—Counseling is conducted in an area that is as quiet, calm, private, and as conducive to concentration as possible (for example, in an automobile, office, home, or outdoor place away from noise or activity).
2. *Comfort*—The comfort of the person in crisis should be addressed. The client is provided warmth, food, and water.
3. *Safety*—A safe environment is essential, not only for the person in crisis but for the crisis worker as well. When a person is potentially dangerous, it is essential that
   - Potential weapons are removed, such as glasses, plates, heavy bookends, and so forth.
   - Access to help has been anticipated (for example, an inconspicuous signal system can be set up in the office).

Referral Service A. **MAKING A REFERRAL**

Whenever crisis resolution requires services beyond the scope of the center, referral is made to other appropriate community resources and follow-up is provided. When referral is needed, the crisis worker considers the following:

1. *Who* is to initiate the referral? (Will the client make the contact, or is the helper to do it?)
2. *What* is the appropriate resource (contact person's name, telephone number)?
3. *Where* is the resource located (address and client's means of transportation)?
4. *When* can referral arrangements be made (date, time of appointment)?
5. *Why* was this particular resource chosen (purpose; anticipated outcome)?
6. Was the contact made?
7. What were the results?
8. Is further intervention needed?

B. **EVALUATING THE REFERRAL SERVICE**

A center's referral service is more effective and efficient when it has[3]

1. Access to a *directory* of community resources
2. Knowledge of the *admission criteria* for each
3. Formal written *referral procedures* and agreements with all agencies involved in crisis work, including a review process
4. Initial and continuing *personal contact* with other agencies so that communication is maintained

Education and Training

Staff Development The purpose of staff development is to assist individuals to fulfill role expectations within the agency and to help them perform competently on the job.[4] Staff development in the crisis center includes training by orientation, followed by on-the-job inservice education designed to build continually upon prior knowledge and skills.

A crisis center's staff may include professionals (both "in-house" and consultant), para- and nonprofessionals, volunteer and salaried personnel, and any combination thereof. It is a mistake to assume that every staff member is working from the same knowledge base or theoretical model. Therefore, *all* staff should be given the same training opportunities, so that everyone is operating under the same set of "rules."[4]

The Nonprofessional
Volunteer

History demonstrates that a center's professional volunteers can contribute significantly to the staff and function adequately as crisis counselors when they have access to professional consultation.[4]

A. **RECRUITMENT**

All segments of the population should be considered potential sources for recruitment of volunteers. Several methods are useful:

1. *Mass Media*—Radio, television, newspaper articles, and local bulletin boards can be used to announce that the center is seeking volunteers.
2. *Nomination*—Community leaders can suggest names of qualified persons.
3. *Group Membership*—Local clubs sometimes will assume the task of staffing the center.

B. **SCREENING AND PREPARATION**

There will be times when a person who volunteers to work in the center simply is not suitable for crisis intervention work. The center decides in advance how to handle such a situation, both in terms of screening before "hiring" and deciding when a volunteer must be let go. The following suggestions may be helpful[4,6]:

1. Characteristics of an unacceptable volunteer are agreed upon ahead of time.
2. The application form includes the person's prior volunteer activities and experiences with people in crisis.
3. An initial screening meeting with the applicant is scheduled during which the volunteer's readiness to help can be assessed.
4. A trial (preparatory) period is built in *before* "official" orientation begins, during which a core group of experienced staffers can evaluate the newcomer, and vice versa. (Sometimes volunteers will recognize themselves as unsuitable and make the decision to leave before being asked to do so.)
5. To obtain additional information, it may be useful to administer psychological tests that describe personality, for example the Philosophy of Human Nature Scale, Myers-Briggs Type Indicators.

C. **MAINTAINING MORALE**

Morale problems are endogenous to any crisis program because of the stressful nature of the work. Ways of alleviating these problems are[4]

1. Volunteers are encouraged to select a coordinator from their ranks to manage their interests.
2. Volunteers organize themselves into a representative body to facilitate their negotiating with other staff members and to give them a voice in decision making.
3. The role relationship and expectations between volunteers and other staff are made explicit.
4. Channels of communication are established.
5. Mailboxes are provided so that messages and announcements are relayed properly.

6. Rewards and recognition are built in so that commitment and involvement are acknowledged and encouraged.
7. Limits are set on work to prevent the possibility of ''burn-out.''

Teaching Principles and Methods of Crisis Intervention

Each center will have its own method of training its staff to develop basic listening and helping skills. (See, for example, the *Trainer's Manual* and the *Counselor Training: Short-Term Client Systems* course developed by the National Drug Abuse Center for Training and Resource Development, 5600 Fishers Lane, Rockville, Maryland, revised May, 1977.)

Accountability Through Record Keeping

Accountability to the community is indicated by the emphasis placed on record keeping. A center's systematic collection, recording, and filing of information about itself and its clients can be useful for a number of reasons:

A. **CONTINUITY OF SERVICE**
Clients who have made prior contact are better served when their records at the center indicate what was tried and found to be effective in the past.

B. **QUALITY OF SERVICE**
Effects of helper's clinical behavior on clients can be documented; individual workers and the center as a whole can profit from this knowledge and be held accountable for their actions.

C. **ASSESSMENT OF NEEDS**
Demographic data may reveal
1. Characteristics and patterns of the population being served by the agency
2. Agency services most in demand, most used by members of the community
3. Adequacy of funding and justification for further funding

D. **ACCREDITATION**
The center is better prepared for external evaluation by various accrediting agencies should it undergo such a process. It should be noted that accreditation carries with it far more than the immediate satisfaction of having proven compliance with professional standards. Beyond protecting the public from substandard care, accreditation may bring to the program
1. Stimulation toward self-improvement
2. Public recognition and prestige
3. Listing in the official directory of the accrediting agency
4. Eligibility for government funding
5. Protection from external pressures, which enables the program to keep legitimate control over its own growth and development

Legal Considerations

Crisis centers must operate within the framework of the law. Therefore, it is essential that crisis workers be familiar with whatever federal, state, and local laws are currently affecting them. Such knowledge enhances the freedoms of both the helper and those being helped. Some issues to be considered are[5]

1. *Responsibility*—What client activities must be reported? (For example, many state laws require the reporting of child abuse.)
2. *Consent*—What are the state laws concerning commitment procedures and standards?
3. *Confidentiality*—What are the current federal laws regarding the protection of confidence of clients (for example, alcohol and drug abusers)?
4. *Duty to Warn*—Under what circumstances is the helper obliged to warn a potential homicide victim?

Precautions In general, there is a certain degree of legal latitude granted to crisis workers. To avoid legal redress, crisis workers who are nurses would be wise to consider these precautions[7]:
1. Base practice on the Standards of Psychiatric–Mental Health Nursing Practice as described by the American Nurses Association (see Appendix A).
2. Be familiar with state laws, including the Nurse Practice Act.
3. Keep accurate and concise records.
4. Maintain the confidentiality of those being helped.
5. Carry malpractice insurance.
6. Consult an attorney should a legal dilemma arise.

Maintaining Relationships with the Community

A center's relationship with other service agencies and with the population it serves must be nurtured as carefully as any other aspect of its role in the community.

Purpose The crisis center advertises its services to the public in order that
1. The availability of the crisis service is announced
2. The quality of service being offered can be evaluated publicly
3. Other service agencies in the community are informed and the way is cleared for interagency referral

Method Any of the following can be used to inform the public of services:

A. **BROADCAST MEDIA (RADIO, TELEVISION)**
   1. Public service spot announcements
   2. Feature programs
   3. Guest spots on "talk" shows
   4. Videotape

B. **PRINT MEDIA**
   1. Newspapers
      • Public service advertisements
      • Feature articles
      • Press releases
      • Article reprints
   2. Telephone book "Yellow Pages" and white pages
   3. Posters, pamphlets, brochures, business stationery, and business cards

        4. Center newsletter
        5. Individual mailings

    C. **PUBLIC PLACES**
        1. Bulletin boards (for example, by time clocks, in lobbies, near entries to grocery stores, in store front windows)
        2. Buses
        3. Billboards
        4. Bumper stickers; pins

    D. **SPEAKERS' BUREAU**
        Center staffers speak to
        1. Service clubs
        2. Informal community support groups (for example, bartenders, cab drivers, motel clerks)
        3. Public servants (hospital emergency room personnel, police officers)

Evaluation   It is always useful to ask clients how they came to hear about the crisis program so that accurate conclusions can be drawn about the effectiveness of advertising efforts and appropriate changes can be made.

References   1. American Nurses' Association: Guidelines for Staff Development. Kansas City, Missouri, ANA, 1976
2. Hemelt MD, Mackert ME: Dynamics of Law in Nursing and Health Care. Reston, Virginia, Reston Publishing Company, 1978
3. Hoff LA: People in Crisis: Understanding and Helping. Reading, Massachusetts, Addison-Wesley Publishing Company, 1978
4. McGee RK: Crisis Intervention in the Community. Baltimore, University Park Press, 1974
5. Resnick H, Ruben H: Emergency Psychiatric Care. Bowie, Maryland, The Charles Press, 1975
6. Silverman P: Helping Each Other in Widowhood. New York, Health Science Publishing, 1974
7. Stuart G, Sundeen S: Principles and Practices of Psychiatric Nursing. St Louis, CV Mosby, 1979

Bibliography   Aguilera DC, Messick JM: Crisis Intervention: Theory and Methodology, 4th ed. St Louis, CV Mosby, 1982
Dixon SL: Working with People in Crisis: Theory and Practice. St Louis, CV Mosby, 1979
Okura KP: Mobilizing in response to a major disaster. Commun Mental Health J 11:136, 1975
Phelan LA: Crisis intervention: Partners in problem solving. J Psychiatr Nurs 17:22, 1979
Wallace MA, Schreiber FB: Crisis intervention training for police officers: A practical program for local police departments. J Psychiatr Nurs 15:22, 1977

6

Designing a Community Health/Mental Health Consultation Program

Shirley TeMaat Hollingsworth

Description A community health/mental health consultation program is carried out by nurses who use the epidemiological model of primary, secondary, and tertiary prevention. By incorporating mental health concepts into this model, nurses enhance the client's adaptation to stress and teach coping mechanisms. The elements of this chapter will focus on primary and secondary prevention.

Definitions A. **PRIMARY PREVENTION**
Primary prevention is the process of strengthening coping mechanisms to deal effectively with crisis events in life, thereby reducing susceptibility to mental disorders.

B. **SECONDARY PREVENTION**
Secondary prevention is the process of facilitating early case-finding and treatment strategies to prevent recurrences of mental disorders and return clients to a productive level of functioning.

Program Goals 1. To raise the level of mental health in a community and reduce mental disorder
2. To provide mental health consultation for community health nurses to exert a widespread effect on the community

Administrative Processes Administrative processes vary in accordance with available resources and geographical locality.

A. **ORGANIZATIONAL STRUCTURE**
1. *Unified Services*—This is provided by a joint collaboration between a large public psychiatric hospital and a local health department, both of whom contract with a community nursing service to administer the mental health program.
2. *Lines of Responsibility*—The state hospital and the health department contract with the community nursing service to provide a mental health nurse consultant and home visits by nurses. The consultant is directly responsible to the director of nurses of the community nursing service. The consultant establishes mechanisms for open communication among all program participants. Figure 6–1 demonstrates the communication process.

B. **FUNDING**
The following costs should be considered:
1. Secretarial service, office space, telephone
2. Consultant's salary and benefits
3. Home visits by the community health nurses (salaries, benefits, transportation)

C. **LINES OF RESPONSIBILITY**
Lines of responsibility within the community nursing service are determined by the definition of consultation.
1. The consultant advises, teaches, and instructs.
2. The consultant does not have explicit authority to hold the consultee accountable.
3. The consultee is free to use or not use the information received.
4. The consultant's authority is the authority of knowledge.
5. The consultant is in a "staff" position as described in Figure 6–2, and advises the other nurses without direct responsibility to or for them.
6. The line position indicates direct responsibility for the agency's work.

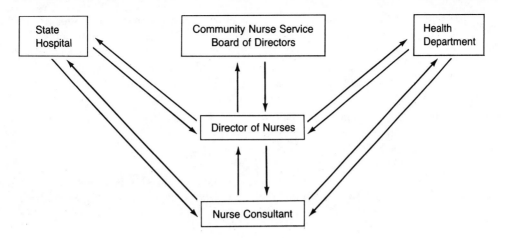

FIG. 6–1 Communication process in organizational structure.

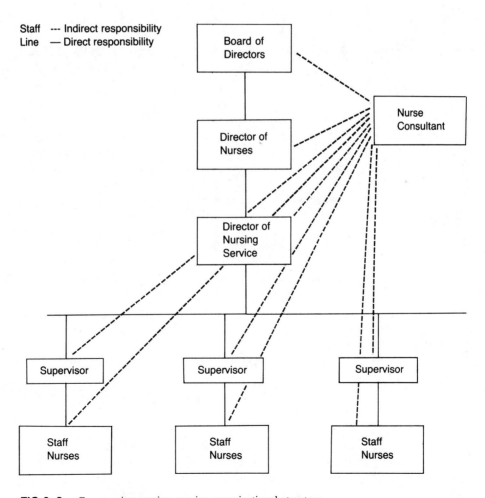

Staff --- Indirect responsibility
Line   — Direct responsibility

FIG 6–2. Community nursing service organizational structure.

Philosophy   It is important that the consultant have strong administrative support. The director of nurses must consider consultation to be of value because this attitude permeates the entire staff and affects the use of the consultant. The consultant should be a nurse with previous experience in community health. The consultant is in a position to understand the experience of the staff nurse and is a role model.

Consultant's Role   To implement program goals the consultant's focus is on the staff nurses and the community. The roles are:

A. VIS-À-VIS THE STAFF NURSE
   The consultant provides consultation and in-service education to the staff nurse.
   1. To broaden the nurse's knowledge of mental health principles
   2. To enhance the nurse's ability to reduce the client's susceptibility to a mental disorder
   3. To increase the nurse's ability to detect early symptoms of a mental disorder and to refer for effective treatment

B. VIS-À-VIS THE COMMUNITY
   The consultant provides consultation for the community.
   1. To develop a referral process and evaluation mechanism between the community health nurse service and mental health facilities
   2. To develop a team relationship with other mental health professionals in the community
   3. To represent nursing on county mental health board planning committees

Consultation Model[1]   Consultation is a process designed to focus on the problems the community health nurse (consultee) cannot solve alone. The consultant's approach may be nondirective or directive, depending on the presenting situation. The consultant uses knowledge that applies to the given consultation situation (for example, developmental stages—Erikson; grief process—Lindemann; transference/countertransference—Freud; enmeshment/differentiation of self—Bowen). Objectives of the consultation process are to
   1. Educate the consultee to be able to handle similar problems more effectively in the future
   2. Develop an understanding of the meaning of human behavior within the context of a nurse–client relationship

Why Staff Seek Consultation   Requests from staff for consultation cover a wide range of problem situations. Some of the common themes are
   1. Feeling inadequate and helpless ("I don't know what else to do.")
   2. Feeling frustrated and blocked because the client/family will not follow the medical regime
   3. Feeling overwhelmed by many social/psychological problems
   4. Lack of knowledge about certain areas
      Examples of cases presented for consultation appear in Table 6–1.

The Consultation Process   The consultee
   1. Defines the problem for which help is required
   2. Examines all aspects of the problem
   3. Reviews attempted solutions

Table 6–1
EXAMPLES OF CASES PRESENTED FOR CONSULTATION

Client, Diagnosis, Age	Problem
Mrs. A., antepartum, 19	Very unstable 7 months pregnant woman. The nurse needed consultation to understand how she could help the client handle her feelings of anxiety and how and where to refer for counseling.
Mr. B., cancer of the bladder, 65	The nurse needed help with her own feelings of grief for this dying client and how she could help the family through the grief process.
Mrs. C., emphysema, 60	Client living with alcoholic husband; argumentative and assaultive toward each other. Nurse had difficulty in understanding the limitations of her role.
Mrs. D., postpartum—fourth child, cancer of uterus, 26	The client seemed to be denying the seriousness of her illness and was unable to understand the need for a hysterectomy. The nurse needed suggestions for different approaches to foster a more realistic appraisal by the client.
Mr. E., pneumonia, aortic stenosis, CHF, anemia, 90	The nurse needed suggestions for communicating with this client who was very angry about being ill, living with his children, and losing his independence. His family had difficulty dealing with him and handling their own feelings of anger and guilt.
Battered child, 3	Appropriate referral resources were discussed as well as coordination with other agencies to help the child and to provide a support system for the boy's 25-year-old mother who had five other children, aged 6 to 13.

4. Explores alternative solutions
5. Discusses possible results of alternative solutions
6. Discusses the plan of action, for example, communication techniques to use with the client
7. Discusses means of evaluating progress
8. Ascertains resolution of goal or need for further intervention
   Table 6–2 illustrates the consultation process.

Indications for Intervention   A. **PREDICTABLE LIFE EVENTS**
   Life events that may cause stress are
   1. Marriage
   2. Parenthood
   3. Developmental stage transitions
   4. Retirement
   5. Death of a significant other/bereavement

Table 6–2
THE CONSULTATION PROCESS

The Consultee	The Consultant
Indicates problem—''Maybe you can help me.''	*Shows willingness to help*—''Let's talk about it.''
Begins to describe the problem—''I visit an elderly couple. . . .''	*Exhibits permissive behavior* (attentive, accepting attitude, nods, agrees with part of the statement)—''You feel caught in the middle because each asks you not to tell the other. . . .''
Adds to or expands upon other areas of the problem—''I don't know what to say when he asks me why he isn't getting better. . . .''	*Encourages expression of frustration, anger, helplessness*—''It is difficult when people can't openly express how they feel. . . .''
Continues description—(solution A didn't work) ''She doesn't want to tell him because he has threatened suicide in the past. . . .''	*Explores other possible solutions*—''Have you tried to ask him what he knows about his illness. . . .?''
Explores solutions B and C—''I thought of trying B or C, but I don't think I'd better (etc)''	*Questions*—''You don't think they would work? What do you think would happen if you did that?''

B. **UNPREDICTABLE SITUATIONAL EVENTS**
Situational events that cause stress are
1. Illness
2. Hospitalization
3. Loss of job or home
4. Separation
5. Catastrophic events

Example of Primary Prevention (Stress of Childbirth) Most parents having their first child do not automatically know how to care for that child. The community health nurse begins to teach parenting skills and to enhance the bonding process in the prenatal period on through the infancy stage of development. The nurse helps the parents identify unrealistic expectations, gives information on child development, physical and psychological needs, and practical skills. This is primary prevention, for if stress is high in the family, all members will be at risk for mental illness, including the new baby.

Chart 6–1 shows an interview guide for expectant parents that gives the nurse information on areas of need in which to plan nursing interventions. The interview provides information about the parents' needs, for example
1. Parents may be comfortable about impending parenthood but may need:
   a. Supportive counseling
   b. Anticipatory guidance
   c. Knowledge of normal growth and development
2. Parents may be ''at risk'' as potential child abusers and thus need
   a. Supportive counseling
   b. Anticipatory guidance
   c. Education about normal growth and development
   d. Referral to an appropriate mental health facility for in-depth counseling, the local child protective services, and parent support groups

Chart 6–1
NURSE ASSESSMENT GUIDE FOR EXPECTANT PARENTS

Nursing Questions	Theoretical Rationale
1. "What is it like to be pregnant?"	1. If the child is planned for and wanted, the parents' level of stress may be lower.
2. "What do you think it will be like when you have your baby?"	2. Rigid expectations may cause problems if the child does not live up to them.
3. "What would you like to have, a boy or a girl?"	3. If parents are eager for one gender, they may be deeply disappointed and anxious if their baby is the opposite gender.
4. "What if it's the opposite?"	4. Desire for one gender only may be indicative of other problems.
5. "What was it like when you were growing up?"	5. The way they were treated by their own parents affects the way they will act as parents. Parents who were battered are at risk of battering their own children.
6. "Who did you want to be like when you grew up?"	6. If they wanted to be like their parents, the quality of parenting was probably good.
7. "How do you get along with your parents?"	7. Positive feelings toward parents may lead to supportive grandparents for the baby.
8. "What do you do when you need help?"	8. An available support system helps new parents cope with stress.
9. "What do you do for fun?"	9. Ability to plan for own individual needs decreases negative effects of stress.
10. "How do you get along with each other?"	10. If the relationship is a close, mutually supportive one, there will be less stress after the baby is born.
11. If not married, "What are your plans for taking care of the baby?"	11. If the client is an adolescent, meeting the needs of an infant and trying to master the tasks of her own developmental stage may cause conflicts.
12. "What do you know about child growth and development? Have you ever taken care of an infant, any younger brothers or sisters?"	12. Knowledge will help the parents be less anxious.
13. "What kind of work do you (or husband) do? What is your income?"	13. Economic stability and no other changes in life-style help reduce stress. The chances of child battering increase with financial problems.
14. "Do you plan on moving just before or soon after the baby is born?"	14. Moving adds additional stress.

Example of Secondary Prevention (Child Battering)

Certain patterns alert the nurse to the possibility of child battering once the baby is born.

A. **IDENTIFIED PATTERNS OF THE BATTERED CHILD SYNDROME**
   1. *Parents*
      a. History of traumatic upbringing
      b. Immature, impulsive
      c. Unrealistic expectations that the child meet parents' needs
      d. Nonsupportive spouse
      e. Poor self-image
      f. Lower socioeconomic and educational status
      g. Isolated, no support system
      h. Abuses alcohol
      i. Distrustful, hostile

2. *Child*
   a. Unwanted
   b. Premature
   c. Disabled
   d. Resembles someone hated
   e. Cries inconsolably
   f. Seen as a "special child"
   g. Scapegoated
3. *Environment*
   a. Emotional crisis
   b. Financial problems
   c. Illness in family
   d. Separation in family
   e. Death in family

When the nurse suspects child battering, the family is referred to a mental health facility or local child protective services.

Advantages and Disadvantages of Being A Consultant

A. **ADVANTAGES**
1. High level of independence to design and implement programs
2. Freedom to interact with many other "providers" in the community
3. Enjoyment of watching staff develop and effect change in the community

B. **DISADVANTAGES**
1. Lack of peers on the job
2. Disappointment when consultee chooses not to use the intervention, resulting in continuation and enlargement of the problem

Evaluation Process

The community health nurse
1. Documents specific short- and long-term goals
2. Evaluates movement toward the goal or need for goal changes
3. Ascertains resolution of the goal or need for further intervention

Reference

1. Caplan G: Concepts of Mental Health and Consultation. Washington, DC, Children's Bureau Publication No. 375, 1959

Bibliography

Bowen M: Family Therapy in Clinical Practice. New York, Jason Aronson, 1978
Caplan G: Principles of Preventive Psychiatry. New York, Basic Books, 1964
Clark CC: Mental Health Aspects of Community Health Nursing. New York, McGraw-Hill, 1978
Erikson E: Childhood and Society. New York, WW Norton and Co, 1963
Ginott H: Between Parent and Child. New York, McGraw-Hill, 1965
Gordon T: P.E.T. in Action. New York, Bantam Books/published by Peter H Wyden, 1978
Lahinica E: The Nursing Process, A Humanistic Approach. Menlo Park, CA, Addison-Wesley, 1979
Lindeman E: Symptomotology and management of acute grief. In Fulton R (ed): Death and Identity. New York, John Wiley & Sons, 1965
Miller J, Janosik E: Family Focused Care. New York, McGraw-Hill, 1980
Palermo E: Mental health consultation in a home care agency. J Psychiatr Nurs 16:21, 1978
Spradley B: Community Health Nursing, Concepts and Practice. Boston, Little, Brown & Co, 1981
Weed L: Medical Records, Medical Education, and Patient Care. Cleveland, Case Western Reserve University Press, 1970

7

Designing a Jail Deferment Program

Jean Moore

It is clear that deinstitutionalization alone will not solve the problems of emotionally disturbed clients who live in the community. The major goal of the 1980s is the development of an organized and integrated system of community resources. Such a system must be responsive to the needs of clients to ensure their survival in the community. One important task is to establish a connection between agencies in the mental health system and agencies in the criminal justice system.

Jail deferment programs provide client-oriented mental health consultation to agencies within the criminal justice system. A mental health consultant serves as the connecting link between mental health and criminal justice agencies. Clinical assessment, collaboration, and negotiation are three key functions of the mental health consultant. A well functioning program should affect not only the systems involved, but also the treatment received by clients in both systems.

A jail deferment program can bridge the gap between two systems and, consequently, prevent clients from "falling through the cracks." Such programs demonstrate the broader role that community mental health nurses and other professionals must now play to promote emotional well-being in the community.

Definition of Terms A. **JAIL DEFERMENT PROGRAM**

The jail deferment program is a community-based service providing client-oriented psychiatric consultation to agencies within the criminal justice system. The purpose is to evaluate mental health needs to prevent inappropriate jailing of clients who are in need of psychiatric treatment.

B. **POPULATION TO BE SERVED**

The population to be served includes clients who have allegedly committed minor infractions of the law and who would benefit more from psychiatric treatment than incarceration. It *excludes* all clients who are found not responsible by reason of mental defect or who are found incompetent to stand trial.

C. **MENTAL HEALTH CONSULTATION**

Mental health consultation is "a provision for technical assistance by an expert to individuals and agency care givers related to the mental health dimensions of their work."[2]
1. Types of mental health consultation[6]
   a. Client-oriented
   b. Consultee-oriented
   c. Situation-oriented

D. **CRIMINAL JUSTICE SYSTEM**

The criminal justice system is "a system for the enforcement of traditional penal laws, analysis of which involve describing the structural interrelationships of legislatures, appellate courts and enforcement and administrative agencies as well as their corresponding processes of decision making from arrest of subjects through charging adjudication, sentencing, imprisonment and release on parole. Criminal justice is mostly concerned with the decisions of the various crime control agencies."[5]

E. **FORENSIC SERVICES**

Forensic services represent the provision of mental health care to persons involved in the criminal justice system, including those presentenced, those acquitted by reason of insanity, and those who have been tried and convicted and are serving sentences in a correctional setting. A jail deferment program is an example of a community-based forensic service.

Rationale for Jail Deferment Program

A. **THE IMPACT OF DEINSTITUTIONALIZATION**
In 1955, the total inpatient census of New York State psychiatric institutions was 93,000; in 1980 it was 23,000.[4] Clients who had spent years living in psychiatric institutions were placed in the community. Years of institutional living left many ill-equipped to confront the daily problems of community living. The initial effort at deinstitutionalization met with failure because the communities also were not prepared to confront the problems engendered by the process.

B. **COMMUNITY RESPONSE TO CLIENT BEHAVIOR**
With psychiatric clients living in the community, the "acting-out" behavior that can accompany emotional disturbance became visible and problematic. The community response to such behavior was either to return the client to the psychiatric institution or to incarcerate the client. Both responses were reactive, not preventive, and were based on lack of information.

C. **CREATING A NETWORK OF SUPPORTIVE COMMUNITY SERVICES**
It has become increasingly clear that the mere placement of clients will not ensure their successful reintegration into a community. It is the role of the community mental health service system to link clients with the necessary resources to support their adjustment to community living and to educate communities to better understand the unique needs of psychiatric clients. The most efficient and effective approach is to create an integrated network of support services within the community.

Assessment of Need

A. **PROBLEMS THAT A JAIL DEFERMENT PROGRAM MAY ADDRESS**
1. *Systems Problems*—Lack of consistent communication and cooperation between a mental health system and a criminal justice system may occur because the systems
   a. Have diametrically opposing goals
   b. Lack common theoretical ground
   c. Do not speak the same language
2. *Client Problems*—The community mental health movement has resulted in growing numbers of clients who receive primarily outpatient psychiatric treatment. Many of these clients "fall through the cracks" between the criminal justice system and the mental health system for the following reasons:
   a. Some clients refuse to comply with outpatient psychiatric treatment, break the law, and get arrested; the stress of jailing results in an acute psychotic episode, which warrants psychiatric hospitalization.
   b. Some clients break the law, but their reputation for "being crazy" exempts them from being treated like anyone else who breaks the law.
   c. Some clients who have never sought mental health services may break the law secondary to a psychiatric problem and could benefit more from psychiatric treatment than from incarceration in a jail.

B. **SYSTEMS BENEFITING FROM JAIL DEFERMENT PROGRAMS**
1. *Police courts*—Because referrals to mental health services could be made directly

2. *Probation departments*—Because probation officers could work in cooperation with a mental health clinician on a case where both services are indicated
3. *County jails*—Because emergency psychiatric hospitalization could be arranged through this program and the police court consultation process would divert (to outpatient psychiatric services) clients who might otherwise be inappropriately jailed
4. *Mental health service systems*—Because it would create a consistent link to agencies involved with psychiatric clients

Establishment of a Program

A. **PROGRAM ENDORSEMENT—AGENCY CONTRIBUTIONS AND COMMITMENTS**

All agencies must endorse the program administratively. Since a jail deferment program involves contributions and commitments from all agencies involved, administrative support correlates directly to the willingness of the agency to contribute to the program.

1. *A mental health system* contributes the mental health consultant (psychiatric nurse) who serves as liaison to the criminal justice agencies involved in the jail deferment program. The mental health system must also contribute psychiatric inpatient beds reserved for emergency admission from police court or jail.
2. *A police court* commits itself both to use the mental health consultant in the assessment of cases in which psychiatric services may be needed, and to follow the recommendations of the consultant as indicated. The mental health consultant coordinates all cases in which a client is already receiving psychiatric treatment and faces legal prosecution.
3. *A probation department* commits itself to use the mental health consultant when referrals for psychiatric services are made for any clients of that agency. The mental health consultant, in turn, collaborates with the probation department on any case in which a client already receiving psychiatric treatment has been placed on probation.
4. *A city or county jail* commits itself to use the mental health consultant in the assessment of jailed clients who are in need of either inpatient or outpatient psychiatric services. The mental health consultant, in turn, works with the jail in coordinating all cases in which a client is already receiving psychiatric treatment.

B. **QUALIFICATIONS OF THE MENTAL HEALTH CONSULTANT**

The mental health consultant is the consistent point of interface between any agencies involved in a jail deferment program. The skills and abilities of the consultant can result in the success or failure of a jail deferment program. For this reason, a mental health consultant should have the following qualifications and experiences:

1. Educational preparation must include a masters degree in a specialty such as psychiatric nursing, which includes in-depth clinical training.
2. At least 3 years' postmasters clinical experience in psychiatric nursing or a similar specialty is also essential. Such experience can adequately prepare a nurse clinician for the clinical assessment aspects of a jail deferment program.
3. Knowledge of systems and strategies for systems negotiations is useful.

C. OBTAINING CONTRACTS OF AGREEMENT

A preliminary step in implementing a jail deferment program is the establishment of written contracts with all parties involved. The mental health consultant should assume responsibility for initiating contracts or agreement.

1. The contract includes
   a. Who will be involved
   b. Where and when services will be rendered
   c. Purpose of service
   d. Duration of service
   e. Plan for evaluation of service
2. An example of a contract of agreement with a police court is shown in Figure 7–1

Dear Judge K,

Per our verbal agreement, I will be attending Albany Police Court each Thursday from 10:00 am to 12:00 pm beginning 2/8/79 to serve as a mental health consultant. As we agreed, I will be available to assess any cases in which the client's emotional stability may be in question and to make recommendations on these cases. Listed below are my objectives for this program:

1. To identify psychiatric treatment needs of any identified Capital District Psychiatric Center client facing legal prosecution
2. To determine the extent to which such legal action may be implemented in accordance with treatment plans of CDPC clients
3. To educate the court system to the special needs of psychiatric clients
4. To promote the concept that "acting out" behavior is not always "sick" behavior but is, at times, illegal behavior
5. To support court efforts toward clients seeking psychiatric treatment, when indicated, as part of the terms for probation
6. To identify those people facing legal charges who may benefit from outpatient psychiatric treatment

After a three-month period, I would like to meet with you to assess the usefulness of this program both for you and Capital District Psychiatric Center.

I look forward to working with you.

Sincerely,

Jean Moore, R.N., M.S.

FIG. 7–1 Sample letter of contract. (From Moore J: Community mental health consultation in police court. Perspect Psychiatr Care 18:206, 1980. Reprinted with permission)

Table 7–1

ROLES, BEHAVIORAL OBJECTIVES, AND GOALS OF THE NURSE IN JAIL DEFERMENT PROGRAMS

Role	Behavioral Objectives	Goals
A. Interview clients at the request of agencies within the criminal justice system	1. To identify the verbal deficits and behaviors that may indicate the presence of emotional distress 2. To determine the extent to which emotional distress may have influenced alleged illegal behavior 3. To establish an accurate history of involvement with mental health services 4. To identify clients' own perceptions of what they need 5. To assist clients in selecting the most appropriate available help	To divert clients from incarceration in the criminal justice system to treatment in the mental health system when appropriate
B. Provide information to agencies within the criminal justice system	1. To communicate to all parties involved (district attorney, public defender, judge, probation officer) recommendations on a case based on a consistent theoretical framework of human behavior 2. To consistently define the limitations of the jail deferment program in order to prevent an influx of inappropriate referrals.	To help agencies within the criminal justice system to recognize psychiatric illness and make appropriate referrals
C. Refer clients to other agencies that offer supportive services as indicated. (for example, Alcoholics Anonymous)	1. To assist clients in obtaining appropriate community resources necessary for survival in the community 2. To develop consistent relationships with other agencies to expedite other referrals 3. To ensure that a client receives consistent treatment from all agencies 4. To educate other community agencies about the unique needs of psychiatric clients	To support the development of a network of supportive community services responsive to the needs of clients
D. Provide case follow-up	1. To follow up on clients referred to other agencies 2. To serve as an advocate for clients who have difficulty accessing needed services from an agency 3. To negotiate change at a systems level with those agencies that fail to follow through in providing needed services to clients 4. To demonstrate consistency in executing collaborative plans with other agencies; to serve as a role model for expected behavior	To develop a mechanism for accountability between systems to ensure that clients are receiving necessary community services and have not "fallen through the cracks" of a referral between systems

Roles of the Mental Health Consultant in a Jail Deferment Program

Table 7–1 shows five major roles of a mental health consultant in a jail deferment program and the behavioral objectives and goals accompanying each role.

Case Example

The case study in Chart 7–1 is an excerpt from a previously published article describing an actual experience in mental health consultation in which the author served as police court consultant.[3]

The diagram in Figure 7–2 describes the process in which a lack of knowledge of psychological factors led to a communication breakdown between the court staff and Louis. Like other similar schemas,[1] it illustrates how the consultative process provides new information which, in this instance, helped the consultee, and Judge K, and the Public Defender to arrive at better understanding of the mental health aspects of the case.

Chart 7–1
CASE STUDY

Clinical Data

Louis, a 22-year-old single man, was arrested 2 days prior to his arraignment for provoking an altercation in a restaurant. He had eaten a meal there, was unable to pay for it, argued with the manager, and subsequently ripped a pay phone off a wall of the restaurant. After his arrest, Louis talked "strangely." I was asked to speak with him before his arraignment. Both Judge K. and a lawyer from the Public Defender's Office commented on how "crazy" this man was. When asked to explain his current circumstances, Louis explained he had extra sensory powers, which enabled him to read minds. He had been reading minds since he was 14, and enjoyed relating at a "cosmic level," but sometimes "got lost." He also said he received public assistance and food stamps, but ate at the restaurant on a day when he had no money or food stamps. He intended to repay the restaurant as soon as he received his monthly food stamp allocation. When asked why he thought he could eat in a restaurant without paying right away, Louis replied that his extra sensory powers gave him extra privileges. When asked what he was doing in jail if this were so, he said that now he realized he was wrong. Louis explained that he had moved to Albany from Florida 6 months before. He had his own apartment, and was a maintenance worker in the work relief program. While in Florida, he had completed 2 years of college, had two brief psychiatric hospitalizations, and about 3 years ago had been arrested under circumstances identical to those that led to his current arrest. He stated that 1 week before the arrest he had voluntarily sought outpatient psychiatric services and was scheduled to be seen for an initial evaluation that day.

Assessment

My assessment of this client was that despite an on-going, chronic thought disorder, he managed extremely well. Louis's description of his power to read minds, and his tendency to sometimes get lost in "cosmic communication" could be interpreted to mean that he had weak ego boundaries and feared losing the boundaries completely under the stress of close interpersonal contact. He therefore tended to "distance" himself from others as a defense. His current situation, that is, establishing himself in Albany, indicated a capacity to care for himself. Another indication of Louis's high functional capacity was his plan to seek psychiatric help 1 week before the acting-out episode occurred (i.e., just before his arrest); he was seeking an appropriate resource to help him maintain emotional control and support his efforts to function independently.

Louis's acting-out behavior did appear to be related to his thinking disorder; therefore, his mental state seemed to contribute to his criminal behavior.

Recommendation

Based on this assessment, I thought that the most appropriate course of action would be for this client to be probated, conditional on his continued involvement in outpatient psychiatric treatment.

In explaining my assessment and recommendation to Judge K. and the Public Defender, I did not refute their position that Louis was "crazy," but merely pointed out that despite his "craziness" he was capable of functioning in a relatively stable fashion. Judge K. and the Public Defender both spoke with Louis, reviewing his past history and examining his current situation. Both concurred with my recommendation for action. Louis was sentenced to 3 years' probation on the condition that he engage in outpatient psychiatric treatment during that time. I offered to follow up on this plan to ensure that Louis was receiving the services he sought.

(From Moore J: Community mental health consultation in police court. Perspect Psychiatr Care 18:204, 1980. Reprinted with permission)

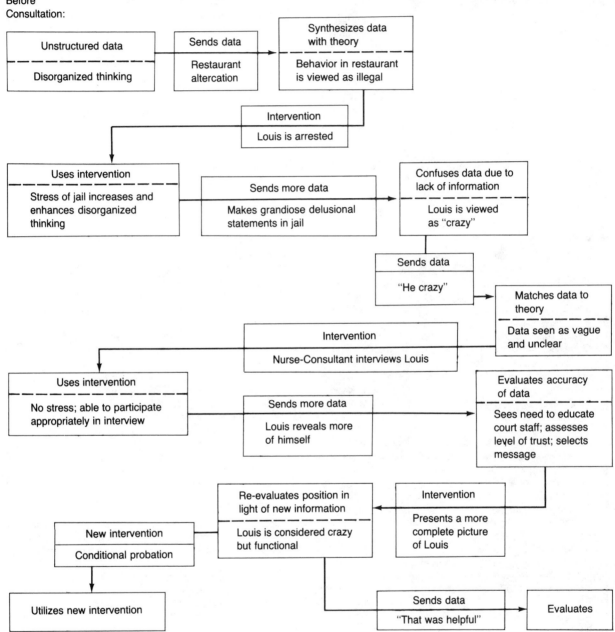

FIG. 7–2 Integration of client, justice system, and client behavior. (From Moore J: Community mental health consultation in police court. Perspect Psychiatr Care 18:208, 1980. Reprinted with permission)

Evaluation of Program Effectiveness

A. **IMPACT ON SYSTEMS**

1. Comparing Program Goals to Program Outcomes
   a. A successful attempt to divert inappropriate jailings is reflected in a reduced number of emergency psychiatric admissions from the jail.
   b. A successful attempt to educate criminal justice agencies in recognizing emotional distress in clients is reflected in the number of appropriate referrals made to the mental health consultant in a jail deferment program.
2. Subjective Information from Agencies Involved
   It is critical to encourage each agency in the program to provide comments on program effectiveness from their perspectives. Such information can be useful in revising program design to meet the needs of agencies involved.

B. **IMPACT ON CLIENTS**

Unfortunately, one of the most important areas of consideration is one of the most difficult to measure. Successful treatment outcomes differ greatly from client to client. While one client may benefit from mental health treatment aimed at learning the consequences of "acting out" illegal behavior, another may be incapable of learning such consequences and needs a protective environment. Given the variability of treatment outcomes, the best approach may be to randomly sample individual clients who received services within the jail deferment program to determine successful treatment outcome.

References

1. DeLoughery G, Gebbie K and Newman B: Community Mental Health Nursing: Consultation and Community Organization. Baltimore, Williams & Wilkins, 1971
2. Mannino F, Maclennan B, Shore M: The Practice of Mental Health Consultation. New York, Gardiner Press, 1975
3. Moore J: Community mental health consultation in police court. Perspect Psychiatr Care 18:204, 1980
4. New York State Office of Mental Health Statistical Services: Changes in the Inpatient Census, a Simplified Description. Unpublished, April 1981
5. Newman D: Introduction to Criminal Justice, 2nd ed. Philadelphia, JB Lippincott, 1978
6. Schwab J: Handbook of Psychiatric Consultation. New York, Appleton-Century-Crofts, 1968

8

Designing a Psychiatric Nursing Liaison Program in a General Hospital

Lisa Robinson

Definition   Psychiatric liaison nursing is a subspecialty of psychiatric nursing that uses nursing process focused on the alleviation of psychological distress in persons with physical illness or who are undergoing treatment of a physical nature.

Scope   Psychiatric liaison nursing uses both verbal communication and laying on of hands to administer direct care to clients, and the consultation method with staff nurses to help them to care for clients. Through these processes, clients who experience anxiety, fear, depression, loss, or any other disturbing emotion are helped to feel an increased sense of well-being. Psychiatric liaison nursing can be practiced wherever people are located who experience psychological pain associated with physical illness or its treatment. Some common settings are
1. General hospitals
2. Outpatient settings
3. Nursing homes
4. Hospices
5. Long-term care settings
6. The client's home

Hospital-Based Psychiatric Liaison Nursing

A. **RECIPIENTS OF SERVICE**
   Recipients of the services of the psychiatric liaison nurse in the hospital include the following:
   1. Direct service
      a. Any person admitted to the hospital for diagnosis or treatment of an illness or for terminal care who experiences a psychological problem
      b. The person's family or associates who experience psychological problems that engender anxiety in the client
   2. Indirect service
      a. Staff nurses who seek consultation or supervision concerning the care of the hospitalized person
      b. Other care-givers, such as physicians and ancillary staff whose functions directly affect the person who is hospitalized

B. **NURSE'S QUALIFICATIONS**
   The psychiatric liaison nurse is a registered nurse who has earned a masters degree in psychiatric nursing and whose course of study includes supervised practice in liaison nursing.

C. **OTHER TEAM MEMBERS**
   1. Other members of the health delivery team may collaborate in direct care if they have either
      a. Closer relationships to the client than the psychiatric liaison nurse has
      b. Greater access to the client, for example, the primary nurse in the labor room, the primary nurse of a client in isolation, the aide who speaks the native language of a non-English speaking client
   2. Other members of the health delivery team may include
      a. The staff nurse
      b. The nursing assistant
      c. The volunteer

     d. A parent or other family member

     e. A significant other to the client

     f. The physician

  3. It is assumed that membership on the health delivery team is voluntary and includes all persons who have skills that will facilitate the client's achievement of improved health *and* persons whose relationship(s) with the client are supportive of psychological well-being.

D. **SPECIFIC INPATIENT SETTINGS**

  1. The general hospital, including medical–surgical units and specialty areas (*i.e.*, ICU, CCU, emergency room, orthopedic units, etc.)

  2. The in-house hospice

  3. The nursing home

  4. The long term care facility such as

     a. Rehabilitation facility

     b. Renal dialysis unit

E. **INFLUENCES**

The design of a psychiatric liaison nursing program is influenced by the following:

  1. Administrative policies

  2. Funding sources

  3. Formal and informal objectives

  4. Physical structure

  5. Client profiles

  6. Philosophy and standards of care

Roles of the Psychiatric Liaison Nurse

A. **THERAPIST**

The psychiatric liaison nurse helps clients to

  1. Clarify their problems

  2. Acknowledge their feelings about the problems

  3. Become less sensitized to their feelings

  4. Alter the problems if this is possible

B. **CONSULTANT**

The psychiatric liaison nurse helps staff members to

  1. Clarify the problem

  2. Separate reality issues of the problem from their own feelings about the problem

  3. Develop options for managing the problem

  4. Become less anxious about the problem

  5. Implement their plan for management

  6. Evaluate the outcome of their actions

C. **SUPERVISOR**

The psychiatric liaison nurse helps staff members to

  1. Understand the dynamics of a selected client's problems

  2. Develop nursing care plans aimed at the alteration of clients' problems or their reaction to the problems

  3. Interact therapeutically with clients

4. Examine interpersonal interaction with clients to help build the staff member(s) skills in performing these nursing activities

D. **TEACHER**
   1. Identifies needs among unit staff for inservice education
   2. Develops teaching modules
   3. Delivers in-service education to staff

E. **RESEARCHER**
   1. Identifies psychiatric nursing liaison problems for which research questions can be formulated
   2. Uses systematic methods for data collection
   3. Analyzes data to answer research questions
   4. Communicates findings to staff and colleagues through ward conferences and articles in appropriate journals

Functions of the Psychiatric Liaison Nurse

A. **THERAPIST**
   1. Clarification of clients' problems begins with awareness that a problem exists. Awareness usually occurs through the client's report of a problem or through behavioral symptoms such as crying, withdrawal, excessive nightmares, inappropriate gaiety, or agitation.
   2. The liaison nurse may choose to see clients for assessment purposes only and then help the staff to design and implement a care plan, or may choose to care for clients directly. To help clients identify the problem and their accompanying feelings, the liaison nurse talks with the clients using open-ended questions that focus on the area of the problem.
   3. Clients are encouraged to describe the problem, identifying its components and their dynamic relationship.
   4. If clients do not spontaneously identify their feelings they are asked to try to name them. If they cannot do this, the nurse suggests broad categories of feelings (for example, mad, sad, glad, and scared) and continues to question.
   5. Clients are taught that feelings are different from thoughts and that energy is trapped in feelings. It is useful to separate thoughts and feelings and to have the energy from feelings available to use for problem solving, which is a thinking process.
   6. Desensitization of feelings is facilitated by ventilation. When clients report their feelings, their impact on the client is lessened. The feelings may have to be described several times, depending on their magnitude. In most cases each telling lessens the degree to which the client experiences them.
   7. Clients are helped to focus on those aspects of the problem that are potentially alterable, and options are identified. If the problem does not have potential for change, clients are helped to recognize this and, if loss or pain is involved, are supported and encouraged to grieve or react in a manner appropriate to the client and the situation. This might include support of the client's defenses, such as denial, sublimation, repression, or compensation.

Example: C.K. is a 19-year-old male who suffered multiple fractures and other internal injuries in a car accident in which he was the driver. His 15-year-old brother, who was a passenger, was killed. The nursing staff requested that this client be evaluated in light of his apparent withdrawal from them. C.K. has been on an intermediate care unit for 2½ weeks since his discharge from the trauma unit. The psychiatric liaison nurse tries to interview this client and finds him unwilling to talk with her. He is taciturn, and when pressed, he becomes hostile. The interviewer respects the client's need for privacy, yet she is concerned about his feelings because she wonders if he is experiencing guilt, depression, horror from flashbacks of the moment of impact, and so forth.

In this case, because she cannot work with the client, the liaison nurse tells him of her continued interest and availability and arranges to meet with his parents. On interview, they seem highly concerned about their surviving son while they simultaneously grieve the loss of the younger son. The liaison nurse suggests to the parents that she is available to them as well as to their son. She tells them that the nursing staff is concerned about their son's feelings and that he seems rather inaccessible to them. The nurse suggests that the boy may be grieving and simultaneously blaming himself, experiencing guilt or numerous other thoughts and feelings that are not immediately evident. She asks the parents if they can help the staff to create an environment in which the boy will feel safe to share his experience with either the parents or a staff member. The liaison nurse then suggests ways in which the parents can communicate to their son that he will be supported and that those concerned about him wish to understand how this experience is affecting him.

B. **CONSULTANT**
1. If a client presents a problem to all those caring for the client, the problem is explored through a staff conference. If only one staff member experiences the problem, that person may consult alone with the liaison nurse. Exploration of the problem is accomplished through identification of the "sensitizing scene" that has caused staff members to believe something is wrong. Various components of the problem are identified.
2. The liaison nurse assists staff members to separate their feelings from their thoughts by encouraging them to identify their feelings. They are then assisted to explore the sources or real objects of their feeling and reactivity and to refocus on the current client, who in most cases, is not the source or object. The liaison nurse encourages staff members to assign their feelings to the real objects and to view the client nonreactively.
3. Staff members are encouraged through discussion of the client's problem to identify means of altering the problem and to plan implementation of one or more options. Implementation is facilitated when specific persons are assigned to carry out identified activities.
4. Evaluation of outcomes may include a meeting or informal talks to discuss changes in the client's behavior.

Example: No one wants to take care of M.A., a 36-year-old female with multiple sclerosis. She has been in the chronic care unit for 10 years. She is paralyzed from midchest down and has had recurring bouts of blurred vision and blindness. The client is bitter, outspoken, and frequently rude to the staff. Nothing seems to suit her. A conference with the whole staff indicates that they are angry with the client. They have tried individually to understand what they might have done wrong. After varying self-explorations, they have not been able to modify the situation and, as a group, have come to the conclusion that this client is "diffi-cult," rude, and irrational. The liaison nurse helps the group to become issue oriented rather than person oriented. They are helped to see this client's life from her perspective: A helpless woman in what should have been the prime of her life, now paralyzed with few hopes. The staff is helped to understand the client's lack of control and helplessness. With the consultant's help they develop a care plan that addresses helplessness, hopelessness, and the need for some gratification using the concepts of territoriality and personal space. Within a short time the client is less angry in her communications with the staff. The latter become less reactive to the client.

C. **SUPERVISOR**

1. As a supervisor, the liaison nurse presents psychodynamic theories at the staff members' level of knowledge to help them understand the reasons for the client's problematic behavior. Usually the focus is on the client's needs and drives to satisfy those needs. When staff members understand the underlying dynamics of the client's behavior, they are usually more accepting of the behavior.

2. After the staff has designed a nursing care plan, the supervisor suggests various ways of meeting the client's needs in a manner that is appropriate to the setting and the client's physical condition. When the client is regressed, the nurse uses the principle of accepting the client's regression without pushing for "mature" behavior.

3. Sequential meetings are scheduled with staff members to hear how the nursing care plan is being carried out, how the staff members feel about the client and the effectiveness of the plan. Suggestions are offered for further nursing actions that will enhance the client's care or that will facilitate the desired change in the client.

Example: C.J. is an 8-year-old boy with leukemia. During his initial hospitaliza-tion, the staff finds that the boy is not communicative. His grandmother, who stays with him, speaks for him and insists on answering questions that they direct to the child. The liaison nurse is asked to intervene. He tries to make an initial assessment and soon understands the staff's problem! He notes that when he speaks to the child, the latter runs around the room with his index finger lightly pressed to the wall. The child does not speak, however.

With staff, a plan is formulated in which the grandmother is to be heavily supported by staff. She will be visited each day by the same nurse who will invite the grandmother to have a cup of coffee with her in the cafeteria. During that time, a child-life worker will be in the room with C.J. The goal of that person's interactions with the child will be to decrease his anxiety about interaction and later to support the child's efforts at direct and appropriate communications with the child-life worker. Both the nurse's work to decrease the grandmother's anxiety and to help her separate from the grandchild, and the child life worker's efforts with the little boy are supervised each day in a late afternoon conference with the liaison nurse. The three staff members share the events of each interaction and evaluate the child and the grandmother's progress. The liaison nurse coaches each staff member in strategies to attain these goals. The grandmother soon expresses her gratitude to the child-life worker for making it possible for her to "get away for a little spell each day.'' The child is able to stop running the perimeter of the room within the first 4 days. He soon begins to speak, although in monosyllables. The child-life worker and pediatric nurse integrate new behaviors into their professional repertoires for helping their clients. The daily contacts of the liaison nurse for supervising the two workers require about 10 minutes each day for 2 weeks. During that time, the child shows consistent ability to communicate directly with the staff.

D. **TEACHER**
1. The liaison nurse evaluates needs of staff for in-service education by observing their communication techniques with clients, by asking for their recommendation for educative programs, and by analyzing trends in problematic behaviors of nursing staff on the unit. The liaison nurse may also provide learning experiences relevant to the types of clients cared for routinely on the unit. Examples of seminars appropriate for a coronary care unit, for instance, might be the client's fear of death, defenses that are used and their behavioral manifestations, or human sexuality teaching following myocardial infarction.
2. Teaching modules may be designed after the median level of nurse education on the unit is identified. Theoretical material is explored and that which is relevant to the nursing staff and clients' needs is presented at the level at which staff can integrate the material and use it in their ongoing nursing care plans. The modules are arranged so that learning is sequential, and classes are offered at times when staff members are least stressed and optimum learning can take place.
3. Timing may require that the liaison nurse present the class more than one time and possibly at irregular hours.

E. **RESEARCHER**
1. The psychiatric liaison nurse is prepared at the masters level or higher, and it is assumed that nursing research will be conducted as one method of solving clinical problems. At present nursing care is often carried out without substantiation that the activities are effective in bringing about identified outcomes. The liaison nurse has many opportunities in direct practice and in the supervision of staff nurses' practices to observe client situations and nursing actions and to raise questions about effective nursing care. Examples of such questions follow:
    a. Should all surgical clients receive preoperative teaching? If not, which patients might be more anxious if they are taught?
    b. Is a protocol that uses reality orientation helpful for postconcussion syndrome clients to reduce their impulsivity and inappropriate behavior? If so, at what point in their rehabilitation is such an intervention most useful?
    c. Which method is most effective in reducing staff nurses' anxiety about clients who are acting out: didactic teaching about the psychodynamics underlying the client's behavior or role playing to model nursing actions?
2. Because psychiatric liaison nursing is a relatively new specialty it is not well researched and much baseline data is needed. For this reason descriptive studies are highly appropriate, and the methodologies that generate data for this kind of study are correct.[2]

3. The liaison nurse shares observations and findings with other colleagues so that peers may either replicate studies of interest or alter their practices to align them with new knowledge. Some journals that publish material that is of interest to psychiatric liaison nurses include
   a. International Journal of Psychiatry in Medicine
   b. Journal of Psychosocial Nursing and Mental Health Services
   c. General Hospital Psychiatry
   d. Perspectives in Psychiatric Care

Models for Psychiatric Liaison Nursing Programs[1]

A. **THE LIAISON NURSE IN A STAFF POSITION UNDER IN-SERVICE EDUCATION**
   1. Functions as a clinical specialist
   2. Is responsible for in-service education and research
   3. Does not have direct responsibility or authority vis-à-vis nursing staff
   4. Functions
      a. Provides consultation to nurses
      b. Intervenes in client crises
      c. Provides in-service education
      d. Refers long-term treatment to the department of psychiatry or social service

B. **THE LIAISON NURSE IN A LINE POSITION UNDER IN-SERVICE EDUCATION**
   1. Functions as a clinical specialist
   2. Has administrative supervisory responsibility for nursing division
   3. Is responsbile to nursing administration and the department of psychiatry
   4. Functions
      a. Makes initial assessments of clients; writes consultation notes
      b. Provides consultation to nurses
      c. Makes weekly liaison rounds with social service, psychiatry, and occupational therapy to ensure continuity of care and to prevent duplication of services

C. **THE LIAISON NURSE IN A STAFF POSITION UNDER NURSING SERVICE**
   1. Functions as a clinical specialist
   2. Is responsible to nursing service (no doctor's order is necessary before consultation is conducted)
   3. Functions
      a. Makes client assessments
      b. Provides short-term therapy
      c. Provides in-service education

References

1. Beraducci M, Blandford K, Garant C: The psychiatric liaison nurse in the general hospital. Gen Hosp Psychiatry 1:66, 1979
2. Diers D: Research in Nursing Practice. Philadelphia, JB Lippincott, 1979
3. Johnson B: Psychiatric nurse consultant in a general hospital. Nurs Outlook 10:728, 1963
4. Nelson J, Schilke D: The evolution of psychiatric liaison nursing. Perspect Psychiatr Care 14:61, 1976
5. Robinson L: Liaison psychiatric nursing. Perspect Psychiatr Care 6:87, 1968

Bibliography

Baker BS, Lynn MR: Psychiatric nursing consultation: The use of an inservice model to assist nurses in the grief process. J Psychiatr Nurs 17:15, May, 1979

Baldwin CA: Mental health consultation in the intensive care unit: Toward greater balance and precision of attribution. J Psychiatr Nurs 16:17, 1978

Davis DS, Nelson JK: Referrals to psychiatric liaison nurses. Gen Hosp Psychiatry 2:41, 1980

Forsland CK, Errickson EA: A behavioral approach to physical rehabilitation: A case study. J Psychiatr Nurs 16:48, 1978

Garrick TR, Stotland NA: How to write a psychiatric consultation. Am J Psychiatry 139:849, 1982

Hackett T, Cassem N (eds): Massachusetts General Hospital Handbook of General Hospital Psychiatry. St Louis, CV Mosby, 1978

Howard JS: Liaison nursing. J Psychiatr Nurs 16:35, 1978

Jackson H: The psychiatric nurse as a mental health consultant in a general hospital. Nurs Clin North Am 4:327, 1969

Jansson D: Student consultation: A liaison psychiatry experience for nursing students. Perspect Psychiatr Care 2:77, 1979

Lange FM: The multifaceted role of the nurse consultant. J Nurs Ed 18:30, 1979

Langman-Dorwart N: A model for mental health consultation in the general hospital. J Psychiatr Nurs 17:29, 1979

Lipowski ZJ: Consultation–liaison psychiatry: Past failures and new opportunities. Gen Hosp Psychiatry 1:3, 1979

Palmateer LM: Consultation and liaison implications of awakening paralyzed during surgery: A syndrome of traumatic neurosis. J Psychosoc Nurs 20:21, 1982

Pasnau RO: Consultation–Liaison Psychiatry. New York, Grune & Stratton, 1975

Robinson L: Liaison Nursing, Psychological Approach to Nursing Care. Philadelphia, FA Davis, 1974

Robinson L: Psychological Aspects of the Care of Hospitalized Patients. Philadelphia, FA Davis, 1976

Severin N, Becker R: Nurses as psychiatric consultants in a general hospital emergency room. Commun Mental Health J 10:261, 1974

Strain JJ: Psychological Interventions in Medical Practice. New York, Appleton-Century-Crofts, 1978

9

Designing a Comprehensive Alcoholism Program

*Linda Barile**

*This work was developed when the author was a clinical specialist on the alcoholism recovery unit at New York Hospital/Cornell University, Westchester Division. Acknowledgment is given to the staff on that unit.

Introduction Each alcoholism program is different and is based on the values of those designing the program. Treatment must take into account the differences as well as similarities among clients and must fit the program to the client. There are, however, basic principles and goals for treating the alcoholic.

Basic Principles
1. Alcoholism is a multifaceted, treatable disease.
2. No one person, discipline or treatment modality is successful with the disease for all clients.
3. A multidisciplinary team of medical doctors, psychiatrists, nurses, psychologists, social workers, alcoholism counselors, clergy, and occupational and recreational therapists using a number of different treatment modalities is the most effective approach.
4. Alcoholics, their families, and significant others are involved in developing and implementing the treatment plan.
5. Treatment is voluntary, supportive, directive, and oriented toward symptom reduction.

Phases of Recovery from Alcoholism[3,7]
1. Admitting one is alcoholic
2. Compliance with alcoholism program
3. Acceptance of the severity of the disease and responsibility for recovery
4. Surrender to the chronic nature of the disease and need for continued help

Goals of Treatment
1. Identify the alcoholic.
2. Detoxify clients in a safe manner (see Chap. 47).
3. Help clients recognize and accept that they have a disease and are responsible for their own recovery.[3]
4. Identify and point out defenses that prevent this recognition.[3]
5. Bring clients to an awarenes of the totality of their situation.
6. Assist clients to be aware of the specific impact of their behavior.
7. Educate clients and significant others about alcoholism.
8. Help clients discover themselves and others as feeling persons.[3]
9. Provide marital, family, and sex counseling.
10. Improve communication between clients and significant others.
11. Teach assertiveness of expression.
12. Provide for resocialization and increased interpersonal relationships.
13. Educate clients to long-term adaptive coping in response to stress.
14. Teach relaxation.
15. Teach clients to reach out to others when help is required.
16. Help clients become more responsible to self, others, and society.
17. Provide behavioral alternatives to alcohol use.
18. Organize a new way of life with new patterns of living and thinking.[3]
19. Provide occupational skills training.
20. Emphasize the necessity of permanent abstinence.

Structure of an Inpatient Treatment Program The treatment program must be orderly, organized, and well structured, and must address the problems of the alcoholic. Alcoholics, while drinking, lose structure in their lives and often become depressed and isolated with little or no socialization. They lose control over themselves and do not assume responsibility for themselves or others. Therefore, there must be careful structuring of the physical and social environment so that every activity, rule, and interaction is therapeutic and addresses these problems. At the same time, involvement, support, and spontaneity are encouraged.

A. OVERALL STRUCTURE

1. The physical structure of the unit is designed to facilitate socialization, encourage clients to be together, and reduce loneliness.
   a. Double bedrooms are provided.
   b. Clients have their meals together in a dining room.
   c. Furniture is arranged in circles to facilitate socialization.
   d. Group rooms and study areas are provided.
2. The structure and routine begins in the morning and lasts through the day. Clients receive a copy of the daily schedule, shown in Chart 9–1.
3. Clients are responsible for personal hygiene and activities of daily living.
4. Punctual attendance and participation in all activities is mandatory.
5. The therapeutic community concept of ward government is encouraged. Clients hold certain positions and assume responsibility for showing new clients around the unit and for maintenance of the unit. Clients can voice complaints, suggest unit policies, and learn socially acceptable ways of influencing their environment, thereby learning to accept responsibility.

B. RULES AND REGULATIONS

1. Telephone calls, visitors, and passes to leave the unit may be restricted early in treatment to enable clients to concentrate on their problems, to provide the needed distance from significant others, and to foster a commitment to treatment. The client is informed of these restrictions and signs an agreement to this effect.
2. Television, record players, outside reading material, and any other distraction or mechanism of avoidance are discouraged.
3. The possession or use of alcohol or any other nonprescribed drug usually results in immediate discharge from the treatment facility. All products containing alcohol, such as aftershave lotion, perfume, and so forth, are restricted.
4. Gambling is prohibited.
5. Close intimate or physical involvement between clients is discouraged because this replaces dependency on alcohol with dependency on another, distracts

---

Chart 9–1
**SAMPLE DAILY ROUTINE IN AN INPATIENT
ALCOHOLISM PROGRAM**

Time	Activity
7:00 AM	Wake-up and personal care
8:00 AM	Breakfast
9–10:30 AM	Small group therapy
10:30–11 AM	Free time/study period
11–12:00 N	Lecture
12–1:00 PM	Lunch
1–2:00 PM	Study group
2–3:00 PM	Free time/individual or family therapy
3–4:00 PM	Occupational or recreational therapy
4–5:00 PM	Free time
5–6:00 PM	Supper
6–7:00 PM	Free time
7–9:00 PM	AA meeting/family meeting

from treatment, and often interferes with the goal of sobriety. In the early stages of recovery, the anxiety associated with interpersonal relations can trigger drinking.

C. **STAFF MEETINGS**

The staff working in an alcoholism program need regularly scheduled staff meetings to maintain the system and facilitate communication. Staff meetings are either client-centered, administrative, educational, or group process meetings. Each meeting has a definite purpose, goal, and objective. The boundaries of the meetings are adhered to whenever possible. Agendas are set in advance and staff has prior notification of the agenda. Meetings are as follows:

1. Client-centered meetings
   a. Morning rounds/daily report
   b. Treatment planning meetings
   c. Client government meetings
   d. Community meetings
2. Administrative meetings
   a. Staff council
   b. Administrative staff meetings
3. Educational meetings
   a. Case presentations
   b. Staff development meetings
4. Group process meetings
   a. Staff-centered
   b. Client-centered

Modalities of Treatment

Didactic groups. Educational groups or lectures are a form of didactic confrontation in which there is direct clarification of the alcoholic's possible misinformation or lack of information about the disease. In this treatment, there is a factual study of the disease, its progressive nature; the physical, social and emotional changes; the methods of treatment and means of achieving sobriety. Clients receive study material, reading lists, and homework assignments. Educational groups help clients to realize that they have a disease and introduce them to the group experience. Didactic groups often do not, alone, result in a permanent behavior or attitude change.

Study groups. Study groups are modeled along the lines of the Alcoholics Anonymous (AA) study group and have been used in a variety of ways. In these groups, clients discuss issues such as philosophy, steps, and sponsorship in AA in more depth, than they have been covered in didactic groups. In some study groups clients are expected to tell their stories as they would in an AA meeting; in other study groups clients receive an evaluation from peers as to their commitment and progress in treatment.

Group therapy. Group therapy is an effective treatment modality for alcoholics. Therapy groups are usually open, and consist of six to ten alcoholics who meet with a professional leader. The group is a microcosm of life situations. Groups facilitate self-discovery, growth, and change by enabling the alcoholics to recognize, accept, and express their own feelings and to recognize responses from other group members. The defense mechanisms that maintain the drinking behavior as well as the client's strengths and resources are explored. Peer relationships within the group influence the individuals' attitudes, values, and social behaviors in a therapeutic way.

Family therapy. Alcoholism is a family disease, and the family requires treatment along with the alcoholic client. Alcoholism has a devastating emotional impact on the family members and family life. The family system, in order to maintain equilibrium and to exist as a family, must change and accommodate to the alcoholic member. The family disease and recovery parallels that of the alcoholic's disease and recovery. Family members' feelings parallel the feelings, attitudes, and behaviors of the alcoholic, and family members experience the same stages of denial, enabling (unconsciously helping the alcoholic to continue drinking), anger, and acceptance. Any appreciable and lasting change of alcoholics can come about only through simultaneous behavior change of the significant people involved with them on a daily basis. The goals of family therapy are to

1. Educate the family about the disease of alcoholism
2. Encourage recognition, acceptance, and open expression of feelings
3. Learn about family roles, routines, and responsibilities that have been incorporated to accommodate to the alcoholic
4. Change relationships, roles, and responsibilities to facilitate sobriety
5. Discuss the threat of change and adjustment required to accommodate the sober alcoholic
6. Improve intimate, sexual relatedness between couples

Alcoholics Anonymous (AA). Alcoholics Anonymous has probably been the most effective modality in helping alcoholic people achieve sobriety. Chart 9–2 shows some slogans used in AA and the reasons behind them.[6]

The group approach for the treatment of alcoholics is also seen in the fellowship of AA. The curative factors of group psychotherapy[9] are evident. AA provides the following assistance to members:

1. Accurate information about the disease
2. Direct advice and guidance
3. Hope through the example of others who have maintained sobriety

---

Chart 9–2
AA SLOGANS AND THEIR RATIONALES[6]

Slogan	Rationale
"Tell your story"	Recognition and acceptance of the disease
"Keep the memory alive"	Acceptance that the disease does not go away
"First things first" "One day at a time" "Easy does it"	Encouragement of patience and tolerance of frustration
"Turn it over" "Let go and let God" "Get out of the driver's seat"	Relinquishment of control to a higher authority
"Make amends for previous wrongs"	Encouragement of self-evaluation, disclosure, and responsible behavior

---

4. Recognition of the universality of feelings
5 A sponsor who provides support and the example of altruism
6. Catharsis of feelings and problems
7. Group cohesiveness in a caring community
8. Development of socialization skills
9. Activities that do not include the use of alcohol

AA offers not only emotional support of its members but also a body of traditions, values, and coping mechanisms, and a specific life-style. AA incorporates the following coping mechanisms for members who encounter problems:

1. Talk the problem over with others.[5]
2. Find out more about the situation by seeking more information.[5]
3. Break the problem up into manageable bits and take first things first.
4. Draw on past experience.[5]
5. Make alternative plans for handling the situation.[5]
6. Take some definite action on the basis of present understanding.[5]
7. Express positive and negative feelings.
8. Work tension off by physical exercise.[5]
9. Use relaxation techniques.
10. Be flexible and willing to change.
11. Tolerate frustration.
12. Believe in a supernatural power who cares about you.[5]

AA has recognized the importance of treating the family in the formation of Al-Anon for the adult relatives, Al-Ateen for teenagers, and Al-Atots for young children of alcoholics. Members of these programs attempt to improve their own lives, which have become unmanageable from living with the alcoholic. Although the purpose of these programs is to help the member and not the alcoholic, they indirectly help the alcoholic as well.

Adjunctive activities (occupational, recreational, and physical therapy). Activities therapy is also a part of any alcoholism program. Goals of activities therapy include

1. Improved physical health through exercise
2. Identification of muscle tension
3. Reduction of stress through relaxation therapy and exercise.
4. Increased socialization, relatedness, and communication
5. Discovery of more about oneself in a casual, social setting
6. Planned participation in activities as a means of socializing and occupying leisure time without the use of alcohol
7. Increased self-esteem through physical activities and successful completion of activities and tasks
8. Exploration of vocational interests and talents; learned readjustment to a work setting

Discharge or aftercare groups. An important component of any inpatient alcoholism program is a well-developed aftercare program. Most programs encourage participation in AA and in an aftercare group for predischarge and discharged clients. The length of these groups varies from 6 weeks to 2 years. For the alcoholic, the first year of maintaining sobriety is the most difficult and the most critical. There is some indication that programs with aftercare groups have lower recidivism rates.[1,8] Goals of the aftercare group are to

1. Help facilitate discharge and reentry to family, employment, and community
2. Provide continued support in the form of group therapy

3. Facilitate and support a new life-style without the use of alcohol
4. Confront stressful life situations with the continued help of the group in developing alternative coping mechanisms
5. Provide for both external and internal control over alcohol

Therapist Characteristics and Role

The therapist treating the alcoholic must display characteristics of empathy, respect, genuineness, concreteness, and confrontation. He must be willing to establish an intensive relationship with the client and be open and honest about his thoughts and feelings. The therapist must be educated and trained in the treatment of alcoholics and must understand the dynamics of the disease. As therapists receive training in alcoholism, they come to view the disease as a physiologic, psychological, social, and behavioral problem, and are effective in treating the alcoholic.

Evaluation of the Program

Program evaluation is included in the design of an alcoholism program. Inpatient programs can evaluate the milieu using Moss's Ward Atmosphere Scale.[4] Clients and families are asked to evaluate the program during and after hospitalization. Staff continually evaluate the program and request consultation and evaluation from experts in the field. Follow-up data and outcome studies are obtained from clients postdischarge to determine sobriety and level of adjustment in the community.

Outpatient Treatment

Outpatient treatment has been effective for the client who does not require inpatient detoxification or the intensive milieu of inpatient treatment.

The same principles, goals, and therapies apply. In outpatient treatment the client must first be detoxified from alcohol and medical management must be provided. A complete assessment of the extent of the drinking problem and its effects on the client's life is obtained. While the client is in treatment, whether individual or group therapy, attendance at AA meetings is encouraged. Significant others are encouraged to attend Al-Anon meetings. Family, couples, or marital treatment is often provided simultaneously. Antabuse may be prescribed as a means of external control over drinking until internalized control is achieved.

The major tasks of outpatient treatment are

1. To stop drinking
2. To understand and work with the transference that the client establishes with the therapist[2]

Prevention and Outreach

Prevention in alcoholism is sorely needed but cost effectiveness and outcome have been difficult to demonstrate. Some educational programs have been financed and undertaken. Prevention starts with educating school children about problem-solving, decision-making, coping mechanisms and the effects of using alcohol to avoid problems. Parents must also be taught early recognition and treatment of alcohol abuse. Goals of prevention are to

1. Educate the community about alcoholism
2. Discourage the abuse of alcohol
3. Reduce the prevalence of alcoholism
4. Provide behavioral alternatives to alcohol use

The National Council on Alcoholism has been active in providing preventive educational programs and outreach to the alcoholic. This group offers educational services and counseling of family members and alcoholics with the aim of getting the person into treatment. There are also organizations that provide education and confrontational meetings with significant others and the alcoholic to ''create a crisis'' and facilitate the alcoholic's seeking treatment. Significant others present to the alcoholic specific behavior and facts that have caused concern. The client is then presented with alternatives or choices that will lead to treatment.

Employee assistance programs have become a part of the work place and are a successful mechanism of outreach. Employers and managers are educated to early signs and symptoms of alcoholism as these are manifested on the job. Methods of supervision, documentation, evaluation and confrontation are taught to managers. The employee is often presented with the alternative of seeking treatment or losing his job. Many companies have medical insurance that pays for hospitalization.

More must be done in outreach and education "through radio, television, news media, in advertising or marketing at sports events, super-markets, on matchbooks, litter bags, balloons, bumper stickers," or any other means that gets the message across and prevents the silent killer.[6] In-service training workshops should be provided to "church groups, educational personnel, judicial system personnel, public health workers and to other community service providers."[6] Goals of an outreach program are to

1. Identify families and individuals with alcoholic problems
2. Establish a relationship with client and family
3. Enable recognition of the disease by family, employer, and client
4. Educate significant others, families, and employers to alcoholism and the enabling process
5. Facilitate "creating a crisis" that results in the client seeking help
6. Refer to community resources for treatment

References

1. Costello RM: Alcoholism aftercare and outcome: Cross legged panel and path analysis. Br J Addict 75:49, 1980
2. Howard D, Howard N: Treatment of significant others. In Zimberg S, Wallace J, Blume S (eds): Practical Approaches to Alcoholism Psychotherapy. New York, Plenum Press, 1978
3. Johnson V: I'll Quit Tomorrow. New York, Harper & Row, 1973
4. Moss RH: Evaluating Treatment Environments. New York, John Wiley & Sons, 1974
5. Sidle A: Development of a coping scale. Arch Gen Psychiatry 20:226, 1969
6. Tiebout H: The ego factors in surrender in alcoholism. Q J Stud Alcoholism 15:610, 1954
7. Tiebout H: Surrender versus compliance in therapy with special reference to alcoholism. Q J Stud Alcoholism 14:58, 1953
8. Vannicelli M: Impact of aftercare in the treatment of alcoholics: A cross-legged panel analysis. Q J Stud Alcoholism 39:1875, 1978
9. Yalom I: The Theory and Practice of Group Psychotherapy. New York, Basic Books, 1970

Bibliography

Vaillant GE: The Natural History of Alcoholism. Causes, Patterns, and Paths to Recovery. Cambridge, Harvard University Press, 1983

10

Designing an Inpatient Program

Rachel Parios

Introduction Psychiatric inpatient treatment is provided for clients who are unable to remain at home or in the community owing to their psychiatric illness. Hospitalization provides security to the client and others by minimizing the potential danger of acute psychopathology.

Purposes of Inpatient Hospitalization

1. To protect the client and others from the client's homicidal or suicidal behavior
2. To safeguard the client's reputation in the community (when behavior is bizarre)
3. To remove the client from an intolerable environment
4. To provide close observation and psychiatric treatment with the availability of specialized procedures
5. To provide rapid administration and professional monitoring of medication schedules too complex for home use
6. To provide observation and assurance that the client takes medication
7. To provide psychotherapies and sociotherapies fostering client participation in assuming social responsibility during hospitalization
8. To allow therapeutic exploration of critical relationships and issues without interference from outside sources
9. To motivate the client and family or significant others toward
    a. Accepting and supporting therapeutic treatment
    b. Making changes in daily living patterns

Disadvantages of Inpatient Hospitalization

1. Social stigma affects the client's view of self; educational, family, and community prospects.
2. Clients are deprived of work and earnings.
3. Upon discharge, clients may have trouble discarding deviant behavior that was considered acceptable in the hospital.
4. Clients may become dependent on the hospital routine and may learn what phrases and symptoms to use for readmission.

Purpose of Therapeutic Milieu Program

1. To enhance open, effective communications between
    a. Clients and staff
    b. Clients and clients
    c. Staff and staff
2. To use the therapeutic community as a social system in which clients and staff reciprocally affect one another and can discuss this process
3. To provide an atmosphere in which transferences and countertransferences can arise and be identified and analyzed in detail
4. To provide activities based on individual client conflicts, needs, interests, skills, and aspirations
5. To allow expression of aggressive and other repressed feelings through varied activities and therapies
6. To include the community outside the hospital in the treatment of clients
7. To allow clients to generalize behaviors learned in the hospital to situations outside the hospital

Design of Therapeutic Milieu Program Guidelines, structure, and appropriate control help clients who are confused and anxious, and feeling out of control. Clients are thereby protected from self-distraction and antisocial behavior. To do this, they are divided into three different groups according to their level of functioning.

A. **GROUP I**

Group I (highest level of functioning) consists of clients with mild symptoms who
1. Have some insight into their illness or problems
2. Understand the goals of the program or treatment
3. Are reality oriented
4. Are motivated to attend groups
5. Attempt to work through their feelings, defense mechanisms, and perceptual problems

B. **GROUP II**

Group II (middle level of functioning) consists of clients with moderate symptoms who
1. Have only slight insight into their illness or problems
2. Are not fully aware of program treatment goals
3. Are in and out of contact with reality
4. Are relatively unmotivated to attend groups
5. Have difficulty acknowledging feelings, defense mechanisms, and perceptual problems

C. **GROUP III**

Group III (lowest level of functioning) consists of clients with severe symptoms who
1. Have no insight into their illness or problems
2. Are not able to establish goals
3. Are usually out of contact with reality
4. Are not motivated to attend groups
5. Are unable to acknowledge feelings, defense mechanisms, and perceptual problems

Staff   Table 10–1 shows an ideal staff for a 30-bed inpatient unit.

Table 10–1
SAMPLE STAFF FOR A 30-BED INPATIENT UNIT

Title and Number	License/Degree	Role
Staff psychiatrists (4)	M.D.	1. Initiates treatment plan 2. Prescribes treatment 3. Provides individual therapy 4. Conducts multidisciplinary rounds and team meetings
Staff psychologists (2)	Ph.D. psychology	1. Provides psychological testing 2. Participates in multidisciplinary rounds and team meetings 3. Contributes to treatment plan
Clinical nurse specialist (1)	M.S. in psychiatric nursing	1. Monitors implementation of the treatment plan 2. Supervises nursing care 3. Provides group therapy 4. Contributes to treatment plan 5. Participates in multidisciplinary rounds and team meetings

(continued)

Table 10–1
(*continued*)

Title and Number	License/Degree	Role
Head nurse (1)	B.S.N.	1. Organizes client care assignments 2. Manages unit 3. Monitors physician's treatment plan 4. Establishes therapeutic objectives that meet individual client needs 5. Promotes client–team collaboration 6. Stimulates staff development
Primary nurse (day shift, 6 R.N., 3 L.P.N.; evening shift, 4 R.N., 1 L.P.N.; night shift, 2 R.N., 1 L.P.N.)	R.N.	1. Provides nursing assessment 2. Establishes goals with clients 3. Initiates nursing care plan 4. Administers individual nursing care to clients 5. Reports symptoms and behavior to psychiatrist, head nurse, or clinical nurse specialist 6. Provides clients with one-to-one therapeutic relationship 7. Participates in team rounds and meetings 8. Monitors client participation in program 9. Documents nursing care
Nurses aides, orderlies, and technicians (2 per shift)	B.A. in Psychology, Nurses Aide Certificate	1. Assists nursing staff with clients 2. Transports clients to treatment areas 3. Attends team rounds and meetings, contributing observations about clients
Psychiatric social worker (1)	M.S.W.	1. Provides family therapy 2. Assists clients with concrete services: (*e.g.,* assists with Social Security insurance or disability application, employment, housing) 3. Arranges aftercare referrals and transportation 4. Participates in team rounds and meetings
Activity therapists (dance, music, occupational, art, recreational—1 of each)	M.A. certification	1. Provides specific therapeutic modalities 2. Monitors clients' verbal and nonverbal expression and behavior 3. Reports changes in clients' behavior to the primary nurse, head nurse or clinical nurse specialist 4. Documents attendance and participation in activity therapy group
Life skills therapist (1)	M.A.	1. Provides clients with activities that teach skills for daily living 2. Participates in team rounds and meetings 3. Documents assessment of clients' capabilities and progress

Table 10–2
SAMPLE NURSING STAFF FOR A 30-BED INPATIENT UNIT

Day shift—7 AM to 3:30 PM
6 R.N. and 3 L.P.N.
Primary Nurses, 9—(L.P.N. is under direction of R.N.)
Nurse/client ratio—1:3 or 4

Evening shift—3 PM to 11:30 PM
4 R.N. and 1 L.P.N.
Primary Nurses, 5—(L.P.N. is under direction of R.N.)
Nurse/client ratio—1:6

Night shift—11 PM to 7 AM
2 R.N. and 1 L.P.N.
Primary Nurses, 3—(L.P.N. is under direction of R.N.)
Nurse/client ratio—1:10

Each shift has
1 nurses' aide
1 orderly or technician

Note: Pattern changes with suicide observation, precaution, and seclusion. 1/1 management is carried out with R.N. or L.P.N.

Nurse Staffing Patterns   Staffing schedules are planned by the head nurse. A typical 24-hour pattern is shown in Table 10–2.

Meetings   A. **MULTIDISCIPLINARY TEAM MEETINGS**
Multidisciplinary team meetings are held weekly to
1. Evaluate treatment planning
2. Discuss client care
3. Provide consistency in client care
4. Discuss discharge planning

B. **NURSING REPORTS AT THE CHANGE OF EACH SHIFT**
Nursing reports are held at the end of each shift to
1. Share information about each specific client
2. Foster communication among staff members, which allows client care to be consistent

C. **WEEKLY STAFF MEETINGS**
Staff meetings are held each week to
1. Allow the head nurse to communicate hospital information to staff
2. Allow staff to participate in unit management

D. **WEEKLY STAFF FEELINGS MEETINGS**
Staff meetings are held each week to
1. Assist staff to identify transferences and countertransferences
2. Reduce staff burn-out

E. **MONTHLY GRAND ROUNDS**
Grand rounds are held each month to
1. Offer clinical presentation for educational purposes
2. Foster staff development

Table 10–3
COMPONENTS, DESCRIPTION, AND RATIONALE FOR THE PHYSICAL FACILITY

Component	Description	Rationale

1. Atmosphere	1. Unit surroundings are
	  a. Bright in color
	  b. Decorated with paintings (without frames)
	  c. Furnished with comfortable lounge furniture
		1. Provides the clients with a relaxing, pleasant atmosphere
		Encourages clients to respect their environment and control impulsive actions

2. Client rooms	2. Fifteen rooms for a 30-bed unit, each containing
	  a. 2 beds (of modern, home style)
	  b. 2 bureaus
	  c. 2 lounge chairs
	  d. 2 closets
	  e. 1 bathroom
		2. Provides privacy and individual space
		Designed to foster a comfortable, ''homey'' atmosphere

3. Client attire	3. Clients wear their own street or home clothes	3. Allows clients to maintain some of their own identity Encourages clients to engage in preparation for daily activities Fosters self-esteem

4. Safety	4. Windows on the unit are protected with
	  a. Shatterproof glass
	  b. Locked screens
		4. Prevents clients from harming themselves
		Allows outside lighting to brighten the unit

5. Dayroom or lounge	5. A multipurpose room for activities requiring space	5. Encourages socialization and larger group participation

6. Dining room	6. Tables and chairs are arranged to seat 4 at a table. Food is served family style.	6. Provides an atmosphere of relaxed dining
		  a. Encourages socialization at mealtime
		  b. Reduces stimuli and acting out behavior

7. Nurses' station	7. An open, centrally located area where
	  a. Nurses are accessible
	
	  b. Medications are contained
	  c. Client care can be monitored and implemented easily
		7. Encourages staff/client interaction
		  a. Fosters communication and interaction
		  b. Provides safety and staff control
		  c. Prevents critical situations from becoming unmanageable

8. Activity rooms	8. Three rooms are designated for client activities.	8. Fosters security and privacy for clients participating in group activities
		  a. Reduces interruption
		  b. Reduces resistance from clients

9. Quiet room (seclusion)	9. A room with soothing color, protection from harm, with a mattress and bathroom for clients who require reduced stimuli and privacy	9. Encourages clients (in an agitated or otherwise uncontrollable state) to gain control and become less frightened
		  a. Ensures protection
		  b. Provides for rapid monitoring of medications

10. Locked area for risk items	10. Locked cabinet for all sharp items, razors, glass bottles, and aerosol cans. Staff monitors distribution and use of items with clients.	10. Reduces risk of self-harm and danger to others

(continued)

Table 10–3
(continued)

Component	Description	Rationale
11. Laundry room	11. A room with a washer, dryer, iron, and ironing board—iron is secured to a wall Clients are supervised when using laundry room equipment.	11. Fosters skill development for daily living needs a. Reduces risk of self-harm and danger to others b. Provides an atmosphere for learning
12. Consultation rooms	12. Six small consultation rooms for psychiatrists, nurses, psychologists, and others to meet with clients on a one-to-one basis	12. Fosters privacy for individual psychotherapy, testing, and counseling to take place without interruption
13. Staff room	13. A staff room for charting, reporting, meetings, and conferences	13. Ensures privacy for staff activities and requirements
14. Staff attire	14. Staff wear street clothes and name pins for identification (lab coats may be worn).	14. Allows clients to identify staff when needed, and provides role modeling for clients

Physical Facility Table 10–3 shows the components, description, and rationale for the physical facility.

Program Schedules A major part of the nurse's role on the inpatient unit involves participating with clients in the daily program. Table 10–4 shows a typical weekday program, and Chart 10–1 a typical weekend program. Table 10–5 lists each component of a milieu program and its theoretical rationale.

Nursing Interventions For each of the activities of the therapeutic milieu there are specific nursing interventions based on theoretical principles. These are shown in Chart 10–2.

(Text continues on page 100)

Table 10–4
TYPICAL WEEKDAY PROGRAM

Time	Monday	Tuesday	Wednesday	Thursday	Friday
8:15 AM	Wake-up	Wake-up	Wake-up	Wake-up	Wake-up
8:30 AM	Breakfast in dining room	Breakfast in dining room	Breakfast in dining room	Breakfast in dining room	Breakfast in dining room
9:30 AM	Preparation for day	Preparation for day	Preparation for day	Preparation for day	Preparation for day
10:15 AM	Community meeting	Community meeting	Community meeting	Community meeting	Community meeting
10:45 AM	Communication/ group 1	Exercise—led by ADL therapist	Exercise—Led by ADL therapist	Exercise—led by ADL therapist	Communications/ group 2
11:15 AM	Arts & crafts	Women's group	Group therapy/1	Creative writing	Current events
12:00	Free	Free	Free	Free	Free

(continued)

Table 10–4
(continued)

Time	Monday			Tuesday			Wednesday	Thursday			Friday		
12:30 PM	Lunch in dining room			Lunch in dining room			Lunch in dining room	Lunch in dining room			Lunch in dining room		
1:15–2:00 PM	1	2	3	1	2	3	1	1	2	3	1	2	3
	Group ther-apy	Move-ment ther-apy	A D L	Group ther-apy	Art ther-apy	Arts & crafts	Planned trip or project groups 1:00–2:30 PM	Move-ment ther-apy	Group ther-apy	A D L	Group ther-apy	Art ther-apy	R T
2:15–3:00 PM	Move-ment ther-apy	Group ther-apy	O T	Art ther-apy	Medi-cation edu-cation	Move-ment ther-apy	Visiting hours	Group ther-apy	A D L	Move-ment ther-apy	Medi-cation edu-cation	Group ther-apy	A D L
3:00–3:30 PM	Free			Free			Free	Free			Free		
3:30–4:30 PM	Women's & men's groups			Movement therapy			Relaxation group (4:00–5:00 PM)	Arts & crafts (4:00–5:00 PM)			Leisure time planning		
4:30–5:00 PM	Free			Free			Free	Free			Free		
5:30 PM	Dinner in the dining room			Dinner in the dining room			Dinner in the dining room	Dinner in the dining room			Dinner in the dining room		
7:00–8:30 PM	Evening activities			Visitors (7:00–8:00 PM) Postvisitors group			Film	Visitors (7:00–8:00 PM) Postvisitors group			Dance or pizza party		

ADL = activities of daily living; OT = occupational therapy; RT = recreational therapy

---

Chart 10–1
TYPICAL WEEKEND PROGRAM

Saturday		Sunday	
8:00 AM	Wake-up	8:00 AM	Wake-up
8:30 AM	Breakfast	8:30 AM	Breakfast
9:30 AM	Preparation for day	9:30 AM	Preparation for day
10:15 AM	Community meeting	10:15 AM	Community meeting
10:45 AM	Plant care	10:45 AM	Recreational therapy or church service
11:15 AM	Movement therapy		
12:00 N	Free	12:00 N	Free
12:30 PM	Lunch	12:30 PM	Lunch
1:15 PM	Occupational therapy	1:15 PM	Activities of daily living
2–4 PM	Visiting hours	2–4 PM	Visiting hours
4:30 PM	Recreational therapy	4:30 PM	Post-visit group
5:30 PM	Dinner	5:30 PM	Dinner
7:00 PM	Games		Free evening

Table 10–5
COMPONENTS OF A MILIEU PROGRAM AND THEORETICAL RATIONALE

Component	Theoretical Rationale
Daily Therapeutic Community Meeting 1. Co-led by nurse or ADL therapist and client 2. Held in morning after doctor's rounds and attended by all staff and clients	1. Provides clients with structured expectations and an atmosphere to make contributions and participate in unit government 2. Attendance indicates importance of the meeting. Clients have the chance for imitation, identification, and social learning from staff. Staff have the chance to assess and evaluate client progress.
Group Psychotherapy 1. Led by clinical nurse specialist 2. Held in the afternoon when interruptions can be prevented	1. Provides the opportunity for clients to verbally interact with others in an atmosphere in which fantasies, feelings, behavior, and interpersonal reactions are verbally expressed, explored, and analyzed. Prevents clients from resisting confrontation 2. Lack of interruptions is important to analysis of group process. It also shows the importance of the therapy.
Activities of Daily Living Group 1. Led by nurse ADL therapist or occupational therapist	1. Motivates, develops, and provides awareness of daily living needs, within and outside of the hospital (*e.g.,* hygiene, grooming, budgeting, nutrition, cooking, housekeeping) 2. Teaches clients skills necessary for daily living 3. Helps clients to assume responsibility for daily living 4. Task-oriented activities help staff to evaluate client abilities, concentration, and capabilities.
Art Therapy 1. Led by a registered art therapist	1. Provides opportunity for clients to reveal themselves through artistic productions 2. Allows clients an art modality whereby conflicts can be symbolically expressed 3. Helps the art therapist to clarify the client's diagnosis and progress based on interpretation of art work
Dance or Movement Therapy 1. Led by a registered dance or movement therapist	1. Provides the opportunity for clients to express themselves and to identify and release emotional inner experiences 2. Provides rhythmic expressive movement whereby positive one-to-one and group relationships evolve 3. Provides changing actions of the group, which foster independence, freedom, self-esteem, and relaxation 4. Provides client control over body and emotions enhancing body image 5. Increases client coordination and feelings of self-confidence 6. Provides a safe, nonthreatening atmosphere for risk taking 7. Helps the movement therapist with client evaluation

(continued)

Table 10–5
(continued)

Component	Theoretical Rationale
Occupational Therapy	
1. Led by a registered occupational therapist	1. Provides selected activities that facilitate learning and concentration based on scientific principles
	2. Restores, reinforces, and enhances social performance with task-oriented activities
	3. Helps client learn skills essential for adaptation and productivity
	4. Provides tasks appropriate to the client's individual needs and goals
	5. Fosters attitudes of assertiveness
	6. Helps the occupational therapist with client evaluation
Recreational Therapy	
1. Led by a recreational therapist	1. Gratifies clients through meaningful play
	2. Enhances creative activities for enjoyment and leisure
	3. Provides clients with approval for pleasurable interactions
	4. Helps with client evaluation
Exercise Group	
1. Led by recreational therapist, movement or dance therapist, or ADL therapist	1. Provides clients with routine for exercise resulting in
	a. Increased circulation
	b. Increased muscle tone
	c. Improved body image
	d. Invigorated feeling
	e. Relaxation

Chart 10–2
NURSING INTERVENTIONS IN MILIEU THERAPY AND RATIONALE

Milieu Program Activities	Nursing Intervention	Theoretical Rationale
Communication Group		
1. Led by nurse	1. Introduce components of communication: a. Speaking b. Listening c. Body language d. Actions	1. Improved use of language leads to increased ability to relate to others.
	2. Help clients learn or relearn how to interpret verbal messages: a. Provide a verbal statement and ask them what it means.	2. Helps the nurse to evaluate and assess client's communicative and interpretive skills with the use of specific examples
	3. Help clients learn to assert themselves verbally: a. Ask each member to express a thought they would like communicated to the group. b. Ask for client responses to what has been said.	3. Provides the opportunity for assertiveness, clarity, and creativity and develops the client's ability to communicate ideas to others

Chart 10–2
(continued)

Milieu Program Activities	Nursing Intervention	Theoretical Rationale

Medication Education Group
1. Led by nurse (see Chap. 65)
	1. Assist clients to learn
	  a. Names of drugs they are taking
	  b. Mode of action
	  c. Side effects
	  d. Importance of compliance
		1. a. Teaches clients about their medications
		  b. Allows clients the opportunity to question medication regime
		  c. Enhances client's awareness of the importance of chemotherapy

Leisure Time Planning Group
1. Led by nurse or ADL therapist
	1. Explore client's present use of leisure time.
	
	2. Discuss passive versus active leisure time planning.
	3. Introduce leisure time activities:
	  a. Theater
	  b. Art
	  c. Sports
	  d. Cultural and historical possibilities
		1. Establishes a baseline and understanding of the client's concept of leisure time activities
		2. Creative use of leisure time reduces tension
		3. Offers exposure to activities and opportunities available within the community for enjoyment

Creative Writing Group
1. Led by nurse and ADL therapist
	1. Introduce opportunity for clients to put thoughts into writing:
	  a. Ask clients to select a theme.
	  b. Help clients to adhere to the theme and write about it.
	2. Organize the printing of material.
		1. a. Enhances client's creative awareness
		  b. Fosters expression of emotions through writing
		  c. Encourages concentration through a task-oriented project
		2. Increases client's self-esteem

Women's/Men's Group
(see Chap. 30)
1. Led by nurse and ADL therapist
	1. Separate men and women.
	
	2. Provide atmosphere in which clients feel free to discuss personal subjects.
	
	3. Introduce topics specific to males or females.
		1. Fosters exploration of
		  a. Identity
		  b. Sexuality
		  c. Intimacy
		  d. Improved social skills
		  e. Body image
		2. Enhances concept of self as male and female and encourages self-assertion through role playing
		3. Reduces anxiety and provides needed information about these topics

Weekly Field Trips 1. Led by nurses and nurses aides/orderlies, ADL therapist, occupational therapist	1. Orient clients to cultural availabilities in the community. 2. Structure trips that encourage clients to walk or use public transportation. 3. Orient clients to places of interest in the community.	1. Encourages clients to gain adaptive functioning and reduce anxiety with independent actions 2, 3. Reduces fear and distorted perceptions about reality within the community through exposure
Postvisiting Group 1. Led by nurse or ADL therapist	1. Encourage clients to gather after visitors leave the unit.	1. Provides an atmosphere in which clients can explore feelings about visitors, while these feelings are still fresh in their minds

(continued)

Chart 10–2
(continued)

Milieu Program Activities	Nursing Intervention	Theoretical Rationale
	2. Allow clients to express feelings about having no visitors, too many, or not the desired ones, or about the visit.	2. Encourages ventilation of feelings and reduces the possibility of acting out behavior after visitors leave
Somatic Therapies (ECT, Chemotherapy)	1. Explain treatment to clients.	1. Provides information and understanding to reduce anxiety
	2. Assist with administration of treatments.	2. Provides specified intervention to reduce symptoms
	3. Coordinate treatment with activity program.	3. Acts in conjunction with other therapies so that the client benefits from the totality of all modalities
Weekly Parties and Films	1. Arrange with local libraries for the use of films.	1. A community resource is used to link the hospital and community to provide mental health service
	2. Organize social programs with hospital administration.	2. Provides approval from administration for expenses
	3. Encourage clients to help with planning.	3. Encourages socialization, increasing self-esteem Increases participation once program starts
Visiting Hours	1. Restrict visitors for the first 48 hours.	1. Prevents the client from being disrupted in treatment by those in the environment from which the client came
	2. Monitor visiting hours.	2. a. Allows assessment of client–family interactions b. Provides structure and supervision of client behavior in critical relationships c. Allows opportunity for intervention should a crisis arise during visiting hours
	3. Provide support to client when visitors are not permitted.	3. Fosters trust and understanding
Telephone Privileges	1. Restrict phone calls for the first 48 hours.	1. Same as visiting hour restriction
	2. Restrict phone calls during group activities.	2. Discourages resistance and acting-out behavior
	3. Encourage phone calls after this.	3. Fosters family/friend interactions and self-esteem
Discharge Planning	See Chap. 66	

Client Crises Because inpatients are often very anxious upon admission, there is the potential for crisis situations such as aggressive outbursts, suicidal gestures, elopements, and so forth. Chart 10–3 shows organized nursing intervention during client crises, including the plan, nursing action, and nursing rationale. During a crisis, the head nurse and clinical nurse specialist remain available as resource persons, interacting wherever needed.

Evaluation The nurse who designs an inpatient program ensures that the American Nurses Association Standards of Psychiatric and Mental Health Nursing Practice are followed (see Appendix A). These standards provide a framework for practice and can be used

Chart 10–3
ORGANIZED NURSING INTERVENTION DURING CLIENT CRISIS

Plan	Nursing Intervention	Nursing Rationale
1. Intervention is organized and assigned daily by the head nurse or charge nurse	1. Assign a coded number to each staff member for direction of action during a crisis.	1. a. Provides structure and organization to a chaotic environment b. Provides safety to the client, other clients, and staff c. Invites a secure environment after a crisis occurs
2. Coded number system is as follows: Staff #1—R.N.	2. a. Assist the client to a quiet area (client's room or quiet room) ensuring rapid intervention. b. Provide direction to staff in assistance.	2. a. Reduces stimuli, allowing the client to gain control, verbalize feelings, and understand behavior b. Avoids duplication of staff responsibility and offers necessary help
3. Staff #2—R.N. or L.P.N.	3. Help Staff #1 with client's needs (preparing medication and/or securing needed equipment).	3. Ensures that treatment measures will be implemented efficiently and rapidly while providing reassurance to the client
4. Staff #3—R.N.	4. Assume telephone responsibility: a. M.D. when necessary b. Security (if needed) c. Other departments (EKG, Code team)	4. Increases efficiency by offering necessary assistance, obtaining needed physician orders, and implementing required treatment
5. Staff #4—R.N., L.P.N., or nurses aide/orderly	5. Help with client in crisis and take direction from Staff #1.	5. Provides assistance with client in crisis and availability to provide needs, relay messages and give support
6. Staff #5—R.N., L.P.N., nurses aide/orderly, or activity therapist	6. Gather other clients and direct them to the dayroom area, encouraging verbalization of feelings about crisis.	6. Fosters clients' ability to cope by establishing a supportive atmosphere in which they can ventilate feelings of fear, anger, anxiety, and insecurity
7. Staff #6—L.P.N., nurses aide/orderly	7. Obtain any supplies, medications, or needs from other departments and assist as needed.	7. Ensures messenger service when needed
8. Staff evaluation of crisis managed by head nurse/charge nurse and clinical nurse specialist	8. Lead meeting to encourage: a. Staff verbalization b. Staff contributions about crisis management c. Ideas for improving future crisis management	8. Reduces staff frustration, encourages ventilation of staff feelings, and encourages improvement in staff actions during crisis

to constantly evaluate practice. While evaluation is done in a systematic way periodically, it is also built into team meetings and staff meetings.

Clients are also included in evaluation of the inpatient program. This takes place informally in therapeutic community meetings and informal conversations. In addition, clients are asked to fill out a questionnaire just before discharge. This is done to elicit suggestions for improvement and general comments about the inpatient program.

Bibliography

Andrews M: Poetry programs in mental hospitals. Perspect Psychiatr Care 13:17, 1975

Anumonye A: Nigerian nursing care and milieu therapy. Nigerian Nurse 11:43, 1979

Benton DW: The significance of the absent member in milieu therapy. Perspect Psychiatr Care 18:21, 1980

Braff DL et al: The therapeutic community as a research ward: Myths and facts. Arch Gen Psychiatry 36:355, 1979

Carser DL: Primary nursing in the milieu. J Psychiatr Nurs 19:35, 1981

Coltrane F, Pugh CD: Danger signals in staff/patient relationships in the therapeutic milieu. J Psychiatr Nurs 16:34, 1978

Costello RM et al: Formative program evaluation and milieu therapy with alcohol abusers. J Clin Psychol 35:449, 1979

Davis C et al: The architectural design of a psychotherapeutic milieu. Hosp Commun Psychiatry 30:453, 1979

Devine BA: Therapeutic milieu/milieu therapy: An overview. J Psychiatr Nurs 19:20, 1981

Ellsworth RB et al: Some characteristics of effective psychiatric treatment programs. J Consult Clin Psychol 47:799, 1979

Feldman R, Cousins A, Grimaldi D: The developmental phases of the nurse/resident relationship on an inpatient psychiatric unit. Perspect Psychiatr Care 19:31, 1981

Gunderson JG: A re-evaluation of milieu therapy for nonchronic schizophrenic patients. Schizophr Bull 6:64, 1980

Jacobs MA: Promoting responsibility and mutual concern through a modified form of patient government. J Psychiatr Nurs 15:30, 1977

Larkin AR: What's a medication group? J Psychosoc Nurs 20:35, Feb., 1982

Leone D, Zahourek R: "Aloneness" in a therapeutic community. Perspect Psychiatr Care 12:59, 1974

Liberman RP: A review of Paul and Lentz's psychological treatment for chronic mental patients: Milieu versus social learning programs. J Applied Behav Anal 13:367, 1980

Malcomson K et al: An evaluation of the effect of nurses wearing street clothes on socialization patterns. J Psychiatr Nurs 15:18, 1977

Miller TW, Lee LI: Quality assurance: Focus on environmental perspectives of psychiatric patients and nursing staff. J Psychiatr Nurs 18:9, 1980

Moran JC: An alternative to constant observation: The behavioral check list. Perspect Psychiatr Care 17:114, 1979

Mosher LR, Keith SJ: Research on the psychosocial treatment of schizophrenia: A summary report. Am J Psychiatry 136:623, 1979

Rasinski K et al: Practical implications of a theory of the "therapeutic milieu" for psychiatric nursing practice. J Psychiatr Nurs 18:16, May, 1980

Romoff V, Kane I: Primary nursing in psychiatry: An effective and functional model. Perspect Psychiatr Care 20:73, 1982

Ryan LJ, Gearhart MK, Simmons S: From professional responsibility to professional accountability in psychiatric nursing. J Psychiatr Nurs 15:19, 1977

Sattin SM: The psychodynamics of the "holiday syndrome." Perspect Psychiatr Care 13:156, 1975

Schanding D et al: A small study on how the staff of an inpatient psychiatric unit spends its time. Perspect Psychiatr Care 20:91, 1982

Sclafani M: Medication classes for the mentally ill. J Psychiatr Nurs 15:13, 1977

Singerman B et al: An evening diversional activity program for psychiatric patients. J Psychiatr Nurs 18:28, 1980

Skinner K: The therapeutic milieu: Making it work. J Psychiatr Nurs 17:38, 1979

Sweeney LJ: Psychiatric patients' perceptions of their milieu therapy program. J Psychiatr Nurs 16:28, 1978

Torkingtow JR: Psychiatric nursing approaches and outcomes. Australian Nurses J 9:31, 1979

Wittman D, Leeman CP: Using creative writing in an activity therapy group on a short-term unit. Hosp Commun Psychiatr 30:307, 1979

Wolf MS: A review of literature on milieu therapy. J Psychiatr Nurs 15:26, 1977

11

Designing a
Day Hospital Program

John Rosato

Introduction A day hospital program is geared to the chronically disturbed client who has experienced long-standing interpersonal and community adjustment difficulties. The day hospital is meant to combine the attention, supervision, and structured program of a hospital with the openness, availability, and cost containment of a community program.

Types of Clients
1. Clients concurrently treated in a full-time hospital
2. Clients in transition from the full-time hospital to the community
3. Clients who have been discharged
4. Clients so seriously impaired that, except for the support and maintenance of a day program, long-term hospitalization would be required
5. Clients who are in an acute crisis, are decompensating, and need the structure of a day hospital to prevent a first hospitalization

Goals The goals of a day hospital program are dependent on the goals and treatment philosophy of its parent community agency. The basic goals of a day hospital program are
1. Facilitation of community readjustment
2. Improvement of clinical status, to maintain optimum level of functioning
3. Prevention of hospitalization

Chart 11–1 indicates goals, nursing actions, and rationale in a day hospital program.

Advantages of Day Hospital Treatment The major advantage is creation of a therapeutic environment for chronic clients. This environment fosters peer support and personality reintegration for clients who might otherwise become institutionalized on the back wards of state hospitals. Other advantages are that day hospital treatment
1. Allows the client to maintain independent activities despite mental illness
2. Discourages the excessive dependency and dehumanization that often develops in the course of full-time hospitalization
3. Allows the client to remain with the family when this is therapeutically desirable

Chart 11–1
GOALS, NURSING INTERVENTIONS, AND THEORETICAL RATIONALE IN A DAY HOSPITAL PROGRAM

Goal	Nursing Intervention	Rationale
1. Prevention of hospitalization	1. a. Weekly medication group	1. a. 80% of chronic client recidivism is related to improper medication use.
	b. Mental health class	b. Understanding of mental illness lessens anxiety about what clients are experiencing.
	c. Interpersonal issues discussion group	c. Understanding of interpersonal anxiety and conflict leads to more satisfying interpersonal relations.
2. Facilitation of community readjustment	2. a. Field trip to grocery store by bus b. Shopping center trips c. Field classes on the use of public transportation	2. Ability to function in the community prevents hospitalization and facilitates employment.
3. Improvement of clinical status	3. a. Individual therapy b. Group therapy c. Family therapy d. Personal and social adjustment group	3. Modes of thinking, feeling, and acting will gradually change through therapy; these changes will improve other areas of adjustment.

4. Offers a more active and varied therapeutic experience than most inpatient services
5. Presents less social stigma than inpatient therapy.
6. Forces clients to be more aware of their strengths and abilities than inpatient programs where pathology is sometimes overly emphasized
7. Makes possible part-time jobs in the evenings and on weekends
8. Capitalizes on the capacities of the paraprofessionals and other clients as helping agents
9. Provides a means of "tapering off" therapy

Disadvantages of Day Hospital Treatment

While day hospital treatment decreases the dependency that chronic clients have on full-time hospitalization, it may become a substitute dependency. This is a disadvantage that can be avoided by the staff's actively encouraging clients to achieve optimum functioning. Other disadvantages are that it[2]

1. Is fatiguing for staff who find it difficult dealing with problems the clients live with. It is trying when clients test staff by attempts to get inpatient care.
2. Is easier for day clients (than it is for inpatients) to drop out of the program if it does not appear relevant to their needs and problems
3. Presents problems of transportation and living arrangements
4. Usually costs more than regular outpatient care.

Staff

Staff can vary greatly, depending on funding and availability. The program should draw on the services of volunteers and students in health professions. With some orientation and training they can provide a viable changing microcosm of personalities that the client will confront in the community. Staff members should, in addition to their professional training, be intuitively sensitive and empathic to the needs of clients and should support, reinforce, and even direct the client's ego functions. Table 11–1 is a suggested staffing mix for 80 clients.

Table 11–1
STAFF, PREPARATION, AND FUNCTIONS IN A DAY HOSPITAL PROGRAM

Staff	Preparation	Function
Administrator	Master's degree in psychiatric nursing with functional major in administration, or master's degree in social work, or doctorate in psychology	Handles personnel matters, administration and public relations; leads group therapy, carries a small caseload
Clinical specialist	Master's degree in psychiatric nursing and ANA certification as adult psychiatric clinical specialist	Provides clinical supervision; provides therapy for acute and newly admitted clients in individual, group, and family therapy; is hospital and physician liaison person; does client teaching; dispenses medication
Physician (half-time)	Psychiatrist	Co-leads medication groups and therapy groups; does client teaching; performs physical evaluations, prescribes medication
Social worker	Master's degree in social work	Carries caseload; leads groups; provides community placement; is liaison person with community agencies; supervises caseworkers; handles public relations.

(continued)

Table 11–1
(continued)

Staff	Preparation	Function
Caseworkers (2)	Bachelor's degree in social work, nursing, or psychology	Carries caseload, leads activities and programs
Recreational therapist	Bachelor of Science degree in health-related field and certified recreational therapist	Coordinates, develops, and leads recreational activities and programs
Occupational therapist	Bachelor of Science degree in health-related field and certified occupational therapist or Master's of science in occupational therapy and certification	Coordinates, develops, and leads occupational therapy activities and programs
Mental health aides (4)	High school diploma	Assists in all program activities
Vocational therapist		Coordinator of vocational program and job placement

Facility An ideal day hospital has a lounge, arts and crafts area, game room, library meeting room, dining area, staff offices, and treatment room. Rooms are attractively furnished to give a homelike quality rather than an institutional air. Calendars, clocks, maps, and mirrors are all aspects of the environment that support realistic functioning and are included in the physical setting of a day hospital.

Table 11–2 provides some suggestions for what could be included in the various areas.

The day hospital should be centrally located with easy access to public transportation. It may be advantageous to locate near the main hospital, since the clients may already know the area and the transit system surrounding it.

Activities Some activities are scheduled and some spontaneous. Groups, socials, and special events form the cornerstone of the therapeutic milieu of a day hospital. Activities in the day hospital provide the psychiatric nurse with rich opportunities to promote feelings of belonging, enhance clients' self-esteem, and encourage assertiveness. All activities are conducted within a context of a planned physical environment, organized schedules, staff support, and reality orientation. Even though the therapeutic effect of

Table 11–2
ROOMS AND FURNISHINGS IN A DAY HOSPITAL PROGRAM

Craft Room	Game Room	Dining Area	Library Meeting Room
Painting	Table games	Dinette-style tables and chairs	Coffee tables and end tables
Clay modeling	Pool table		
Weaving	Table tennis	Refrigerator	Large, comfortable chairs
Typing	Table shuffleboard	Electric coffeepot	
Woodworking		Kitchen cabinets	Lamps
Leather craft		Sink	Books and magazines
String art		Stove	
Decoupage			

these activities will overlap, it is helpful to identify what activities will have the most beneficial effect on which symptoms. The clinical nurse specialist gives team guidelines in designing a program for each client.

Ideally each client is assigned a case manager who helps to engage the client in the program. If the client attempts to drop out of the program, it is the case manager who offers support and encouragement to keep the client involved. According to the amount of resistance and the client's interest, the case manager and client work out the client's program together.

Table 11–3 illustrates some activities aimed at relieving certain schizophrenic symptoms.

Programming Clients are given every opportunity to take control and make decisions in their treatment plans. Ultimately the day hospital program is aimed at strengthening the ego functioning of individuals who have given up or lost control of their lives. The day hospital fosters the acceptance of responsibility for control in such a way that it can

Table 11–3
SCHIZOPHRENIC SYMPTOMS AND THERAPEUTIC ACTIVITIES

Symptom	Activity
Sense of emptiness, diffusion; poor reality testing; loose thought processes; confusion; poor memory; overwhelming anxiety	Garden group Relaxation training Exercise class Bowling Dancing Leather work Sewing Cooking Singing group Art group Drama group
Unawareness of own or others feelings; low frustration tolerance; labile moods; poor impulse control; inappropriate behavior	Group therapy Cognitive restructuring group Spontaneous guided group discussions Psychodrama
Identity as a sexual, psychological, and social being absent or distorted; poor self-concept; inability to form relationships; inappropriate dress, talk, and behavior	Assertiveness training Socialization groups Weight watchers Grooming classes Games Parties Women's awareness groups Men's awareness groups Social club
Not responsible; unmotivated; unable to initiate or persist in an activity or interaction; poor work habits and skills	Vocational rehabilitation Patient government membership Voter registration Community outings Individual responsibility for specific day hospital functions

be generalized in the community at large. This is best accomplished through individual responsibilities, goal setting, group process, and peer support. *The most effective milieu is one that uses clients as therapeutic agents for one another. This function can be enhanced as staff learn how to tap the client's ability to exert pressure on and provide support for others.*[3]

The day hospital should be organized and structured just enough to make an efficient program but not so much as to make it rigid, stagnant, and unresponsive to the changing needs of the client. Most day hospitals operate Monday through Friday 8 AM to 5 PM, with evening programs once or twice a week and, if possible, an outing one weekend a month. For organizational efficiency the day is scheduled into segments of time for various groups and activities. Since clients are not required to attend full time, they can choose schedules according to their interests and needs. Table 11–4 is a sample of a week's schedule, with responsibilities for the activities assigned to particular staff members.

Description of Program Activities

A. **GROUP THERAPY**
Each group has 8 to 10 members, and meets for two 1-hour sessions per week.

B. **COOKING**
Cooking includes menu planning, budgeting, shopping for bargains, preparing the meal, group dinners, and clean-up.

C. **BOWLING**
A field trip to a local bowling alley is arranged during business hours for special rates.

D. **PERSONAL SOCIAL ADJUSTMENT**
Lecture, role playing, and group discussion are employed to cover an assortment of topics such as interpersonal relations, problem solving, decision making, values clarification, and budgeting.

E. **EMOTIVE–EXPRESSIVE GROUP**
The emotive–expressive group employs a variety of techniques, such as group water color collage, to stimulate the expression of emotions.

F. **ARTS AND CRAFTS**
Arts and crafts includes leather work, sewing, clay work, painting, decoupage, and so forth.

G. **JOB PREPAREDNESS**
Job preparedness includes class instruction and role play in job interviews, job hunting, and completing applications, and learning about W-2 forms, social security cards, and so forth.

H. **MEDICATION GROUP**
The weekly medication group is led by a psychiatrist and clinical nurse specialist. All new clients are seen in this group until stabilized on medications and then are seen at regular intervals for medication review.

I. **ETHNIC GROUP**
Social adjustment problems of minorities are open for group discussion

J. **SOCIALIZATION GROUP**
Dances or other social activities are aimed at getting clients from various community mental health programs together in an informal recreational setting.

K. **STRUCTURED LEISURE TIME**
Clients play pool, table tennis, cards, scrabble, checkers, chess, and other table games.

Table 11–4
TYPICAL WEEKLY SCHEDULE IN A DAY HOSPITAL

Monday	Tuesday	Wednesday	Thursday	Friday
9:30–10:30 Large group (all staff)	9:00–11:30 Personal social adjustment (David)	8:30–10:30 Staffing (all staff)	9:00–10:30 Group therapy (David)	9:00–11:30 Personal social adjustment (David)
10:00–11:00 Arts & crafts (Donna)	9:00–11:45 Emotive–expressive group (Donna)	10:30–12:00 Medication group / Structured leisure time	9:30–10:30 Structured leisure time (Donna, Diane)	9:30–12:00 Individual therapy appointments & socialization
10:00–12:00 Cooking (Alicia)	10:45–11:45 Arts & crafts (Donna)		10:45–11:45 Personal social adjustment (Alicia) Women's group (Donna, Diane)	
12:00–1:00 Lunch	12:00–1:00 Lunch	12:00–1:00 Lunch	12:00–1:00 Lunch	12:00–1:00 Lunch
1:00–3:00 Bowling (Donna, Alicia)	1:15–2:15 Group therapy (Diane) Crafts (Donna, Alicia)	1:15–3:15 Arts & crafts (Donna)	1:00–2:00 Soap opera group (Kevin, Alicia)	1:00–5:00 Charting Follow-up/follow along Program planning
	2:30–3:30 Job Preparedness (Alicia)	1:30–2:30 Group therapy (Diane)	1:15–2:15 Values clarification (Donna)	
Bowl-a-rama	6:00–8:30 Personal social adjustment (David)	2:00–3:30 Group therapy (David)	2:30–3:30 Weight control (Donna, Diane) Supervised activities (Alicia)	
		2:30–3:30 Ethnic group (Alicia)	6:15–8:15 Group therapy (Diane) Personal social adjustment	
		4:00–6:00 River City Junction socialization group		

L. **SOAP OPERA GROUP**
The soap opera group uses the characters and situations on television soap operas to stimulate discussions of real-life dilemmas by nonverbal or withdrawn clients.

M. **VALUES CLARIFICATION**
Lecture, role play, and discussion are used to aid clients in developing and structuring their values.

N. **WEIGHT CONTROL**
Peer support group for weight loss and improved self-esteem is provided.

Nursing Techniques   The activities of a day hospital are designed to elicit the clients' typical maladaptive behaviors in a therapeutic environment. Once the maladaptive behaviors emerge, the staff can work with clients, offering corrective experiences. As clients become comfortable with new adaptive ways of interacting in a setting that resembles the community at large, with an added degree of safety, they begin the process of generalizing what has been learned to the environment outside the day hospital.

The techniques in Chart 11–2 are typical occurrences in a day hospital. These techniques can be used in various settings, and more than one can be applied during the same activity.

Medication   A day hospital revolves around two basic classes of therapy, psychotherapy and psychopharmacology—one without the other has limited usefulness in a day hospital. The very nature of the chronic schizophrenic client dictates the judicious use of neuroleptic drugs and timely therapeutic interventions directed at a reintegration of the personality. It is the responsibility of the psychiatric nurse to see that the whole individual gets treated, and that the biochemical as well as the psychological aspects of the client are addressed. Specifics about neuroleptics can be found in Part VI.

Chart 11–2
NURSING TECHNIQUES AND EXAMPLES IN A DAY HOSPITAL TREATMENT PROGRAM

Nursing Technique	*Example*
Support—individually applied to allay anxiety by giving encouragement, reassurance, and direct assistance	A client states that he is no good at cooking and always fails when he tries. The nurse reassures him that it is the effort that counts and goes on to work directly with the client to prepare brownies.
Direction and guidance—includes role modeling and giving advice on what, when, or how to act	The nurse conducts a grooming class for female clients and discusses proper hygiene.
Environmental manipulation—arranging settings and circumstances in the physical and social environment in ways thought likely to have a beneficial effect on behavior	Chairs in lounge are always arranged in small circles. A donated television is refused because it is felt that it would deter maximum social interaction.
Positive reinforcement—the selective use of verbal recognition and approval when a client exhibits a positive adaptive behavior. This is done consistently, immediately, and directly in order to encourage repetition and generalization of the desired behavior.	The nurse praises a normally disheveled client for appropriate personal grooming. A client is cited as an example in group for exhibiting appropriate communication of anger. Peer support and praise are elicited for a withdrawn client participating in a group game.
Extinction—purposeful inattention to maladjustive behavior	A client repeatedly walks up to staff and says, "You are going to take away my Social Security disability because you hate me." This has been explored in group, and the staff ignores the behavior.
Redirecting—diverting diffusely expended energies into more focused, productive channels	A client who builds up tensions and then explodes by hitting the wall and throwing ashtrays is directed to the gym for vigorous activities.
Role playing—the acting out of different roles in a therapy situation to rehearse and reduce anxiety in the real situation	A client practices a job interview situation with the therapist. The therapist plays an irresponsible landlord and the client practices being assertive.
Catharsis—ventilation of feelings. The nurse acts as a sounding board and uncritical listener to promote self-understanding and an atmosphere of trust.	Pent-up feelings surface in a group activity or a bull session between the nurse and client. The nurse encourages the client to say what he is thinking and feeling.

Public Relations   Referrals and funding are greatly affected by what the community, individual professionals, and other agencies know of the day hospital. Staff members must clarify their own thinking about theoretical concepts and practices in the day treatment program and then communicate this clearly in order to achieve optimum use of the day hospital. "The general community and the medical and psychiatric professions must be well informed about its (day hospital) purpose, how it works, and how it compares and what relates to other treatment methods and facilities."[1]

It is to the advantage of the nurse administrator to maintain a positive liaison with funding agencies and state and community mental health officials. Maintaining a high profile with documentation of cost effective and efficient treatment that is unique and serves a perceived need is the best way to keep a viable program funded.

Evaluation   Depending on the individual client's goals the day hospital program is considered a success if
1. The chronic client is able to remain outside the hospital
2. The client in transition from hospital to community is able to obtain a job and be weaned from the day hospital
3. The acute client is able to avoid hospitalization, become stabilized, and return to usual activities.

References

1. Barnard R: Achieving optimum use of the day hospital. Mental Hospitals 12:18, 1961
2. Glasscote RM, Kraft AM, Glassman DM, Jepson WW: Partial Hospitalization of the Mentally Ill: A Study of Programs & Problems. Washington, DC, The Joint Information Service of the American Psychiatric Association and the National Association for Mental Health, 1969
3. Gross R: A conceptual outline for day treatment center practice. Compr Psychiatry 12:437, 1971
4. Rosato J: Unpublished study, 1977

Bibliography

Aron KW, Smith S: The Bristol psychiatric day hospital. J Ment Sci 99:564, 1953

Barnard R: The day hospital is an extension of psychiatric treatment. Bull Menninger Clin 16:50, 1967

Bradshaw WH: PASST (primary attending and socialization skills training): Filling the gap between hospital and community for chronic schizophrenics. Int J Partial Hospitalization 1:59, 1982

Brooks D: Creating a day hospital. Psychiatr Communication 12:23, 1970

Butts H: The organization of a psychiatric day hospital. JAMA 56:381, 1964

Cararino JP, Wilner M, Maxey JT: American Association for Partial Hospitalization (AAPH) Standards and Guidelines for Partial Hospitalization. Int J Partial Hospitalization 1:5, 1982

Craft M: Psychiatric day hospital. Am J Psychiatry 116:251, 1959

Edwards MS: Psychiatric day programs: A descriptive analysis. J Psychosoc Nurs 20:17, 1982

Guidry LD, Winstead ML, Eicke F: Evaluation of day treatment effectiveness. J Clin Psychiatry 40:31, 1979

Herz MI: Partial hospitalization, brief hospitalization, and aftercare. In Kaplan HI et al (eds): Comprehensive Textbook of Psychiatry, 3rd ed. Baltimore, Williams & Wilkins, 1980

Herz MI: Research overview in day treatment. Int J Partial Hospitalization 1:33, 1982

Lefkowitz PM: The assessment of suitability for partial hospitalization: The Day Therapy Appropriateness Scale. Int J Partial Hospitalization 1:45, 1982

Luber RF (ed): Partial Hospitalization: A Current Perspective. New York, Plenum Press, 1979

Mosher L, Keith S: Research on the psychosocial treatment of schizophrenia: A summary report. Am J Psychiatry 136:623, 1979

Ozasin L: Community alternatives to institutional care. Am J Psychiatry 133:69, 1976

Shepherd G: Day care and the chronic patient: What we have here is the same old problems in different places. Int J Partial Hospitalization 1:23, 1982

Talbott J: Deinstitutionalization: Avoiding the disasters of the past. Hosp Community Psychiatry 12:621, 1979

12

Designing a Deinstitutionalization Program

Rachel Parios

OVERVIEW

Introduction
Purpose
Design of Deinstitutionalization Programs
Physical Facility
Staff
Staff Meetings
Admission Criteria
Referral Process
Initial Intake Evaluation
Client Preparation
Program Hours
Phases of Deinstitutionalization
Nursing Intervention
Program Evaluation

Introduction   Deinstitutionalization programs are designed to help psychiatric clients with adjustment during their transition from an institution or family to the community. Programs are divided into four phases (each phase of no more than 6 months' duration), which incorporates a philosophy of progression toward more advanced functioning. At the end of 2 years, clients are able to live independently within the community.

Purpose   Deinstitutionalization programs help clients to

1. Develop technical, personal, and academic skills necessary for community living, continued education, and entry into a vocational career
2. Pursue activities that provide personal satisfaction and immediate gratification
3. Generate initiative, motivation, and values necessary to live creatively in urban, suburban, or rural settings
4. Learn about themselves and how they interact with other people, other cultures, and their environment
5. Foster and maintain trusting relationships in the community
6. Experience therapeutic benefits derived from socialization and prevocational experiences
7. Live in a sheltered setting when they can reside in the community but cannot function in the employment market

Design of Deinstitutionalization Programs   Community-based psychosocial rehabilitation services are offered to psychiatric clients through structured activities, with appropriate controls. Funding is provided by city, state, and federal monies or through private sponsorship.

Physical Facility
1. Types. Two kinds of structures are used:
   a. Buildings are converted into residences or "group homes" where clients live in small groups (8–10 clients) in Phase I.
   b. Furnished apartments are rented by the program for clients' use in Phase II of the program.
2. In both phases the client pays rent to the program. After 1 year, when clients enter Phase III, they find and rent their own apartments and pay their landlords directly.
3. Requirements. The facility must be located near public transportatin. The residence or apartment should provide a bedroom for each client plus a living room, dining area, and kitchen. The residence usually has a staff bedroom where residence counselors sleep at night.

Staff   Table 12–1 shows the staffing needed in a deinstitutionalization program.

Staff Meetings
A. DAILY MORNING MEETING FOR ALL STAFF
   1. Discuss events of past evening or weekend
   2. Discuss plans of the day, including staff assignments
B. WEEKLY STAFF MEETING FOR ALL STAFF
   1. Review and evaluate program and change as needed
   2. Discuss feelings about working with the clients
C. MONTHLY STAFF MEETING FOR ALL STAFF
   Guest speakers provide continuing education.
D. WEEKLY RESIDENT COUNSELORS MEETING
   1. Discuss issues of the residence
   2. Plan weekly activities for clients

Table 12–1

TITLE, QUALIFICATIONS, AND ROLES OF STAFF IN A DEINSTITUTIONALIZATION PROGRAM

Staff Title	Discipline License/Degree	Role
Director (1)	*One* of the following: Psychiatrist—M.D. Psychologist—Ph.D. Clinical nurse specialist—masters degree in psychiatric nursing Social worker—M.S.W.	1. Directs and supervises program and staff
Psychiatrist (1)	M.D.	1. Initiates treatment plan and monitors implementation 2. Prescribes treatment 3. Consults with staff
Intake coordinator (1)	Clinical nurse specialist or social worker	1. Is liaison between agency, client, and institution 2. Provides agency with initial intake evaluation
Life skills coordinator (1)	Vocational rehabilitation—M.A.	1. Coordinates daily life skills program and activities 2. Collaborates with primary counselors 3. Supervises life skills assistants and resident counselors
Life skills assistants (2)	Psychology/vocational rehabilitation—B.A.	1. Assists life skills coordinator with implementation of activities.
Housing coordinator (1)	Social worker—M.S.W.	1. Is liaison between program and rental agencies. 2. Initiates and secures federal housing assistance funding (H.U.D.). 3. Assists clients with all areas of housing.

Primary counselors (5)	Clinical nurse specialist
	Social worker
	Psychologist (M.A.)
		1. Assists clients with clinical aspects of their transition into the community and program including
		    a. Finances
		    b. Housing
		    c. Leisure time planning
		    d. Personal needs
		    e. Health maintenance
		    f. Training on public transportation
		2. Provides individual psychotherapy
		3. Leads evening and weekend programs

Registered nurse (1)	B.S.N.	1. Collaborates with M.D., clinics, and health care facilities for client referrals 2. Assesses clients' health needs 3. Teaches health management 4. Provides emergency treatment during program time 5. Collaborates with primary counselors about clients' health

Table 12–1
(continued)

Staff Title	Discipline License/Degree	Role
Resident counselors (6)	Psychology—B.A. Social work—B.A.	1. Supervises clients at the residence 2. Collaborates with the primary counselors, life skills coordinator, and nurse about needs of residents 3. Participates as a role model in daily living at the residence

Vocational rehabilitation counselor (1)	Vocational rehabilitation—M.A.	1. Helps clients develop prevocational and vocational skills
		2. Collaborates with clients' primary counselors
		3. Is liaison between program and vocational agencies:
		  a. Sheltered workshops
		  b. Division of Vocational Rehabilitation
		  c. Transitional employment
		4. Is liaison between program and educational facilities:
		  a. High school equivalency exam (G.E.D.)
		  b. College/university

Secretaries (3)	High school graduate who has attended secretarial school or medical secretary school	1. Types and files agency records 2. Types interagency communications

E. **EMERGENCY STAFF MEETINGS**
Staff discuss crisis situations as they arise.

F. **COMBINED STAFF AND CLIENT MEETING**
Staff and clients share information about changes in the program that affect clients and staff.

Admission Criteria Clients must
1. Have a psychiatric history, not necessarily including hospitalization
2. Be discharged from the hospital (if they have been inpatients) or about to be discharged
3. Be evaluated and cleared for
   a. Signs of active psychosis
   b. Suicidal or homicidal behavior
   c. A history of arson
4. Have the potential for independent community living

Referral Process The client's record upon referral must include

1. Written consent from the client authorizing transfer of information
2. Admission intake summary, including client history and hospital discharge summary
3. Hospital treatment plan
4. Summary of psychological testing
5. Medication regimen
6. Social Security Insurance, Social Security Disability, Medicaid, or Medicare application or acceptance, or proof of personal finances
7. Description of the client's level of functioning
8. The client's agreement to enter the deinstitutionalization program

Initial Intake Evaluation Interviewing and screening includes introducing the client to the concept of deinstitutionalization and the program, as well as making a clinical assessment of the client's potential for

1. Benefit from the deinstitutionalization program
2. Successful adjustment to independent community living

The staff then makes a decision to accept the client based on

1. Client's history, experience, and background
2. Current level of functioning
3. Thorough knowledge of client's strengths and limitations

Client Preparation Once clients understand the deinstitutionalization program and goals, they enter the program voluntarily agreeing to

1. Assume the responsibility for self-medication
2. Meet the deinstitutionalization fee schedule
3. Abstain from alcohol and drugs
4. Demonstrate productive activities toward independent living and prevocational training
5. Attend six to eight predischarge group meetings with other clients entering the program
6. Make 3 or 4-day visits to the deinstitutionalization program prior to entry

See Chart 12–1 for a typical residence contract.

Program Hours
1. Monday through Friday, 9:00 AM to 3:00 PM—day program
2. Monday through Wednesday, 7:00 PM to 9:00 PM—evening programs
3. Saturday, 9:00 AM to 12:00 PM—weekend program
4. Monday through Friday, 9:00 AM to 5:00 PM for staff*

Phases of Deinstitutionalization Deinstitutionalization is divided into four phases, each lasting 6 months. Phase I introduces clients to group life in the community. Each phase after that carries clients further into the community, weaning them slowly from the program and providing vocational, educational, and social skills needed for life outside the institution or family. Whenever possible, the client receives psychotherapy in each phase. At the end of the 2 years, the client is referred to a clinic or community mental health center for continued psychotherapy. If clients want to and are able to move more quickly through these phases they may do so. Tables 12–2, 12–3, 12–4, and 12–5 show each of the four phases, including the components, staff intervention, and theoretical rationale.

(Text continues on p. 122)

*Staff monitors a beeper on rotating weekends for emergencies at the residence.

Chart 12–1
RESIDENCE CONTRACT FOR PHASE I

Resident's contract:

While you live at the supervised residence you must follow certain regulations in order to safeguard the health and welfare of yourself and fellow residents.

The following behaviors cannot be tolerated in group living situations *and will result in immediate suspension:*

1. Assaultive behavior or any behavior harmful to others.
2. Destruction of property.
3. Use of guns, knives, or other dangerous instruments or weapons.
4. Bringing alcoholic beverages or illegal or unprescribed drugs on the premises.
5. Lending or borrowing of medications.

In addition to the above, expectations are as follows:

1. Take prescribed medication regularly, as directed.
2. Pay your rent regularly and on time.
3. Be responsible for your room key.
4. Take complete care of your room and help with all household chores, including food preparation, service, dishwashing, and keeping common areas clean and orderly.
5. Keep yourself, your clothing, your bed linens, and towels clean and neat. Staff will assist you in learning skills to meet these responsibilities.
6. Be productively occupied during the day with a job, school, training or day program, volunteer work or other activities that foster independence. Staff will help you obtain such a placement.

7. Get along with other people, especially your fellow residents and nearby neighbors.
8. Be careful with your own property and respectful of other people's property.
9. Notify staff whenever you want to plan an overnight absence from the residence or program.
10. Learn to make decisions and plan your own life. Ask for assistance whenever necessary.
11. Attend all regularly scheduled community meetings and meetings arranged with staff.
12. Lending or borrowing money is not helpful to either party and should not be done.
13. Abide by the rules of the residence or phase of the program in which you're involved.
14. Try your best to benefit from what the program offers so that you can progress to the next phase as expected.

> *Note:* Failure to live up to these expectations will indicate an unwillingness or inability to participate in the deinstitutionalization program and will be reason for staff to re-evaluate your continued stay in the program.

I have read and understand the above rules and regulations.

Client's signature _____ Date _____

Staff signature _____ Date _____

(Reprinted with permission of Transitional Services of New York, Inc., Queens Village, NY)

Table 12–2
PHASE I PROGRAM—RESIDENTIAL LIVING

Component	Staff Action Intervention	Theoretical Rationale
Housing Supervised residential living	1. Ensure that client has his/her own room.	1. a. Establishes client's territory outside the institution or home b. Encourages client's feelings of belonging

	2. Supervise client's responsibility for upkeep of room.	2. Promotes client's skill development for
		   a. Cleaning
		   b. Bedmaking
		   c. Organization
		   d. Tidiness

	3. Supervise meal planning, food shopping, and meal preparation.	3. Fosters development of skills for
		   a. Cooking
		   b. Meal planning
		   c. Nutrition
		   d. Kitchen utensil use

(continued)

Table 12–2
(continued)

Component	Staff Intervention	Theoretical Rationale
	4. Supervise client participation in responsibilities of shared rooms: a. Living room b. Dining room c. Kitchen d. Bathrooms	4. Develops lines of responsibility, cooperation, satisfaction and self esteem in activities of daily living
	5. Supervise client's budgeting, including a. Rent b. Personal needs c. Banking	5. a. Develops responsibility and self control of finances b. Fosters self-esteem
	6. Supervise client's self-medication regimen: a. Dispense medication for 7 days b. Review daily medication schedule with client	6. Fosters independence in daily living
Task Oriented Activities Horticulture Woodworking Sewing Gardening Meal preparation Shopping Banking Grooming Prevocational groups Voting and registration Bazaar preparation Using public transportation Participation in sponsored community functions	1. Ensure that clients attend program and activities.	1. Fosters client's motivation and skill development for the following: a. Meeting time requirements b. Following specific instructions c. Dressing appropriately for work/ activity performance d. Vocational initiative e. Sharing work tasks f. Sharing work breaks
Evening Activities, Phase I Monday evening, 7–9 PM— community living group	Led by 2 primary counselors 1. Discussion prompted by guest speakers: Police department Fire department YMCA Telephone company Consumer education group Social security office Legal aid society Town council Board of education Local merchants	1. a. Provides clients with information about community living b. Enhances clients' understanding, security, and transition into community living
Tuesday evening, 7–9 PM— health group	Led by registered nurse and clinical nurse specialist	1. a. Provides clients with information and understanding about health issues and needs

Table 12–2
(continued)

Component	Staff Intervention	Theoretical Rationale
	1. Health teaching (use audiovisual aids and guest speakers): American Cancer Society American Heart Association Planned Parenthood American Dental Association American Respiratory Association American Diabetic Association Kidney Foundation Nutritionist Sexuality—male/female	b. Motivates clients to attend to their own health responsibilities
Wednesday evening, 7–9 PM—social evening	Led by 2 primary counselors 1. Provide activities of a social nature: Music Dance Theater Parties Games with prizes	1. Encourages clients' social interaction, leisure time planning, enjoyment and increased self esteem.

Table 12–3

PHASE II PROGRAM—SUPERVISED APARTMENT LIVING WITH PREVOCATIONAL TRAINING

Component	Staff Intervention	Theoretical Rationale
Housing Temporary, supervised, furnished apartment living Toward the end of Phase II, staff members help client to find an apartment in the community for Phase III.	1. Introduce clients to temporary apartment 3 weeks prior to move. 2. Discuss with clients their choice of co-tenant and proceed with choice. 3. Set up two weekly meetings with both clients and both counselors to establish guidelines: a. Budget for two b. Housekeeping responsibilities c. Program responsibilities d. Guests 4. Help clients move to the temporary apartment. 5. Establish regular weekly meetings with both clients and both counselors to discuss a. Budgeting b. Shopping c. Meal planning d. Laundry e. Personal needs	1. Allows clients time to prepare for move and change 2. Provides clients with participation in decision-making process 3. Fosters clients' understanding of new life-style and roles 4. Reduces client anxiety level and confusion associated with moving 5. Provides structure for client's understanding of self-management
Clients live in apartments which they rent in the community.		

(continued)

Table 12–3
(continued)

Component	Staff Intervention	Theoretical Rationale

Task Oriented Activities
Prevocational and vocational groups (attendance, 9 AM–3 PM)
	Led by vocational rehabilitation counselor
	
	1. Help clients learn vocational responsibilities:
	  a. Job interview
	  b. Proper attire
	  c. How to locate employment
	  d. Personal interests and related employment
	  e. Resume writing
	  f. Employment preparation
	2. Set up "model" business operation (for example, horticulture) and have clients learn each aspect:
	  a. Purchasing
	  b. Potting, pruning, propagating
	  c. Sales
	  d. Telephone management
	  e. Bookkeeping
	  f. Quality control
	  g. Maintenance
	  h. Advertising
	3. Explore with clients
	  a. Volunteer jobs
	  b. Sheltered workshops
	  c. Transitional employment
		1. Fosters clients' development of
		  a. Vocational initiative
		  b. Personal growth
		  c. Crystallizing job goals
		
		2. a. Provides a secure environment in which clients can learn varied skills for vocational future
		  b. Establishes self worth, confidence, and esteem in the vocational setting
		
		3. Provides clients with a vocational experience before permanent employment

Evening Activities, Phase II Monday and Wednesday evenings, 6:30–9:00 PM—field trips	Led by two primary counselors 1. Meet in alternate client apartments. 2. Plan, organize, and establish trips to community functions, after selecting a client leader.	1. Encourages socialization to begin in the home rather than the program 2. Fosters clients' awareness and participation in community sponsored functions, while developing leadership abilities

Table 12–4

**PHASE III PROGRAM—UNSUPERVISED APARTMENT LIVING WITH
VOCATIONAL TRAINING OR EMPLOYMENT AND COMMUNITY SOCIAL LIFE**

Purpose
1. To promote a more sophisticated community life for the client
2. To foster separation from the program and integration into vocational, educational, and social activities in the community.

Component	Staff Intervention	Theoretical Rationale
Housing Community apartment (see Chap. 29 for ADL—housing)	1. Help client locate and apply for a community apartment. 2. Assist client with moving, locating furnishings, and transition into apartment.	1. Provides support to client and encouragement necessary for independent apartment living 2. Lessens client's anxiety level and confusion about change in life-style
Vocational/Educational	1. Assist client with securing employment if level of functioning warrants such. 2. Help client to apply for vocational training at the Division of Vocational Rehabilitation. or 3. Help client to secure permanent or temporary volunteer work. or 4. Help client to apply for GED (high school equivalency exam)	1. Fosters client's independent financial security and opportunity 2. Provides those clients who need special career training with an opportunity to obtain it; uses a community resource rather than the deinstitutionalization program 3. a. Provides client with a nonthreatening work environment b. Prepares client for employment or interest development for work when the client is ready to advance in the future 4. Provides client the opportunity for basic education needed for further education or employment
Leisure Time Activities	1. Encourage client to branch out into community social resources.	1. Integrates client into mainstream of society and provides the opportunity for clients to establish new friends.

(During this phase of the program, the client becomes a role model for other clients participating in earlier phases.)

Table 12–5
**PHASE IV PROGRAM—APARTMENT LIVING WITH EMPLOYMENT,
EDUCATION (IF DESIRED), AND ACTIVE COMMUNITY INVOLVEMENT**

Component	Staff Intervention	Theoretical Rationale
Housing Same as Phase III	1. Act as a resource person for client.	1. a. Promotes client's independence in the community b. Fosters the weaning of clients from the program
Vocational/educational	1. a. Ensure that client is actively involved in employment, volunteer work, or school. Educational programs that combine classroom learning and work experience are encouraged so that clients gain specific skills and knowledge together. b. Communicate that adults residing in the community work and support themselves.	1. a. Encourages client's motivation and self-esteem b. Discourages client's possible regression

Nursing Intervention   The client who is moving from the hospital or family out into the community is faced with the usual anxiety one experiences at periods of separation. However, these are more pronounced than usual because of the poorly developed egos of these clients. The nurse recognizes that these clients often have anxiety about

1. Independent actions
2. Progressing too fast
3. Relinquishing old behavior patterns or family roles
4. Success
5. The unknown
6. Gratification and pleasuare

Examples of behaviors that result from clients' intense anxiety, and appropriate nursing interventions are shown in Chart 12–2.

Program Evaluation   Evaluation includes the following aspects:

1. Client progress through the deinstitutionalization program
2. Program/staff interventions generating client skill development for community living, continued education, or entry into a vocational career
3. Client ability at the end of each 6-month program phase

All staff members are involved in program evaluation. Nurses use the ANA Standards of Psychiatric and Mental Health Nursing Practice to evaluate their work.

Chart 12–2
COMMON BEHAVIORS OF DEINSTITUTIONALIZED CLIENTS AND NURSING INTERVENTIONS

Behavior	Example	Intervention

1. Resistance
  a. Withdrawal
  b. Isolation
  c. Tardiness
  d. Absenteeism
  e. Detachment
  f. Inability to complete tasks
  g. Noncompliance with medications
	1. Client remains in room at residence or apartment for long periods, is unusually quiet at activities, arrives late at program, seems preoccupied or does not attend program. Client becomes hostile, angry, and uncooperative.	1. a. Confront the client and investigate behavior.
		  b. Provide individual therapy.
		  c. Assist client in making connections between behavior and progress in program.
		  d. Include other staff members in supportive interventions.
		  e. Encourage client to participate in the program.
		  f. Hospitalize client briefly if needed.

2. Acting out	2. a. Client exhibits deviant behavior (drinking, drugs, and stealing and may invite police action).
	  b. Client attempts suicide or homicide.
	  c. Client demonstrates exhibitionist behavior.
	  d. Client becomes aggressive and destructive and damages property.
	  e. Client is disruptive.
		2. a. Confront client and investigate actions.
		
		  b. Ensure that clients face charges brought against them.
		  c. Provide individual therapy.
		
		  d. Collaborate with other staff in treating client.
		  e. Remove client from living situation if needed.

3. Delusions and hallucinations	3. a. Client becomes paranoid or has extreme irrational fears.
	  b. Client has persecutory, grandiose, and immobilizing delusions.
	  c. Clients believe that they can assume responsibilities beyond their capabilities.
		3. a. Confront client with reality.
		
		  b. Refer client to M.D. for evaluation (alter medication regimen, change treatment plan, hospitalize if necessary).
		  c. Alter client goals in collaborating with other staff members.

4. Obsessive-compulsive behavior	4. a. Client exhibits irrational obsessive-compulsive behavior, including
	    Cleaning
	    Washing
	    Eating
	    Dressing
	    Shopping
	    Rituals
		4. a. Point out obsessive-compulsive behavior and investigate actions.
		  b. Analyze actions and intervene, pointing out how behavior retards progress toward independence.
		  c. Provide constructive alternatives for compulsive behavior.

5. Regression	5. Client exhibits the following:
	  a. Dependency
	  b. Helplessness
	  c. Infantile behavior
	  d. Insatiable need for attention
		5. a. Discuss observable behavior with client.
		  b. Encourage client to understand that regression interferes with progress.
		  c. Discuss client's goals and unreadiness to attain them and offer alternatives.
		  d. Hospitalize if necessary for a brief period.

Bibliography

1. Adams PE: Brief hospitalization: One effective approach in the treatment continuum. Hosp Community Psychiatry 26:199, 1975
2. Altschul AT: A multidisciplinary approach to psychiatric nursing. Nurs Times 69:508, 1973
3. Bassuk E, Gerson S: Deinstitutionalization and mental health services. Scientific American 238:46, 1978
4. Batey SR et al: Medication education for patients in a partial hospitalization program. J Psychosoc Nurs 20:7, 1982
5. Battle EH, Halliburton A, Wallston KA: Self medication among psychiatric patients and adherence after discharge. J Psychosoc Nurs 20:21, 1982
6. Beedson RD: The Psychiatric Halfway House: A Handbook of Theory and Practice. Pittsburgh, University of Pittsburgh Press, 1978
7. Buckwalter KC, Kerfoot KM: Teaching patients self care: A critical aspect of psychiatric discharge planning. J Psychosoc Nurs 20:15, 1982
8. Craig AE, Hyatt BA: Chronicity in mental illness: A theory on the role of change. Perspect Psychiatr Care 16:139, 1978
9. Davies MA: Continuing care unit: A model of services for chronic psychiatric patients. J Psychosoc Nurs 19:42, 1981
10. DeFalco ML: The rehospitalization of discharged schizophrenic patients. Perspect Psychiatr Care 13:130, 1975
11. Hjorten MK: A volunteer support system for the chronically mentally ill. Perspect Psychiatr Care 20:17, 1980
12. Ishiyama T: Transitional program for ex-mental patients: Final Report. Washington, DC, NIMH, Mt-14843, 1969
13. Jansson DP: Return to society: Problematic features of the re-entry process. Perspect Psychiatr Care 13:136, 1975
14. Katz RC, Wooley FR: Criteria for releasing patients from psychiatric hospitals. Hosp Community Psychiatry 26:33, 1975
15. Krauss JB: The chronic psychiatric patient in the community—A model of care. Nurs Outlook 28:308, 1980
16. Krauss JB, Slavinsky AT: A model for advanced nursing preparation in chronic psychiatric care. Perspect Psychiatr Care 19:10, 1981
17. Lantz JE: Adlerian community treatment with schizophrenic clients. J Psychosoc Nurs 20:25, 1982
18. Lyon GG, Hitchens EA: Ways of intervening with the psychotic individual in the community. Am J Nurs 79:491, 1979
19. Moyer AA: Involving boarding home owners in the clinical process: A case study. Int J Partial Hospitalization 1:99, 1982
20. Nolan BS: Dustin House: An expression of concern. J Psychiatr Nurs 15:16, 1977
21. Roets GA, Good DW: Group home program. J Psychiatr Nurs 14:15, 1976
22. Rogers J, Grubb P: The VA psychiatric patient: Resocialization and community living. Perspect Psychiatr Care 17:72, 1979
23. Schneggenburger C, Nolan BS: Diet teaching at Dustin House. J Psychiatr Nurs 15:18, 1977
24. Slavinsky AT, Krauss JB: Mutual withdrawal . . . or Gwen Tudor Will revisited. Perspect Psychiatr Care 13:194, 1980
25. Talbott J: Deinstitutionalization: Avoiding the disasters of the past. Hosp Community Psychiatry 12:621, 1979
26. Wilson HS: Deinstitutionalization: Residential Care for the Mentally Disordered. New York, Grune & Stratton, 1982

13

Designing an Outpatient Therapy Program

Sheila Rafter Webster

OVERVIEW

Legal Mandates   Administrators of outpatient therapy programs must first consider legal regulations that will affect their agencies. The following jurisdictions have laws, rules, and regulations that affect mental health clinics and their operations:

A. FEDERAL
1. Mental Health Systems Act (P.L. 96–398), which lists criteria for federal grants to *initiate* a community health center and services that must be provided
2. Medicare rules and regulations

B. STATE
1. Fire and safety laws
2. Laws governing voluntary and involuntary admissions to the state mental institutions, including court commitments
3. Medicaid and welfare laws
4. Laws governing who shall practice and professional licensure laws
5. Pharmacy law
6. Civil service law
7. Operational licenses—often issued by the department of health or other state level department

C. LOCAL
1. Zoning laws
2. Laws regarding police or sheriff assistance in an emergency
3. Laws regarding transportation of clients to a state institution in an emergency
4. Civil service laws

D. OTHER
Mental health centers often elect to voluntarily seek certification from specific groups and organizations. These groups may have specific requirements that are not necessary for the legal operation of the center, but are necessary for certification. These special certifications may affect third-party reimbursements. Examples are accreditation by the Joint Commission for the Accreditation of Hospitals (JCAH) and Blue Cross/Blue Shield certification.

Administrative Objectives   A. GENERAL
Administrators are generally responsible to
1. Carry out the organization's unique task
2. Monitor and audit the accomplishments of the organization's task
3. Create an environment that fosters the vocational development and expertise of each provider

B. SPECIFIC
Administrators are specifically responsible for
1. Administration of agency programs—planning and implementing service delivery
2. Budget
3. Personnel administration

Budget   The administrator must be aware of each of the following considerations:
1. Cost to maintain current services
2. Salaries

3. Maintenance and upkeep of the physical facility
4. Employee benefit programs
5. Funding sources
6. Grant monies
7. New monies needed to meet goals and objectives
8. Inflation

Guidelines for a New Administrator

The new administrator
1. Meets with each staff person to determine goals, backgrounds, and special interests
2. Asks the staff members what they see as problems in the agency.
3. Determines who has the informal power
4. Learns the strengths and weaknesses of the staff members
5. Reviews all personnel and several clinical records to become familiar with the staff and the agency's record keeping
6. Is available to the staff
7. Does not let the need to be liked lead to quick decisions or relaxations of rules and regulations
8. Attempts *no* change until sure what must be done, and by whom

Staff Qualifications and Functions

Table 13–1 shows ideal qualifications for program administrators and staff members, Table 13–2 the functions of the professional staff, and Table 13–3 the qualifications and functions of the adjunctive staff.

Physical Facility

A. **GENERAL CONSIDERATIONS**
   The facility
   1. Must be in the neighborhood of the population being served. One building may meet agency needs, or satellite offices may be necessary.
   2. Should be located near public transportation and have adequate parking facilities for staff and clients
   3. Must meet requirements for access by the handicapped or elderly

B. **CLINICAL CONSIDERATIONS**
   1. Each site or facility must have a reception area large enough to house the receptionist and a waiting area.
   2. Each clinician should have a private office, desk, and at least six comfortable chairs. This enables a clinician to see individuals and small families with a minimum of scheduling difficulties. (Suggested room size is 8′ × 10′ or 10′ × 12′.)
   3. Depending on the size of the agency, a number of larger rooms should be set aside for group therapy, large family sessions, and administrative committee meetings. These rooms require only chairs and a few small tables for ashtrays and miscellaneous items. They must comfortably seat 10 to 12 persons. (Suggested size is 12′ × 15′.)
   4. A large staff room is necessary for staff meetings, employee breaks, and so forth. It must comfortably seat the entire staff.
   5. Any special functions served by the facility may require special space considerations. For example
      a. Day treatment programs—large group rooms, kitchen, client lounge, supply storage, and so forth
      b. Staff training—''one-way mirror'' rooms, video rooms, and so forth
      c. Children—play area, toy storage

Table 13–1

IDEAL QUALIFICATIONS FOR PROGRAM ADMINISTRATORS AND STAFF MEMBERS

Position Title	Degree/ License	Years of Experience	Comments
Program Administrator			
1. Chief Administrator			
a. Psychiatrist	M.D.	5–8	3 years of clinical
b. Psychologist	Ph.D.	5–8	experience and 5
c. Social Worker	M.S.W.	5–8	years of administrative
d. Nurse clinician	M.A./M.S.N./R.N.	5–8	or supervisory
e. Administrator	M.P.A., M.H.A.	5	experience is desirable. If the person lacks clinical background, a "clinical" associate administrator should be hired.
2. Assistant or Associate Director	As above	3–5	3 years of clinical experience; 2 years of supervisory experience
Staff Members			
1. Psychiatrist	M.D.		Must be licensed; should be eligible for board certification
2. Psychologist	Ph.D.		Should be licensed
3. Social worker	M.S.W.		Should be certified
4. Clinical nurse specialist	Master's degree or doctorate		Must be licensed; should be ANA certified at specialist level
5. Clinical supervisors	a-b-c-d above	3	Clinical experience Demonstrates clinical competence
6. Program Directors	a-b-c-d above	3	Clinical experience; demonstrates clinical competence and possesses administrative talent

    6. Clerical functions must be provided adequate space. These include secretarial, medical records, client billing, and agency bookkeeping.

    7. Pharmacy services must be provided a secure location in the facility.

C. **BASIC EQUIPMENT**

    1. Comfortable, durable, functional, and easy-to-maintain furniture

    2. Reading material in waiting room

    3. Toys to entertain small children

Clinical Considerations in Providing Therapy

1. All appointments begin and end on time.
2. Generally, individual sessions last 45 to 60 minutes, family sessions last 1 hour to 1½ hours, and group sessions last 1 hour to 1½ hours. The clinician tells the client how long sessions last and adheres to this schedule.

Table 13–2
FUNCTIONS OF THE PROFESSIONAL CLINICAL STAFF

Professions	Functions*
Psychiatrist	1. May do psychiatric assessments 2. Prescribes medications 3. May provide psychotherapy 4. May supervise other staff 5. Commits involuntary clients to the hospital 6. Offers consultation and education
Psychologist	1. Does psychometric testing 2. Provides psychotherapy 3. May supervise other staff 4. May have legal authority in some states to commit involuntary client to hospital 5. Offers consultation and education
Social worker	1. May be liaison with other agencies and institutions 2. Provides psychotherapy 3. May supervise other staff 4. Offers consultation and education
Psychiatric nurse clinician	1. Administers medication 2. Provides psychotherapy 3. May supervise other staff 4. Offers consultation and education

*Lists do not include all possible functions.

Table 13–3
QUALIFICATIONS AND FUNCTIONS OF THE ADJUNCTIVE STAFF*

Staff Member	Formal Preparation	Functions
1. Rehabilitation or vocational rehabilitation counselor	Master's degree	Works with clients having vocational problems; may do training placements and lead groups or sheltered workshops
2. Music, dance, and art therapist	Master's degree	Works with individuals or groups; helps clients express feelings in specific art forms and interprets feelings seen in specific art form
3. Recreation counselor	Master's degree	Helps clients plan and develop recreational activities
4. Paraprofessional	Bachelor's degree	May lead task-specific group, *i.e.,* cooking, sewing, exercise, and so forth
5. Nonprofessional	None	Assists in recreational activities
6. Clerical	None**	Reception, secretarial, medical records, and other office functions
7. Maintenance and janitorial	None	Maintenance and upkeep of facility

*Varies with size and scope of agency. Personnel needed will depend on programs.
**Certification as medical-record clerk may be desirable.

3. Clients wait in the waiting room until their appointment and are not permitted to wander through halls or wait in vacant offices.
4. Clients calling to cancel sessions must speak with their respective clinicians. Messages to cancel are not left with the receptionist. The receptionist tells clients that the clinician will return the call if the clinician is not available to talk to the client at that moment.
5. Clinicians do not accept calls during sessions.
6. Each clinician has a place to pick up phone messages and may then return calls.
7. Receptionists should always be aware of where clinicians are located when they are away from their desks.
8. Emergency evacuation procedures are posted conspicuously.
9. There is a procedure familiar to all staff for handling violent and threatening clients. Nonprofessional and clerical staff do not intervene directly.
10. No clinical records leave the office or are kept in clinicians' desks. They are kept in a central location and returned at night.
11. All medications are kept in a secure location away from client access.
12. Clients who arrive intoxicated for appointments are not seen until they are sober. If there is concern about the client's well-being, a family member or a friend is called to take the client home.
13. When there is concern about clients' physical condition, they are referred for medical treatment.
14. At the close of business, all clients and staff vacate the premises.
15. No staff member remains alone with clients in a building.
16. Supervision is provided to all clinical staff.
17. All staff members dress appropriately, since their dress reflects the professionalism of the agency.

Programs A. **INDIVIDUAL PSYCHOTHERAPY**
Time—45 to 60 minutes
1. Psychoanalytic psychotherapy
2. Supportive psychotherapy
3. Cognitive behavior therapy and behavior modification
4. Other kinds of psychotherapy, depending on staff preparation and client appropriateness, for example, rational emotive therapy, transactional analysis, and so forth

B. **GROUP PSYCHOTHERAPY**
Time—1½ hours
1. Psychoanalytic group therapy
2. Couples groups
3. Various support groups, for example, groups of single parents, recently divorced persons, elderly, victims of violent crimes, overweight people, and so forth
4. Adolescent groups
5. Multifamily groups

C. **FAMILY THERAPY**
Time—1 to 1½ hours
1. Marital counseling
2. Family psychotherapy
3. Sexual counseling

D. **SPECIFIC PROGRAMS**

Specific groups provide services to a client or groups of clients with unique needs.

1. Cultural and ethnic programs—offer psychotherapeutic services to various cultural and ethnic groups in the community, for example, Spanish speaking group psychotherapy.
2. Substance abuse programs—offer specialized services to drug and alcohol abusers.
3. Victims of violent crimes programs—offer support and counseling to victims of crimes, for example, rape counseling.
4. Geriatric and children's programs—offer services designed to meet the needs of specific age groups.
5. Rehabilitation programs—provide rehabilitative and vocational guidance and counseling to all clients.
6. Aftercare programs—provide service to those discharged from psychiatric institutions. Generally these services include, but are not limited to, music, dance, art, recreation, and occupational therapy, skills groups such as socialization, and activities of daily living.
7. Crisis intervention programs—provide service to those in crisis, for example, suicide prevention.
8. Chemotherapy programs—provide medication including psychotropics, antidepressants, and tranquilizers.

E. **CONSULTATION AND EDUCATION**

1. Provide case consultation to agencies in the community including schools, churches, hospitals, nursing homes, welfare departments, police departments, and so forth
2. Provide in-service training for community groups
3. Provide information to the general public through brochures, pamphlets, speeches, and other means.

Meetings Table 13–4 shows the administrative and clerical meetings needed to keep the outpatient program running smoothly. Minutes are taken at all meetings and kept for future reference.

Supervision A. **ADMINISTRATIVE**

Administrative supervisors are responsible for hiring and firing, time off, employee problems, assignments, and so forth.

B. **CLINICAL**

Clinical supervisors are responsible for clinical teaching of psychotherapeutic skills, transference issues, countertransference issues, case management, treatment planning, and all other clinical issues. Some professions require that unlicensed members who wish to become licensed be supervised only by a licensed person in that same profession. An agency or program may decide to assign supervisors on that basis.

Methods of Clinical A. **BEGINNING SUPERVISEES**
Supervision
1. The same client is used for supervision. This enables the supervisor and the supervisee to work on specific techniques and issues that occur during various treatment phases. It also aids the supervisee in developing sequential strategies, and the supervisor can monitor the outcome of the therapeutic interventions.

Table 13–4
ADMINISTRATIVE AND CLINICAL MEETINGS IN AN OUTPATIENT PROGRAM

Meeting	Who Attends	Purpose
Administrative		
Program Directors (weekly)	All program directors and clerical persons	Plan for growth, coordination of client care, general communication
Policy & Procedure (monthly)	Representative staff from all levels; usually chaired by agency director or assistant and clerical person	Plan agency policy and set up procedures concerned with agency operation
Medical Records (monthly)	Representatives of clinical professional staff, medical records clerk, and clerical person.	Review and update the format of agency medical records
Program Staff (weekly)	Entire program staff	Discuss program concerns and issues
General Staff (weekly)	Entire agency staff	Discuss agency concerns, issues, and changes
Clinical		
Case Conference (weekly)	All treatment staff	Formulate treatment plans
In-service (monthly)	As many treatment staff as possible	Expand the knowledge of treatment staff

2. Audio or audiovisual tapes are used. This enables the supervisor to monitor such things as tone of voice, body posture, and so forth. It also prevents the supervisee from eliminating important segments of sessions either consciously or unconsciously.

B. **EXPERIENCED SUPERVISEES**
1. One or many clients are presented at the supervisee's discretion. One client may be followed through a difficult or complex clinical course, or several clients may be presented over time. The issues discussed in supervision focus more on transference and countertransference and less on technique.
2. Audio or audiovisual tapes may be used. If many clients are being discussed this may not be feasible or practical.

C. **GROUP SUPERVISION**
May take place in small groups. This provides more opinions and ideas and can help staff members to get to know and appreciate one another.

Outside Supervision   Outside supervisors may be hired part-time to supervise experienced clinicians, or beginning clinicians either at the agency or in their own offices. This has the following advantages:
1. The agency may not have experienced supervisors on staff.
2. An outside supervisor is not involved in agency "politics" and can be objective.
3. An outside supervisor has no administrative responsibility and can concentrate entirely on clinical issues. Staff members may feel freer to be open with a supervisor who has no administrative control over them.

Evaluation Evaluation of mental health services is difficult because it is hard to define mental health. Evaluation usually starts with the belief that what the agency offers benefits clients; therefore, the more clients served, the more people benefited.

A. STATISTICAL METHODS
  1. Individual therapist productivity—The number of clients seen and the amount of time spent doing so are calculated.
  2. Program or unit efficiency—The cost per client hour is calculated.
  3. Client satisfaction surveys—Clients evaluate the treatment received in various categories on a numerical rating scale.

B. QUALITY ASSURANCE
  1. Peer review—Staff members review the treatment plan of a representative sample of clients for appropriateness of treatment. Any questions about treatment are referred to the program director for resolution. Peer review may be done by discipline (for example, nursing, social work) or by program (for example, prolixin program).
  2. Audit—may be combined with peer review. This procedure assesses the completeness of the medical record.
  3. Utilization review—reviews the length of treatment for clients. Generally, appropriate length of stay is based on the "average" for the client diagnosis. In some agencies the length of treatment is rigidly set by predetermined regulations. In others clinician recommendations for length of treatment are followed.

Bibliography

Bennis WG, Benne KD, Chin R: The Planning of Change, 2nd ed. New York, Holt, Rinehart, & Winston, 1969

Irion LA: Community health nurses in administration. In Archer SE, Fleshman R (eds): Community Health Nursing. North Scituate, Duxbury Press, 1975

Pardes H: The Mental Health Systems Act and Its Implementation, Memorandum to Programs, Cities, Counties, States and Organizations Interested in the Mental Health Systems Act. Washington, DC, National Institute of Mental Health, 1981

Sheinfeld SN, Weirish, TW: Ideology and performance: Service delivery in a community mental health center. Pub Adm R, 41:63, 1981

Smith ML, Glass GV: Meta-Analysis of psychotherapy outcome studies. Am Psychol, 32:752, 1977

14

Designing an Adolescent Inpatient and Day Program

Candy Dato

The types of therapeutic programs that are helpful for adolescents are varied. Planning a treatment program requires an assessment of the community and a general philosophical framework.

Community Assessment

A. **COMMUNITY NEEDS OR PREFERENCES**
The community is defined (for example, drug-addicted adolescents), priorities of needs or preferences are determined, and existing programs are examined.

B. **AVAILABILITY OF SUPPORTS OUTSIDE THE PROGRAM**
Administrative, community, or political support is sought. Related services (aftercare, halfway houses, group homes, transportation for clients, schools, and so forth) are considered, along with existing programs. In addition, sources of funding are determined, potential physical facilities are examined, and potential staffing resources are investigated.

Philosophy

The philosophy of the program spells out its goals and purposes within a theoretical framework for viewing individual behavior and psychic structure. It is a blueprint for program decisions. A philosophy includes

A. **HOW THE INDIVIDUAL ADOLESCENT IS VIEWED AND TREATED**
Examples
1. Emotional growth arises from insight and intrapsychic reorganization.
2. Behavior is a response to external pressures and conditions and must be modified.
3. A dynamic orientation places emphasis on individual treatment plans, encouraging emotional expression and insight.

B. **HOW THE FAMILY IS VIEWED AND TREATED**
The family may be seen as the client or as a source of the adolescent's difficulties, or more neutrally.

C. **HOW THE COMMUNITY IS VIEWED AND TREATED**
The community may be seen as casual, supportive, or minimally involved.

Staff Qualifications and Roles

A. **PROFESSIONAL QUALIFICATIONS**
Multidisciplinary roles and qualifications are shown in Table 14–1. Nursing staff roles, responsibilities, and qualifications are shown in Table 14–2.

B. **PERSONAL QUALIFICATIONS**
1. Willingness to learn and discuss personal reactions and feelings as they pertain to the treatment of an individual or group of clients
2. Ability to respect others and work with them
3. Ability to both fulfill and accept the role, including the role of authority figure
4. Ability to be empathic, sensitive, patient, warm, consistent, and clear
5. Ability to relate to other professionals and work as a member of a team

C. **TOTAL STAFF GROUP CHARACTERISTICS**
1. Mixture of ages—Older staff may provide wisdom and perspective,[1] whereas younger staff may provide greater enthusiasm, energy, and empathy.
2. Balance of men and women

Table 14–1
STAFF TITLES AND QUALIFICATIONS

Title	Qualifications
Administrative	
1. Unit Chief—inpatient unit	1, 2. Certified psychiatrists, one of whom
2. Assistant Unit Chief—inpatient unit	has had training in child psychiatry, with both clinical and administrative experience
3. Director, Co-Directors, Assistant Directors—day program	3. Psychiatrist Psychologist with doctorate Nurse with master's degree or doctorate Social worker with master's degree or doctorate M.P.H. With both clinical and administrative experience
Clinical	
1. Therapist	1. Psychiatrist Clinical nurse specialist Psychologist Social worker Trainees in above fields
2. Case manager, client administrator, hospital therapist Case coordinators	2. Psychiatrist Clinical nurse specialist Psychologist Social worker Trainees in above fields
3. Family therapist Multiple family group therapist Group therapist	3. Psychiatrist Clinical nurse specialist Psychologist Social worker Trainees in above fields
4. Occupational therapist	4. Registered occupational therapist OTR student OT assistant
5. Recreational therapist	5. Recreational therapist, students, assistants, physical education teacher
6. Creative arts, expressive arts, activities	6. Dance/movements therapist Art therapist Artist, student assistant
7. Educational staff—administrative— school principal, director, teachers, aides	7. Teachers (and educational administrators) with appropriate qualifications; may include special educational background

3. Wide variety of racial, social, socioeconomic, and life-styles to provide more opportunities for models for identification
4. Mixture of professional, educational, and work experiences

Physical Setting 1. Bedrooms for two clients per room
2. Rooms for meetings, and individual, group, and family sessions
3. Places for activities that are developmentally appropriate for adolescents, such as recreational, social, athletic, and academic pursuits

Table 14–2
NURSING STAFF TITLES, RESPONSIBILITIES, AND QUALIFICATIONS

Nursing Staff Titles	*Responsibilities*	*Qualifications*
Leadership		
Nursing Care Coordinator; also known as Head Nurse, Nursing Supervisor, Clinical Nurse Specialist	Provides 24-hour-services (8 hours for day programs) Supervises nursing staff Shares administration of the total program with other disciplines Represents nursing with other discipline heads	Registered professional nurse with a specified amount of experience and educational preparation. This varies in relation to community availability; generally a master's degree and 2 years' experience
Assistant Nursing Care Coordinator; also known as Charge Nurse, Senior Nurse, Team Leader, Administrative Group Leader	Is responsible for nursing care for a specific time period or for a specific part of the program Supervises less experienced or nonprofessional staff	Registered professional nurse; as above, generally a B.S. degree and 2 years' experience
Nursing staff		
a. Staff nurses b. Paraprofessionals	a. Supervise paraprofessionals and carry out activities below b. Manage the unit under the leadership above Directly supervise individual and groups of clients Are major figures in the therapeutic milieu Are members, multidisciplinary team Share responsibility for consistently seeking to understand the meaning of verbal and nonverbal communications among themselves and the clients Are role model for clients Act as a parent (including therapeutic use of authority, confrontation, limit setting, providing emotional support) Establish, maintain, and terminate therapeutic relationships Provide for normal developmental needs	a. Registered professional nurses—may not require specific educational background or work experience Licensed practical nurses Licensed psychiatric technicians b. Mental health worker Psychiatric aides Psychiatric assistants Special educational preparation is usually not required.

4. There may be a need for a seclusion room, locked doors, or the capacity to lock the unit.

Therapeutic Milieu A. **DEFINITION**

The therapeutic milieu is the total environment of the program and is the direct outgrowth of the philosophy. Adolescents in a day program are part of the program therapeutic milieu as well as the milieu where they live. This may be a therapeutic milieu in the case of group homes or halfway houses. The therapeutic milieu includes

1. All formal and informal interactions among clients, staff, family, and others
2. Physical features
3. Relationship of the program to the larger community, especially related agencies

4. Staff attitudes toward clients and their behavior
5. Staff attitudes toward other staff, administration, families, and other agencies
6. Rituals

B. **ADMINISTRATIVE STRUCTURE**
Overall purpose—The formal organization of authority to provide leadership, direction, and decision making
1. Internal—The administrator
   a. Provides effective, clear, well-defined channels of communication at various levels
   b. Provides consistent, clear, effective decision making
   c. Establishes and maintains internal role boundaries
      • Staff roles
      • Clear lines of authority within each discipline
      • Supervisory structures
   d. Provides clear leadership
   e. Intervenes in interdisciplinary struggles
   f. Provides ongoing exploration and evaluation of the therapeutic structure
2. External—The administrator
   a. Provides a link to the "outside" (upper levels of administration, organization, other agencies)
   b. Represents, explains, supports, and defends the program
   c. Provides the proper client population as determined by the program philosophy.

C. **MEETINGS**
Table 14–3 shows meetings, who attends each, primary purpose, and secondary purpose.

D. **THERAPEUTIC STRUCTURE**
The therapeutic structure is the entire gamut of therapeutic modalities provided for the psychological, behavioral, and ongoing developmental needs of the clients.
   1. *Psychotherapy*
      a. *Individual psychotherapy* is used to bring about understanding of the meaning of past and present behavior. It may involve discussion of current and past relationships, transferential feelings, unconscious and conscious motivations, and dreams.
      b. *Group therapy* is used to provide a social framework for the exploration of behavior and its impact on others. It also provides an important forum for peer relationships, including varying degrees of peer pressure and support.
      c. *Family therapy* may be provided for an individual family with one or more therapists. It may also be a multiple family therapy group with more than one family meeting with one or more therapists. The purposes range from information gathering to ongoing exploration of family dynamics.
   2. *Community meetings* are large group meetings of all staff and all clients for the purpose of discussing issues that affect life and work together. Clients and staff coming and going, administrative changes, and external changes that affect the program are discussed here. It is a forum to explore large group dynamics and pressures.

Table 14–3
MEETINGS, ATTENDANCE, AND PRIMARY AND SECONDARY PURPOSES

Meeting	Attendance	Primary Purpose	Secondary Purpose
Team meeting Rounds Client planning Treatment review Client discussions Client status reviews	Multidisciplinary staff, various levels Clients generally not present Sometimes staff from other agencies may be included (for example, school, group home)	Review clients' progress and effectiveness of staff interventions Plan short-term and long-term goals of treatment	Enhance staff morale, staff education/development Explore countertransference
Staff meetings	All staff from the program	Formal, organizational boundaries maintained through announcements of new staff arrivals, leavings, vacations, changes Formal announcements of policy changes, administrative decisions	Enhance staff group cohesiveness Prevent or reduce possibilities of destructive large group processes
Case conference	Multidisciplinary staff of the unit, outside consultants	Discuss an individual client a. If early in treatment, primarily for evaluation and diagnosis b. If later in treatment, used to evaluate the effects of treatment c. Interdisciplinary involvement d. Staff education/development	Provide staff education/development Enhance staff morale
Change of shift report	Generally nursing staff May include most staff from both off-going and on-coming shifts or may include only 1 or 2 representatives	Communication about the previous shift(s) may include 8 or 16 hours for the purpose of providing continuity of care, follow-up Changes affecting the program Problem identification and exploration	Identify and solve problems Provide supervision Reduce ambiguity and situations of inconsistency
Sector meetings (for example, nursing, therapy, school, OT/RT)	All staff from a specific sector	Discuss common problems and issues; problem solving Administrative channel Maintenance of boundaries	Form group identity Provide emotional support
Supervisory structures	All levels, all disciplines	Oversee staff approaches to clients Maintain agreed-upon performance standards	Provide emotional support to staff
Administrative group meetings	Section heads and unit chief and/or director	Program planning and education Review of on-going issues	Provide mutual support

3. *Client government* is an organization of clients under some (usually minimal) staff guidance that provides a client voice in the distribution of authority though staff veto power and overall responsibility remains.
   a. Provides for the use of peer authority, which is generally more acceptable and less threatening and for client input into program policies and plans.
   b. A substructure of committees may exist, for example, clean-up, activities, party, outings, welcoming, and so forth.
   c. Regular channels of communication to administration are available and used.
4. *Spontaneous groups* are usually small (2–6) groups of clients with one or more staff who meet for a single or time-limited series of meetings with a specific task.
   a. These groups encourage the adolescent to work with peers constructively and discourage the formation of antitherapeutic groups by fostering the alliance of staff and clients.
   b. They are used to discuss interpersonal issues that are often intense, such as friction, fighting, sexuality, jealousy, acting out, violence, separation, rejection, loss, suicide attempts, elopements, depression, use of space, anger, drug use, and responsibility.
5. *Nursing relationships* with clients range from formal to informal, individual to group encounters. The relationships vary in intensity and usefulness to a particular patient at a particular time. The nurse points out the client's behavior and its impact on the nurse, the staff, and other clients through direct discussion, labeling, and intervention. The nursing relationships are heavily linked to parental authority, parental nourishment and support, and struggles for independence versus dependence.
6. *Client management relationships* (also called client administrators, case managers) are the relationships between a member of the staff and a client.
   a. Relationships may be identical to nursing relationships described above. Non-nursing staff might also be involved in these relationships, or the functions might be carried out in a small group of staff and clients.
   b. Functions may include decision making; sharing of decisions regarding medications and other treatments; information sharing; liaison to significant others such as school, family, or friends; determination of restrictions, punishment, family visits, and so forth.
7. *Other groups* may be used to enforce, support, and clarify specific boundaries. Examples include:
   a. A morning meeting to welcome each client to the program, enhance group cohesiveness, identify problems, plan activities
   b. A wrap-up group to end the day's activities, allowing each person to voice whatever they have left unsaid
   c. A discharge group to share feelings about upcoming discharge plans, often including former clients for a limited time as a transition
   d. An orientation or newcomers group
   e. A family orientation group
   f. Separate men's and women's groups.
8. *Developmental activities*
   a. School
   b. Creative arts
   c. Occupational therapy

d. Vocational guidance
e. Social skills training and development
f. Daily life activities
g. Outings
h. Social events

9. *Controls*
   a. Medications, usually neuroleptics, are used to help maintain behavioral control and to make the client more accessible to therapy.
   b. Locked unit, or an open unit with a capacity to be locked, may be used as a means of providing external controls and limits.
   c. Limit-setting techniques are many and varied, and are used with both individuals and groups.
   d. Rewards and punishment are used to control behavior.
      • Privileges such as walking freely off the unit, unaccompanied to and from the program, staying in or out of specified areas.
      • Restrictions (as above)
   e. Seclusion is used to provide a secure, safe environment for limited periods of time.
   f. Physical restraints provide for safety.
   g. Time out or use of an open quiet room can be used by adolescents of their own accord or by staff request.
   h. Boundaries of time and space are established and maintained to provide clear standards of acceptable behavior. See Chart 14–1 for a sample daily schedule.

10. *Rituals* develop that become an important part of the therapeutic structure as symbols of the group culture and values. Examples include
    a. Manner in which introductions are made, often involving a go-round of names at a community meeting
    b. Parties for leavings, birthdays, special events, holidays
    c. Gift giving
    d. Special meal planning and preparations
    e. Repetitions of certain events on certain days
    f. The way chores are done
    g. Nicknames

Chart 14–1
SAMPLE DAILY SCHEDULE

Time	Activity
8–8:30 AM	Breakfast/entry for day clients
8:30–9 AM	Morning meeting
9–12 N	School/individual therapy
12–12:30 PM	Lunch
12:30–3 PM	School/OT/individual therapy
3–4 PM	Community meeting—3 times a week, group therapy 2 times a week
4–5 PM	Wrap-up group for day clients, special groups, RT
5–6 PM	Dinner and free time
6–7 PM	Visiting
7–9 PM	Recreation/family therapy or family groups
9–10 PM	Wrap-up/snacks
10–11 PM	Bedtime

Evaluation   Evaluation of the program should be built into the framework of the program and conducted at regular intervals. It includes
1. Individual case reviews with the entire staff
2. Review of all treatment structures
A quality assurance program may be used to determine whether the program is attaining its goals.

Reference   1. Meeks J: The Fragile Alliance, 2nd ed. Huntington, New York. Robert E Krieger, 1980

Bibliography   Buchanan DM, Rogers AS: A comprehensive adolescent treatment program: An inpatient, interdisciplinary approach. J Psychiatr Nurs 18:42, 1980
Jurgenson K: Limit setting for hospitalized adolescent psychiatric patients. Perspect Psychiatr Care 9:173, 1971
Parker G, Gibson C: Development of the hospitalized adolescent anxiety tool. J Psychiatr Nurs 15:21, 1977
Rinsley DB: Treatment of the Severely Disturbed Adolescent. New York, Jason Aranson, 1981
Walker P, Brook BD: Community homes as hospital alternatives for youth in crisis. J Psychiatr Nurs 19:17, 1981

15

Designing a Methadone Maintenance Program

Thomas A. Sherwood

Philosophy	The philosophy of the methadone maintenance program must include a professional attitude toward the problem free of moralizing and with a primary goal of rehabilitation, rather than elimination of the drug.[5]
History	Methadone is an opiatelike synthetic narcotic invented by the Germans during World War II. It became a drug for the treatment of narcotic addiction when it was accidentally discovered that, unlike morphine, the use of which causes the addicted client to be functionally immobilized in the research setting, methadone allows the addicted client to function and be creative.[2] With the substitution of methadone for heroin, the client has an opportunity for control over the addiction and can lead a "normal" life, free from the constant pursuit of heroin.

Hospital-Based Programs

A. INPATIENT PSYCHIATRIC UNITS

(Staff controls client.) Clients are restricted to the ward. Purposes may be any or all of the following:

1. Detoxification and methadone maintenance for clients addicted to barbiturates, opiates, meperidine hydrochloride (Demerol), and methadone
2. Diagnosis and treatment of medical problems
3. Diagnosis and treatment of psychiatric problems

B. AMBULATORY CARE SETTINGS

(Staff and client control client.) This setting allows the client to achieve medical and psychiatric stability within the acute care setting. The purposes are

1. Medical supervision and close addictive services supervision for the client who is drug free, in maintenance, or requires follow-up after an acute hospitalization.
2. The initiation of community-based support systems in preparation for discharge including[6]
   a. Ongoing medical supervision
   b. Drug counseling
   c. Health education
   d. Vocational counseling

Private Store-Front Clinics

The privately owned "store-front" outpatient methadone maintenance treatment clinic is a common approach to serving clients. Professional nurses must be aware of the limitations of these store-front settings, especially since their professional status may lend a credibility to the service, which may not be deserved. In the store-front services funded through third party payors such as Medicaid, financial profit may have priority over community service.

The store-front clinics found in large metropolitan areas often have many clients (some have over 1000) and small staffs with limited services. While meeting a community need, standards and regulations in the interest of quality care must be upheld. Therefore, before assuming any responsibility in the store-front setting the professional nurse must consider the following:

A. QUALITY CONTROL

The clinic should have

1. A license to operate
2. Legal regulatory relationships to
   a. Municipal, state, and federal government
   b. Voluntary regulatory agencies and acts such as

- Joint Commission on Accreditation of Hospitals (JCAH)
- Occupational Safety and Health Administration (OSHA)
- Drug Enforcement Act (DEA)
- State Department of Health
- State Department of Social Services
- Federal Food and Drug Administration

B. **BACK-UP AND SUPPORT SYSTEMS**
  1. Possible emergencies that could occur include
     a. Cardiac arrest
     b. Respiratory arrest
     c. Overdose
     d. Shock
     e. Psychotic episode
  2. Necessary back-up systems
     a. Neighborhood hospital with emergency room
     b. Ambulance service
  3. Necessary emergency equipment
     a. Ambu-bags
     b. Endotracheal and laryngeal airways
     c. Suction equipment
     d. Cardiac resuscitation equipment
     e. Emergency medications
  4. Surrounding community should be aware of clinic's existence in the event of
     a. Fire
     b. A public health problem
     c. An environmental safety problem
     d. Any situation that the community may regard as an endangerment[4]

Nursing Responsibilities   A. **EXAMINATION OF PERSONAL BELIEFS**
Nurses must be sure that they are able to work with methadone clients without conscious prejudice. This is not always easy, since these clients frequently engage in antisocial and manipulative behavior. Nurses who are aware of their feelings and react in a direct, honest, open way to clients are best suited to work in methadone programs.

B. **KNOWLEDGE OF THE DRUG CULTURE**
The nurse should have a good understanding of the milieu in which these clients live daily. Many are deeply disillusioned with their lives, and have felt helpless to change them. They have developed a way of life geared to the constant pursuit of drugs to make life bearable. This pursuit has involved antisocial and often violent behavior, cunning, and manipulation. For this reason, the client views the nurse with mistrust, and tests the credibility of the nurse and other team members for some time.

C. **KNOWLEDGE OF METHADONE**
Methadone is a powerful synthetic narcotic that satisfies clients' craving for heroin, and in the proper dosage makes it impossible to induce euphoria by injecting heroin or any other narcotic.[7]
  1. *Potentiating effects*—In combination with other narcotic drugs, methadone can lead to respiratory depression, hypotension, circulatory collapse, and coma.

2. *Synergistic effects*—In combination with wine or other relaxing drugs methadone can produce euphoria different from that received by each alone.
3. *Inhibition effects*—Side effects include constipation, inhibited ejaculation, and decreased sexual libido.

D. **INITIAL ASSESSMENT OF THE CLIENT**
   1. Epidemiological factors that put these clients at high risk include the fact that these clients often
      a. Have poor nutrition and lack of sleep
      b. Ignore health maintenance
      c. Use contaminated needles and other equipment[3]
      d. Engage in prostitution to support their habit
      e. Engage in violence to get money or drugs
      f. Are poorly educated
   2. Diseases seen in these clients include
      a. Tuberculosis
      b. Hepatitis
      c. Gonorrhea
      d. Syphilis
      e. Rheumatitis
      f. Arthritis
      g. Nephritis
      h. Infections and abscesses
      i. AIDS (acquired immune deficiency syndrome)
   3. Medical evaluations should include
      a. Complete blood count and differential
      b. Routine and microscopic urinalysis
      c. Liver function profile
      d. Australian antigen-antibody testing
      e. Routine tests for sexually transmitted diseases
      f. Chest x-ray
      g. Tuberculin skin testing
   4. Psychological assessment—The American Psychiatric Association lists three criteria for the diagnosis of substance abuse[1]:
      a. Pattern of pathological use
      b. Impairment in social or occupational functioning due to substance use
      c. Minimal duration of disturbance of at least 1 month

E. **TREATMENT PLANS AND RECORD KEEPING**
   1. Treatment plans are based on the nursing process including assessment, nursing diagnosis, planning for care, implementation of the plan, and evaluation[6] (see also Chap. 48).
   2. Treatment plans include the specific rationale for dispensing methadone.
   3. Careful records are kept of all methadone dispensed.
   4. The nurse is liable for medication given and recorded, unless a pharmacist has been assigned this responsibility.

F. **CONTRACTS**
   Clients sign contracts saying that they will not fail to comply with decisions made by a multidisciplinary team, which includes the patient. Such contracts may include statements that the client will not
   1. Sell methadone

2. Abuse drugs
3. Miss or arrive late for therapy
4. Submit dishonest urine specimens
5. Use violence
6. Fail to comply with medical decisions

G. **ASSESSMENT OF CLIENT BEFORE DISPENSING DRUG**
1. Clinical signs that the client is taking other drugs or alcohol, requiring that methadone be withheld include
   a. Slurred speech
   b. Pupil constriction
   c. Distorted gait
   d. Altered status of consciousness
   e. Skin changes
   f. Other changes in usual behavior
2. Urine testing—Each month urine is analyzed for opiates, amphetamines, cocaine, barbiturates, or other drugs as indicated, to determine if they are being ingested. The urine testing does not alert the nurse to alcohol abuse. The urine is analyzed for methadone content to be sure the client is taking the methadone.

H. **DELAYING ADMINISTRATION**
If the nurse determines through clinical observation or urine testing that the client is under the influence of other drugs, the nurse delays giving the drug and tells the client why. The nurse then refers the client to the physician and drug counselor. A team meeting is held to determine further treatment for the client. Usually the dosage of methadone is reduced.

I. **PICK-UP SCHEDULE**
Initially clients come daily and take the methadone in the presence of staff. If clients cooperate and make a good social adjustment, they come three times per week and take medication home for the remaining days. Schedules are worked out by the team, under the supervision of the physician.

J. **PSYCHOTHERAPY**
Maximum benefit is seen when methadone maintenance is combined with time-limited psychotherapy. Clients often enter therapy displaying negativistic, self-centered, angry behavior.
Therapy is often characterized by[7]
1. Initial anger or rage at the methadone program
2. Anxiety in therapy sessions
3. Attempts to intimidate the therapist by communicating that the anger and anxiety cannot be controlled (when this fails, respect for the treatment follows)
4. Overestimation or idealization of the therapist
5. Testing of therapeutic boundaries (lateness, missed sessions)
6. Insistence by the therapist that appointments be kept, and time limits followed
7. Ongoing resistance to engaging in a relationship
The resolution of therapy occurs when the therapist communicates, and the client understands
1. The client's desire for a state of mind that will allow some measure of inner peace[7]
2. The impracticality and lack of satisfaction in a life dominated by seeking relief[7]

References

1. American Psychiatric Association: Diagnostic and Statistical Manual of Mental Disorders, d 3. Washington, DC, American Psychiatric Association, 1981
2. Brecher EM (ed): Licit & Illicit Drugs. Mount Vernon, NY, The Consumers Union Report, 1972
3. Committee on Alcoholism & Drug Dependence, Herbert A. Raskin, MD, Medical Complications of Drug Abuse. Washington, DC, Special Action Office for Drug Abuse Prevention, 1974
4. Department of Health and Human Services: Methadone for treating narcotic addicts; Joint revision of conditions for use: The Federal Register, Vol 45, No 184. Washington, DC, U.S. Government Printing Office, September 19, 1980, p 62717
5. Dole VP: In the course of professional practice. NY State J Med 7:931, 1965
6. The Nursing Theories Conference Group, Julia B. George, Chairperson, Nursing Theories: The Base for Professional Nursing Practice, Englewood Cliffs, NJ, Prentice-Hall, 1980
7. Smith TM: The dynamics in time-limited relationship therapy with methadone-maintained patients. Perspec Psychiatr Care 1:28, 1978

Bibliography

Dy AJ et al: The nurse in the methadone maintenance program: Expansions and transitions in role. J Psychiatr Nurs 13:17, 1975

Walker L: Methadone maintenance. J Psychiatr Nurs 12:25, 1974

Walker L: Nutritional concerns of addicts in treatment. J Psychiatr Nurs 13:21, 1975

16

Designing a "Prolixin" Clinic

Joan Cunningham

OVERVIEW

Problem   Research has demonstrated that 30% to 40% of chronic schizophrenic clients experience recurrence of psychotic episodes requiring hospitalization. Studies have shown that noncompliance with oral medication is a major reason for relapse and hospitalization.[7] Some reasons for noncompliance include the following:
1. Clients forget.
2. Clients feel well, so they believe that they no longer need to put up with pill taking and side effects.
3. Clients' families tell them that they no longer need medication.
4. Clients cannot keep track of multiple medications.
5. Clients want to be in complete control of their lives.
6. Clients see medication as proof that they are sick.
7. Clients are too disorganized and decompensated to take medications.

Description of Prolixin   Fluphenazine decanoate and fluphenazine enanthate (both known under the trade name Prolixin) are long-acting injectable neuroleptics, or major tranquilizers. Fluphenazine decanoate and enanthate slowly release fluphenazine in the body and provide the client with a constant therapeutic level of the drug. The differences between the two drugs are the following:
1. Decanoate acts more quickly and slightly more effectively than enanthate.
2. Decanoate has longer duration of action and less severe extrapyramidal effects.[2]

A. **EFFECTS OF PROLIXIN**
Therapeutic effect occurs at lower blood levels than most neuroleptics. There is almost immediate sedation, and thinking may improve within 24 hours. The effect of the medication may last up to 2 weeks or longer in some clients.

B. **DOSAGE**
The usual initial injection is 0.5 ml (12.5 mg), with 1.00 ml (25 mg) administered at intervals of 4 weeks. The dosage should be individualized for each client. Reduction of dosage is begun when the client is comparatively free of symptoms and when employment and home circumstances are at an optimal level. Normally, reduction is not contemplated for 3 to 4 months after discharge from the hospital. This allows for readjustment after discharge.

C. **ADVERSE EFFECTS**
The adverse effects most commonly found are hypotension, blurred vision, dry mouth, and drowsiness. Extrapyramidal effects frequently evident are tremors, restlessness, rigidity, parkinsonism, and dystonia.[9] These reactions are more severe when higher doses are used or when the interval between injections is short. (Prophylactic antiparkinsonian medication does not prevent the occurrence of extrapyramidal symptoms but may reduce their severity.[4]) To be certain of clients' health status while taking Prolixin they should have an annual
1. Physical examination
2. Complete blood count and hemoglobin
3. SMA-12 (liver function test)

D. **ADVANTAGES OF LONG-ACTING NEUROLEPTICS**[3-5]
1. Effectiveness in controlling the clinical disease
2. Long duration of action
3. Low incidence of significant side effects

4. No delayed or cumulative toxicity
5. Elimination of problems of absorption from the gut
6. Avoidance of premature deactivation by bypassing the liver
7. Good control of symptomatology with a much lower dose of medication than with an equivalent oral neuroleptic
8. Reduced cost of treatment
9. Careful control of the client's dosage
10. Reduced relapse rate

Clients Who Require Long-Acting Neuroleptics

1. Chronic schizophrenic outpatients who require continuous treatment with a neuroleptic drug to prevent relapse
2. Clients who have a history of failure to take medications after being discharged from the hospital
3. Quiet, delusional, rigid paranoid clients who refuse to take any pills for several weeks
4. Homicidal, delusional paranoid clients who have recovered from psychosis through pharmacotherapy. These clients are no longer homicidal as long as they remain on medication.
5. Clients who have made a good remission, are symptom free, and are back home, working, and on maintenance therapy.

Establishing an Outpatient Clinic

A. OBJECTIVES[3]
1. Provide continuity of care for chronic schizophrenics after discharge
2. Ensure quality care at a minimal cost
3. Decrease or prevent recurrent psychiatric episodes in a group of chronic schizophrenics
4. Ensure continued improvement and social functioning of the clients
5. Provide maximal use of scarce professional personnel

B. PROFESSIONAL STAFF
1. A psychiatrist to evaluate clients and to establish dosage schedules
2. A registered nurse to administer the injections and assist in evaluating the client's progress
3. A psychiatric social worker to assist the nurse in working with other agencies
4. A pharmacist to keep a medication profile
5. A psychiatric clinical nurse specialist to provide group therapy and client and family teaching

C. AUXILIARY STAFF
1. Specially trained paraprofessionals to monitor a crisis line, which is available 24 hours a day
2. Vocational rehabilitation counselors to help clients develop skills for securing employment, develop good work habits, and confront the stresses of everyday living

D. FACILITY
1. A room where clients can be seen individually for evaluation and administration of medication
2. A meeting room for group sessions
3. A laboratory to do periodic blood work, or access to a laboratory

E. **SCHEDULING**

Clients are scheduled for a 20-minute session with the nurse when they come in for their injections. This allows for evaluation of mental and physical status and possible side effects, adjustment of dosage, and administration of the medication. Extra time is provided if a client is having difficulties, and additional sessions are scheduled until the problem is resolved. Scheduling is somewhat flexible to accommodate the client. The therapist takes care that clients are seen at the scheduled time, since tardiness on the part of the therapist may lead clients to believe that they are not important or that the therapist does not care.

F. **ATTENDANCE**

For clients who do not keep their appointments, a telephone follow-up is done to reschedule. For clients who habitually fail to keep their appointments, a home visit may be necessary.

Nursing Intervention   A. **AFTERCARE PROGRAMS**

Aftercare programs help clients remain in the community after discharge. The nurse coordinates the program, which focuses on problem solving, social adjustment, living arrangements, obtaining employment, and complying with maintenance drug therapy.

B. **GROUP THERAPY**

Group therapy is especially helpful with chronic schizophrenic clients. Positive results are obtained when treatment is oriented toward support and rehabilitation rather than toward deeper psychological understanding.[10] See Chart 16–1 for common themes in groups of these clients, nursing interventions, and theoretical rationale.

C. **EDUCATION OF CLIENTS AND FAMILIES**

Families and clients are educated about schizophrenia, with emphasis on the concept that it is not a curable disease but an illness that can be controlled. Several books have been written to educate families and clients about schizophrenia.[1,8,11] The following guidelines are useful in counseling clients and their families:

1. To lessen stress, the client should try to get at least 7 to 8 hours of sleep and should avoid shift work. It is important to spread out stressful events as much as possible (for example, avoid several job interviews in one day). It is unwise to plan major changes in life all at the same time. If events can be stretched out over a period of several months, the client will find it easier to deal with them.
2. The client should avoid heavy use of coffee and cigarettes because they act as stimulants.
3. The client should avoid the use of hallucinogens such as LSD, PCP, and amphetamines, which can trigger a schizophrenic episode. Marijuana has also been found to precipitate a schizophrenic episode, as well as heavy use of alcohol.
4. Pregnancy should not be considered unless the schizophrenia is under control. The client should know that the safety of Prolixin during pregnancy has not been established. Genetic counseling is provided.
5. Clients are taught to recognize side effects of Prolixin and are advised to tell the therapist about them when they occur. These are explained to clients in terms they can understand.

Chart 16–1
COMMON THEMES IN GROUPS OF PROLIXIN CLIENTS, NURSING INTERVENTIONS, AND THEORETICAL RATIONALE

Themes	Nursing Interventions	Theoretical Rationale
Social isolation	Arrange for the clients to attend outpatient social groups.	Being home all day with nothing to do can contribute to clients' withdrawal.
	Explore with clients the reasons for their isolation.	Fear of lack of social skills may increase clients' anxiety to such a state that they become immobilized.
	Help clients examine different ways of interacting socially.	Permits clients to choose ways of interacting that are appropriate and provide success. This approach also enables the clients some control over their lives.
Inability to work or trouble keeping a job	Refer clients to a sheltered workshop.	Provides a structured environment within which the client can improve work habits, establish new patterns of behavior, and receive emotional support
	Explore with clients their fears and anxieties about being employed.	Allowing clients to verbalize their fears will decrease anxiety and provide clients the opportunity to examine their feelings. In a group setting clients interact with one another and are able to gain emotional support. Clients discover that other members may share their same feelings.
Desire to stop taking medication	In a noncritical way determine the reason(s). Point out to clients that they are feeling better because of the medication and stress the importance of continuing to take the medication. Emphasize that the clients' illness is something that can be controlled so that they can lead normal lives.	Taking medication is a reminder to clients that they are ill. Resistance to medication may be a way of denying the illness. Chemotherapy can alleviate symptoms and improve social functioning.
Stress	Help clients identify those things at home or work that put pressure on them. Encouage group discussion and support.	This permits clients to put in their own words the things they find stressful. Group participation encourages clients to relate to one another, providing them with a sense of belonging and assisting them to solve problems and to make decisions.

6. Female clients are told that some women skip menstrual periods when taking Prolixin. Pregnancy must be ruled out before attributing this to the medication.

7. Clients and families are taught to recognize early signs of decompensation. For most clients, relapse is not abrupt and sudden, and it is possible to provide effective crisis treatment. One of the earliest signs of relapse is sleeplessness. If clients cannot sleep for several nights in a row, they should contact the nurse. Unusual tension and anxiety may also alert the client to impending relapse. Relatives who have gone through an episode of schizophrenia with a family member should be alert for the same signs and symptoms which were evident in the previous relapse. Family members should also alert the nurse if the client is more tense than usual, eating less, and having trouble concentrating and sleeping.

See Chart 16–2 for problems of families, nursing interventions, and theoretical rationale.

Chart 16–2
PROBLEMS OF FAMILIES OF PROLIXIN CLIENTS, NURSING INTERVENTIONS, AND THEORETICAL RATIONALE

Problems	Nursing Interventions	Theoretical Rationale
Lack of knowledge about schizophrenia	Educate the family that schizophrenia is a disease that can be controlled.	Educating families relieves anxiety and fear of the unknown, and provides hope that the client can be helped.
Inability to handle unusual behavior	Teach family members practical management techniques for unusual behavior. Techniques that can be taught are	
	Refusal to eat—Family members should not let this become a reason for nagging the client. Lack of food for 1 or 2 days will not be detrimental.	Nagging will only precipitate a power struggle.
	Withdrawal—Teach family members not to go to extremes in an attempt to correct the behavior. They should avoid overconcern or false cheerfulness; converse with the client only when the client is in the mood to talk; sit quietly with the client; and avoid breaking in on the client's privacy.	Clients sometimes want to be alone with their thoughts. Sitting quietly with the client conveys acceptance and respect for privacy as well as the client's right to be a separate person.
	Refusal to wash—Family members should simply encourage the client to wash, without nagging.	Forcing the issue will create a power struggle and more resistance. The struggle keeps the client tied to the family.
	Hearing voices—Encourage family members to notify the client's therapist immediately.	The client may be decompensating and may require additional medication or hospitalization.
	Manifesting aggressive behavior—Teach family members to encourage the client to verbalize feelings, without reprimanding the client for the feelings.	Free expression of feelings prevents the aggression caused by "bottling up" feelings. Reprimanding clients may cause them to lose control.
Family members are unrealistic about what the client can or cannot do.	Discuss with the family members appropriate expectations for the client.	Unrealistic expectations increase the family's and the client's feelings of helplessness and futility.
Lack of knowledge about community resources	Identify community resources and help family members to get in contact with appropriate agencies.	This will encourage family members to participate in the client's care, increasing their self-esteem.

Signs of Relapse[6]   It is important for the nurse to be aware of the signs of relapse. In schizophrenic decompensation five stages have been identified. The first two stages are nonpsychotic.

A. **OVEREXTENSION**
The client begins to feel overwhelmed. Persistent anxiety, irritability, and distractability are present.

B. **RESTRICTED CONSCIOUSNESS**
Limitation of the individual's range of thought is evident.

C. **DISINHIBITION**
Relatively unmodulated impulse expression appears.

D. **PSYCHOTIC DISORGANIZATION**
Destructuring of the external world (increasing perceptual and cognitive disorganization), destructuring of self (loss of self-identity), and total fragmentation (complete loss of self and control) occurs.

E. **PSYCHOTIC RESOLUTION**
Less anxiety, and psychotic reorganization, either of a delusional system or massive denial of unpleasant affect and responsibility occurs.

Evaluation The success of a Prolixin clinic is based on the following:
1. Reliability of the clients in keeping return visits
2. Decrease in the number of rehospitalizations
3. Compliance with medication regimen
4. Success of referrals to sheltered workshops and other community agencies
5. Decrease in the clients' need to depend upon the therapist to solve problems for them
6. Ability of clients to function in an independent fashion in general

References
1. Arieti S: Understanding and Helping the Schizophrenic: A Guide for Family and Friends. New York, A Touchstone Book, Simon and Schuster, 1979
2. Chien CP et al: Antiparkinsonian drugs and depot phenothiazines. Am J Psychiatry 131:86, 1974
3. Continuity: The Key to Schizophrenic Maintenance. ER Squibb & Sons, 1979
4. Corbett L: Techniques of fluphenazine decanoate therapy in acute schizophrenic illness. Dis Nerv Syst 36:573, 1975
5. Grozier ML: Why a long-acting neuroleptic? Fluphenazine decanoate. Psychosomatics 12:56, 1971
6. Herz MI, Melville C: Relapse in schizophrenia. Am J Psychiatry 137:802, 1980
7. Hogarty GE et al: Fluphenazine and social therapy in the aftercare of schizophrenic patients. Arch Gen Psychiatry 36:1283, 1979
8. Hyde AP: Living with Schizophrenia. Chicago, Contemporary Books, 1980
9. Idzorek S: Antiparkinsonian agents and fluphenazine decanoate. Am J Psychiatry 133:81, 1976
10. May P: Rational treatment for an irrational disorder. What does the schizophrenic patient need? Am J Psychiatry 133:1009, 1976
11. Seeman MV et al: Living and Working with Schizophrenia. Toronto, University of Toronto Press, 1982

Bibliography Hafford KA: Community mental health: A course for caretakers. J Psychiatr Nurs 18:26, 1980

17

Designing an Outreach Program in an SRO Hotel

Joan Smith Winter

| Introduction | Providing for the mental health needs of a community requires the articulation of many systems and a wide range of modalities. The availability of a central health care agency, such as a hospital, serves those within the population who accept the medical model and who actively seek care from this system. However, a portion of the population is unable, or unwilling to use this system, while exhibiting a need for mental health care. Outreach programs in single room occupancy hotels (SROs) are designed to serve this population. |

Community Community is defined in various ways, depending on the purpose[4] of those defining.[3] In this chapter, community is defined as a geopolitical community within a catchment area of a major hospital center.

Outreach

A. **THE CONCEPT**

Outreach evolved from a growing social concern and sense of responsibility for those community members in need of health care, but unable to use the established, central-hospital system. Outreach describes the effort on the part of the mental health worker to make extrainstitutional contact with a community member who is actually or potentially at risk, for the purpose of providing therapeutic intervention.

B. **CHARACTERISTICS**

Outreach

1. Is geared to the needs of the population, rather than to the needs and norms of the hospital
2. Implies intervention within the client's own territory rather than agency territory
3. May be initiated by telephone, amil, or a visit to the person's home
4. May include psychiatric clients, their relatives, neighbors, landlords, or other community agencies.

C. **THE POPULATION**

The population in need of mental health outreach tends to possess one or more of the following characteristics:

1. A tendency to be passive in using health services
2. A lack of adequate support systems, such as families, or friends
3. A lack of skills or resources to deal with predators
4. A minimal or unclear understanding of services that are available to them
5. An inability to use traditional systems

Outreach services cover the entire span of acute and chronic care, from crisis intervention to ongoing treatment, and encompasses the three levels of health care (see Table 17–1).

Outreach programs can potentially encompass all aspects of community life. However, in order to be manageable, a program must set a narrow focus and reasonable limits. The SRO hotel program is one type of outreach program, which is here examined in detail.

The SRO Hotel Almost every American city has its share of run-down, single-room occupancy hotels, commonly known as SROs. The term SRO has become synonymous with ''welfare hotel,'' largely because hotel clientele tend to be primarily a public assistance/supplemental security income population of single people.

Table 17–1
LEVELS OF CARE AND EXAMPLES OF OUTREACH

Level of Health Care	Examples of Outreach
1. Primary prevention—maintaining wellness, avoiding onset of illness	1. a. Offering an alcoholism education program at a local elementary school b. Organizing a retirement education program within a senior citizens' apartment complex c. Conducting a widows' group for information sharing and mutual support at a community center
2. Secondary prevention—early case finding and treatment of acute problems	2. a. Reviewing emergency room reports and contacting those at risk b. Assisting a client to enter the available care systems of the community c. Treating clients in the appropriate therapeutic mode (for example, individual therapy)
3. Tertiary prevention—rehabilitative, retarding the development of further complications arising from the existing condition	3. a. Establishing or expanding the support system of a chronic client by building a trusting relationship over time b. Helping chronic clients to learn to use the many social systems on which they depend c. Helping a client to enter a vocational or social rehabilitation program

Many of these hotels were at one time elegant, fully serviced hotels with thick carpeting, potted palms, and crystal chandeliers in the ballroom. Now, the frills have been removed, suites and dining rooms divided into tiny cells, and desk clerks wear guns instead of livery. The descriptions presented here apply to many SROs.

A. GENERAL CHARACTERISTICS
   The SRO hotel
   1. Is usually privately owned
   2. Offers minimal services (heat, water, cleaning, and clean linen)
   3. Has substandard building security and structural maintenance
   4. Often provides rooms that lack refrigeration, cooking facilities, and bathrooms. Use of a communal kitchen or a hot plate in the room carries an extra charge.
   5. Has drab walls and poorly lit hallways
   6. Generally has a poor level of hygiene. Accumulated garbage, cockroaches, and rats are plentiful.
   7. Offers easy access to communal areas, such as bathrooms, which sometimes renders them unsafe
   8. Provides minimal room furnishings (bed, closet, chair, dresser)
   9. Is noisy, with loud talk, radios, arguments, dogs barking, pipes clanging, doors slamming
   10. Tolerates a high degree of deviant behavior

11. Charges a monthly rental that may seem undeservedly high, but is within the realm of public assistance allowances

B. **MANAGEMENT**[4]
1. Consists of owner or manager, desk clerks, maids, porters, security guard (one person may fill more than one of these roles)
2. May have full control of telephones and mail boxes, sometimes located within a glass or wire-mesh cage of the desk area
3. May use elaborate precautions to protect themselves and their safe: electronically operated doors, bullet-proof glass, weapons such as baseball bats and firearms in anticipation of any sort of trouble
4. Employs desk clerks as gatekeepers, determining entrance to and mobility within the hotel
5. May cash tenants' public assistance checks, which arrive in the mail, and extract a month's rent, before tenants can take their checks elsewhere
6. Establishes the rules (which may not be consistent) regarding credit, visitors, general behavior that will not be tolerated, and punishments for breaking the rules
7. May avoid bringing in any outside authorities; trouble is "handled" internally, by management, either alone or in collusion with tenants

C. **TENANTS**
Many SRO tenants are known to be isolated, dysfunctional, and distrustful, although some are employed. They feel helpless and frustrated in dealing with social systems. The tenant population includes large numbers of chronic mental patients, alcoholics, and the elderly. The "choice" of living in an SRO is "forced," based on economic necessity, lack of appropriate housing, and personality type (most often schizotypal personality disorders).

Some of the most common "reasons" for living in an SRO are as follows:
1. Some have lived in the hotel before it became rundown, and now do not want to leave familiar surroundings.
2. Most depend on a limited, fixed income (Social Security, public assistance, disability, or small pension), which allows little choice. These hotels are often rent controlled, that is, the law permits landlords to raise rents only at a small, fixed percentage rate.
3. Some exhibit behavioral problems related to psychiatric disorder or alcoholism, which would not be accepted or tolerated elsewhere.
4. Many were placed in the hotel upon discharge from state psychiatric hospitals, and are not resourceful enough to move elsewhere.

D. **NEEDS OF THE SRO TENANT**
The needs of most SRO tenants could be said to echo the needs of most chronic clients. These include[1]
1. Room
2. Board
3. Enrichment and socialization experiences
4. Medical, social, and vocational therapy

The systems depended upon to meet these needs are fraught with problems and a problem in any one system has an effect on all other systems. Table 17–2 shows some of these problems and examples.

Table 17–2

SYSTEMS AND PROBLEMS FOR THE CHRONIC CLIENT/TENANT IN THE COMMUNITY

System Needed by Chronic Clients/Tenants	*Examples of Problems Generated*
1. Housing System a. Clients need housing that is furnished and fits their limited income, where they will be tolerated. This usually means an SRO. b. Housing often has no cooking or refrigeration facilities. c. Clients are seen as suspect, contagious, and unwanted by others in the surrounding community.	a. Clients become intimidated and victimized by other tenants and hotel management. This leads to further isolation and sense of helplessness. b. Clients are forced to buy premium-cost foods in small portions or to patronize a local coffee shop, which charges exorbitant prices. c. Clients stay home to avoid open rejection and humiliation by community and to guard personal property in room.
2. Financial Assistance System a. This includes public assistance, Social Security, supplemental security income, food stamps, and medical insurance systems (Medicare and Medicaid). b. This involves much bureaucratic red tape and requires considerable energy, time, and resourcefulness to negotiate.	a. If clients' monthly income check fails to arrive or is stolen, and if they lose the Medicaid card, clients are unable to "buy" shelter or health care. Credit is generally not extended for either. b. The maze of systems and subsystems, through which clients must travel to correct the situation, is intimidating. They may give up, and live on the street.
3. Transportation System a. Public transportation can be confusing and costly but is necessary for travel to agencies, to untangle errors of assistance systems, and for recertification for services. b. Public transportation is difficult for clients with mobility problems such as physical limitations, fear of strangers, thought disorders, and apathy.	a. When clients are unable to travel to an assistance agency for the requisite "face-to-face" interview, assistance is discontinued. b. Clients with mobility problems are forced to take a taxi to the Medicaid office, then cannot afford to eat for a few days.
4. Health Care System—Subsystems a. *State hospital aftercare system*—Outpatient clinic may be distant from home, offer medication follow-up, but lack the resources for effective outreach services. b. *General hospital emergency room*—This may entail a long wait for "noncritical" care. Clients may be seen briefly and referred back to clinics on subsequent days. The client may be viewed as an unwanted abuser of emergency services. c. *General Hospital Outpatient Clinic*—These clinics may have a waiting list for appointments, usually require clients to arrive on time, and pay for sessions in advance. The clinics are often specialized, requiring that clients return for lab tests and other specialty clinics.	a. Aftercare may be inaccessible to clients who have little motivation to pursue it. Clients eventually run out of medication and decompensate. b. Clients with a low frustration tolerance may be unable to wait to be seen, or unable to postpone treatment to the clinic date. So they seek health care only when they feel in crisis. Negative attitudes of care-givers reinforce noncompliance to follow-up care. c. Clients may become discouraged and give up because these requirements may be too complex, rigid, or alien to a person with a noncompulsive life-style. Disorganized clients may be labeled as resistant.

The Mental Health Outreach Team in the SRO Hotel

A. **GENERAL DESCRIPTION**

The mental health outreach team is a multidisciplinary team of mental health professionals and paraprofessionals, affiliated with a larger health care institution. The team is based on site in the SRO, 5 days a week, to provide a variety of services to the hotel population.

B. ORIGIN OF CONCEPT

The outreach concept developed in response to increasing awareness of the high concentration of people living in the SRO who were in need of community mental health services, while having difficulty obtaining them.

C. OVERALL GOAL

The overall goal is to assist the SRO tenant to gain or sustain maximum functioning within the community. Emphasis is on the individual becoming as autonomous as possible, and developing a working social support network. See Table 17–3 for specific program objectives.

D. CONTRACT WITH SRO HOTEL

It is necessary to have a contractual agreement between the SRO landlord and the sponsoring health agency. This contract
1. Allows the agency to rent or use work space within the SRO

Table 17–3
SRO PROGRAM OBJECTIVES AND RATIONALE

Objectives	*Rationale*
1. To identify those tenants who are in need of health care; formulate a treatment plan (with tenant cooperation); implement and evaluate it	1. Tenants may not identify themselves as having problems, or may be unable to solve problems without assistance. Successful treatment may help them avoid hospitalization, and promote their autonomous strengths.
2. To intervene in situations of acute mental or physical distress and, whenever possible, assist the tenant to remain in the community while obtaining treatment	2. Tenants' sense of self-control and self-esteem may be enhanced by the team's response to their distress and the team's willingness to coordinate treatment in the community.
3. When necessary, facilitate psychiatric or medical hospitalization, collaborate with the inpatient treatment team, and assist with discharge planning for follow-up care	3. The many systems obstacles to hospitalization for the SRO tenant may be more effectively surmounted by an "inside" health worker–tenant advocate, who has acknowledge of the system.
4. Assist tenants to use other outpatient and social agencies in the community.	4. Tenants' dependence on the team and others decreases as tenants' knowledge of available resources, and how to use them, increases.
5. Help tenants take a more active and autonomous role in their dealings with hotel management, each other, and on-site health workers.	5. This helps tenants learn to manage their own affairs, increasing self-esteem and satisfaction.
6. Help to build a "sense of community" among hotel tenants.	6. This provides stability and durability in tenant interpersonal relationships.
7. Help tenants to expand their "community" to include other area residents, local planning boards, and block association, through responsible representation of tenants at these association meetings.	7. Effective communication and understanding between area residents, politicians, and SRO tenants makes for a stronger, more integrated community.

2. Allows access to tenant areas of building for outreach workers
3. Indicates a degree of cooperation between the landlord (including hotel workers) and the health agency (the on-site health workers)
4. Ideally allows health workers to screen prospective tenants

Team Structure   A. **TYPICAL COMPOSITION**
1. Psychiatric/mental health clinical nurse specialists
2. Psychiatric social workers
3. Alcoholism counselor
4. Community mental health aide
5. Psychiatrist (part-time)

B. **ADDITIONAL MEMBERS, AS PROGRAM FUNDS PERMIT**
1. Recreational therapist
2. Clinical psychologist
3. Night counselor
Part-time staff for minimedical clinic in SRO consists of a general practitioner physician and a public health nurse.

C. **NONSALARIED OTHERS**
Students of nursing, social work, psychology, and psychiatry, are generally a welcome, if temporary, addition to team strength. Their participation tends to revitalize mental health workers as well as tenants. Their fresh outlook on chronic problems tends to enhance others' investment in problem resolution.

Volunteers from the community may be successfully used, provided confidentiality concerning client information is not breached.

Team Leadership   The team leader or ''project coordinator'' is a clinician and a full-time professional member of the team (nurse, social worker, or psychologist). This person is appointed on the basis of clinical and leadership ability. The coordinator
1. Acts as team advocate/liaison between sponsoring agency administrators and the team
2. Acts as primary representative of the team to other systems (hotel management, tenant groups, outside agencies, news media)
3. Is responsible for assigning tenants to the appropriate team member(s)
4. Leads team clinical supervisory conferences and passes on pertinent information to all members
5. Acts as a stimulator for team members to expand practice and attempt innovative projects

Team Function   The functions of team members tend to be role blended as well as role specific, depending on the members' areas of expertise and the identified needs of tenants. Thus, while any professional team member may assess a tenant's mental status, the nurse may be consulted to further assess physical complaints in relation to mental status. The psychiatrist is the only member who may prescribe medication, or sign legal authorization for a tenant's involuntary hospitalization.

The types of services offered by the team cover a range of traditional therapeutic activities, as well as innovative approaches which are consonant with mental health principles. Basically, services can be categorized as
1. Individual, group, and family therapy or counseling
2. Crisis intervention

3. Psychiatric evaluation
4. Medication
5. Alcoholism education and treatment
6. Advocacy services concerning basic needs
7. Socialization and facilitation of social support systems
8. Assistance in developing a sense of community

Table 17–4 shows team functions and examples in an SRO program.

Problems of Mental Health Workers in the SRO

Because outreach reverses the traditional flow in which the consumer seeks out the professional, it poses unique problems for the workers "in the field." Chart 17–1 offers problems, examples, and interventions.

Characteristics of the Nurse on the SRO Team[2]

To work in this unusual setting, the clinical nurse specialist must possess a variety of professional and personal attributes. *The nurse*

1. Is a skilled clinician, capable of independent judgment
2. Is willing to accept considerable responsibility
3. Possesses leadership skills to coordinate conflicting systems
4. Has a high degree of flexibility in working with other disciplines and defining a role

Table 17–4
TEAM FUNCTIONS AND EXAMPLES IN AN SRO

Team Functions	*Examples*
1. Works to gain acceptance as a visible, identifiable resource within the SRO	1. Put up posters, talk to tenants in the lobby, knock on doors to explain the team's presence and to offer services
2. Establishes informal relationships with tenants and management, while retaining professional identity	2. Approach hotel manager, porters, and tenants for information on "how things work here," that is, knowledge of the formal and informal processes in the hotel
3. Directly approaches tenants who have been identified as having problems. Referrant may be a hotel clerk, another tenant, a friend, or a team member.	3. Knock on tenant's door, identify self as a team member, explain that others were concerned, and offer to help; encourage tenants to talk about their problems
4. Identifies and assesses the underlying systems problems that are further obstructing a tenant's functioning, and directs the intervention there.	4. Tenant states problem as lack of money; you assess tenant as being extremely disorganized and unable to budget his current income. Intervention is geared to tenant's reorganization.
5. Assumes role of tenant advocate in dealing with systems in situations in which tenants are unable to cope by themselves	5. Approach hotel manager with the tenant to help tenant explain that his rent will be paid as soon as tenant receives his overdue assistance check
6. Provide a consistent support system that encourages tenants' efforts at effective cooperation as a group	6. Initiate and guide the development of a tenant "steering committee" to deal with hotel management concerning problems in the building; help tenants to assume leadership roles

5. Is able to give and receive support, confront conflicts, share, teach, and learn with others on the team
6. Is able to achieve satisfaction with achievement of limited goals
7. Maintains expectations that tenants have the ability to change
8. Is available to clients, reacts to them openly and spontaneously, and deals with them in a variety of settings
9. Has a high tolerance for ambiguity and for deviant behavior
10. Is capable of self-direction, and actively seeks challenges

---

Chart 17–1
POTENTIAL PROBLEMS FOR NURSES IN THE SRO, EXAMPLES, AND INTERVENTIONS

Area of Potential Problems	Examples	Interventions
1. *Territoriality*—is not under health workers' control, but is the "home turf" of hotel management and tenants.	a. Management suddenly denies team and tenants access to kitchen area, where a lunch program has been established.	a. The nurse tries to find out informally (from porters and tenants) why this is happening. He approaches management diplomatically with a tenants' committee representative.
	b. Tenant asks you not to knock on his door again.	b. The nurse must respect tenant's territorial rights. He may try leaving a note in his mailbox, or phoning his room, if further outreach is indicated.
2. *Resistance of tenants*—may be related to tenant's fear of exposure, authority figures, the (traditional) health care system.	a. Tenant is ill or broke, but refuses to accept help. The nurse may become concerned, but feels helpless and inadequate.	a. The nurse confers with the team for support and to develop problem-solving strategies. Constructive manipulation of systems can be effective. If the tenant's friends and hotel management become concerned, they may exert pressure on the tenant to accept help.
	b. Tenant is "crisis oriented;" he accepts help when in crisis, but refuses help designed to prevent crises.	b. The nurse relies on her own skill and ingenuity to form a relationship with the tenant, and then uses any possible opportunity for health teaching.
3. *Negotiations with hotel management*—is an ongoing necessity for health workers, for space and for improvement of services.	a. Management views the nurse alternately as intruder, troublemaker, or peer and is inconsistent in dealings with tenants.	a. The nurse tries to determine the motivation behind actions of management, then deal accordingly. While management may make the final decision, they can be influenced, especially if the nurse's desired outcome is presented as meeting the manager's needs, as well. Health teaching with management may mean a positive change in the treatment of workers and tenants!
4. *Unique nature of the setting*—lack of external work structures and the broad range of needs presented may be disorienting to the health worker who is trying to define a professional role.	a. Tenant feels helpless and distraught when management removes her cat to the pound. Tenant has been a responsible pet owner, but management has decided that all pets must go. Nurse questions his "professional role" in this case.	a. The nurse confers with the team using a systems reference for assessing the problem. He recognizes the meaning of the pet, and the many negative consequences to the tenant when a beloved pet is removed.

Chart 17–1
(continued)

Area of Potential Problems	Examples	Interventions
5. *Multidisciplinary nature of the team*—each member comes from a discipline with certain preconceived notions or role functions; conflicts may arise regarding role definitions.	a. A solitary nurse is without discipline peers on the health team. Every physical complaint of tenants is referred to the nurse. Often, tenants already know the cause of the symptom, and the recommended treatment for the problem.	a. The nurse addresses this issue in the team meeting, clarifying her role, her strengths, and her limitations. Discussion may reveal that non-nurse members feel fearful or inadequate when confronted with tenants' dramatic complaints. Review of assessment skills may help these members shift more responsibility to themselves, and to the tenant.
6. *Supervision*—lack of on-site supervisor may increase the nurse's feelings of helplessness.	a. Situations involving all of the above examples may lead the nurse to doubt his own professional judgment.	a. A supervisor is always available by telephone. Conferring on the phone, requesting a site visit, or arranging supervision at the sponsoring agency, are helpful. Peer/team supervision is of the utmost importance for the on-site health worker; this process generally serves to increase team cohesiveness and mutual support.

Evaluation   The criteria used to determine whether or not program objectives have been met are varied; most frequently they are determined by the nurse's on-going assessment of the client's response to program treatment. Evaluation is related to previously stated program objectives: Tenants identified as being in need of treatment have successfully been engaged in treatment, and are attempting to collaborate and cooperate in the implementation of their treatment plans. Specifically, there is

1. A decrease in the recidivism rate for a significant number of chronic clients and an increase in tenant acceptance of home care and health teaching about physical illness
2. Increased acceptance of brief inpatient treatment, and more follow-up care
3. A decrease in the chronic use and abuse of the emergency room and, instead, use of other community services
4. Growing mutual responsibility among clients, that is, more awareness of neighbors who need assistance and willingness to "get involved" in order to help them
5. Increased self-advocacy and cooperation among clients in planning for shared goals and positive response of management to tenant requests.
6. A more positive and less fearful regard of the client by the community so that local groups ask for tenants' opinions and cooperation in local matters

References   1. Huessy HR: The chronic psychiatric patient in the community: Highlights from a Boston conference. Hosp Community Psychiatry 28:287, 1977
2. Rosamilia JD: Community mental health nursing in an urban setting. Paper presented at the Psychiatric–Mental Health Nursing Practice Conference Group Program at the New York State Nurses Association Convention, October 14, 1977

3. Sarason B: The Psychological Sense of Community: Prospects for a Community Psychology. San Francisco, Jossey-Bass, 1974
4. Siegal HA: Outposts of the Forgotten: An Ethnography of New York City's Welfare Hotels and Single Room Occupancy (SRO) Tenements. Ph.D. dissertation, Yale University, December 1974

Bibliography

Bohm E: Interdisciplinary teamwork in a community SRO. J Psychiatr Nurs 16:23, 1978

Flagg JM: Consultation in community residences for the chronically mentally ill. J Psychosoc Nurs 20:30, 1982

Mealey A: Provision of a multi-range program for clients in a downtown hotel by baccalaureate nursing students. J Psychiatr Nurs 19:11, 1981

Sweeney D et al: Mapping urban hotels: Life space of the chronic mental patient. J Psychosoc Nurs 20:9, 1982

18

Designing a
Private Practice

Suzanne Lego

Introduction It is estimated that over one thousand psychiatric–mental health nurses prepared at the masters level or above are now offering psychotherapy in private practice. Most of these nurses hold full-time or part-time jobs as well,[6] but many now support themselves in full-time private practices.

A number of factors may account for this, including the following:

1. A general dissatisfaction with institutionalized settings among nurses
2. Consumer and women's liberation movements[6]
3. Changes in nurse practice acts that foster autonomy equal to accountability in nursing practice[6]

One study has shown that clients experience the same level of satisfaction with nurse psychotherapists as with physicians.[15]

Advantages Private practice of psychiatric–mental health nursing provides the following advantages:

1. Control of the scope of practice—Nurses can select the kind of clients with whom they like best to work, and their modality and theoretical framework. They can determine how many hours per week to devote to direct care, and how many to lecturing, consultation, writing, community work, and so forth. They can choose their own supervisors.
2. Flexibility of hours—Nurses can schedule office hours according to their own preferences, and can arrange days off and vacations as they see fit.
3. Financial remuneration—Nurses are generally paid more per hour for private practice than they would receive in institutional practice.

Disadvantages Some nurses shun the idea of private practice or become anxious upon entering private practice because private practice may generate fear about autonomy, independence, separation, individuation, and aggression.[2,10] These internal feelings, which nurses experience consciously or unconsciously, are based on the following reality factors about private practice:

1. The practitioner is solely responsible and accountable for the practice. No therapeutic team is available to share a decision and its attendant responsibility.[17]
2. There is no backup for a professional judgment. Decision making must therefore be a highly refined skill.[17]
3. The private practitioner is involved in a contractual one-to-one relationship with the client and does not go "off duty" at five o'clock.[17]
4. There is no social service or occupational therapy department to which the practitioner can turn. The only resources are in the home and community.[17]
5. The client setting may be undesirable, and no other setting may be available. Very few home environments are "therapeutic communities."[17]
6. The practitioner does not have a vast pool of clients from which to select a compatible or special group for group therapy.[17]
7. The practitioner does not have daily contact with colleagues. Some practitioners report loneliness in their daily work.

Qualifications **Certification.** It is generally agreed that nurses who practice psychotherapy privately should be certified or in the process of becoming certified as a Clinical Specialist in Adult Psychiatric and Mental Health Nursing or a Clinical Specialist in Child and Adolescent Psychiatric and Mental Health Nursing. Criteria for this American Nurses Association (ANA) certification include[5]

1. Current licensure as a registered nurse in the United States or its territories
2. Current involvement in direct clinical nursing practice at least 4 hours per week

3. A master's or higher degree in nursing, with a specialization in psychiatric and mental health nursing (special consideration may be given to nurses with a bachelor's degree in nursing and a master's or higher degree in a related field, or a master's or higher degree in nursing plus a diploma in nursing and a bachelor's degree in any field). The master's degree must be from a nationally accredited institution of higher learning.
4. Postmaster's practice in psychiatric and mental health nursing with direct client contact for either
   • 8 hours per week for 2 years, or
   • 4 hours per week for 4 years
   Candidates whose master's or higher degree is in nursing with a specialization in psychiatric and mental health nursing may substitute two academic semesters or three quarters of supervised clinical experience for 1 year of this requirement.
5. Access to clinical supervision or consultation
6. Experience in at least two different treatment modalities
7. At least 100 hours of postmaster's supervision or consultation by a member of the core mental health disciplines (master's prepared clinical specialist in psychiatric and mental health nursing, master's prepared social worker, psychiatrist, or doctorally prepared psychologist). Individual, group, and peer group supervisor or consultation are equally considered. A mental health professional who is not a member of the core mental health professions is given consideration as a supervisor/consultant upon petition by a candidate, if the mental health professional holds certification in a related mental health area.
8. Successful completion of a written examination.

The state nurses' associations in New Jersey and New York also offer certification in clinical specialization in psychiatric and mental health nursing, requiring similar criteria.

Continuing education. Although the private practitioner may be licensed and certified, and hold advanced degrees, professional education does not end there. Because knowledge in the field of mental health is constantly expanding, the professional must keep abreast of current knowledge. A number of states now require continuing education for relicensure, and the ANA requires that certified specialists earn a specified number of continuing education units over each 5-year period of recertification. Most colleges and universities and many private companies provide continuing education programs in the mental health field.

Personal psychotherapy[12]. The clinical specialist who conducts psychotherapy as a private practitioner functions best when personal psychotherapy is a part of the preparation as psychotherapist. This is because the practice of psychotherapy requires a close, intimate relationship over time with the client, who will present a wide range of irrational behaviors. This often touches off in the nurse an equally wide range of irrational thoughts and feelings. Through personal psychotherapy, nurses are helped to understand their own irrationalities so that they can avoid acting out, and can increase their useful, growth-promoting responses to clients.

Financial Considerations in Starting the Practice

At the start of the practice, money is needed for two main reasons[8]:

A. **START-UP COSTS**
   Start-up costs include initial purchases such as
   1. Furnishings and rugs for office and waiting room

2. Stationery, including
   - Announcements of practice (see Fig. 18–1)
   - Letters and envelopes with letterhead
   - Business cards
   - Bills (see Fig. 18–2)
3. An answering machine (if answering service is not used)
4. Legal fees for incorporation

B. ONGOING OPERATING COSTS
   1. Office rent
   2. Phone, electricity, heat
   3. Answering service (if answering machine is not used)
   4. Insurance
   5. Supervision
   6. Accountant fees for filing taxes and financial planning
   7. Magazine subscriptions for office magazines

The Fee At the time of this printing, clinical specialists in psychiatric–mental health nursing charge an average fee of $40 to $50 per session. Sessions are from 45 to 60 minutes. Most clinical specialists allow some low-cost sessions per week or offer a sliding scale for clients who cannot afford the usual fee.

Third Party Reimbursement Nurses are beginning to gain eligibility for third party reimbursement by private insurance companies. In Maryland a law provides the same measure of reimbursement for nurses as for other health care providers.[6] In California insurance companies based in the state are prohibited from discriminating against nurses who provide psychotherapy.[6]

Through the efforts of the ANA Council of Specialists in Psychiatric and Mental Health Nursing, nurses' clients are now eligible for CHAMPUS reimbursement for nurse psychotherapists' services. The council has issued a position statement on reimbursement and has initiated a Blue Cross/Blue Shield Peer Review Committee Project composed of certified psychiatric and mental health specialists appointed by the council.[6]

In a few situations, clients have been reimbursed after the nurse therapist painstakingly proved professional competence and privilege to provide mental health ser-

---

SUZANNE LEGO, Ph.D., R.N., C.S.

announces the relocation of her New Jersey office

to

550 PIERMONT ROAD
DEMAREST, N.J. 07627

New York Office:	Telephone:
One Christopher Street	212 929-5970
New York, N.Y. 10014	201 767-6821

FIG. 18–1 Sample announcement of practice.

Suzanne Lego, Ph.D., R.N., C.S.

550 Piermont Road   One Christopher Street
Demarest, N.J. 07627   New York, N.Y. 10014
(201) 767-6821   (212) 929-5970

FOR PROFESSIONAL SERVICES CONSISTING OF CONTINUING PSYCHOTHERAPY SESSIONS:

1   2   3   4   5   6   7   8   9   10   11   12   13

14   15   16   17   18   19   20   21   22

23   24   25   26   27   28   29   30   31

UNDERLINED DATE(S) INDICATE INDIVIDUAL THERAPY SESSIONS(S)

CIRCLED DATE(S) INDICATE GROUP THERAPY SESSION(S)

FIG. 18–2 Sample bill.

vices. While the situation is not resolved for nurse psychotherapists, it looks more hopeful than in the past.[9]

When submitting bills for third party reimbursement, it is helpful to use a bill with a ''calendar'' as shown in Figure 18–2. The client can then underline or circle the dates to indicate the service received on that date. Insurance companies will usually *not* reimburse for two services on the same day, for example individual and group therapy on the same date. DSM III diagnostic categories are used to describe the client's problem or diagnosis.

The Setting   Whether the nurse's office is in the home or in another location the following provisions are made:

A. **A PRIVATE WAITING ROOM**
   The waiting room should have a comfortable temperature, pleasant decor, quiet surroundings, a bathroom, a coatrack, and reading materials. If it adjoins the consultation room, privacy is maintained through soundproofing or a white noise machine.

B. **A PRIVATE CONSULTATION ROOM**
   The consultation room should be comfortable, pleasant, and quiet. Distractions such as phone calls, deliveries, pets, and other interruptions are avoided.

C. **A LOCATION**

The office should be close to public transportation or have adequate parking facilities.

Personal Image and Attire

A recent study showed that the personal image of the therapist is very important in determining which therapists clients chose.[1] Some of the qualities that appealed to clients were

1. Warmth, liking, caring, support
2. A feeling that the therapist approved, appreciated, and respected them

Therapists who were rejected were described as

1. "Cold fish"
2. Too distant
3. Ungiving

Some descriptions of office decor that clients found unappealing were

1. "Motel" furniture
2. Plastic plants

The researcher concluded that the manner in which the therapist dresses as well as the choice of objects in the office setting are clues to what sort of person the therapist is.[1] Nurses should take care that professional surroundings and attire communicate to clients just what they wish to communicate.[9,13,14]

Practice Promotion Strategies

A recent survey of practice promotion strategies used by psychiatric nurses in private practice generated the following list of strategies. The first 40 are listed with their rank according to their business-producing potential.[7]

1. Developing and maintaining mental health services that otherwise would not be available locally
2. Facilitating third party payment for your clients
3. Providing services at times convenient to the work schedule or life-style of clients
4. Meeting individually with ministers, school counselors, law enforcement agents and court/juvenile authorities to explain the role/scope of practice
5. Meeting individually with physicians to explain the role/scope of practice
6. Reciprocal referral of clients to those persons who refer clients to you
7. Providing classes/workshops directed toward consumer health needs
8. Being willing to negotiate a professional fee with a client
9. Independently providing continuing education workshops for health professionals
10. Appearing as an expert guest on radio/television programs
11. Sending notes/letters of thanks to referral agents
12. Reporting client progress to referral agents
13. Writing consumer-oriented magazine articles or books
14. Providing continuing education workshops sponsored by colleges/agencies
15. Voluntary consultation to nonprofit, community-based health agencies
16. Organizing or advising local support groups (for example, a stroke patient organization)
17. Speaking before civic groups and organizations
18. Exchanging consultation services with other health professionals
19. Distributing professional business cards to other health professionals
20. Writing a health column for a local newspaper
21. Speaking about role/scope of practice before groups of other health professionals
22. Providing a reduced fee schedule for nurses and other health professionals
23. Presenting self at all times to the public as a "healthy person"
24. Organizing and conducting nurse peer support groups
25. Presenting research/scholarly papers before other health professionals

26. Meeting with administrators of local hospitals, community health agencies, private health organizations to explain the role and scope of practice
27. Taking referral agents to a restaurant to discuss your role/practice
28. Mailing announcements of new practice to physicians/other health professionals
29. Locating your office in a medical building
30. Mailing announcements of new practice to others who might refer clients: ministers, school counselors, law enforcement agents, court/juvenile authorities
31. Actively participating in mental health organizations (nonnursing)
32. Actively participating in professional organizations
33. Meeting individually with other nurses to explain the role and scope of your practice
34. Employing a marketing consultant to develop marketing strategies
35. Providing guest lectures at schools and colleges without a fee
36. Giving or mailing a brochure describing your role or practice to potential clients
37. Asking clients to report their satisfaction with your services to referral agents
38. Sponsoring an open house when practice is initiated
39. Advertising in the yellow pages
40. Becoming actively involved politically in issues affecting nursing and mental health

Collaboration with a Psychiatrist

When clients require prescriptions or hospitalization, the clinical specialist usually refers them to a psychiatrist. It is helpful if the therapist and psychiatrist have a good working relationship and similar philosophies of care, for example, if both agree that a minimal amount of medication should be given to help the client function so that psychotherapy can proceed, or that hospitalization should be avoided if possible. Some insurance companies reimburse for services of a nurse psychotherapist if a psychiatrist supervises the therapy or monitors the client's progress on a regular basis. Legislation along these lines was recently proposed in New York state but was opposed by the New York State Nurses Association on the grounds that nurse psychotherapists need not practice under the direction of a physician, but rather collaboratively as needed.

Taxes and Retirement Plans

Since taxes are not withheld by an employing agency, it is up to the nurse to pay quarterly estimated taxes. An accountant determines what the quarterly payments should be, based on the previous year's earnings. If the nurse is not incorporated, these taxes are paid January 15, April 15, June 15, and September 15.

When the nurse's income reaches a certain point, incorporation can provide advantages, such as a medical plan, retirement plan, automobile expenses, and much higher limits on nontaxable retirement contributions. Incorporation laws vary from state to state.

Private practitioners must also plan their own retirement benefits using Individual Retirement Accounts (IRAs) in which $2,000 per year or 100% of annual earned income (whichever is less) can be invested tax free, or Keogh plans in which up to $15,000 or 15% of annual earned income (whichever is less) per year may be invested. These retirement funds can be invested in bank accounts, insurance plans, investment trust funds, and so forth. An accountant is valuable for filing taxes and for providing information about deductions and financial plans.

Insurance

For the private practitioner, a number of kinds of insurance are necessary:

A. **HEALTH AND LIFE INSURANCE**
Since there is no employing agency providing these, the nurse must contract independently for health and life insurance. Some companies provide policies

wherein individuals become members of existing "groups" and pay group rates. The nurse will probably want to carry Blue Cross, Blue Shield, and major medical insurance. Life insurance is available through the ANA at group rates.

B. **DISABILITY INSURANCE**
Disability insurance provides monthly payments should the nurse become disabled through sickness or accidents. This kind of policy is available from private companies or at group rates through the ANA and other professional groups such as the American Orthopsychiatric Association.

C. **MALPRACTICE INSURANCE**
Malpractice insurance provides coverage for damages or court costs should the nurse be sued. It is available through private companies or the ANA.

D. **PROPERTY AND CASUALTY INSURANCE**
Property and casualty insurance provides coverage for damages or court costs should someone sue for damages as the result of an accident on the nurse's property (for example in the waiting room or consultation room). If the office is in the home, "home owners" insurance can cover this if endorsed for professional use.

E. **FIRE, THEFT, MALICIOUS MISCHIEF**
If the nurse rents an office outside the home, fire, theft, and malicious mischief insurance may be desirable, and is fairly inexpensive in most locations. If the office is in the home, "home owners" insurance can cover these claims if endorsed for professional use.

Legal Considerations   Whether a nurse may practice psychotherapy is determined by the state's nurse practice act. Many states are changing or attempting to change their nurse practice acts to allow for the legal practice of psychotherapy by the prepared clinical nurse specialist. In New Jersey, for example, the nurse practice act reads

> The practice of nursing as a registered professional nurse is defined as diagnosing and treating human responses to actual or potential physical and emotional health problems, through such services as case finding, health teaching, health counseling, and provision of care supportive to or restorative of life and well-being, and executing medical regimen as prescribed by a licensed or otherwise legally authorized physician or dentist.

This definition is believed to be broad enough to cover the practice of psychotherapy, although it has not yet been tested in court.

Record Keeping   Records of client visits are kept for the following reasons:

A. **ASSESSMENT AND CONTINUING EVALUATION**
Sometimes nurses keep records of early sessions and notes as sessions progress to record the client's progress.

B. **SUPERVISION OR PEER REVIEW**
For supervision or peer review, a nurse will probably tape-record sessions or take notes during sessions or afterwards. If tape recordings are made, it is a good idea to have the client sign a simple release form stating that the nurse has the client's permission to tape-record for professional use.

C. BILLING

A record of sessions is kept for billing the client each month.

D. TAXES

The nurse keeps a record of all income and expenses for tax purposes. A bound ledger is required for this purpose.[11] Records must be retained for 3 years to be used in the event of a tax audit.

Accountability   Nurses in private practice are accountable to clients and to themselves in the following ways:

1. Nurses provide services as contracted with the client, keeping in mind the elements of the ANA Statement on Psychiatric and Mental Health Nursing (see Appendix A).[3]
2. Nurses are students of the problems that arise in the psychiatric–mental health field, checking and rechecking their assumptions and preconceptions, keeping an open and active mind, and laying aside their own needs so as to recognize and help resolve the needs of clients.[16]
3. Nurses maintain an ongoing, regular, formal consultative relationship with a professional colleague.[3]

Evaluation   The success of a private practice for the nurse therapist may be measured in three ways:

1. The reduction of symptoms and emotional disturbance in the majority of clients
2. The satisfaction and growth of the nurse psychotherapist
3. Financial success

References

1. Albin RS: Therapists choosing therapists: What they look for. New York Times, September 15, 1981
2. Alkon N: Preparing to individuate from team members to independent practitioner. J Psychiatr Nurs 15:31, June 1977
3. American Nurses Association, Division on Psychiatric and Mental Health Nursing Practice: Standards of Psychiatric and Mental Health Nursing Practice. Kansas City, MO, American Nurses Association, 1982
4. American Nurses Association, Division on Psychiatric and Mental Health Nursing: Statement on Psychiatric and Mental Health Nursing Practice, Kansas City, MO, American Nurses Association, 1976
5. American Nurses Association: Take the Extra Step . . . Become a Certified Nurse. Kansas City, American Nurses Association, 1983
6. Colliton MA: Independent practice. In Haber J et al (eds): Comprehensive Psychiatric Nursing. New York, McGraw-Hill, 1982
7. Durham JD: Practice Promotion Strategies Used by Psychiatric Nurses in Private Practice. Unpublished study, Outreach Nursing Service, PO Box 74, Fairbury, IL 61739
8. Edmunds M: Financial planning for independent practice. Nurse Practitioner 35, Sept–Oct, 1980
9. Geller JC: Starting a private practice of psychotherapy. Perspect Psychiatr Care 18:106, 1980
10. Herron W, Rouslin S: The psychodynamics of entering private practice. In Herron W, Rouslin S: Issues in Psychotherapy. Bowie, MD, Robert J Brady, 1982
11. Larkin M, Crowdes NE: A systems approach to private practice. J Psychiatr Nurs 13:5, 1975
12. Lego S: The clinical specialist and the client in individual and group therapy. In Critchley DL, Maurin JT (eds): The Psychiatric Mental Health Clinical Specialist: Theory, Research, and Practice. New York, John Wiley & Sons, 1984
13. Malloy JT: Dress for Success. New York, Warner Books, 1975
14. Malloy JT: The Women's Dress for Success Book. New York, Warner Books, 1975
15. Meldman MG et al: Patient responses to nurse psychotherapists. Am J Nurs 71:6, 1971
16. Peplau HE: The psychiatric nurse—accountable? To whom for what? Perspect Psychiatr Care 18:128, 1980
17. Wilson HS, Kneisl CR: Psychiatric Nursing. Menlo Park, CA, Addison-Wesley, 1979

Bibliography

Gibson KW, Catterson JS, Skalka P: On Our Own. New York, Avon, 1981

Goldman CD, Stricker G (eds): Practical Problems of a Psychotherapy Practice. Springfield, IL, Charles C Thomas, 1971

Goodspeed HE: The independent practitioner—can it survive? J Psychiatr Nurs 14:33, 1976

Hendrickson DE, Janney SP, Fraze JE: How To Start Your Own Private Practice. Muncie, IN, Professional Consultants Associates, 1977

Koltz CJ: Private Practice in Nursing: Development and Management. Aspen, CO, Aspen Systems, 1979

Lewin MH: Establishing and Maintaining a Successful Professional Practice. Rochester, NY, Professional Development Institute, 1978

Pressman RM: Private Practice—A Handbook for the Independent Mental Health Practitioner. New York, Gardner Press, 1979

Randolph GT: Experiences in private practice. J Psychiatr Nurs 13:16, 1975

Riccardi BR, Dayani EC: The Nurse Entrepreneur. Reston, VA, Reston, 1982

Shimberg E: The Handbook of Private Practice in Psychology, New York, Brunner-Mazel, 1979

Sills GM: The Role and Function of the Clinical Nurse Specialist. In Chaska NL (ed), The Nursing Profession: A Time to Speak, New York, McGraw-Hill, 1983

Smalkowsky Sr MF: A year later: An independent practitioner looks back, J Psychiatr Nurs 14:35, August, 1976

19

Designing a Clinical Experience in Psychiatric Nursing for Undergraduate Students

Marie McGillicuddy

OVERVIEW

Description   A course in psychiatric–mental health nursing is expected to provide a broad-based understanding of mental health concepts and the behavioral aberrations that occur in mental illness. Moreover, the course teaches students to analyze the health care system, with a specific critical view of the resources available to the mentally ill. Based on knowledge of growth and development and biopsychopathology, nursing activities are identified and implemented. The basis for intervention is the nurse–client relationship. This requires development of sophisticated skills in the use of self for therapeutic communication and interpersonal relationships. There are opportunities for students to enter into collaborative working relationships with clients and to use the nursing process in a psychiatric setting.

The Nursing Process   The nursing process model adopted in the baccalaureate program should meet the following criteria[5]:

1. Provide knowledge for students to make the judgments inherent in the nursing process
2. Be as dynamic as practice itself, that is, the model should permit dynamic movement back and forth between steps in the process
3. Be applicable to nursing in general and not only to specific clinical settings
4. Be compatible with ethical standards for nursing practice
5. Be consistent with scientific findings on human behavior in health and illness

   The social and cultural aspects of mental illness are covered by emphasizing the impact by and on the family and the community. The ultimate goal is to teach the student to assist the patient and his family to achieve their optimal level of functioning within the community and to support patient (and family) strengths in the maintenance of total health.

Placement of Course   The combined theory and clinical course being described in this chapter might be offered in the fourth or fifth nursing course, within the context of a modified integrated baccalaureate nursing program, that is, in a program not integrated in the pure sense of the term, but containing various patterns or threads that run throughout the total curriculum. For example, the community health thread may be worked into the psychiatric–mental health course by having each student make a home visit and do a family and community assessment; *or* the student could spend a day in an outpatient setting and do a similar assessment.

Course Objectives   In writing the course objectives, the nurse educator takes into account

1. The undergraduate program objectives, so that *course* objectives contribute to the achievement of overall *program* objectives
2. The course description or intent, so that the objectives fulfill the intent of the course as it fits into the overall curriculum plan
3. The student behaviors necessary to function in the clinical area and the content necessary to develop those behaviors

Other guidelines include:

1. The conceptual framework of the program are clearly understood by the faculty and well articulated in the objectives of the course.
2. Overall curricular threads are identified and integrated in the course objectives.
3. ANA Standards of Psychiatric and Mental Health Nursing Practice are reflected in the objectives (see Appendix A).
4. Previous learning is reflected in course objectives, for example, mental health concepts that have been integrated in the nursing courses taught before this. The concepts are as follows:

a. Normal psychological, emotional, and physical development at various life stages

b. Normal life processes (birth, adolescence, death, and so forth) as maturational crises

c. Interrelatedness of components of human functioning

d. Normal patterns of need fulfillment (importance of work, sexuality, recreation)

e. Stress, trauma, illness, and hospitalization as precipitating disequilibrium and crises

f. Dynamics of family life and the functions of the family as a societal unit

g. One's own personality as a determinant of the nurse–patient relationship

h. Use of interpersonal skills in assisting the individual/family to maintain total health

i. Use of group dynamics as a therapeutic tool

j. Inclusion of data or major health problems of a psychosocial nature in health assessments

Sample Objectives* At the end of the course, the students will be able to

1. Examine their attitudes toward mental health, mental illness, and the mentally ill

2. Demonstrate an awareness of their own behavior and its effect on others in the environment

3. Demonstrate knowledge of the dynamics of human behavior in individual, group, and family settings

4. Demonstrate knowledge of the major manifestations of mental illness in this culture

5. Demonstrate an ability to assess the mental and emotional status of an individual

6. Demonstrate the ability to plan and implement intervention with clients

7. Identify factors that inhibit as well as encourage growth and change in individuals, families, and social systems

8. Demonstrate an ability to perceive themselves as potential change agents with problems of individuals, families, and social systems

9. Relate theories of social, economic, cultural, and familial aspects of mental illness in planning client care

10. Demonstrate an ability to function on the health care team with professional colleagues and peers

Course Schedule A. **ORGANIZATION**

This course follows the standard academic calendar. It has the following configuration:

1. Length of course—one semester (14 weeks)

2. Lecture—2 to 4 hours weekly

3. Clinical experience—6 to 7 hours weekly

4. Supervision seminar—2 to 3 hours weekly

5. Prerequisites or concurrent supportive courses

a. General psychology

b. Sociology

c. Growth and development, or developmental psychology

*Sample mental health concepts and course objectives have been adapted from the nursing program at Herbert H. Lehman College, City University of New York, New York, New York.

B. **LECTURES**

Week 1—Orientation to course; criteria of mental health; principles of psychiatric nursing

Week 2—Concepts of transference and countertransference

Week 3—Schizophrenia

Week 4—Schizophrenia

Week 5—Family dynamics

Week 6—Test no. 1; depression/mania; crisis intervention; suicide/homicide

Week 7—Depression/mania; crisis intervention; suicide/homicide

Week 8—Psychoneurosis

Week 9—Psychoneurosis

Week 10—Drug and alcohol abuse

Week 11—Test no. 2; anti-social personality/sexual deviations

Week 12—The psychiatric hospital as a social system

Week 13—Acute and organic brain disorders

Week 14—History of psychiatric nursing

Clinical Experience   The weekly clinical experience includes a 1-hour preconference and a 1-hour postconference.

A. **PRECONFERENCE**

The preconference time is used to supplement and reinforce lecture material, particularly as it relates to the clinical setting. Examples of client behaviors familiar to most of the students are used as illustrations, and specific nursing interventions are discussed. The weekly schedule remains flexible so that the week-to-week student experiences and concerns determine the topic for discussion. (For example, two students are working with severely depressed clients, and the other students have observed these clients on the unit. Readings are assigned and discussed even though the topic has not yet been presented in lecture.)

B. **STUDENT ACTIVITIES DURING THE CLINICAL DAY**

In the course of each clinical day the students will

1. Meet for ½ hour with a client whom they have chosen as their primary client for the semester

2. Tape-record this session for later supervision

3. Accompany this client through his/her daily routine, including group meetings, occupational therapy, recreational therapy, therapeutic community meetings, and so forth

4. Collaborate with other students in a group project (either activity-based or a talking group)

5. Interact with other clients, taking care to seek out clients presenting a variety of behaviors

6. Collaborate with other health professionals on the unit by sharing pertinent data and seeking them out for consultation

7. Seek out new experiences to enrich their education, for example, attending an admission conference, making rounds with the nursing supervisor, observing an initial nursing assessment

C. **POSTCONFERENCE**

The postconference time is used for students to share their experiences and mutual concerns. The group process is analyzed as part of the learning experience.

Selection of Clinical
Agencies

A. **FLEXIBILITY**
There should be flexibility in selection of clinical sites so that students are exposed to a variety of settings.[3]

B. **PROVISIONS**
The clinical agency provides
1. A setting in which objectives can be met
2. Availability of role models in the agency
3. A client population reflective of a broad socioeconomic range and a variety of behavioral dynamics
4. Available treatments that cover a range of modalities
5. Follow-up or aftercare in the community
6. Ample opportunity for students to collaborate with other professionals on the health team

C. **TYPES OF FACILITIES**
1. State hospitals
2. Private psychiatric hospitals
3. Psychiatric units in general hospitals
4. Community mental health agencies
5. Partial hospitalization programs or outpatient units. (It is usually difficult for this type of facility to absorb a typical clinical group of ten students.)
6. If arrangements can be made, it is ideal for students to have some exposure to other than inpatient settings, although some inpatient experience is always included.

Supervision of the
Student

A. **PURPOSE**
The purpose of supervision is to help students
1. Become aware of their impact on clients
2. Understand the client's communication
3. Clarify and validate their own communication, thoughts, and feelings

B. **INDIVIDUAL SUPERVISION**
1. The student comes prepared with verbatim notes, taped sessions or process records of nurse–client interaction.
2. Supervision occurs on a regularly scheduled weekly or biweekly basis. Proponents of individual (as opposed to group) supervision believe that it "provides the student with the security and freedom she needs to develop as a compassionate, flexible and thinking person."[2]

C. **PEER GROUP SUPERVISION**
1. Group usually meets weekly for 2 to 2½ hours with four scheduled presentations.
2. Instructor provides guidance.
3. Presentors cite actual dialogue between themselves and the client.
4. Presentors receive both positive and negative comments from peer group on clinical performance.
5. Different reactions (perceptions) to the same material help clarify for the presenting students.
6. The students soon begin to look at their own performance more critically.
7. The group process is examined, as well as the process between the student and the client.

Teaching and Learning Aids	A. **SELECTION OF TEXT(S)** Selection of text(s) is consistent with the intent and philosophical approach of the course.

B. **BIBLIOGRAPHY**

Bibliography is organized around topics so as to facilitate its use. (Journal articles serve to familiarize the student with nurse authors and researchers and provide up-to-date material.)

C. **TEACHING STRATEGIES**

Teaching strategies or operations are planned so that they meet the following criteria[1]:

1. Are consistent with the theoretical framework of the school of nursing, especially the accepted learning theories
2. Provide for the level of concreteness or abstractness of the learner's thinking processes (style)
3. Consider the learner's learning tempo (rate)
4. Are appropriate to the target behaviors

D. **PASSIVE LEARNING**

Passive learning occurs through the use of lecture, films, tapes, television, writing, and reading.

E. **CONVERTING PASSIVE LEARNING TO ACTIVITY[1]**

1. Weekly process recordings and presentations of this material under supervision
2. Nursing assessments and interventions based on problems identified in process recordings. Students may role play interventions, as well as actually carry them out with clients.
3. Detailed mental–emotional assessments
4. A group of two or three students devise a project involving a group (three or more) of clients. Students prepare objectives with accompanying rationale and carry out the projects. Students examine the process of the student group, as well as the client group.
5. A paper is written about a particular theoretical concept, using examples from the clinical area as well as other events in the student's personal experience.

Evaluation of the Student	A. **PURPOSE[1]**

1. To determine student attainment of the behaviors established as objectives
2. To assess the success of the instructional delivery system and all of its components
3. To predict professional success, for example, with state boards and in the work world
4. To determine grades. Grading is done to provide the learner and others insights into his/her achievement either in relation to the course goals or in comparison with peers.

B. **METHODS**

1. Paper and pencil tests.
2. Direct observation in clinical setting. Clinical competence is difficult to assess and often causes consternation among faculty. Assumptions made in assessing clinical competence are as follows[4]:

a. Evaluation of clinical competence by direct observation in the clinical laboratory presupposes that the nursing student has had the opportunity to learn before being evaluated on performance.

b. Competence in the actual clinical situation presupposes sufficient knowledge to take appropriate action.

c. The total milieu of the real-life setting cannot be replicated in a simulation situation.

d. Paper and pencil tests can measure only the cognitive aspects of the total constellation of behavior inherent in the practice of nursing.

e. The answers selected in a paper and pencil test reflect only what the student chose in that particular instance and cannot be interpreted to mean that the student would take that action in a real-life situation.

Rating scales and checklists are particularly helpful in evaluation by observation; the tool must contain the discrete observable behaviors broken down from the course objectives.[1]

3. Videotapes
4. Simulation or games[4]

a. Mock-up type—Student is presented with a mock situation with problems to solve.

b. Oral or role-playing type—Student is asked to role play to demonstrate how problem would be handled.

c. Written type—Student is asked to solve problem on paper and pencil test.

d. Computer type—Student is asked to solve problem on computer with immediate feedback and direction.

Evaluation of the Course   There must be continuous ongoing evaluation of individual courses, as well as the program as a whole. The faculty must engage in the ongoing examination of course material and teaching methods. Some tactics suggested to obtain information about course effectiveness are[1]

1. Student rap sessions or discussions
2. Teacher rap sessions
3. Performance test checklist (actually the task objectives derived from course objectives), filled out by the students
4. Tests to compare current student group to other comparable groups (for example, the NLN Achievement Test in Psychiatric Mental Health Nursing)
5. Course evaluation filled out by students. Questions are geared to students' ideas, feelings and experiences about the course. Some areas to consider in such a questionnaire are

a. Overall appraisal of course
b. Whether course met course objectives
c. Students' opinions about
   • Text(s)
   • Bibliography
   • Required reading
   • Lectures
   • Seminars/supervisory sessions
   • Assignments (evaluate each one separately)
   • Grading
   • Clinical experience
   • Faculty, hours, preconferences and postconferences.
d. General comments . . . "What did you like best?" "What would you like to see changed?"

A scaled questionnaire form yields richer responses and provides more pertinent information. The data gathered from these methods should lead to course changes that will provide more effective and efficient teaching.

References

1. Bevis EO: Curriculum Building in Nursing—A Process. St Louis, CV Mosby, 1973
2. Gregg DE, Bregg EA, Spring FE: Individual supervision: A method of teaching psychiatric concepts in nursing education. Perspect Psychiatr Care 3:115, 1976
3. National League for Nursing, Baccalaureate and Higher Degree Programs Council: Characteristics of Baccalaureate Education in Nursing. (Publ. No. 15-1958) New York, The League, 1979
4. Schneider HL: Evaluation of Nursing Competence. Boston, Little, Brown & Co, 1979
5. Twelker PA: A basic reference shelf on simulation and gaming. In Zukerman DW, Horn RE (eds): The Guide to Simulation Games for Education and Training. Cambridge, MA, Information Resources, 1970
6. Walker L, Nicholson R: Criteria for evaluating nursing process models. Nurse Educator 5:8, 1980

Bibliography

Davidhizar RE: Simulation games as a teaching technique in psychiatric nursing. Perspect Psychiatr Care 20:8, 1982

Feather R, Bissell B: Clinical supervision versus psychotherapy: The psychiatric/mental health supervisory process. Perspect Psychiatr Care 17:266, 1979

Geach B: The problem-solving technique: As taught to psychiatric students. Perspect Psychiatr Care 12:9, 1974

Jansson DP: Student consultation: A liaison psychiatric experience for nursing students. Perspect Psychiatr Care 17:77, 1979

Marley MS: Teaching and learning in a psychiatric–mental health clinical setting. J Psychiatr Nurs 18:16, 1980

Price JL et al: Value assumptions in humanistic psychiatric nursing education. Perspect Psychiatr Care 12:64, 1974

Sayre J: Common errors in communication made by students in psychiatric nursing. Perspect Psychiatr Care 16:175, 1978

20

Designing a Graduate Program in Psychiatric Nursing

Anita Werner O'Toole / Viola Morofka

OVERVIEW

Description   Graduate education in psychiatric mental health nursing prepares nurses through specialization in one area. Specialization at the master's degree level helps the nurse acquire expertise in the knowledge and practice of psychiatric–mental health nursing. Graduate education provides students with the opportunity to use an investigative approach as they develop breadth and depth in their understanding of theory and increased competence in nursing practice and research. Curiosity and critical thinking are nurtured as students examine issues and question current nursing beliefs. Learning experiences increase in complexity as students move from learning to work with individuals, groups, and families to communities.

Doctoral level graduate education provides expertise in research and theory development in the field. Learning increases in both complexity and specialization as the student investigates phenomena within the field.

Students entering graduate programs in psychiatric mental health nursing are heterogenous; they bring with them a variety of experiences, attitudes, and interests. Recognition of what students bring with them and exploration of their needs are essential for the formulation of meaningful learning experiences.

A cooperative teacher–student relationship is essential, since a primary function of a teacher is the facilitation of students' learning and development. The teacher is responsible for developing an environment in which students have freedom and responsibility for self-direction and self-evaluation of their learning experiences in the program.[6]

Major Processes   Experiences emphasize process as well as content. Content of knowledge and the nature of roles change; therefore, it is impossible to learn in any given program all one might need to know in the future. However, many educational processes have far more enduring characteristics; they may be described as follows:

A. **INDUCTIVE**

The inductive process of theorizing from clinical and empirical data, whereby concepts and categories arise from the data instead of being superimposed upon the data

B. **DEDUCTIVE**

The deductive process of theory development, whereby theories are applied to empirical data and revised accordingly

C. **EXPERIENTIAL**

The experiential learning process, whereby one learns as one does. Like the inductive process of conceptualizing, experiential learning is based upon the examination of the data of one's experience. In psychotherapy, clients learn new forms of behavior by examining current and past behavior and its antecedents and consequences. Likewise, in learning therapeutic skills, students are encouraged to apply theory and examine its usefulness in bringing about the desired outcome.

D. **SUPERVISORY**

The supervisory process, whereby students examine their clinical work over time with supervisors and peers to guide the learning process

E. **THERAPEUTIC**

The therapeutic process, whereby students learn to *be* therapists which includes values inherent in the professional role of a psychotherapist

1. The process of therapeutic intervention which is applicable to any type of clinical situation, for example, intervention on an inpatient unit
2. The process of providing psychotherapy

F. **RESEARCH PROCESS**
   The research process, which is a logical, systematic approach to problem solving

Values Perhaps the most enduring outcome of an education experience is the acquisition of new values. Graduate students in psychiatric–mental health nursing should learn to value
1. Their own intellectual and interpersonal competence
2. Nursing as a major profession in the mental health field
3. Professional development throughout one's career, including ongoing clinical practice, research, and publication

Content Table 20–1 shows the course content that should be included in master's and doctoral programs in psychiatric–mental health nursing

Master's Degree Education

A. **GENERAL AIMS**
   1. Specialization in psychiatric–mental health nursing
   2. Preparation in a functional area, such as clinical specialization, education, or administration

B. **BEHAVIORAL OBJECTIVES**
   1. *Clinical courses*
      a. Therapeutic modalities—individual, group, and family therapy. The master's level student learns to
         1) Assess the status and dynamics of selected clients using various personality concepts and theories

Table 20–1
CONTENT OF CURRICULUM FOR MASTER'S AND DOCTORAL EDUCATION

Course Area	M.S.N.	Ph.D.
Clinical courses	Individual, group, family therapy; consultation, community work	Selection of one modality or one problem area for advanced clinical specialization
Theory	Examination and critique of nursing theories	Development of new theories with emphasis on utility for specialty area
Research	Research methodology, statistics, theses project	Advanced research methods, advanced statistical methods, dissertation
Cognates	Psychiatric, psychological, and sociological theories relevant to psychiatric–mental health nursing	Study in cognates that have a direct relevance to research or clinical problem area
Functional area	Clinical specialization, education, or administration	May select problem in a functional role for research
Electives	Nursing and cognate electives to broaden knowledge	Nursing and cognate electives to support research problem area

2) Apply formulations of individual, group, and family therapy theories appropriately to those demonstrating dysfunctional behaviors
3) Analyze the rationale for the selection of the therapeutic modality
4) Identify and analyze processes in and provide individual, group, and family therapy
5) Assess the theory underlying nursing intervention
6) Examine crisis intervention as it prevents mental disorders and provides reorganization at a higher personality level
7) Assess research findings applicable to the therapeutic modalities

b. Indirect services
1) Consultation
   a) Analyze various approaches to consultation
   b) Identify and examine process in mental health consultation with various categories of health care workers in selected settings
   c) Identify and evaluate resources
   d) Evaluate performance as a consultant and consequences of consultation
2) Community work
   a) Identify and assess mental health needs of an agency or a community
   b) Formulate solutions to problems and issues of the agency or a community
   c) Evaluate success of the intervention

2. *Core courses*
   a. Nursing theory
      1) Define concept, theory, and levels of theories
      2) Analyze and critique conceptualizations and theories in nursing and in fields relevant to nursing
   b. Research courses
      1) Statistics
         a) Identify assumptions underlying statistical measures
         b) Perform statistical tests
         c) Interpret and evaluate statistical measures used in research[5]
      2) Research methodology
         a) Define and develop researchable problems relevant to nursing
         b) Critique nursing research
         c) Assess application of findings
         d) Develop beginning skills in testing and expanding nursing knowledge through research

3. *Cognates and electives*
   a. These courses support the clinical major and the functional area by
      1) Providing theoretical perspectives from other disciplines
      2) Adding breadth of knowledge for the development and expansion of theories and practice skills in nursing
      3) Providing a foundation for functional roles (clinician, educator, administrator)
   b. An essential cognate is a course that addresses personality theories and theories of psychopathology
      1) Knowledge and theory facilitate students' conscious decisions about application to practice and assist them to move beyond the intuitive level of practice
      2) Knowledge of various theories of psychopathology and personality development offers conceptualization for
         a) Comprehending meanings of behavior

        b) Describing how change occurs

        c) Explaining directions for corrective growth and development

        d) Developing increased self-understanding

    3) Evaluation of the usefulness and limitations of any one theory is necessary. When selecting theoretical formulations to apply to practice, students consider

        a) Their own beliefs, values, and needs

        b) The fit between the theoretical formulations and techniques and their personality

        c) The fit between dimensions of theories and techniques, and each client's personality and psychopathology[3]

4. *Functional area—Clinical specialization, education, and administration*

    a. Student chooses one functional area for in-depth study

    b. General objectives for the functional area—The student learns to

      1) Collaborate with others in nursing and in other disciplines

      2) Integrate theory, research, and clinical practice in a leadership role

    c. Since clinical practice is viewed as the primary focus for specialization at the master's level, additional objectives for clinical specialization are that the student learns to

      1) Examine concepts and behaviors associated with clinical specialization

      2) Analyze roles and relationships of the clinical specialist in different types of health settings

      3) Examine subroles of the clinical specialist—Psychotherapist, liaison, consultant, collaborator, mental health educator, and independent practitioner

      4) Negotiate with agency staff for desired position and learning experiences within an organization

      5) Develop proficiency in performing the role of clinical specialist

      6) Analyze problems in the performance of the role and develop approaches to manage these

      7) Use self-evaluation to assess and improve professional skills

C. **EXAMPLE OF A MASTER'S LEVEL CURRICULUM**

Chart 20–1 shows a sample curriculum in a 2-year master's level program in psychiatric–mental health nursing.

Chart 20–1

EXAMPLE OF A MASTER'S CURRICULUM IN PSYCHIATRIC–MENTAL HEALTH NURSING

Fall	*Spring*
First Year	
Theoretical Formulations in Nursing (3)	Family Psychotherapy (6)
Personality Theories and Theories of Psychopathology (3)	Research Methodology (4)
Individual and Group Psychotherapy (6)	Cognate/Nursing Elective (3)
Statistics (3)	
Second Year	
Evaluation Research and Consultation (6)	Practicum in Functional Areas (5)
Seminar in Functional Area (3)	Thesis or Project (3)
Thesis or Project (3)	Cognate/Nursing Elective (3)

Note: Numbers indicate credits.

Clinical Supervision   A. **TYPES**

1. *Individual supervision*—An intense learning experience in which students learn psychotherapy by interacting with their individual supervisors[1]
2. *Group supervision*—Ideas about and performance with clients are shared, examined, and evaluated by peers and supervisor.

B. **PURPOSE**

1. To evaluate the use of self as a therapeutic variable
2. To assess intrapsychic and interpersonal processes that promote and impede communication
3. To develop psychotherapeutic skills with individuals, groups, and families
4. To demonstrate knowledge and skills of the client–student relationship.

C. **STYLES**

1. *Variations in supervision*
   a. Differences exist in what supervisors teach and in methods used.
   b. Differences are related to the supervisors' perspectives of mental illness and health, definition of what is relevant knowledge, and teaching style.
2. *Approaches to supervision* focus on
   a. Meanings of client–student verbal and nonverbal behaviors
   b. Client's childhood and past experiences
   c. Symptoms as an expression of unconscious conflicts
   d. Interactional patterns of client and student during sessions
   e. Theoretical formulations and helpful interventions
   f. Techniques used by students with examination of meanings
   g. Students' feelings and attitudes toward client[1]

D. **PROCESSING SESSIONS**

1. Student develops own style for recording client sessions and own method for reporting during supervisory sessions.
2. Student writes detailed notes on main ideas discussed.
3. Student and supervisor listen to sections of taped recording of sessions with client.
4. Student processes sessions according to guidelines prior to supervisory session. See Chart 20–2 for a guideline for supervision of one session.

Chart 20–2
SUPERVISION GUIDELINES

1. If first session, include presenting problem from the intake session.
2. State theme(s) of session.
3. State problem(s) presented.
4. Identify functional and dysfunctional behaviors.
5. State medicines prescribed, briefly identify actions, and evaluate effects on client(s).
6. Analyze and evaluate interventions that impeded or facilitated progress. Include one or more nontherapeutic interventions and one or more therapeutic interventions.
7. Provide theoretical rationale for interventions.
8. Comment on transference as it occurred.
9. Comment on countertransference as it occurred.
10. Plan modifications in interventions and rationale. (that is, what will you do next time?)
11. If session is tape-recorded identify sections of tape you want supervisor to focus upon with specific questions/comments.

E. **PERSONAL PSYCHOTHERAPY**

Personal psychotherapy is desirable for all graduate students to

1. Experience the client's side of the therapeutic alliance
2. Become aware of unresolved conflicts and resistances
3. Broaden students' range of self-awareness
4. Investigate factors underlying inappropriate responses to self, clients, and others

F. **COMPARISON OF PSYCHOTHERAPY AND SUPERVISION**

Similarities exist between psychotherapy and clinical supervision in that both are learning experiences. A comparison of supervision and psychotherapy is shown in Table 20–2.

Clinical Placement A. **AGENCY REQUIREMENTS**

The agency must have available the types of experiences that permit the student to meet the course objectives.

B. **SETTINGS**

Since graduate students have different past experiences and future goals, they choose the settings that meet their needs. Settings may include

1. Inpatient psychiatric unit in a general hospital
2. Inpatient psychiatric hospital
3. Community mental health center
4. Family service center
5. Child guidance and counseling center

Table 20–2

COMPARISON OF SUPERVISION AND PSYCHOTHERAPY

	Supervision	*Psychotherapy*
Objectives	1. Enhance quality of educational experience in relation to course objectives and learning needs 2. Learn therapy skills and dynamics of behavior 3. Become a psychotherapist	1. Achieve resolution of personal problems over time 2. Achieve self-awareness and self-knowledge over time
Focus	Assess, intervene, and evaluate work with clients	Explore personal experiences and resolve personal problems
Responses	Identify self-responses (thoughts, feelings, and behavior) that affect client positively and negatively	Identify self-responses (thoughts, feelings, and behavior) that affect self positively and negatively
Change	Identify and change behaviors that interfere with the therapeutic alliance	Explore and resolve personal problems
Evaluation	Assess work with client(s); expect a minimum learning level for the course	Assess degree of change in self and in response to others; progress occurs over time with no time limit

C. NEGOTIATION WITH STAFF

1. Students are given a list of agencies faculty have previously contacted or which have been used in the past.
2. Students select an agency from the list or choose another agency on the basis of current professional interests, future goals, and geographic proximity.
3. Students contact agency staff and discuss clinical experiences in relation to course objectives, performance expectations, and clinical hours (ideally 12–16 hours per week).
4. As needed, the clinical supervisor meets with agency staff to verify the student's status in the program, discuss the graduate program, and discuss the student's performance at the agency.

Evaluation of Clinical Experiences

Student and supervisor evaluate student's progress together in relation to the course objectives and student's goals. The student's ability to perform the following activities is evaluated:

1. Identify themes and problems within the client–student interaction
2. Identify functional and dysfunctional behaviors
3. Provide therapeutic interventions
4. Provide theoretical rationale for interventions
5. Analyze and evaluate the effectiveness of interventions
6. Plan modifications, as needed, in interventions and goals for treatment
7. Assess effects of medications on client
8. Participate with agency staff by communicating activities with clients and sharing knowledge at staff meetings

Doctoral Education

A. DESCRIPTION

Psychiatric nurses pursue doctoral education in one of three different programs:

1. Ph.D. or Ed.D. in education
2. Ph.D. in a related science, promoted in the 1960s by "nurse scientist" funds
3. Ph.D. or professional degree (D.N.S., D.N.Sc.) in nursing. This section will outline the elements for a Ph.D. in nursing, which is traditionally considered a research degree.[3]

B. GENERAL AIMS

1. Preparation of researchers
2. Advancement of theory in psychiatric–mental health nursing
3. Advanced preparation in clinical practice

C. CURRICULUM

This curriculum builds on the 2-year clinical master's degree in psychiatric mental health nursing described previously.

1. *Research preparation*—The student
   a. Selects a particular phenomenon, diagnosis, age group, intervention, and so forth as the basis for specialized study. For example, the student might focus on the event or situation of crisis, or the phenomenon of hallucinations, or an intervention, such as group therapy.
   b. Selects appropriate courses in related disciplines to provide an interdisciplinary approach to the problem
   c. Continues clinical practice to refine the problem

```
┌─────────────────────────────────────────────────────────────────┐
│  Chart 20–3                                                        │
│  EXAMPLE OF A DOCTORAL CURRICULUM IN PSYCHIATRIC–MENTAL HEALTH     │
│  NURSING                                                          │
└─────────────────────────────────────────────────────────────────┘
```

Fall	Spring
First Year	
Theory Development in Nursing (3)	Theory Development in Psychiatric–Mental Health Nursing (3)
Statistics (3)	Statistics or Computer Science (3)
Cognate (3)	Cognate/Nursing Elective (3)
Second Year	
Advanced Practicum (6)	Advanced Practicum (6)
Research—Problem Formulation (3)	Research—Design (3)
Cognate/Nursing Elective (3)	Data Analysis (3)
Third Year	
Dissertation (9)	Dissertation (9)

Note: Numbers indicate credits.

    d. Completes preparation in methodologies and statistics, including computer science

    e. Completes and orally defends a dissertation

2. *Theory development*—The student

    a. Develops knowledge of current nursing theories along with the ability to critique them

    b. Develops the ability to formulate theory from practice and research

    c. Develops knowledge about the formal structure of theories

3. *Clinical practice*—The student

    a. Develops advanced skills in a specialized area and objective study of clinical phenomena

    b. Completes eligibility for national certification by the end of the program

An example of a doctoral level curriculum in psychiatric–mental health nursing is shown in Chart 20–3.

References

1. Bruch H: Learning Psychotherapy: Rationale and Ground Rules. Cambridge, MA, Harvard University Press, 1974
2. Clark CC: Learning to negotiate the system. Nurs Outlook 1:39–42, 1977
3. O'Toole AW: Doctoral study for psychiatric nurses. Perspect Psychiatr Care 4:161–164, 1973
4. Passons WR: Gestalt Approaches in Counseling. New York, Holt, Rinehart, & Winston, 1975
5. Stetler C, Marram C: Evaluating research findings for applicability in practice. Nurs Outlook 9:559, 1976
6. Stiles L: Student self-direction and assessment. In Mathis BC, McGagie WC (eds): Profiles in College Teaching. Evanston, IL, Center for Teaching Professions, Northwestern University, 1972

Bibliography

Feather R, Bissell B: Clinical supervision versus psychotherapy: The psychiatric/mental health nursing process. Perspect Psychiatr Care 17:266, 1979
Martin EJ, Finneran MR: A teaching design: Standards of practice as a basis for peer review. Perspect Psychiatr Care 18:242, 1980

Part III

Therapeutic Modes

21

Individual Therapy

Suzanne Lego

OVERVIEW

Definition
Settings
Qualifications
Types
Role of the Therapist
Goals
Appropriate Clients
Phases
Key Concepts
Evaluation

Definition   Individual therapy is characterized as a relationship between two persons who engage in a confidential and primarily verbal series of interactions over a relatively prolonged period, with the agreed-upon purpose of change in the behavior of one participant.[2]

Settings   Nurses practice individual therapy in
1. Inpatient units
2. Outpatient clinics
3. Day hospitals and day treatment centers
4. Outreach settings
5. Private practice

Qualifications   The nurse who practices individual therapy
1. Is certified as a clinical specialist in psychiatric and mental health nursing or is in the process of becoming certified (see Chap. 18)
2. Is undergoing personal psychotherapy or has done so
3. Is participating in peer review or other supervision

Types   Three types of individual therapy have been described[4]:

A. **SUPPORTIVE**
Supportive therapy includes techniques such as guidance, reassurance, and relaxation with the aim of reinforcing strengths in the personality and helping clients to discover better control mechanisms and to adopt some kind of acceptable behavioral functioning.

B. **REEDUCATIVE**
Reeducative therapy includes behavior therapies and nondirective therapies with the aim of remodeling attitudes and behaviors in such a way as to increase the client's effectiveness.

C. **RECONSTRUCTIVE**
Reconstructive therapy includes exploratory, investigative, and psychoanalytic techniques designed to promote personality growth, alteration of the character structure, awareness of important unconscious conflicts, ego strengthening, emotional and interpersonal maturation, and the creation of new enabling potentials.
Since the first two categories are covered in other chapters of this book, the remainder of this chapter will refer to reconstructive therapy.

Role of the Therapist   The role of the therapist is to help the client to experience consciously those aspects of life that are unconscious or dissociated, but that appear in the form of symptoms or unsatisfactory life patterns. This is done through the establishment of an intimate professional relationship between the client and nurse over time.

Goals   A. **THE THERAPIST'S GOALS**
The therapist's goals are to[10]
1. Remove, modify, or retard existing symptoms
2. Mediate disturbed patterns of behavior
3. Promote positive personality growth and development

B. **THE CLIENT'S GOALS**
Clients usually begin therapy because of painful symptoms or because of dissatisfactions in their relationships with others or with their work. Therefore, their

general goals will be symptom relief or increased satisfaction with life. It is not a good idea in reconstructive therapy to set more explicit, specific goals than these for the following reasons[5]:

1. Clients do not always enter therapy for the reasons they state (and believe to be true).
2. Clients are often unable to formulate why they have come for therapy.
3. Clients often have very specific goals consciously, which are for a time unobtainable, owing to unconscious factors.
4. Goal setting implies a mechanical, problem solving approach, which can impede the process of exploring human experience.
5. Goal setting is antithetical to the natural process of the development of ongoing intimate relationships (of which the client–therapist relationship is one).
6. Goal setting implies a kind of "closure" about life which is limiting in itself.

Phases A. **INTRODUCTORY PHASE**[7]

In the introductory phase, which may last several months, the client and therapist examine one another closely to assess the "boundaries" of the relationship. The therapist is alert to the problems of the client and the characteristic ways of handling them. At the same time the client's strengths and attributes are being measured.

The client, in turn, is closely watching the nurse's ability to hear and understand what is being said. Both are aware of one another's ways of relating and are making the slight adjustments necessary to make each understood to the other. Once this method of communicating openly is established, the working phase of the relationship begins.

B. **WORKING PHASE**[7]

In the working phase, the client comes to the session prepared to talk about what is bothersome that day. This may include something that is currently happening, a memory of a past event or relationship, a recent dream, a recent fantasy, or thoughts or feelings about the therapist.

Anything the client brings up is considered "grist for the therapeutic mill." That is, all thoughts, feelings, dreams, and fantasies offer an entré into the client's unconscious or dissociated experience. By talking about them, clients become aware of wishes, feelings, conflicts, and desires of which they were not wholly aware. Over time, this material fits into a general pattern, which becomes clear to the nurse long before it is so clear to the client, by virtue of the fact that the nurse is an objective, though participant observer. As the pattern becomes clear, the nurse helps the client to see how the pattern manifests itself.

C. **TERMINATION PHASE**

1. The client and therapist agree that the client has reached maximum benefit (mutual termination)
2. The nurse must cease treating the client owing to geographical move, job change, and so forth (forced termination)
3. The client decides to stop treatment prematurely owing to resistance (premature termination)

During this period if the first or second reasons are responsible, the sessions may be concerned with separation, and the reawakening of early painful separations. If the client is stopping therapy prematurely, the nurse attempts to explore the reasons for the resistance.

Charts 21–1, 21–2, and 21–3 show client behaviors, interventions, and theoretical rationale in the introductory, working, and termination phases of individual therapy.

Key Concepts   The following are definitions of key concepts in individual therapy:

A. **CONTENT AND PROCESS**
   The content of a therapy session includes all that is *said,* and the process, all that is *done*. Elements of process include the sequence of topics, body language, voice level and tone, and so forth.

B. **TRANSFERENCE**
   Transference is the attribution to the therapist of feelings, wishes, and attitudes, originally felt *toward* or *by* the client's parents or significant others.

C. **COUNTERTRANSFERENCE**
   Countertransference occurs when the therapist experiences irrational, exaggerated, or unrealistic feelings toward the client, based on the therapist's own past life or current conflicts.[7]

Chart 21–1

POSSIBLE CLIENT BEHAVIORS, INTERVENTIONS, AND THEORETICAL RATIONALE IN THE INTRODUCTORY PHASE OF INDIVIDUAL THERAPY

Client Behavior	Intervention	Theoretical Rationale
1. The client enters the room and sits down, looking expectantly at the therapist.	1. The therapist suggests that the client tell why he/she is there. "Why don't you tell me what brings you here today" or "Tell me what has happened to bring you into the hospital."	1. Clients are very anxious at this time and need structure and a task to help them to begin and to relax.
2. The client tells about the symptoms or problems that have led to the need for treatment. (This may continue for weeks or months.)	2. The therapist mostly listens but may ask clarifying questions from time to time, and carefully observes the client's demeanor, attitude, level of anxiety, and ways of relating, carefully assessing the situation (see Chap. 1, 2, and 3).	2. Observations in the first session are very important, because they are "fresh" or "pure," that is, uncontaminated by the client's unconscious conformity to what is "expected."
3. The client asks explicitly or implicitly if there is any hope for change in the situation.	3. The therapist states that individual therapy is indicated and can be helpful. "I believe that by talking over what you are going through, things can change for the better. I suggest you come once a week".	3. The client's anxiety is reduced somewhat on learning that the situation is not terribly unusual and can be improved with therapy.
4. The client needs to know the practical details of therapy.	4. The therapist tells the client the time, place, and fee for therapy as well as how the therapist can be contacted. The client is told that it is important to attend sessions every time and to inform the therapist 24 hours in advance of any cancellation.	4. A professional "contract" conveys to the client the importance of the endeavor upon which they are about to embark, and clarifies mutual responsibilities.

D. RESISTANCE

Resistance occurs when powerful, often unconscious factors prevent clients from giving up defenses and distortions, often when the client is on the brink of insight.[7] Examples include silence, missed sessions, lateness, excessive intellectualization, and abrupt change of subject.

E. ACTING OUT

Acting out occurs when the client relives or reproduces through actions rather than words, the feelings, wishes, or conflicts operating unconsciously.[6]

F. INSIGHT

Insight occurs when the client connects unconscious feelings, wishes, and conflicts to conscious behavior.[6] This connection is emotional and experiential, not merely intellectual.

Chart 21–4 shows an example of each of the key concepts, the intervention, and theoretical rationale.

Chart 21–2

POSSIBLE CLIENT BEHAVIORS, INTERVENTIONS, AND THEORETICAL RATIONALE IN THE WORKING PHASE OF INDIVIDUAL THERAPY

Client Behavior	Intervention	Theoretical Rationale
1. The client begins the session by discussing • Symptom • Problem • Dream • Fantasy • Recent occurrence • Thoughts or feelings about the therapist	1. The therapist listens carefully, eliciting information as needed, for example • The client's notion of the meaning of the dream, symptom, and so forth • The client's associations to the dream, symptom, and so forth • What happened right before or on the day of the dream, symptom, and so forth	1. The therapist is vigilant not to take over the session or make premature interpretations. The less active the therapist, the more active the client. The therapist does offer associations and connections that are not readily available to the client by virtue of the client's resistance.
2. The client falls silent	2. The therapist gently encourages the client to verbalize thoughts and feelings.	2. The therapist demonstrates that the time is used to discuss any thoughts or feelings, even uncomfortable ones.
3. The client demonstrates in relating to the therapist the interpersonal problems that have brought the client into therapy (for example, manipulation or intimidation).	3. The therapist is careful not to fall into the client's pattern, but rather points out what is happening, even though this may cause the client to become angry, for example, "Are you trying to manipulate me now into doing what you want?"	3. The therapist is often the only person in the client's life who can be honest, straight, and direct with the client, since the therapist has no vested interest, that is, nothing to gain or lose by being honest.
4. The client demonstrates transference, resistance, acting out, and insight and may elicit countertransference responses.	4. See Chart 21–4.	4. See Chart 21–4.

Chart 21–3

POSSIBLE CLIENT BEHAVIORS, INTERVENTIONS, AND THEORETICAL RATIONALE IN THE TERMINATION PHASE OF INDIVIDUAL THERAPY

Client Behavior	Intervention	Theoretical Rationale
Mutual Termination The client's symptoms have disappeared, interpersonal relationships are satisfying, work is rewarding, and the client is able to change things that need to be changed and let alone those that cannot be changed. The client looks forward to the future with pleasure.	The therapist reinforces the client's accomplishments, pointing out that "ups and downs" may occur as a natural part of life, but that the client will be able to handle these.	No one is ever totally free of all irrationality, and to expect this will lead to disappointment and frustration.
Forced Termination The client may experience strong positive feelings along with negative feelings toward the therapist for leaving.	The therapist encourages the expression and exploration of both, connecting these to earlier feelings. "You must feel abandoned by me and very angry," and then, "Does this remind you of an earlier time?"	The therapist's leaving is bound to arouse earlier feelings of actual separation or emotional abandonment. The client profits from expressing these feelings and "surviving" them and from seeing that separation can also be survived.
Premature Termination The client states that therapy is not working or that another therapist or another kind of therapy would be better. Often the client states, "I need a vacation from therapy."	The therapist helps the client to explore the client's feelings in great detail, alert to the signs of unconscious resistance. Attention is paid to what has been discussed recently and to what has been happening in *process* between the client and therapist.	Premature termination is usually caused by resistance. Resistance occurs when the client is on the brink of change or insight. If this prospective change can be examined and allowed to happen, the client may not need to terminate. Sometimes clients are reluctant to change and grow in front of one therapist and must move on to the next. This is because the client fears the withdrawal of parental love if separation and growth occur.

Evaluation   The nurse is constantly evaluating the client's progress throughout therapy. Evaluation is tricky because the relief of symptoms does not always mean the client is "better" and an increase of anxiety does not always mean the client is worse. Typically the therapy runs the following course:

A. **HONEYMOON STAGE**

A honeymoon stage occurs, during which the client feels amazingly better. This is caused by the feeling of relief at being heard and understood and the richness of honest, open communication.

B. **AGGRESSIVE STAGE**

During an aggressive stage, the client experiences long buried anger and resentment, which may be expressed toward the therapist or significant others.

C. **REGRESSIVE STAGE**

During a regressive stage, the client begins to give up defenses that have warded off anxiety and begins to feel very anxious and almost "raw."

Chart 21–4
KEY CONCEPT, EXAMPLE, INTERVENTION, AND THEORETICAL RATIONALE IN INDIVIDUAL THERAPY

Example of Concept	*Intervention*	*Theoretical Rationale*
Content and Process Interplay The client complains in her session that her husband is always mad at her for her irresponsibility and that he constantly demeans her and treats her like a child. In process, she is late for every session, often misses sessions, forgets her insurance forms, forgets to pay the therapist, and so forth.	The therapist points out that the client portrays for the therapist the very behavior she is describing that annoys her husband. An attempt is made to help the client figure out how she learned to use this childlike behavior in earlier life and how it continues to serve her unconsciously now in her adult life. The therapist is careful not to pass judgment on the behavior, or to urge the client to stop.	It is inevitable that the client exhibit in the nurse–client relationship those behaviors that have brought the client into treatment. If the therapist has a stake in getting the client to stop acting a certain way, the client will either conform simply to please the therapist or will rebel. Neither behavior is growth promoting.
Transference (positive) The client tells the therapist that he was kind to the therapist in a past session because he did not want to hurt or disappoint the therapist. His mother was a hysterical, erratic person who frequently used guilt to control the client.	The therapist points out that the client is treating the therapist as though she were his mother, and questions whether this occurs in other situations.	Because the therapist is seen as an authority figure by the client, the situation is reminiscent of the parent–child relationship. The inevitable distortions, when analyzed in therapy, help the client to recognize the distortions that occur in all aspects of the client's life.
Transference (negative) The client accuses the therapist of disliking her and treating her meanly because she holds a different opinion from the therapist. The client had an overbearing mother.	1. The therapist points out that this behavior would be in keeping with the mother's usual behavior, and that the therapist is not aware of any such feelings. There is an examination of how this might occur in other situations. 2. The therapist is always careful to entertain the possibility that there may be some truth to the client's assertion. If there is, and countertransference does occur, this is explored in the manner described below.	1. It is both inevitable and useful when the client distorts the therapist's behavior in line with the past behavior of parents or significant others. It is through this distortion and its exploration that the client begins to see a pattern of distortions in all relationships. Early longings, fears, and other strong feelings are brought to light in the process. 2. Clients who are schizophrenic or borderline are acutely attuned to the therapist's unconscious.
Countertransference (positive) The therapist finds herself being overly protective and "helpful" to the client, and feels happy when the client appears to appreciate her.	1. The therapist examines why it is important to her that the client appreciate and love her. 2. She is alert to the behaviors in the *client* that elicit this kind of helping behavior. For example, does the client seem helpless in situations when he is not? She does not hide her reaction if it has been observed by the client.	1. Positive feelings from the client often supply narcissistic gratification for the therapist, and provide needs that the therapist missed early in life. 2. However, it is useful for the client to see how his behavior affects others in a situation in which the therapist is open and direct.

(continued)

Chart 21–4
(continued)

Example of Concept	Intervention	Theoretical Rationale

Countertransference (negative)
The therapist becomes exasperated and angry when the client acts narcissistic, provocative, and controlling. These are all behaviors the therapist has struggled to give up himself with some but not total success.
	1. The therapist examines internally and with a therapist, supervisor, or colleague, the meaning of his overreaction to the client's behavior. He realizes that he is resentful that the client is still able to "get away" with this behavior that he is working so hard to overcome. He is mad at the "unfairness" of the situation and at being reached by the client, and reminded of his *own* humaness.
	2. He examines with the client the meaning of the client's behavior vis-à-vis their relationship. For example, what does it mean to the client? He does not attempt to deny his reaction when it has been observed by the client.
		1. Therapists become irrationally angry at clients when clients
		  a. Display behavior they are displeased with in themselves
		  b. Display the therapist's own defenses or unconscious behavior in a clumsy, transparent way
		  c. Display behavior toward the therapist reminiscent of behavior the therapist's parents or significant others displayed
		2. The therapist tries to represent a stable, realistic reference point uncontaminated by the therapist's distortions. However, it is useful for the client to see how his behavior affects others, in a situation in which the therapist is open and direct.

Acting out
The client, who is struggling in therapy with ambivalent feelings about her parents and strong sibling rivalry, enters an affair with her college professor.
	The therapist helps the client to recognize those feelings that are being acted upon, without attempting to stop the client's acting out.
	
	As the feelings are explored and openly experienced by the client, the acting out stops.
		Acting out provides excellent grist for the therapeutic mill. As it progresses, feelings are brought to the surface for exploration.
		
		If the therapist attempts to stop the acting out, the client
		  a. Is deprived of valuable analytic material
		  b. May conform or rebel and leave treatment. Neither is useful.

Insight The client tells of an incident that in the past would have intimidated him and caused much anxiety. He reports that instead he was able to handle it in an adult, direct way by simply stating his needs and how he planned to proceed. "I found I didn't need to act like a scared child. I could be an adult and no harm came to me."	The therapist reinforces this positive behavior and brings up any other aspects of the situation that could be further explored.	Insight is the anticipated end result of reconstructive therapy. True emotional insight has occurred when, by and large, the problem behavior or symptoms stop. However, regressions occur from time to time, an no one is ever perfectly "healthy" or absolutely "cured."

D. **ADAPTIVE STAGE**

During an adaptive stage, the client has begun to resolve major problems and is trying out new kinds of behavior.

"Evaluation" at any of these stages could be misleading.

Freud once said that therapy is successful if the client is able to love and to work. This remains a good general criterion for positive outcome in individual psychotherapy.

References

1. American Nurses Association, Division on Psychiatric and Mental Health Nursing Practice: Standards of Psychiatric and Mental Health Nursing Practice. Kansas City, MO, American Nurses Association, 1982
2. Ford DH, Urban HB: Systems of Psychotherapy. New York, John Wiley & Sons, 1964
3. Fromm-Reichman F: Principles of Intensive Psychotherapy. Chicago, University of Chicago Press, 1950
4. Herron WG, Rouslin S: Issues in Psychotherapy. Bowie, MD, Robert J Brady, 1982
5. Lego S: Explicit goal setting: Is it appropriate in psychotherapy? Proceedings of Second Southeastern Regional Conference of Psychiatric/Mental Health Clinical Specialists, Charleston, SC, April 1980
6. Lego S: Group psychotherapy. In Haber J et al (eds): Comprehensive Psychiatric Nursing, 2nd ed. New York, McGraw-Hill, 1982
7. Lego S: The clinical specialist and the client in individual and group therapy. In Critchley DL, Maurin, JT (eds): The Psychiatric Mental Health Clinical Specialist: Theory, Research, and Practice. New York, John Wiley & Sons, 1984
8. Searles HF: Collected Papers on Schizophrenia and Related Subjects. New York, International Universities Press, 1965
9. Sullivan HS: Schizophrenia as a Human Process. New York, WW Norton & Co, 1962
10. Wolberg LR: The Technique of Psychotherapy, 3rd ed. New York, Grune & Stratton, 1977

Bibliography

Bruch H: Learning Psychotherapy. Cambridge, MA, Harvard University Press, 1974

Field WE (ed): The Psychotherapy of Hildegard E. Peplau. New Braunfels, TX, PSF Productions, 1979

Lego S: An anxious young man. In Riffle K (ed): Rehabilitative Nursing Care Studies. New York, Medical Examination Publishing Co, 1979

Lego S: Treatment of the Acting Out Borderline Patient in Private Practice. Clinical and Scientific Sessions, Nashville 1979. Kansas City, MO, American Nurses Association, 1979

Lego S: Beginning resolution of the oedipal conflict in a lesbian who is about to become a "parent" to a son. Perspect Psychiatr Care 19:107, 1981

Lego S: The Nurse Psychotherapist and the Advanced Nurse Practitioner. Presented at Perspectives in Psychiatric Care '80. Available on tape cassette, Teach 'em, 160 East Illinois Street, Chicago, IL 60611

Lego S: The one-to-one nurse–patient relationship. Perspect Psychiatr Care 18:67, 1980

Slipp S (ed): Curative Factors in Dynamic Psychotherapy. New York, McGraw-Hill, 1982

22

Group

Therapy

Suzanne Lego

Description	Intensive or reconstructive group psychotherapy is a method of therapeutic intervention based on the exploration and analysis of both individual and intrapsychic structures and the group process. As individuals interact in a group over time, they are able to observe their own and each other's secret wishes, conflicts, and motivations. An understanding of these unconscious processes and the way they are acted upon with others can help clients to adopt more satisfying modes of interaction. In intensive group psychotherapy, members' behavior is continually examined, keeping in mind that the group is a microcosm of the larger world.

Other Types of Group Psychotherapy

A. **EDUCATIVE THERAPY**

Leader presents fixed content in lectures or written material, which is then discussed by clients (for example, medication education or women's awareness groups).

B. **SUPPORTIVE THERAPY**

Supportive therapy uses clients' present ego strength and further strengthens it through support and encouragement in order to help clients repress problems more successfully.

Selection of Members

A. **NUMBER**

Seven has been found to be the ideal number for maximum interaction in a therapy group. It is helpful to select ten clients, because some attrition will occur. If there are more than ten members, the group tends to subdivide.

B. **HETEROGENEITY**

The more heterogeneous the group, the better. Members should vary in age, gender, and psychodynamics. Exceptions to this rule are psychotic, alcoholic, and drug-addicted clients.

1. *Age*—Members should be 20 and over. When clients come from different "generations," there is a greater likelihood of transference of feelings about their own parents or children.
2. *Gender*—Interaction with both genders helps clients to recognize and work through feelings about both men and women.
3. *Psychodynamics*—A variety of styles helps members to view their own lives from different vantage points and to help one another do so.
4. *Difficult clients*—In the past, schizophrenics and borderline clients have been considered inappropriate for group psychotherapy. This is not necessarily so.[2,4] However, it is recommended that beginning therapists refrain from treating borderline clients in group, since they present many challenging problems. Sociopathic clients are not appropriate for group psychotherapy because they are often disruptive to the group and are unable to relate in a way helpful to themselves.

Creation of the Group

Chart 22–1 lists nursing actions in organizing a psychotherapy group and gives a theoretical rationale for each action.

Group Leadership

A. **ROLE**

The role of the group leader is to stimulate group interaction and the group's analysis of the interaction. This is done by making observations of individual dynamics and group dynamics. The leader never does anything for the group that

Chart 22–1
NURSING ACTIONS AND RATIONALE WHEN ORGANIZING PSYCHOTHERAPY GROUPS

Nursing Action	Theoretical Rationale
All prospective members are seen at least once individually before admission to the group. (The more times they are seen, the better.)	A libidinal tie will develop between the client and nurse. This tie helps clients to remain in the group later, when they become anxious.
Clients are not seen in group only, without individual sessions as well.	Group psychotherapy produces anxiety, which spills over at times outside the group. This anxiety can motivate clients to explore their reactions in individual sessions.
Before entering the group, the client is not prepared for what happens in the group or who will be there. Only a general statement is made such as, "The group is a place to discuss feelings, problems, or reactions."	If the client knows a great deal about the group in advance, spontaneous reactions are lost to exploration. These spontaneous reactions are "grist for the therapeutic mill."
Group members are not told about new members before they appear.	Their spontaneous or irrational response to the new member is useful to explore (for example, this may be reminiscent of the birth of a sibling).
Group members sit in chairs in a circle. No table is used, nor does anyone sit on the floor.	All members should be visible to one another. This increases anxiety slightly, which leads to more irrational behavior and its subsequent observation. It also aids in the observation of nonverbal communication, which can then be explored.
The leader changes seats each session, causing other members to shift seats.	Members should not be able to find a comfortable "niche" in which to hide.
Weekly sessions last 1½ hours, and daily sessions last 1 hour.	When groups meet only once a week, resistance builds between sessions, and it may take 45 minutes for work to begin. When groups meet daily, the resistance is less.
Sessions begin and end on time.	Clients pace their reactions according to this time frame. This pacing in itself is interesting to note, for example, when a client reports in the last 5 minutes that he has quit his job.
The same leader leads the group.	Group process is based on a balance of forces that takes the leader into account. Changing leaders seriously changes this balance and makes interaction more superficial.
Observers do not sit in the group.	This disturbs the ongoing balance and process, causing more superficiality.
Open-ended groups are more effective than time-limited groups. The group continues indefinitely, with replacements made as members leave.	When members know there are only a certain number of sessions left, they remain more controlled and superficial.

members can do for themselves. For example, members are not called upon by the leader to speak or introduced to one another. Instead of asking, "John, why don't you tell us about yourself?" the leader would wait several sessions for John to speak. If he failed to do so, the leader would comment, "John, I notice you seem to have trouble talking here. Do you have any idea why?" The principle here is that, rather than being a boss or guide, the leader is a stimulator. Table 22–1 shows the relationship between the leader's behavior and the group's development.[3]

From this table it can be seen that the leader must remain somewhat behind the scene in regard to what happens in the group. The first session sets the stage for this. The leader lets the group begin on its own, instead of suggesting introductions or describing the purpose of group therapy. In this way, members will

Table 22–1
RELATIONSHIP BETWEEN LEADERSHIP OF GROUP AND GROUP'S DEVELOPMENT

Type of Leader	Group Interaction Phenomena	Production Range of the Group
Boss: Plans, controls, directs, and decides autocratically.	Group submits, conforms when told what to do, has little influence on things except in a passive way.	From nothing useful to support of leader's irrational needs.
Guide: Plans, controls, and steers, usually subtly and indirectly.	Group can register differences, initiate complaints, and make requests. Group participates in thinking and forming opinions, makes minor decisions. Group has some active influence, but little responsibility.	Limited to leader's capacity.
Stimulator: Educates, facilitates production and communication, balances group forces, and shares leadership.	Group generates ideas, sets limits, and establishes methods. Group sets no limits on productivity and development of members. Group has primary responsibilities, uses self-evaluation, has healthy group spirit, is creative and productive.	Can be expected to go beyond leader's capacity to members' maximum potential.

(From Lego S: Group psychotherapy. In Haber J et al (eds): Comprehensive Psychiatric Nursing, 2nd ed. New York, McGraw-Hill, 1982. Reproduced with permission.)

catch on from the beginning that the group is their responsibility. The leader avoids an ''I am the expert'' attitude and comments only with observations that no one else has made or seems ready to make. Table 22–2 shows leader's behaviors that inhibit growth and those that promote growth.[3]

B. **QUALIFICATIONS**
1. The American Nurses Association suggests that nurses who practice group psychotherapy should hold a master's degree in psychiatric nursing.
2. Nurses who are group psychotherapists should be certified as clinical nurse specialists, or should be in the process of becoming certified.
3. As a part of graduate study, certification, and professional development in general, nurses will find these activities helpful in their preparation:
   a. Didactic preparation—Courses in group theory and group psychotherapy theory
   b. Ongoing intensive supervision over time
   c. A personal group experience over time

C. **LEADER'S EXPECTATIONS OF CLIENTS**
The leader has certain expectations of clients, some of which are voiced by the leader at the outset and others which are discussed as the event occurs. This is because giving a list of ''rules'' at the beginning creates an authority–subordinate ''atmosphere'' and because the expectations might cause undue anxiety in the clients. Chart 22–2 shows leader's expectations of clients, possible client behavior, and appropriate leader interventions.[3]

Table 22–2

GROWTH-INHIBITING BEHAVIORS (TO BE AVOIDED BY LEADERS) AND GROWTH-PROMOTING ALTERNATIVES

Growth-Inhibiting Behaviors	Growth-Promoting Behaviors
Starting sessions by introducing members or explaining the purpose of group therapy.	Waiting for members to begin on their own. Avoiding lengthy explanations of anything.
Bringing food or drink for group members.	Exploring dependency needs in the context of the group and the members' lives outside the group.
Calling on specific members to talk.	Allowing silences to continue until a group member breaks them, or after a few minutes, commenting on the silence. Allowing other members to deal with consistently silent members.
"Going around" the group, requiring that each member talk in turn.	Allowing members to talk at random as they please.
Pushing for closure on a topic or summing up sessions at the end.	Realizing that there is no "final solution." Allowing issues to be discussed, explored, examined by anyone in the group, with interest and respect shown to all. Allowing sessions to end "up in the air," with some members feeling anxious.

(From Lego S: Group psychotherapy. In Haber J et al (eds): Comprehensive Psychiatric Nursing, 2nd ed. New York, McGraw-Hill, 1982. Reproduced with permission.)

Chart 22–2

LEADER'S EXPECTATIONS OF CLIENTS, POSSIBLE CLIENT BEHAVIOR, AND LEADER INTERVENTION

Expectation	Possible Client Behavior	Appropriate Leader Intervention
Members will attend every session or tell leader beforehand if they must miss one. (Voiced by leader.)	Leave message with another client, secretary, or answering service.	Tells members they must speak to leader directly. Explores need to avoid leader in this case.
	Miss sessions without notice.	Asks members about absence. Explores meaning if appropriate.
	Call to cancel with vague excuse ("I'm not feeling up to it.").	Strongly encourages members to come anyway, pointing out that not feeling well may be related to feelings about the group.
Members will be as open as possible. (Not voiced by leader.)	Conscious deception. Members feel one way (for example, angry) but act another (for example, sweet).	Point out inconsistency: "You look angry, but you're acting sweet."
	Unconscious deception. Member seems to feel one way but does not seem aware of it and acts another.	Point out inconsistency or question in a gentle way: "Are you sure you're not angry?"
No physical violence will occur. (Not voiced by leader.)	Members threaten violence.	State that physical violence is not allowed, but encourage verbal exploration of reason for violent feelings.

Chart 22–2
(continued)

Expectation	Possible Client Behavior	Appropriate Leader Intervention
Members will not discuss group matters outside the group with those who are concerned in these matters. (Not voiced by leader.)	Members break group confidentiality.	Explore this in the group.
Members will not meet outside the group, or if they do, they will discuss their meetings in the group. (Not voiced by leader.)	Two members form a sexual relationship.	Intensive exploration in the group of the meaning of the relationship vis-a-vis the group itself, the leader, and past relationships with significant others.
	Two members of the group appear to be attracted to one another.	Intensive exploration of the relationship in the group, as above, in order to "nip it in the bud" and deal with the motivation rather than have it acted out.

(From Lego S: Group psychotherapy. In Haber J et al (eds): Comprehensive Psychiatric Nursing, 2nd ed. New York, McGraw-Hill, 1982. Reproduced with permission.)

D. **PROBLEMS OF BEGINNING LEADERS**

Beginning leaders often feel anxious. This anxiety is reflected in a need to maintain a good self-image and the need to maintain control of the group. Table 22–3 lists ways in which each of these irrational needs may be expressed in the leader's behavior. Supervision is helpful in working through these problems.[3]

Phases of Development   The growth of a group follows four stages of development. There is sometimes overlap, but in general the group moves through phases of uncertainty, overaggressiveness, regression, and adaptation. When new members join an ongoing group, they move through these phases as individuals.

Table 22–3
COMMON IRRATIONAL AND NONPRODUCTIVE NEEDS OF BEGINNING GROUP PSYCHOTHERAPISTS

Need to Maintain a "Good" Self-image
  Need to be liked
  Need to avoid exposing self as "human"
  Need to impress group with knowledge and authority

Need to Maintain Control of the Group
  Need to prevent group disintegration
  Need to prevent regressive behavior
  Need to prevent resistance
  Need to prevent expression of hostility
  Need to prevent acting out
  Need to avoid "taboo" topics
  Need to prevent intensive, multiple transference reactions
  Need to prevent the examination of individual or subgroup problems
  Need to restrict process that does not "go through" the therapist

(From Lego S: Group psychotherapy. In Haber J et al (eds): Comprehensive Psychiatric Nursing, 2nd ed. New York, McGraw-Hill, 1982. Reproduced with permission.)

Chart 22–3
BEHAVIOR, EXAMPLES, AND LEADER INTERVENTION IN THE UNCERTAINTY PHASE

Behavior	Example	Leader Intervention
Initial anxiety	Pacing the floor. Leaving and returning. Hallucinations and delusions. Excessive intellectualization. Organization of a "group plan".	Comment about the anxiety. Question what members fear happening in the group.
Demands on leader to explain purpose or provide structure	"Do we begin now?" "What is supposed to happen here?" "How does this work?"	Communicate to members that it is their group. ("Let's see how things go.")
Competition	Comparison among members of past group experience, past number of years of psychotherapy, knowledge of the leader, and so forth.	Point out that competition is taking place, being careful to communicate that it is not wrong and should not necessarily stop just because it is noted.
Excessive politeness	Members feel anxious and angry about the lack of structure from the leader, but they are afraid to show this. Instead, they react with inappropriate kindness. To a monopolizer: "You certainly are talkative today."	Note the covert feeling and ask if it is present. ("Are you a little irritated by all that talking?") Encourage openness rather than politeness.
Silence	All members sit for 5 minutes staring at the floor or occasionally glancing at each other.	Comment on the silence: ("I guess everyone is afraid to start.") Comment on some nonverbal behavior. ("Mary, I notice you're staring at John. Do you wish he'd speak?")
Questions about the leader's personal life, qualifications, and competence	Member asks: "Are you a mother?"	"No. Are you afraid I won't know how to care for you because I'm not?"
	Member asks: "Are you an MD?"	"No, I'm a psychiatric nurse. Are you afraid I won't know enough to do things right?"
Avoidance of involvement in the group	Schizophrenic member talks to voices instead of other group members. Members intellectualize about their problems. Members adopt roles which were used in their families to reduce anxiety but which are not appropriate in the current group (for example, the buffoon, the boss, the incompetent person, the ingenue).	Comment that these are methods to avoid reacting emotionally to the current group. Explore why this is feared and avoided.
Strong, irrational reactions to the leader	The leader is seen as a "savior" with all the answers.	Explore why a "savior" is necessary.
	The leader is seen as using power to manipulate or humiliate members and as having a secret reason for every comment or move.	Explore the meaning of these ideas in the context of the members' lives.

(From Lego S: Group psychotherapy. In Haber J et al (eds): Comprehensive Psychiatric Nursing, 2nd ed. New York, McGraw-Hill, 1982. Reproduced with permission.)

Uncertainty (1–20 sessions). In this phase, group members are anxious and attempt to carve out a place for themselves in the group. Many demands are made on the leader to provide structure. When the leader does not give in to these demands, members become angry. Chart 22–3 shows typical client behaviors and leader interventions with each.[3]

Overaggression. In this phase, members have begun to understand how the group operates. As a defense against the regression and adaptation soon to follow, the members become aggressive toward one another and toward the leader. Often the aggression expressed toward one another is actually meant for the leader. In this phase, members also begin to feel attracted to one another. This, in turn, leads to aggression, for members unconsciously fear the closeness that may result from the attraction. See Chart 22–4 for behaviors and leader interventions in the overaggressive phase.[3]

Chart 22–4
BEHAVIOR, EXAMPLES, AND LEADER INTERVENTION IN THE OVERAGGRESSIVE PHASE

Behavior	Example	Leader Intervention
Criticism of one another	One member who is very lonely but who leads the life of the happy, sophisticated swinger is critical of another member whose isolation and loneliness are all too stark and evident.	Ask whether the "swinger" is reminded of herself by the isolated member. Explore their similarities and the resultant anxiety.
	One member becomes enraged when another acts stubborn and inpenetrable.	Ask whether there was someone else in the member's life that he could not "get through" to.
Anger at one another for using their own defenses in a clumsy way	One obsessional member begins sentences with "Please don't think I'm trying to be controlling but . . ." Another obsessional says "Don't warn us so obviously. It only calls our attention to the fact that you are!"	Point out the dynamic that people feel their own defenses should be used only in their own unique way and are spoiled or "exposed" if used "incorrectly."
Ganging up	One member who is secretly anxious about almost everything arrives late to group each week, giving various weak excuses. He refuses to acknowledge that he might have wanted to miss part of a session or that he may have wanted to stir everyone up.	Examine and explore both sides of the process, why the member is so provocative as well as why members cannot resist being provoked.
Hostility toward the leader	Clients distort the leader's behavior: ("You do nothing to help us.") Clients point out real eccentricities of the leader. ("You are too compulsive!")	Accept their hostility in a nondefensive way. Avoid a win–lose approach. Weaknesses and eccentricities may be acknowledged freely. It is often a great relief to members to see that the leader is human and does not mind if this shows.

(From Lego S: Group psychotherapy. In Haber J et al (eds): Comprehensive Psychiatric Nursing, 2nd ed. New York, McGraw-Hill, 1982. Reproduced with permission.)

Regression. At this point in group development, earlier defenses are put aside and members experience pure anxiety, anger at more primitive sources, dependency, fear, longing, envy, jealousy, and other forms of pain. Members no longer feel the need to be in control (although there may still be unconscious resistance). Regression is no longer used as manipulation, but rather occurs spontaneously. Members are often surprised at the emotional reactions that they experience when others regress. Members who regress are often surprised at the support they receive, because they have previously believed that to lose control would be disastrous. In this phase, the leader comes to be seen as a resource person and as a human being.[3]

Adaptation. Members in this phase accept one another in spite of their weaknesses and faults. As a result, defenses are lowered, and in this atmosphere of acceptance, members are able to explore their conflicts more openly. This mutual acceptance can be a disadvantage because members may become ''immune'' to one another's neuroses. This is why the leader must continue to ''stir up the dust'' and poke at members' defenses. Open-ended groups are advantageous in that new members are occasionally admitted and bring a fresh perspective to old patterns.[3]

Group Cohesiveness   Group cohesiveness is a feeling of ''belonging'' which is very important in group life. Cohesiveness has been described as ''the resultant of all factors which act on members to remain in the group.''[1] Forces to remain in the group may come from the following:

1. The group members tend to encourage one another to remain in the group. All want to believe that the group is right for them and must validate this by convincing one another.
2. The tie to the leader acts upon members to keep them in the group. This tie may have both healthy and neurotic aspects.
3. Significant others outside the group may urge the members to continue, observing that the group is having a positive effect on the member.
4. The client may experience internal pulls based on the satisfactions felt in the group.

When group cohesiveness has occurred, there are observable signs. These appear in Table 22–4.[3]

Group cohesiveness cannot be artificially produced through exercises that are designed to move members quickly through the phases of development. Positive and negative emotions must be experienced in their own good time as they emerge naturally. There are, however, ways to promote cohesiveness within the natural group process. These are listed in Table 22–5.[3]

Content and Process   The *content* in group psychotherapy consists of all that is *said* in a session, and the *process* is all that *occurs*. Examples of process include

1. All nonverbal communication, such as body posture, who speaks to whom, and so forth
2. The order in which topics are brought up

Clients often act out in process what they have described in content. For example, a client may present herself as a ''victim'' in her relations with her family. However, as she talks and interacts in the group it becomes clear through process that she unconsciously sets up situations in which she plays the victim role, although actually she powerfully controls events. The group therapist is alert to this interweaving of content and process and carefully points this out when it is appropriate.

Table 22–4
SIGNS OF GROUP COHESIVENESS

Meetings outside the group	Members want to go for coffee after meetings.
Resentment of new members	Old members act closer than usual and discuss, without an explanation, matters which are unknown to new member or that are sexually or highly emotionally charged.
Rescuing the leader when under attack	When one member is critical of the leader for giving ''bad advice'', other members point out that it was not advice but rather exploration.
Control of monopolizers	When one member monopolizes, the others point this out and do not permit it to continue.
Looking down on those outside the group	Members state how lucky they are to be in this particular group.
Acceptance of other members even though they are disliked	One member is domineering. The others work around her bossiness and, without strong hostility, cheerfully tease her about it.

(From Lego S: Group psychotherapy. In Haber J et al (eds): Comprehensive Psychiatric Nursing, 2nd ed. New York, McGraw-Hill, 1982. Reproduced with permission.)

Table 22–5
WAYS TO PROMOTE COHESIVENESS, WITH EXAMPLES

Ways to Promote Cohesiveness	*Examples*
Make group personally rewarding.	Clarifying observations about group or individual behavior which help members understand themselves better. Pointing out to members that they seem healthier or different.
Promote usefulness of other members whether they are liked or not.	Pointing out that an unpopular member is only a symbol of significant other or oneself and therefore useful in helping work out one's own conflicts. Pointing out the ''good'' qualities of an unpopular member.
Make activities attractive.	Subtly rewarding clients for helping others to recognize distortions or clarifying issues by saying, ''Mary has a good point,'' and so on.

(From Lego S: Group psychotherapy. In Haber J et al (eds): Comprehensive Psychiatric Nursing, 2nd ed. New York, McGraw-Hill, 1982. Reproduced with permission.)

Central Concepts of Group Psychotherapy   There are four central concepts that are crucial to the practice of group psychotherapy. They are transference and countertransference, resistance, acting out, and insight. In Chart 22–5 each concept is defined, an example is given, and guidelines for intervention are presented.

Termination   Termination ideally occurs when both the client and the therapist believe that the client has reached maximum benefit. Freud once stated that this is when the client is able to "love and work." Prior to termination, clients usually relate to others in a

---

Chart 22–5
CONCEPT, EXAMPLE, AND INTERVENTION IN GROUP PSYCHOTHERAPY

Example of Concept	*Example of Intervention*
Transference	
The client says that the therapist prefers all the other members over her. In reality, this has never entered the therapist's mind, and on reflection, she does not believe this to be true.	The leader asks the client what this is all about. As other members explore this with the client, it is learned that she had a "Cinderella" role in her large family. When the client's distortion is questioned by a group of people who do not believe the distortion, the client is able to view the situation more realistically.
Countertransference	
The therapist experiences the client as hostile, or very special, or inadequate, and feels strongly about these attributes.	The leader explores silently, or with a therapist, supervisor, colleague, or so forth, what this is about. It is likely that the client does show some of these attributes and that these serve some neurotic purpose for the client. This should be explored openly in the group, for example: "Mary, you seem to be trying to control what happens here today." The strong emotional reaction of the leader to the client must be worked through by the leader, apart from the client.
Resistance	
The client begins to miss sessions or to come late just after the birth of her first child. She tells the group that she is so happy at home with her husband and new baby that she hates to come to group and get all "stirred up" again.	The leader encourages a discussion of the resistance in the group. Most members enter into discussion because this is a familiar feeling. It is revealed that the client identifies with the new infant's own narcissism and omnipotence and is especially sensitive to the disruptions of this fantasy world that occur in group sessions. This discussion continues for a few sessions, and the resistance passes.
Acting Out	
A client secretly desires a close, special relationship with the therapist. Instead, she enters an affair with a group member.	The leader brings this matter up in the group or encourages the members who are involved to do so. The meaning of the behavior is explored and analyzed by the group. As this is discussed, members become aware consciously of the real feelings, wishes, and conflicts that were previously only acted on without an understanding of their meaning. The acting out loses its "kick" as understanding occurs, and the acting out stops.
Insight	
A client has been very angry at her husband, whom she loves and admires. She is puzzled by the anger because she experiences him as loving and kind. She finds herself picking on him for no reason.	The client describes the situation in group, saying, "I thought that marriage to a wonderful person would make my life complete. But it hasn't. He hasn't! He has let me down by not giving me total fulfillment!" As she tells this, she is very moved, as are all the group members. This insight into her irrational anger is further enhanced by continuing discussion of her experience.

nondefensive way and show other signs of healthy self-esteem. There is satisfaction with life on the whole and a realization of those unsatisfying areas that cannot be changed. There is contentment in self-directed pleasures as well as happiness in relationships with others. Group members can be helpful to clients who want to terminate by pointing out resolved as well as unresolved areas.[3]

References

1. Cartwright D: The nature of group cohesiveness. In Cartwright D, Zander A (eds): Group Dynamics. New York, Harper & Row, 1960
2. Geller JJ: Group psychotherapy in the treatment of schizophrenic syndromes. Psychiatr Q 63:1, 1963
3. Haber J et al (eds): Comprehensive Psychiatric Nursing, 2nd ed. New York, McGraw-Hill, 1982
4. Lego S: Treatment of the acting out borderline patient in private practice. In Clinical and Scientific Sessions, Nashville, 1979, Kansas City, MO, American Nurses Association, 1979

Bibliography

Greenfield RC: Trial by fire: Rites of passage in psychotherapy groups. Perspect Psychiatr Care 12:152, 1974

Hankins-McNary L: The use of humor in group therapy. Perspect Psychiatr Care 17:228, 1979

Horowitz JA: Sexual difficulties as indicators of broader personal and interpersonal problems (as reflected in the psychotherapy group). Perspect Psychiatr Care 16:66, 1978

Joyce C: The religious as group therapists: Attitudes and conflicts. Perspect Psychiatr Care 15:112, 1977

LaSor B, Phanidis J, Webster MS: Point: Bring those outside observers in, Counterpoint: Don't bring those outside observers in. Perspect Psychiatr Care 20:13, 1980

Lego S: The clinical specialist and the client in individual and group therapy. In Critchley D, Mavrin J (eds): The Psychiatric Mental Health Clinical Specialist: Theory, Research and Practice. New York, John Wiley & Sons, 1984

Light N: The "chronic helper" in group therapy. Perspect Psychiatr Care 12:129, 1974

Sattin SM: The psychodynamics of the holiday syndrome. Perspect Psychiatr Care 13:156, 1975

Ward JT: The sounds of silence: Group therapy with non-verbal patients. Perspect Psychiatr Care 12:13, 1974

White EM, Kahn EM: Use and modifications in group psychotherapy with chronic schizophrenic outpatients. J Psychosoc Nurs 20:14, 1982

23

Marital

Therapy

Cynthia M. Taylor

Description	Marital therapy is not merely another method of therapeutic intervention. It is a way of conceptualizing a client's problem in which the focus is on the marital relationship rather than on intrapsychic forces. Behavior is analyzed in the context of the relationship. Traditionally, the term marital therapy is used when a therapist works with a couple together. However, there are several variations:

1. The therapist may see the partners separately.
2. A different therapist may see each spouse with collaboration between the two therapists.
3. The couple may be seen together in group therapy.
4. The couple may be part of a couples group.

Regardless of the particular arrangement, the therapist who works with a married client is involved in marital therapy to some extent. One partner cannot change without affecting the other person, and hence the relationship as a whole changes.

Indications for Marital Therapy[1] Table 23–1 shows indications for marital therapy and a rationale for each indication.

Types of Marriages[3] Marriages are divided into three types:

1. A pure united-front marriage
2. A pure underadequate/overadequate marriage
3. A pure conflictual marriage

In actual clinical practice, there are only a few marriages that could be called pure types; most are combinations of these types. Table 23–2 describes each type.

Table 23–1
INDICATIONS FOR MARITAL THERAPY AND RATIONALE

Indication	Rationale
1. When a client's onset of symptoms coincides with a marital conflict	1. Sometimes symptoms are used to deny or distract from marital problems.
2. When it is requested by a couple that is in conflict	2. When one spouse requests marital therapy, the other will usually come, because if one partner is under stress the other is too.
3. When it appears that improvement in the client will result in divorce or symptoms in the spouse	3. If a client with severe symptoms claims that the marriage is ideal and the spouse concurs, it is likely that improvement in the client will lead to divorce or a distressed spouse. Therapists have a responsibility to the relatives of a client if they bring about a change.
4. When methods of individual psychotherapy have failed	4. Often, a client is involved in a marital relationship that is inhibiting personal improvement and perpetuating stress to a point that individual therapy cannot effect change.
5. When methods of individual psychotherapy cannot be used	5. Clients sometimes offer no information about feelings or about their lives in general. Bringing the spouse into the session will increase communication and information sharing. Partners will feel a need to provide their own versions of the relationship's problems.

Table 23–2
DESCRIPTION AND PURPOSE OF THREE TYPES OF MARRIAGES

Description	*Purpose*
United Front	
Partners indicate that their marriage is wonderful, but that there is a problem with a third factor (for example, one of the children). All of their conversation is focused on the other factor, distracting them from any problems with one another. There is a fear that if they were to fight, something terrible would happen (for example, the marriage would dissolve).	1. Provides a sense of ''closeness'' 2. Avoids conflict between the spouses 3. Avoids contact with each other; children always present
Underadequate/Overadequate	
One partner is dominant, stronger, and healthier. The other is weaker, sick, and unable to cope. One spouse has symptoms or problems, and the other claims to be without symptoms or problems (for example, a marriage in which one partner is an alcoholic).	1. Provides each person with a way to deal with feelings of inadequacy 2. Assures that underadequate spouse does not make decisions, hence is not responsible; overadequate spouse feels in control 3. Reinforces underadequacy of the other spouse because children will usually side with the overadequate spouse
Conflictual	
Couple fights overtly much of the time. Process of arguing is what is important. Arguments tend to be repetitive, and much blaming takes place. These couples do not feel any relief after a fight because major issues are not addressed.	1. Avoids dealing with major issues by always fighting about ''little things'' 2. Avoids affectionate display of intimacy; contact is achieved instead by fighting 3. Maintains chaos in the relationship, thereby avoiding intimacy 4. Prevents exchange of feelings, thereby avoiding intimacy

Major Theoretical Issues It can be seen from the description of these three types of marriages that two major issues underlie most marital problems:
1. The fear of being separate and adult
2. The fear of intimacy

Assessment of the Marital Relationship At the onset of treatment, it is important for the therapist to complete an assessment of the marital relationship. Many times, a couple enters therapy in a time of crisis and desires immediate relief, including advice and direction from the therapist. The therapist is empathetic to the couple's situation, but is never persuaded to eliminate the assessment phase of therapy. Areas to be assessed include
1. Manner in which the couple solves problems
2. Level of intimacy
   a. Companionship
   b. Sexual relationship

3. Commitment to the relationship
4. Family history from each individual, focusing on the client's perception of the parent's marital relationship

Marital Conflict   Dealing with the marital conflict quickly becomes the focus of therapy with any couple, regardless of the indication for therapy or the type of marriage. Conflict in a married couple can arise in several areas:

1. Conflict over what kind of rules to follow in dealing with each other and what type of relationship to have
2. Conflict over who is to set the rules
3. Conflict over the process of working out conflicts
4. Conflict in the sexual relationship. Sexual relations tend to become a way of demonstrating the conflicts in a relationship. Sexual problems do not necessarily need to be worked on in marital therapy, because as the couple works out conflicts in other areas, the sexual ones are also resolved. However, if an assessment is made and a true sexual dysfunction is found, the therapist must consider integrating sex therapy techniques[2] or referring the couple to a sexual-dysfunction clinic.

Couples coming into marital therapy have difficulty solving problems and conflicts. Instead, they demonstrate behavior that increases or sustains the conflict. Table 23–3 shows some of the most common behaviors exhibited by couples in conflict.

The therapist points out these behaviors as they occur during a conflict and redirects the couple to make different statements and to try new behaviors, at times demonstrating these for the couple. These new behaviors are aimed toward more separate, adult behavior, leading to increased intimacy. The goal of the therapist is to get the *couple* to identify the marital conflicts, talk openly about them, apply problem-solving techniques, and ultimately achieve a resolution to the conflicts.

Table 23–3
TYPICAL BEHAVIORS OF COUPLES IN CONFLICT

Behavior	*Example*
1. Hostile, nonverbal behavior	1. Sneering, inattentive posture
2. Global problem statements	2. "I *never* do that"; or "You *always* say that."
3. Personal attacks	3. "Anyone who would do that is a terrible person." "That's a stupid thing to say."
4. Intention labeling	4. "You want to hurt my feelings."
5. Sidetracking	5. Bringing up another issue with a loose connection to the one being discussed
6. Stating problems in negative terms rather than in positive terms	6. "I hate it when you do that." rather than "I would like it if you could . . ."
7. Cross complaining rather than listening to each other	7. "I don't like it when you . . ." "And, *I* don't like it when you . . ."
8. Blaming the other person rather than accepting one's own part in the problem	8. "It's your fault we never . . ." "No, it's *your* fault."
9. Rigidly insisting that one's view be accepted by the other	9. "It absolutely has to be done this way."

Therapeutic
Interventions in
Marital Therapy
The nurse uses a variety of techniques in working with a couple toward resolution of the marital conflict, that is, toward increased adult behavior and intimacy. Some of the common interventions used with couples in marital therapy are shown in Chart 23–1.

Chart 23–1
COMMON INTERVENTIONS IN MARITAL THERAPY

Intervention	Rationale
1. Redirect communication.	1. Couples in conflict are unable to communicate effectively. It is helpful for the nurse to point out destructive patterns in their communication and redirect them whenever possible.
2. Direct the couple to behave differently.	2. When control is an issue for the couple, the nurse can often temporarily resolve this by giving directions to the couple, thereby assuming control. Such directions should be in areas in which the conflict is minor or in which it is likely a spouse would like to behave that way but is just waiting for an excuse. Mere advice to a couple to treat each other in a different way is rarely followed.
3. Direct the couple to continue to behave in the same way as they have been behaving (paradoxical interventions).	3. Directing a couple to behave in their usual way is paradoxically one of the most rapid ways to bring about change. When the nurse encourages usual behavior, the person tends to discontinue it as its absurdity becomes clear. This technique also puts the therapist in control and lays the groundwork for a later shift, at the same time taking advantage of any rebellious urges in the spouses. The anger may then become focused on the nurse, and can be examined in the context of the nurse–client relationship.
4. Provoke a couple to fight.	4. When partners are unable to fight and bring up what is on their minds, they are avoiding intimacy. With these couples the nurse encourages the partners to say what is on their minds directly, so that they will learn that no harm results. Eventually, this sharing leads to intimacy.
5. Encourage less interaction between the couple and have them talk instead to the nurse.	5. This slows down the conflictual process by discouraging blaming and encouraging the couple to talk about themselves, instead of each other.
6. Split the balance in the relationship (especially with underadequate/overadequate couples).	6. The underadequate partner is helped to see personal strengths and get some support. The overadequate spouse is allowed to feel less responsible and acknowledge dependency needs. Each feels supported.
7. Encourage the parents to have a relationship separate from the children (especially with united-front marriages).	7. This forces them to move the focus of their conflict from the children to one another.
8. Role playing	8. When spouses assume each other's role in an argument they can "experience" the conflict from their partner's position.
9. Contracts including each partner's expectations of the relationship, their psychological and biological needs, their perception of the problems in the marriage, and what each partner feels he/she can give in the relationship. Contracts can be used at the beginning of therapy and evaluated and revised throughout therapy.[4]	9. This gives couples a chance to verbalize their expectations and needs to one another. Each can see the rational and irrational aspects of their own as well as the other's expectations.

Resolution of the Marital Conflict Couples learn and adopt constructive ways of handling conflict through successful marital therapy. Some specific behavior changes that can be seen are

1. Body language changes, such as an attentive posture
2. Active listening
3. Sticking to one issue
4. Statements about specific behaviors that have improved
5. A willingness to share responsibility
6. A willingness to search for compromises

It can be seen that these behaviors show a general move toward adult behavior and intimacy.

Not all successful marital therapy will terminate with the couple exhibiting the above behaviors and continuing to grow in their relationship. There will be successful marital therapy that terminates in a decision to divorce. When this is the outcome, it is not uncommon for the novice marital therapist to feel that he or she has failed the couple. However, the decision to obtain a divorce can be the result of seeking marital therapy once the decision had already been made to divorce, or may be the result of having learned through therapy that the partners were incompatible. In either case, marital therapy can help a divorcing couple to leave the relationship without feelings of failure or guilt.

References

1. Haley J: Marriage therapy. In Haley J: Strategies of Psychotherapy. New York, Grune & Stratton, 1963
2. Kaplan HS: The New Sex Therapy. New York, Brunner/Mazel, 1974
3. Kramer C et al: The Theoretical Position: Diagnostic and Therapeutic Implications. Beginning Phase of Family Treatment, The Family Institute of Chicago, 1968
4. Sager C: Marriage Contracts and Couple Therapy. New York, Brunner/Mazel, 1976

Bibliography

Ellis A: Techniques of handling anger in marriage. J Marriage Fam Counsel 10:305, 1976

Freidman D: Blaming: An impasse in marital conflict—Strategies for intervention. J Psychiatr Nurs 19:8, 1979

Padberg J: Bargaining to improve communications in conjoint family therapy. Perspect Psychiatr Care 13:68, 1975

Sager C, Kaplan HS: Treatment of marital and sexual problems. In Sager C, Kaplan HS (eds): Progress in Group and Family Therapy. New York, Brunner/Mazel, 1972

Wile: Couples Therapy—A Motivational Approach. New York, John Wiley & Sons, 1981.

24

Family

Therapy

Susan L. Jones

Introduction   The purpose of family therapy is to remove family system pathology and to improve the functioning of the family as a working interdependent group, while removing individual pathology and helping each member to function as an individual. The family is seen as a system instead of a group of separate individuals. Individual symptoms are viewed as by-products of relationship struggles. Interventions are therefore geared toward understanding individual behavior patterns that arise from, and feed back into, the family system. All family therapists agree that the first purpose of family therapy is improvement of family functioning, although they disagree on how this may be accomplished.

Assessment of the Family   A. **PURPOSE**
1. To observe and collect data on the family interactional patterns
2. To observe and collect data on the "identified" client or clients in relation to the family as a whole
3. To formulate a "working hypothesis" to explain the family's pathological functioning
4. To assist the family to understand what interpersonal factors are operating to maintain the problem behavior by the family as a whole and by any individual family members

B. **DESCRIPTION**
A family assessment is an account of the family systems through at least two generations, together with current information relevant to the identified client's presenting problem. It has advantages of providing a great deal of information in a short amount of time for the therapist and at the same time being therapeutic for the family. Invariably, family members find out information about each other that was not known before.[26,27]

C. **THE GENOGRAM**
A family genogram is a pictorial representation of the role structure, relationship structure, and demographic data of a family.

The family genogram is used for gathering structural data. It has the advantage of helping to organize visually complex material about the family structure, which can then be reviewed by the therapist and family. Organization of the genogram is shown in Figure 24–1 and instructions for drawing the genogram are in Chart 24–1.

D. **FAMILY ASSESSMENT GUIDE**
The family assessment guide is a conceptual outline used to organize data and to indicate where some key problem areas in the family reside.[26] The family assessment guide is modified according to the role structure and the presenting problem of the family. The guide is shown in Chart 24–2.

Indications and Contraindications   A. **INDICATIONS**
1. Whenever the therapist evaluates or the family indicates that the family system is involved to a significant degree in some type of psychosocial problem, or when significant psychopathology is present (for example, schizophrenia or depression)
2. When the family has difficulty functioning
3. When a child is the identified client and is seen to be the "symptom bearer" of a more general family problem, such as an unresolved marital issue

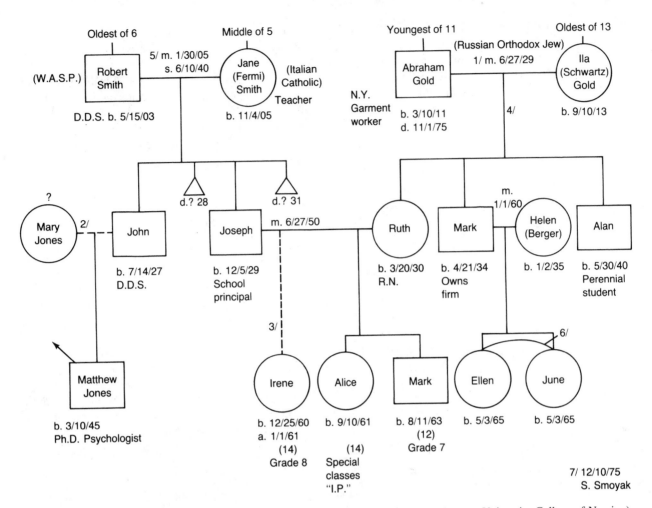

FIG. 24-1 Three generational genogram. (Genogram drawn by Dr. Shirley Smoyak, Rutgers University College of Nursing)

Chart 24–1
INSTRUCTIONS FOR DRAWING A THREE-GENERATIONAL GENOGRAM

General

Divide paper horizontally into 3 levels.
Begin in the middle, with husband on left.
Designate males as squares and females as circles.
Aborted fetuses, too early to determine sex, are triangles.
Place birthdates below symbol, prefaced by a "b".
Place deathdates below symbol, prefaced by a "d;" mark an X through identity symbol.
Place marriage date, preceded by "m" on the paired solid line. Separation = "s," divorce = "d."
Indicate adoption date as "a."
For first generation (the grandparents), indicate the sibling structure by "oldest of _____," or "youngest of _____."
Indicate occupation and ethnicity of first generation alongside symbols.

Indicate occupation of middle generation.
Indicate school year or occupation of third generation (children of major couple).

Notations

(Illustrated on genogram and marked 1/, 2/, and so forth.
1/ Solid horizontal line linking man and woman indicates marriage.
2/ Broken horizontal line linking man and woman indicates nonmarriage relationship.
3/ Broken vertical line indicates adoption.
4/ Solid vertical line indicates children of the couple.
5/ Broken brackets indicate divorce, separation.
6/ "Rocker" between children indicates twins, triplets, and so forth.
7/ Date genogram constructed and clinician's name.

Chart 24–2
FAMILY ASSESSMENT GUIDE

A. Family structure (using family genogram)
 1. Parents of nuclear family
 2. Children—ages and ordinal position
 3. Personality description of each individual
 4. Level of education
 5. Individuals in nuclear home and outside of home
 6. Grandparents
B. Family in relation to the community
 1. Ethnicity
 2. Socioeconomic class, educational level
 3. Religion
C. Presenting problem
 1. Each family member's perception of the problem(s)
 2. Each family member's perception of how he/she would like things to change
 3. Each family member's perception of the positive aspects of the family
D. Communication patterns
 1. Who speaks to whom, when, and in what manner of tone
 2. Family themes and values
 3. Emotional climate
 4. Manner by which hostility and anger are expressed

E. Family roles
 1. Which members are supportive, antagonistic, critical, scapegoated, rescuers, victims?
 2. Are there family coalitions, pairings, splits, triangles?
 3. What is the seating arrangement of members?
 4. How does each person feel about his/her relationship with each member of the family?
F. Developmental history
 1. Of family in general
  a. History of family of origin of each parent
  b. History of courtship of parents
  c. History of birth and general rearing of each child in nuclear family
 2. Of presenting problem
  a. Early behavioral symptoms of the problem
  b. Persons involved in the problem
  c. Behavioral patterns involved in the problem
G. Family's expectations of therapy

4. Some therapists believe that whenever there is a child who is symptomatic before puberty, family treatment is indicated, since the child's symptomatology is directly related to marital conflict.

5. Family therapy is the treatment of choice when the identified client has been in individual therapy and the individual therapy fails. Failure may be related to family factors such as poor communication between family members. A clue in such a situation is that the individual client seems unable to use individual sessions and spends most of the therapy sessions talking about a family member. A common situation is that one marital partner comes into therapy and talks only about the other partner.

6. When improvement of one family member's functioning (for example, that of the identified client) results in another family member becoming dysfunctional. For example, if a mother is unable to function and psychologically needs to take care of her son who will not go to school.

7. When the client is an inpatient and is ready for discharge. Improvement during the course of hospitalization often is totally negated when the family member returns home *unless* family members have been involved in the treatment for more than last-minute discharge planning.

8. Some family therapists take the extreme position that family therapy is the treatment of choice in all conditions in which psychotherapy is indicated.

B. **CONTRAINDICATIONS**
 1. When key members of the family are unavailable or are unwilling to come to sessions
 2. When one family member is so severely disturbed that the family approach is unworkable because this member is disruptive of sessions

Arranging for Therapy   A. **WITH THE FAMILY**

The entire family, including parents and children, are present for the family assessment. After the assessment, arrangements are made concerning who shall attend the therapy, how often sessions will be held, and for how long. Although some family therapists contend that the entire family should attend all sessions over the course of therapy[12–14] and others contend that family therapy can take place with one person,[6] most use various combinations of persons attending the sessions over the course of therapy.

B. **WITH THE CHILDREN**

Children over 4 are usually included for most if not all of the family therapy sessions. These children are excluded when sensitive issues such as sex are discussed. Children under four may attend some early sessions to evaluate child–parent interactions, but do not come to every session during the middle phase of therapy. Meetings with the adults alone are scheduled to focus on the marital dyad and to help parents see themselves as marital partners rather than as just parents.[19–21]

C. **IF THE IDENTIFIED CLIENT IS A CHILD**

When the identified client is a child (for example, a 12-year-old bed wetter), the child may still be excluded from some sessions to allow the parents to focus on the marital dyad. This practice stems from the belief that individual problems with the child are related to and partially a product of the marital dyad.[3–5]

Location   A. **OFFICE**

Some therapists prefer to see the family in the office to create a more professional and formal atmosphere for the meeting.[19–21]

B. **FAMILY'S HOME**

Some therapists prefer to see the family in the home. The advantage of this is that the therapist can evaluate the family in the natural environment in which the family is more relaxed and perhaps more honest.[17,28]

Theoretical Orientations to Family Therapy   A. **PSYCHOANALYTIC FAMILY THERAPY** (Ackerman, Boszormenyi-Nagy, Framo, Spark, Paul)

1. *Description*—The traditional view is taken that psychopathology results from internal, intrapsychic forces that are manifested in the ways people in close relationships interact with and affect each other.[1,2,7,8,24,29]
2. *Goals of therapy*—The goal is deep reconstructive change in personality. The change in personality comes about through a "working through" of the unconscious transference distortions of each family member with each other family member and with the therapist. This therapy takes place over an extended period of time, and clients explore the connections between past relationships and current problems.[2]

B. **BOWEN APPROACH TO FAMILY THERAPY** (Bowen, Guerin)

1. *Description*—Pathology is viewed as a by-product of a larger family system. This view of the family as a system is similar to the interactional orientation. Bowen differs, however, in that he considers communication to be only part of a wider system of relationships in the family,[3–6] whereas the interactionalists view communication as the primary system.[10]

2. *Goal of therapy*—The goal is differentiation of self from the family system. The therapeutic process focuses on the family of origin of one or both spouses. The intense emotional problems that occur within the nuclear family are resolved only by resolving undifferentiated relationships with one's family of origin.[3-6,11]

C. **STRUCTURAL APPROACH TO FAMILY THERAPY** (Minuchin, Fishman)
   1. *Description*—Pathology is viewed as resulting from both internal and external forces. "Man in his social context" is the therapeutic unit. Crucial to this approach is avoidance of the artificial dichotomy that exists between individuals and their social context. Pathology results when the family cannot adapt to change. One of two possible dysfunctional systems results: an enmeshed family system (overly close emotionally) or disengaged family system (isolated emotionally).[19-21]
   2. *Goal of therapy*—The goal is to transform the family structural patterns. Such a transformation is defined as a change in the position of each family member vis-à-vis each other family member so that there is a change of their complementary demands and interactional patterns. The transformation is significant for all family members, but particularly so for the identified client, who is freed from the deviant position.[19,20]

D. **INTERACTIONAL APPROACH TO FAMILY THERAPY** (Haley, Hoffman, Jackson, Madanes, Satir, Watzlawick, Weakland, Wynne)
   1. *Description*—The starting point for the interactional approach is rejection of the psychoanalytic constructs in the assessment and treatment of human problems.[10] Instead, the unit of analysis is derived from the dynamics of interchange between individuals. Basic to this perspective is the assumption that psychiatric problems result from the way people behave with each other in the context of a particular organization such as a family. The locus of pathology is seen to be external to the individual—although these family therapists contend that they do not completely deny the existence of intrapsychic mechanisms that influence family functioning.[12-16,18,25,30,31]
   2. *Goals of therapy*—The goals are clarification of family rules,[16] initiating of behavior change within family members,[12-15] clarification and functional reconstruction of the family's communication patterns.[30]

E. **BEHAVIORAL APPROACH TO FAMILY THERAPY** (Patterson)
   1. *Description*—According to the behavioral family therapists, all behavior is learned or, conversely, no behavior is intrapsychically determined. These therapists differ in the extent to which they include the entire family unit as a focus for treatment; however, they all define the family as a system of interlocking *behaviors*. Each individual "learns" how to respond to each other individual within the family.[22,23]
   2. *Goal of therapy*—The goal is to change the contingencies of reinforcement so that the family members give social reinforcement for desired behavior instead of maladaptive behavior. Through this process, the family members "unlearn" maladaptive behavior and "learn" functional behavior in relation to each other.

F. **RELATIONSHIP OF THEORETICAL APPROACHES AND FAMILY THERAPY TECHNIQUES USED**
   Research shows that, in general, family therapists endorse a systems approach of

some kind, although many therapists claim to have an "eclectic" theoretical orientation. Therapists who endorse a given theoretical model generally endorse the expected goals of this model and the model's views toward the therapy process.[9] Although therapists endorse different theoretical orientations and corresponding goals, therapists with *different theories and goals use similar family therapy techniques.*[9]

Major Techniques

A. **FOCUSING ON HERE-AND-NOW INTERACTIONS**

1. *Description*—Focus on here-and-now interactions means that the therapist has family members focus on *present* feelings and behaviors rather than past feelings and behaviors. They believe that this method arouses a much deeper response in an individual than dealing with feelings described in retrospect. Nearly all family therapists focus on here-and-now feelings, although those of the psychoanalytic school use this technique to work through *past* relationships.

2. *Examples*

   a. To work through a *present* relationship—Mr. Smith, a single parent, and his 14-year-old daughter are in family therapy with the presenting problem of acting-out behavior by the adolescent. During one session, the daughter screams at the father to leave the room, and he ignores her behavior. The therapist interjects, "Mr. Smith, your daughter just told you to get out of the room, yet you smiled and ignored her statement and then got angry about something else. What were your feelings when your daughter screamed at you? Talk with your daughter about these feelings."

   b. To work through a *past* relationship—Mr. and Mrs. Jones are in family therapy because of marital conflict. The marital conflict is related to Mrs. Jones's family of origin. After observing an interaction in therapy, the therapist responds, "You say, Mrs. Jones, that your husband will not talk, but every time he tries to get a word in edgewise here, you interrupt him or finish his sentence. What was the marital relationship like between your parents?"

B. **RESTRUCTURING FAMILY TRANSACTIONAL (INTERACTIONAL) PATTERNS**

1. *Description*—Basic to this intervention is the notion that it is more beneficial to enact family interactional patterns than to describe them. Therapists assist the family to transact, in their presence, ways in which they naturally resolve conflicts, support each other, enter into alliances and coalitions, diffuse stress, and so forth. Reenacting transactional patterns helps family members to experience their own behaviors with heightened awareness. From the therapists' point of view, it also helps them see family members in action, and it is through such observations that the family structure becomes apparent.

2. *Examples*

   a. "Talk with your father about that."

   b. "Discuss with your husband the curfew rules for Johnny."

   c. "Talk about the budget now and try to come to a decision."

C. **CLARIFYING COMMUNICATIONS**

1. *Description*—Dysfunctional communications exist when family members do not differentiate the verbal and nonverbal levels of communication; consequently, a different message may be given on each level of communication. By pointing out or investigating with individuals their meanings on each level

of communication, the therapist allows family members to send and receive accurate communications.

 2. *Examples*

  a. Report (verbal message) and command (nonverbal message)—A marital couple is in therapy because of marital conflict. A central issue in the conflict is the husband's domination of the wife. The couple is discussing the possibility of the wife beginning college now that the children are getting older. The husband responds, "I really don't care whether you go back to school, if you think you can still run the household. You make the decision." The report level of communication is "yes" go back to school. However, the command level of communication, based upon past experience in the marital relationship and other subtle cues is "No, don't go back to school because it will disrupt the household."

  b. *Communication (verbal message) and metacommunication (nonverbal message)*—A marital couple is in therapy because of marital conflict. At the beginning of a session, the husband asks the wife if she has just gotten a permanent wave (verbal message) when it is quite obvious she had just gotten her hair cut and curled. The nonverbal message is "I don't like your new hairdo." At this point the therapist has the couple discuss this further to allow the incongruent message to become obvious. Another therapeutic alternative for the therapist would be to gently point out the seeming incongruence between the husband's verbal and nonverbal message.

D. **RELABELING OR REFRAMING**

 1. *Description*—The therapist renames seemingly dysfunctional behavior as reasonable and understandable. The goal is to emphasize the positive aspects of interpersonal feelings and behaviors.

 2. *Examples*

  a. A mother and daughter in therapy are talking when the mother begins to cry. Because the daughter is seen to be aggressive, she is assumed to be the cause of the mother's crying. The daughter confirms this unwritten assumption by stating that she did not mean to hurt her mother. The therapist relabels the hurt and calls it "touching closeness" to take away the negative motive for the act.

  b. A marital couple is in therapy because of marital conflict. A central issue in the conflict is the intrusion of the husband's mother. Particular conflict exists between the wife and mother-in-law. During a discussion between the husband and wife about the mother-in-law's "intrusiveness" into their life, the therapist interjects by relabeling the intrusiveness as "caring" by the mother-in-law.

E. **PARADOXICAL TECHNIQUES**

Paradoxical interventions in family therapy are somewhat controversial. Some therapists are reluctant to use them, whereas others consider them ingenious ways to force a person to abandon old, dysfunctional behavior. These techniques, in general, are based on the interactional theoretical formulation.

 1. *Description*—Paradoxical techniques are directives given the family by the therapist which the therapist hopes the family will resist and, in so doing, change its behavior. Through the assignment, the therapist is asking the family not to change while at the same time covertly telling them that they should

change. These techniques are based on the assumption that families who come for help are also resistant to the help being offered, providing potential for a power struggle.

    2. *Examples*
        a. Prescribing the Symptom
            1) Description—The therapist "orders" the family members (or individual) to continue and perhaps increase the symptoms. The rationale is that whereas the symptoms previously may have seemed out of anyone's control, after the therapist gives the directive, the symptoms begin to lose their autonomy, mystery, and power. They appear to come under the therapist's control. The participants in the behavior become more conscious of them, and the dysfunctional behavior may disappear.
            2) Example—A marital couple that has engaged in nonproductive arguing now finds that the therapist has asked them to continue fighting and to increase it. The couple is told to fight about the menu before dinner so that they can enjoy the food. This injuction jars the continuing process and they may rebel against the outsider's orders.
        b. *Reductio ad absurdum*
            1) Description—This is a technique in which the symptom is reduced to the absurdity by discussing it to a point of absurdity.
            2) Example—A mother and father are in family therapy with their acting-out 14-year-old daughter, who is the identified client. The primary conflict is between the mother and daughter. The therapist commiserates with the mother about the cross she bears and the scientific fact that anyone else would have been completely crushed by it. The goal is to force the mother to say, "I didn't say it was that bad!" The point is to show her that she is not as vulnerable as she seems.

F. **FAMILY SCULPTING**
    1. *Description*—Family sculpting is a technique whereby the relationships between family members are recreated in space through the formation of a physical tableau. The tableau or sculpture symbolizes the emotional position of each member in the family in relation to other family members. By using their bodies to create an actual representation of specific relationships, family members are using the physical space during the session to recreate the emotional space between them. Because sculpting involves activity and bodily movement during the creation of the sculpture, it can be a useful means of engaging children for whom nonverbal models of expression are natural.
    2. *Example*—The Smith family, consisting of mother, father, and three children is in therapy because the 12 year old wets the bed repeatedly. During one session, the therapist introduces sculpting. She first outlines the nature of the activity, then chooses the sculptor (the identified client), and then instructs all of the family members to move out of their seats so that the sculpting can begin. The sculptor physically arranges each member of the family in relation to each other member. During this time, the therapist encourages the identified client, observing and commenting on the manner by which he sculpts each person. After the physical activity is complete, the entire family talks about how they felt during the activity, the extent to which they agree with the sculptor's physical representation of the family, and how they might have sculpted the family differently. At times, it is helpful to have more than one family member sequentially sculpt the family and to go through the same process as described previously.

Termination in Family Therapy

A. **PURPOSE**
1. To allow the family to share their overall experience in the therapy process
2. To provide closure for the therapy process
3. To have the family members evaluate their success in handling old problems
4. To have the family members evaluate their ability to handle existing concerns

B. **DESCRIPTION**
A formal termination session consists of all family members meeting to "terminate" therapy. When the session is arranged, it is understood that this will be the final session of the therapy process.

C. **EXAMPLE**
Mr. and Mrs. Smith and their two teenage sons have been in therapy for 6 months. The acting-out behavior of the youngest son has decreased over the past several months, and the family and therapist agree that therapy may be terminated. A termination session is arranged. The therapist first has each family member discuss the *most beneficial* and *least beneficial* aspects of the therapy. Then the family is asked to discuss changes that have taken place over the course of therapy. Here, the family discusses changes that have occurred on the individual level and on the family systems level. The final item, before closing the session, is when the therapist gives the family members an invitation to return in the future if they feel they need help.

References

1. Block D, Simon R: The Strength of Family Therapy: Selected Papers of Nathan W. Ackerman. New York, Brunner/Mazel, 1982
2. Boszormenyi-Nagy I, Spark G: Invisible Loyalties: Reciprocity in Intergenerational Family Therapy. New York, Harper & Row, 1973
3. Bowen M: Family psychotherapy with schizophrenia in the hospital and in private practice. In Boszormenyi-Nagy I, Framo J (eds): Intensive Family Therapy. New York, Harper & Row, 1965
4. Bowen M: The use of family theory in clinical practice. In Haley J (ed): Changing Families: A Family Therapy Reader. New York, Grune & Stratton, 1971
5. Bowen M: Theory in the practice of psychotherapy. In Guerin P (ed): Family Therapy: Theory and Practice. New York, Gardner, 1976
6. Bowen M: Family Therapy in Clinical Practice. New York, Jason Aronson, 1978
7. Framo J: Rationale and techniques of intensive family therapy. In Boszormenyi-Nagy I, Framo J (eds): Intensive Family Therapy. New York, Harper & Row, 1965
8. Framo J: Symptoms from a transactional viewpoint. In Sager C, Kaplan H (eds): Progress in Group and Family Therapy, New York, Brunner/Mazel, 1972
9. Green RG, Kolevzon MS: Three approaches to family therapy: A study of convergence and divergency. J Mar Fam Ther 8:39, 1982
10. Greenberg GS: The family interactional perspective: A study and examination of the work of Don D. Jackson. Fam Process 16:385, 1977
11. Guerin P (ed): Family Therapy: Theory and Practice. New York, John Wiley & Sons, 1976
12. Haley J: Strategies of Psychotherapy. New York, Grune & Stratton, 1963
13. Haley J: Control in psychotherapy and schizophrenics. In Jackson, D (ed): Therapy, Communication, and Change. Palo Alto, Science and Behavior Books, 1973
14. Haley J: Problem Solving Therapy. San Francisco, Jossey-Bass, 1976
15. Hoffman L: Foundations of Family Therapy. New York, Basic Books, 1981
16. Jackson DD (ed): Therapy, Communication and Change. Palo Alto, Science and Behavior Books, 1973
17. Jones SL: Family Therapy: A Comparison of Approaches. Bowie, MD, RJ Brady, 1980
18. Mandanes C: Strategic Family Therapy. San Francisco, Jossey-Bass, 1981
19. Minuchin S: Families and Family Therapy. Cambridge, Harvard University Press, 1974
20. Minuchin S, Fishman HC: Family Therapy Techniques. Cambridge, Harvard University Press, 1981
21. Minuchin S, Rosman B, Baker L: Psychosomatic Families: Anorexia Nervosa in Context. Cambridge, Harvard University Press, 1978

22. Patterson G: Families: Applications of Social Learning to Family Life. Champaign, Research Press, 1975
23. Patterson G: Professional Guide for Families and Living with Children. Champaign, Research Press, 1975
24. Paul NL, Paul BB: A Marital Puzzle. New York, WW Norton, 1975
25. Satir V, Stachowiak J, Taschman H: Helping Families to Change. New York, Jason Aronson, 1976
26. Smoyak S (ed): The Psychiatric Nurse as a Family Therapist. New York, John Wiley & Sons, 1975
27. Smoyak S: Family systems: Use of genogram as an assessment tool. In Clements IM, Buchanan DM (eds): Family Therapy: A Nursing Perspective. New York, John Wiley & Sons, 1982
28. Smoyak S: Homes: A natural environment for family therapy. In Hall J (ed): Distributive Nursing Practice: A Systems Approach to Community Health. Philadelphia, JB Lippincott, 1977
29. Spark G: Grandparents and intergenerational family therapy. Fam Process 13:225, 1974
30. Watzlawick P, Weakland JH (eds): The Interaction View: Studies at the Mental Research Institute. Palo Alto 1965–1974. New York, WW Norton, 1977
31. Wynne LC, Cromwell RL, Matthysse S (eds): The Nature of Schizophrenia: New Approaches to Research and Treatment. New York, John Wiley & Sons, 1978

Bibliography

Barash DS: Dynamics of the psychological family system. Perspect Psychiatr Care 17:17, 1979

Benton DW: Family therapy: Problems encountered in defocusing the identified patient. J Psychiatr Nurs 17:28, 1979

Clement J: Family therapy: The transferability of theory to practice. J Psychiatr Nurs 15:33, 1977

Clements IW, Buchanan DM (eds): Family Therapy: A Nursing Perspective. New York, John Wiley & Sons, 1982

Collison CR, Futrell J: Family therapy for the single parent family system. J Psychosoc Nurs 20:16, 1982

Danziger S: Major treatment issues and techniques of family therapy with the borderline adolescent. J Psychosoc Nurs 20:27, 1982

Fife BL, Gant BL: The resolution of school phobia through family therapy. J Psychiatr Nurs 18:13, 1980

Floyd GT: Managing member silence in family therapy. J Psychiatr Nurs 11:20, 1973

Gunderson SS: Advocacy in family therapy. J Psychiatr Nurs 18:24, 1980

Hartman K, Bush M: Action-oriented family therapy. Am J Nurs 75:1184, 1975

Herman SJ: Divorce: A grief process. Perspect Psychiatr Care 7:108, 1974

Impey L: Art media: A means to therapeutic communication with families. Perspect Psychiatr Care 19:70, 1981

Jones SL, Dimond M: Family theory and family therapy models: Comparative review with implications for nursing practice. J Psychosoc Nurs 20:12, 1982

Koehne-Kaplan NS: The use of self as a family therapist. Perspect Psychiatr Care 14:29, 1976

Lansky MR, McVey GG, Wendahl N, Keyes V: Family treatment training for psychiatric nurses: A report on serial in-service workshops. J Psychiatr Nurs 16:19, 1978

Lantz JE: Family therapy: Using a transactional approach. J Psychiatr Nurs 15:17, 1977

Lantz JE, Treece N: Identify operations and family treatment. J Psychosoc Nurs 20:20, 1982

Mealy AR: Sculpting as a group technique for increasing awareness. Perspect Psychiatr Care 15:118, 1977

Miller SR, Wintead-Fry P: Family Systems Theory in Nursing Practice. Virginia, Reston, 1982

Miller V, Mansfield E: Family therapy for the multiple incest family. J Psychiatr Nurs 19:29, 1981

Monea HP: A family in trouble. Perspect Psychiatr Care 7:165, 1974

Morgan SA, Macey MJ: Three assessment tools for family therapy. J Psychiatr Nurs 16:39, 1978

Padberg J: Bargaining: To improve communications in conjoint family therapy. Perspect Psychiatr Care 18:68, 1975

Sedgwick R: Family Mental Health: Theory and Practice. St Louis, CV Mosby, 1981

Seeger PA: A framework for family therapy. J Psychiatr Nurs 14:23, 1976

Sharp L, Lantz J: Relabeling in conjoint family therapy. J Psychiatr Nurs 16:29, 1978

Siegel E: Scapegoating: Manifestation and intervention. J Psychiatr Nurs 19:11, 1981

Soderberg SJ: Theory and practice of scapegoating. Perspect Psychiatr Care 15:153, 1977

Tousley MM: The use of family therapy in terminal illness and death. J Psychosoc Nurs 20:17, 1982

Whall AL: Nursing theory and the assessment of families. J Psychiatr Nurs 19:30, 1981

25

Crisis Intervention

Ardis R. Swanson

Introduction   A concept of crisis, as distinguished from stress and emergencies, is the foundation stone of crisis intervention. Crisis intervention is dependent on nurses' underlying assumptions about the capacities of people in crisis and about the nurse's role with persons in crisis. There are many events that can provoke a crisis and several techniques other than the face-to-face interview that facilitate the resolution of crises. These techniques are based on clinical research with people in crisis.

Basic Concepts   A. **STRESS**

Stress is tension, but tension is not necessarily disorganizing to human systems. On the contrary, degree of stress appears to be a prerequisite to growth and change. One way of measuring stress is, by counting life change events with weightings that have been established for the amount of stress each event typically gives a person (see Holmes and Rahe scale, Table 1–1). There is a correlation between a high score on life changes and crisis, but not a perfect correlation. People differ in their capacities to deal with change, and each event has a different meaning for every person.

B. **EMERGENCY**

An emergency is a situation in which immediate action is essential for the survival of the system. A crisis is not an emergency except on rare occasions, and ought not to be mistaken for one. If crises are treated like emergencies then clients may be denied the opportunity for growth and change in resolving the crisis themselves.

C. **CRISIS**

Crisis occurs when more change is required of clients than they are capable of negotiating at the time. Facts and misperceptions about crisis appear in Table 25–1.

Table 25–1
FACTS AND MISPERCEPTIONS ABOUT CRISIS

Fact	Misperceptions Corrected
1. Crisis is a state of human systems (individual or groups).	1. Crisis is not merely an event (for example, a flood is not a crisis except in terms of its real or perceived threat to human systems).
2. In crisis the entire human system is disorganized, with internal ramifications. There is anxiety, inadequate problem solving, and erratic behavior.	2. A crisis is *not* displayed psychologically, somatically, or in overt actions alone.
3. For a period of time the outcome is uncertain; however, inevitably the system will change to a. Disintegration b. The precrisis state, or close to it c. A state superior to the precrisis state, owing to growth, greater strength, and learning	3. A crisis is *not* a period of time. Rather, the nature of human systems is such that the crisis period cannot continue indefinitely.

Characteristics of Crisis Intervention

Crisis intervention differs from other traditional types of intervention, for example, counseling and psychotherapy, in the following ways:

A. **CRISIS INTERVENTION IS ACTIVE**
   1. The nurse uses active listening techniques and actively connects the person(s) in crisis to network support systems.
   2. The *client* is called upon to be active in all steps of the crisis intervention process. This means that the client is a participant in clarifying the problem, in verbalizing feelings associated with the situation, in identifying goals and options for reaching the goals, in decision on a plan, and on a timetable for carrying out the plan.

B. **CRISIS INTERVENTION IS FOCUSED**
   Focus in on the immediate problem in the present or near-present, not all the problems and their roots in the past. Only data that are directly related to the problem are allowed focus. Other data distract and dilute the focus.

C. **CRISIS INTERVENTION HAS A TIME STRUCTURE THAT IS UNIQUE TO EACH CRISIS SITUATION**
   1. Crisis intervention begins immediately.
   2. A given session may be brief and still be effective. A client may be seen once only.
   3. Subsequent appointments may be scheduled, sometimes in fairly quick succession (for example, three sessions within 2 to 5 days), but the total number of sessions is fewer than 12, and sessions do not extend beyond 4 to 6 weeks.

Assumptions about People in Crisis

One of the myths about crisis intervention is that people in crisis are helpless and lack the capacity actively to participate in a treatment plan; therefore, the crisis worker bears full responsibility for the plan and the outcome. This is antithetical to crisis intervention theory, which actively involves the client. Other myths and facts about people in crisis are presented in Table 25–2.

Developmental and Situational Crises

A developmental crisis occurs when the client enters a new stage of life development and is unable to make the changes necessary to function in this new stage. Examples are inability to change with marriage, birth of a child, or death of a parent.

Situational crises are unexpected occurrences that necessitate change in the person because they involve a severe threat to self-esteem or physical safety. Examples are rape, muggings, natural disasters, or illness.

Commonalities of developmental and situational crises are
1. There is a suddenness about nearly all crises. Often there is no warning whatsoever, and there is inadequate prior preparation for such an event.
2. The crisis is experienced as life-threatening, either realistically or unrealistically.
3. Communication with significant others is cut off or decreased.
4. There is some displacement from familiar surroundings or significant loved ones.
5. All have an aspect of loss. The loss may be actual or perceived and may involve a person, an object, an idea, or a hope.

The Initial Contact

Caution should be exercised against falling into models of assessment more appropriate for short-term or long-term psychotherapy. Crisis assessment is not a traditional diagnostic process, which emphasizes history and expects that responsibility and decision making rests with the therapist. Instead, crisis assessment focuses on the nurse

Table 25–2
ASSUMPTIONS ABOUT PEOPLE IN CRISIS

Myths[1]	Facts
1. Crisis intervention is only for responding to psychiatric emergencies.	1. Crisis intervention is practiced and can be effective in a wide variety of settings and in response to all sorts of upsets and turning points along life's path.
2. Crisis intervention is a "one-shot" form of therapy.	2. Crisis intervention often has the continuity and follow-through of two to eight sessions during a period when the system is open to the help of a crisis worker.
3. Crisis intervention is a form of therapy practiced only by paraprofessionals.	3. Crisis intervention has become respected and practiced by extensively trained as well as lay paraprofessionals. The full sophistication of psychodynamic theory can be brought to bear on crises although the theory is used differently than in long-term analytically oriented psychotherapy.
4. Crisis intervention represents only a "holding action" until longer-term therapy can begin.	4. Crisis intervention may be the treatment of choice, especially for persons who have a precrisis level of functioning that is productive.
5. Crisis intervention is effective only for primary prevention programs.	5. Crisis intervention is applicable in primary, secondary, and tertiary prevention.
6. Crisis intervention does not produce lasting change.	6. Crisis intervention has been shown to be effective in preventing future crises.
7. Crisis intervention requires no special skills for the well-trained therapist.	7. Crisis intervention includes responses not typical of other therapies.

and the client's definition of the problem, plan of action, and so forth. The client is an active participant throughout the process. Strengths are noted as well as client-perceived failures.

A. **GENERAL GUIDELINES**
1. Listen carefully to both the content and the affective quality of the client's presentation.
2. Use a direct, straightforward approach to elicit the fullness of the situation, including what is thought, what is felt, and what has been happening. Keep the focus on the present. (With this step the person is helped to begin reorganization while assessment is still in progress.)
3. Listen without condemnation or judgment.
4. Give clients frequent validation that you have heard them and that you understand the situation.
5. Use language to demonstrate your active listening, or paraphrase. Allow space for clients to correct your reflected perceptions when they are not congruent with what they are trying to express.
6. Avoid overinvolvement (enmeshment with the person[s] and the problem) and on the other hand, avoid detachment. Keep boundaries between the nurse and client clear, not diffuse and not rigid.

B. **SPECIFIC GUIDELINES**
   1. If the person is clearly on the verge of total collapse or self-destructiveness (see also Chap. 62), institute emergency interventions, but only for as long as is necessary to sustain life.
      a. Be authoritative: "I want you to do as I say."
      b. Be directive: "Tell me your plans."
      c. Involve others (by calling a family member or agency into contact with the client, or by directing the client to call another).
   2. If the client is clearly distressed but not in danger of death
      a. Have the client further clarify and focus on the major current problem.
      b. Elicit from the client experience that might successfully be applied to the current situation.
      c. Support the client's idea if it is a feasible one.
      d. Mutually decide upon a timetable for appointments and action on the problem.
      e. Elicit ideas from the client about possible action.

Continuing Contacts   The nurse must connect emotionally with the person in crisis, because the client borrows or draws from the ego of the nurse. From the stand-point of biological rhythms, the nurse's organization and rhythmicity act as an organizer of the client's disorder, like the heartbeat that settles a crying infant.

   If the client is not in full-blown crisis but is rather concerned about some behavior or worried about what might develop, help the individual and family to understand what to expect as a result of developmental events and changes. Know that any change requires other changes in the individual's family and environment. Help the client(s) to weather each transition in order to strengthen the system and mitigate against future crises. Each successful transition provides learning, growth, and confidence for moving through subsequent transitional stages.

Techniques Other Than Interviewing   Crisis intervention does not always take place in a consultation room. Chart 25–1 shows some other accepted models of crisis intervention.

Chart 25–1
MODELS OF CRISIS INTERVENTION OTHER THAN INTERVIEWING

Intervention	Nursing Action	Example
Environmental crisis intervention	The nurse manipulates the client's environment to provide a chance for the client to reorganize in an environment of less stress.	Moving a family from unsafe quarters following a flood Providing shelter for a battered wife
Generic crisis intervention	The nurse teaches clients to weather a change by using material or strategies shown helpful to others in similar situations.	Preparing clients for surgery that involves body image changes, for example, mastectomy Teaching classes for new mothers
Network development	The nurse helps clients to connect with others who can help prevent crisis or facilitate resolution of crisis in progress.	Leading a discussion of family members in an ICU waiting room Leading a group of parents whose children have cancer

Evaluation There are two ways of evaluating crisis intervention. The first is to determine whether the crisis has been resolved and the client returned to a precrisis condition, or perhaps a higher level of functioning. The second is to determine whether similar provocation leads the client back into crisis or whether the client handles the provocation using strengths obtained through previous crisis intervention.

Reference

1. Burgess AW, Baldwin BA: Crisis Intervention Theory and Practice. Englewood Cliffs, NJ, Prentice-Hall, 1981

Bibliography

Aguilera DC, Messick JM: Crisis Intervention: Theory and Methodology, 4th ed. St Louis, CV Mosby, 1982

Dixon SL: Working with People in Crisis: Theory and Practice. St Louis, CV Mosby, 1979

Finkelman AW: The nurse therapist: Outpatient crisis intervention with the chronic psychiatric patient. J Psychiatr Nurs 15:27, 1977

Hatch C, Schut L: Description of a crisis-oriented psychiatric home visiting service. J Psychiatr Nurs 18:31, 1980

Hoff LA: People in Crisis: Understanding and Helping. Menlo Park, CA, Addison-Wesley, 1978

Imig DR: Accumulated stress of life changes and interpersonal effectiveness in the family. Fam Relations 30:367, 1981

Morris P: Loss and Change. New York, Pantheon, 1974

Okura KP: Mobilizing in response to a major disaster. Comm Mental Health J 11:136, 1975

Phelan LA: Crisis intervention: Partners in problem solving. J Psychiatr Nurs 17:22, 1979

Wallace MA, Schreiber FB: Crisis intervention training for police officers: A practical program for local police departments. J Psychiatr Nurs 15:22, 1977

White HL: Crisis intervention vs. family therapy. Am J Fam Ther 9:87, 1981

Wicks RJ: Crisis Intervention: A Practical Clinical Guide. Thorofare, NJ, Charles B Slack, 1978

26

Individual Therapy with Children

Sheila Rouslin Welt

241

Introduction   Individual psychotherapy with children, aged 4 to 12, takes varying forms. These include play therapy, drawing, and mutual storytelling. Central to any psychotherapeutic treatment of the child is the notion that play is a naturally occurring phenomenon throughout child development.[34] Its purpose in development and in treatment goes beyond "having fun," which indeed is important in development. Play serves as a significant vehicle for growth and maturation and is thus a major tool in psychotherapeutic work with children.

Assessment of the Child   A. **PURPOSE**
1. To ascertain the child's problem and to establish how the problem is impeding or may impede development; to provide a "developmental profile."[14,25] At such time, treatment possibilities can be explored.
2. To give the child an opportunity to get a feel for the therapist and the office and how it feels to be together
3. To give the child an opportunity directly to present his or her situation to the therapist through interview and drawings without a parent present

B. **ASSESSMENT GUIDE**
A child assessment guide is presented in Chart 26–1.

C. **ASSESSMENT THROUGH DRAWINGS**
Paper at least 8″ × 11″ is provided, along with crayons and pencils. Then the child is asked to
1. Draw something, "anything"
2. Draw a person
3. Draw a person of a sex opposite to the one drawn previously
4. Draw the family
With each picture, the child is asked to talk about the contents. The pictures[7,8,21] and the child's "stories" about the pictures serve as succinct projections of the child's inner reality, the perceptions of external reality.

Assessment of the Family   A. **PURPOSE**
The family is assessed in order to determine the predominant patterns of interaction within the family, and how the child fits into the mode of interaction. The nurse is also interested in how the family relates to "outsiders" (herself or himself).

B. **PLACE**
The family may be seen
1. In the office consulting room[10]
2. In the playroom[10]
3. In the family home[13]

C. **WHOM TO INCLUDE**
There are a number of ways to assess the family. Some of these are to
1. See the entire family together, including the child who has been referred
2. See the parents, each alone and then together
3. See the child with his/her siblings

Chart 26-1
CHILD ASSESSMENT GUIDE

Identifying Data:

1. Age
2. School and grade
3. Family members and ages

Presenting Problem

The therapist first tells his or her understanding of the problem as it has been told by the parent and then asks how the child sees the situation.

School Life

The therapist asks the child to tell about his/her
1. Classmates
2. Teachers
3. Subjects

Interpersonal/Emotional Life Questionnaire

A. *Purpose*—The therapist uses this guide to learn
   1. The patterns of parent–child attachment[1,5,6,18,31]
   2. The state of self and self in relation to others
   3. The developmental and pathologic dimensions of aggression[28]
   4. The healthy and pathologic use of fantasy[4,20] and imagination[30]
   5. The state of impulse control
B. *Questions*
   The order here is suggested but may vary, depending on the interpersonal context.
   1. If you could have three magic wishes, what would they be?
   2. What is your ambition when you grow up?
   3. Do you ever think about what it would be like to leave home?
   4. What would you do with $1, with $100?
   5. What is the best thing that has happened to you?
   6. What is the best thing that could happen to you?
   7. What is the worst thing that has happened to you?
   8. What is the worst thing that could happen to you?
   9. What is the thing you like best about kids?
   10. What is the thing you would like to change about kids?
   11. What is the thing you like best about adults?
   12. What is the thing you would like to change about adults?
   13. What is the thing you like best about yourself?
   14. What is the thing you would like to change about yourself?
   15. If you could be an animal, which one would you like to be?
   16. What animal would you never want to be?
   17. When do you get angry? How do you show it?
   18. When do you get sad? How do you show it?
   19. When do you get happy? How do you show it?
   20. When do you get nervous? How do you show it?
   21. When do you get upset? How do you show it?
   22. What are you afraid of?
   23. Who is your best friend? What do you like about him or her? What do you dislike about him or her?
   24. What do you and your friends do together?
   25. Are you on any teams? In any clubs?
   26. What would you say are some problems you have with your sisters or brothers?
   27. What would you say are some problems you have with your mother?
   28. What would you say are some problems you have with your father?
   29. If you could change your life, what would you have it be?

Arranging for Therapy A. **WITH THE CHILD**

At the end of the assessment session(s) (1–2 hours), the therapist tells the child that visiting the therapist would be a chance to (depending on the child's age and personality)

1. Talk things over
2. Figure things out
3. Help him/her feel better
4. Have an adult outside the family to spend some time with

The child is then asked "And what do you think about that?" An appointment time is suggested, and the child is told that the therapist will be checking the arrangements with the parents and discussing future plans. Confidentiality is discussed, but only when it comes up, either in the initial evaluation session or in later sessions.

B. WITH THE PARENTS

Although arranging for the initial evaluation of the child may have included an interview with the parent(s), after the child's individual evaluation and any additional evaluation deemed useful, the parent(s) are seen in order to:

1. Discuss the child's problem areas
2. Advise a treatment plan
3. Arrange the time
4. Establish the fee and payment procedure
5. Discuss parental treatment needs
6. Discuss protecting the child's confidentiality

The therapist tells the parents that if the child draws them into his or her reluctance to coming, it is best to refer the child to the therapist, since it is between the child and therapist to decide what to do. Parents often feel consciously relieved to hear this.

The Role of the Parents in the Child's Treatment   This varies according to

A. THE THERAPIST

Some therapists believe that the parents should have almost no part in the child's treatment. Most believe, however, that periodic progress reports should be made.[31] It is very important that the therapist maintain a positive relationship with the parents.

B. THE NEEDS OF THE PARENTS

Some parents who are involved in their children's lives, but not in a pathologic way, want to be involved in their treatment. Frequently, as the child begins to change (for example, to become more openly angry at the parents), the parents become angry at the treatment, fearing that it is making the child "worse." At these times, the parents need support from the child's therapist.

C. THE CHILD'S PROBLEM

The following children should be seen alone with minimal family involvement:

1. The abused child[29]
2. The child caught between hostile, divorcing parents[29]
3. The drug-and substance-abusing child
4. The child with gender ambiguity[29]
5. The child whose parents are highly intrusive

   Periodic sessions may be held with the parents to discuss parental problems with the child and, in general, any issues that may have come to the parents' attention or issues that the therapist needs to explain or explore with the parents about the child. Some therapists[15] arrange to have parents see someone else to "collect data" about the child's life, which is then shared with the therapist on a weekly or other time arrangement basis.

Developmental and Therapeutic Functions of Play   Play is used

1. To work out problematic experiences[12]
2. To learn about interpersonal relations[35]
3. To learn to compete, cooperate, and collaborate[32]
4. To assimilate and gain mastery over unpleasant and new experiences[5]
5. To learn about the culture[33]
6. To act out an uncomfortable emotion symbolically or gradually enough so that, ultimately, it can be felt

7. To represent an absent object—people or things[26]
8. To represent an observation of a part of the external world
9. To represent an observation of a situation in the external world
10. To represent the internal world—a thought or a feeling, a wish, an attitude
11. To accommodate to reality[26]
12. To organize experience[29] privately and with others
13. To develop the capacity to gratify oneself and to delay gratification
14. As an expression of cognitive status[33]
15. As a contributor to the character of cognition[33]
16. As a bridge between concrete experience and abstract thought[26]
17. As a creative act[26]

Kinds of Play Therapy

A. **PSYCHOANALYTIC PLAY THERAPY**

Play is seen by some theorists[22] as a symbolic function, the activity being interpreted or "translated" as it relates to the child's life: events, fantasies, dreams, and wishes. However, many therapists[15] see play in therapy as multifunctional; therefore, use of interpretation is more selective.

B. **RELEASE THERAPY[23]**

Acting out in an exaggerated form through repeated therapist-structured play activities is the crux of release therapy. The symptoms, preferably of short duration, though based on a past specific event, are "played out" and may or may not be interpreted, depending on the child's personality and age. This technique is often used in combination with other approaches.

C. **RELATIONSHIP THERAPY[2,3]**

Play is used as a vehicle to relate to the therapist. The activity is selected by the child, who expresses experiences and relations through the play. The child relates to the therapist by using the therapist in the activity. Play content is seen as secondary to the child–therapist relationship, though the therapist privately acknowledges links to past experience.

D. **BEHAVIORAL THERAPY**

Operant techniques are often used with hyperactive children[9] to reduce the activity and organize the play.

Materials

Since play therapy's inception, techniques have included the use of dolls, doll houses, sandboxes, water, games, clay, story books, stuffed animals, bean bags, and various toys such as soldiers, guns, and figures of various sizes and types. Materials do not have to be numerous and should not be overwhelming in presentation so that the child has trouble choosing from a vast hoard. Materials should be clinically useful and be appropriate for a range of ages. "Fussy" equipment such as elaborate doll houses and fancy dolls may be too "untouchable" for the child.

Major Techniques

A. **DRAWING AND PAINTING AND MUTUAL DRAWING[36] AND PAINTING**

1. *Description*—In drawing or painting, the child expresses inner reality and outer reality that may otherwise be difficult to know or to express.[7,8,21] The child benefits from the creation and the expression itself, which, in addition, is sometimes a replacement for verbal communication and contact. In mutual drawing or "squiggle"[36] and painting, the therapist draws a squiggle, which the child makes into something, and the child makes a squiggle, which the therapist develops into something, and so on. It is a means of having contact

with the child in a highly collaborative way, making use of the child's and the therapist's inner experience through interpersonal and projective means.

2. *Typical Case*—Andrew is an 11-year-old boy who has a good deal of trouble making friends and much difficulty using his considerable intelligence. He even has trouble leaving the house on weekends when he is "free" and is afraid of almost everyone outside the family.

3. *Typical Dialogue*—Since drawing or painting of any kind is used as a mode of expression in itself, there is most often little or no dialogue, particularly for someone like Andrew, who is afraid of his aggression in any physical or verbal form. The communication must be the production itself, without seeking verbal expression and without interpretation, which would serve only to stop the communication. For example, Andrew drew an idyllic monochromatic picture of a house on a lake, but with a red bomb buried under the ground. It was not until a year later that he could talk about his anger and fear of "breaking out."

B. **STORYTELLING AND MUTUAL STORYTELLING**[17]

1. *Description*—Storytelling is used when other means of expression are difficult for the child. The story is a vehicle for communication of felt or unfelt needs, wishes, or concerns. In mutual storytelling,[17] the child tells a story. The therapist, privately abstracting the psychodynamic meaning, then tells "the story," introducing healthier ways of dealing with the child's difficulties inherent in the story. This method combines indirect interpretation and collaboration by using a vehicle the child understands.

2. *Typical Case*—Paul is an 8 year old who has been very anxious in school and at home. His father is perfectionistic and demanding, particularly with Paul.

3. *Typical Dialogue*

Nurse: [Speaking into tape recorder] Today we have with us a very special guest, Paul Brown, who will tell a story.

Paul: It was Christmas Eve, and the family was gathered in the living room waiting for Santa. Suddenly they heard his sleigh on the roof. Santa yelled, 'Rudolph! Watch out for that chimney!' and then CRASH! Santa shouted 'Rudolph, how can you be so clumsy and stupid? Can't you do anything right?' That's the story [laughing].

Nurse: My turn now. [Repeats Paul's story up to the point of the crash] Then Santa said, 'Oh, dear, too bad that happened. It's okay, Rudolph—nobody's perfect!'

C. **PUPPETS**[19]

1. *Description*—Puppets are useful for children who have difficulty formulating or expressing their inner lives directly or by other play means, or feel too old to play with "toys" or dolls. Puppets may be recognizable (for example, television or comic-strip figures) or anonymous figures. They invite a wide field of projections.

2. *Typical Case*—Annie's parents are divorced and her father remarried. He and his new wife had a baby daughter a year ago. Lately Annie has felt angry at her father for not living with her and her mother. Also, although she likes and enjoys her half sister, she has been pushing and hitting her whenever she can.

3. *Typical Dialogue*—[After making the puppets into a mother and a baby daughter]

Annie (the mother): You're a bad girl. You wet and have no teeth and cry. I hate you!

Nurse (the baby daughter): I think Annie hates me. I feel bad about that, but it sure is hard after 10 years to have me come around and hog the show. Anybody would be awfully mad.

D. **SPONTANEOUS PLAY, INCLUDING "MAKE BELIEVE" PLAY**[26]

1. *Description*—This is the play that arises at any time in a given session and is often of short duration. Directly or indirectly, the child calls on the therapist to join in and take a role. It is initiated by the child for any number of reasons:
    a. To have the therapist communicate on the child's level
    b. To serve as a needed defense against or reprieve from uncomfortable material
    c. To express an uncomfortable thought, feeling, or action indirectly, once removed
    d. To "try out" one's own and a therapist's response to a thought, feeling, or action, once removed
    e. As a sign of or vehicle for closeness, or both.
    It is best for the therapist to move in and out of spontaneous play, usually without interpretation, which tends to negate the significance of the interaction.
2. *Typical Case*—Sandy is a 5-year-old girl whose mother is so highly rational that anything that is not "real" is debunked and not tolerated.
3. *Typical Dialogue*
    Sandy: [Whispering] I have to turn out the lights. [She does] Sh-h-h-h. The ghost is in the room next door. He's talking now. . . .
    Nurse: Oh my, what's he saying? Is he going to come in with us?

E. **FORMAL GAMES**
Like drawing, the games themselves are the expression and the communication; thus, although there is verbal exchange, there is often no dialogue apart from the game itself. The meaning behind that dialogue is not discussed, and the meaning of the choice of game is often a mixture of personality features and personal concerns.

1. *Games of Physical Skill*[27]—Emphasize achievement. Bean bags, basketball, football kicking, batting baseballs, jump rope, hopscotch, jacks, tag, racing, climbing, gymnastics, darts, and marbles are examples in which the outcome is determined by the player's motor activity.
2. *Games of Chance*[27]—Imply high responsibility training, the belief that supernatural beings are benevolent or coercible, and the belief that initiative is punishable. Die tossing, card games such as war or poker or slap-jack, card and board games such as Candyland, bingo, coin matching, and guessing games are examples in which the outcome is determined by an uncontrolled artifact external to the play or by guessing.
3. *Games of Strategy*[27]*—Emphasize and imply cultural complexity and obedience training. Card games such as bridge and gin rummy, checkers, chess, Parcheesi, Trouble, Sorry, backgammon, Monopoly, dominoes, Triominoes, pick-up sticks, marbles, Ping-Pong, tic-tac-toe, Clue, and Twenty Questions are games in which the outcome is determined by rational choices among various possible actions.

---

*These games are not all "pure" strategy; some involve a good deal of chance or physical skill, but to do well, high strategy maneuvers are necessary.

Transference "Affectionate attachment"[16] or positive transference serves both an educational and a therapeutic purpose in the treatment of children. Therapists become new love objects, coexisting with parents upon whom the child is still dependent. From a developmental standpoint, the therapist is more than a transference object; the therapist is a kind of additional parent. Negative reactions must not be seen, therefore, simply as "transference," to be experienced and interpreted, but as posible detriments to the positive attachment necessary for growth through the relationship. With children, such sustained reactions must be addressed quickly in order to move forward.

Countertransference Despite the age of the child, the countertransference problems that arise are no different from ones that occur when the client is an adult, often to the surprise of the therapist. However, the following manifestations are particularly prominent:

1. Overidentification with the child
2. Competition with the parents
3. Competition with the child; the need to be "right"; the need to win or the need to lose
4. Hatred, anger,[24] and disgust, and defenses against these feelings
5. Overconcern about the child's "productions"
6. Too much or too little limit setting regarding play behavior: cheating, hitting, breaking, spitting, changing game rules
7. Engaging in power struggles with the child to "straighten him or her out"
8. Engaging in power struggles with the parents to "straighten them out" (actually or in fantasy)
9. Control of the child: fear of parental anger and disapproval or fear of the child's anger and disapproval
10. Control of the child through interpretation of behavior
11. Control of the child through control of the direction of the session: lack of therapist–child resonance
12. Control of the child through control of the child's direction or vehicle of expression: fear of the child's loss of control
13. Intrusiveness: lack of respect for the child's needs and desires
14. Emotional detachment: lack of therapist–child resonance or anxiety about the "nonintellectual" approach
15. Feeling fraudulent: anxiety about the "nonintellectual" approach

Countertransference reactions are not necessarily detrimental to treatment, especially those reactions induced by the child rather than the therapist's unconscious.[20,24]

The Office It has been traditional to provide a playroom for the child, that is, as distinguished from the consulting room. There are rational reasons for this, such as having access to a sink (often a low sink) and storage space, and the virtues of a child having an "own room." On the other hand, the needs of the therapist for neatness and order in the "real" office have probably contributed to building the tradition.

Space considerations, economics, and mixed adult and child therapy practices have caused some therapists to reconsider the use of a playroom. For children in a mechanically minded society[11] devices such as tape recorders, dictaphones, typewriters, and telephones are features of standard offices, which children may find useful tools for expression, once removed, of their concerns and interpersonal competencies and difficulties. In addition, their use in an adult setting sets a "home" context for interpersonal involvement and growth.

The child may also find the homelike environment useful for testing out spontaneous activity and play with matches, curtains, tables and chairs, mirrors, knickknacks, and other typical furnishing. The therapist's response as an additional love object can be readily compared by the child with that of the parents, thus easily introducing the notion of differences between parents and other adults and in adult–child relations.

Evaluation Evaluation procedures for children vary. Periodic assessment is made of the child's drawings and other productions to note the variation and development throughout the therapeutic process. Verbal behavior, game behavior, and how the child is dealing with school, family, and friends are assessed on an ongoing basis. When it is ascertained that termination is appropriate, treatment is most often tapered off, on a timetable primarily set by the child and eventually resulting in contact that might occur a few times a year until the child no longer wants the contact.

References
1. Ainsworth MDS et al: Patterns of Attachment: A Psychological Study of the Strange Situation. New Jersey, Lawrence Erlbaum Associates, 1978
2. Allen FH: Psychotherapy with Children. New York, WW Norton, 1942
3. Axline V: Play Therapy. Boston, Houghton Mifflin, 1947
4. Bateson G: A theory of play and fantasy. In Bruner JS et al (eds): Play: Its Role in Development and Evolution. New York, Basic Books, 1976
5. Blashki S, Schutz S, Puckering C: Influences on the development of attachment in mothers. In Anthony EJ, Chiland C (eds): The Child in His Family: Preventive Child Psychiatry in an Age of Transition. New York, John Wiley & Sons, 1980
6. Bowlby J: Attachment. New York, Basic Books, 1969
7. DiLeo JH: Children's Drawings as Diagnostic Aids. New York, Brunner/Mazel, 1973
8. DiLeo JH: Child Development: Analysis and Synthesis. New York, Brunner/Mazel, 1977
9. Doubros SG, Daniels GJ: The reduction of overactive behavior. In Schaefer C (ed): Therapeutic Use of Child's Play. New York, Jason Aronson, 1979
10. Dreschsler RJ, Shapiro NJ: A procedure for direct observation of family interaction in a child guidance clinic. Psychiatry 24:163, 1961
11. Durfee MB: Use of ordinary office equipment. In Shaefer C (ed): Therapeutic Use of Child's Play. New York, Jason Aronson, 1979
12. Erikson EH: Studies in the interpretation of play: In clinical observation of play disruption in young children. Genet Psychol Monogr 22:557, 1940
13. Freeman RD: The home visit in child psychiatry. J Am Acad Child Psychiatr 6:276, 1967
14. Freud A: Assessment of childhood disturbances. Psychoanal Study Child 17:149, 1962
15. Freud A: Normality and Pathology in Childhood. New York, International Universities Press, 1965
16. Freud A: The role of transference in the analysis of children. In Schaefer C (ed): Therapeutic Use of Child's Play. New York, Jason Aronson, 1979
17. Gardner R: Therapeutic Communication with Children: The Mutual Storytelling Technique. New York, Science House, 1971
18. Goode M et al: Attachment processes in fathers. In Anthony EJ, Chiland C (eds): The Child in His Family: Preventive Child Psychiatry in an Age of Transition. New York, John Wiley & Sons, 1980
19. Hawkley L: Puppets in child psychotherapy. In Schaefer C (ed): Therapeutic Use of Child's Play. New York, Jason Aronson, 1979
20. Herron WG, Rouslin S: Issues in Psychotherapy. Maryland, Robert J Brady, 1982
21. Kellog R: Analyzing Children's Art. California, Manfield, 1970
22. Klein M: The Psycho-analysis of Children. New York, Delacorte Press/Seymour Lawrence, 1975
23. Levy DM: Release therapy. In Schaefer C (ed): Therapeutic Use of Child's Play. New York, Jason Aronson, 1979
24. Marshall RJ: Countertransference in the psychotherapy of children and adolescents. Contemp Psychoanalysis 15:595, 1979
25. Nagera H: The Developmental Approach to Childhood Psychopathology. New York, Jason Aronson, 1981
26. Piaget J: Play, Dreams and Imitation in Childhood. New York, WW Norton, 1962
27. Roberts JM, Sutton-Smith B: Child training and game involvement. Ethnology 1:166, 1962
28. Rouslin S: Developmental aggression and its consequences. Perspect Psychiatr Care 13:170, 1975
29. Sidelau BF, Light N: Point/Counterpoint: Family treatment for the disturbed child, Perspect Psychiatr Psychiatr Care 2:78, 1981

30. Singer JL: The child's world of make-believe: Experimental studies in imaginative play. New York, Academic Press, 1973
31. Smale S et al: Evolving concepts of attachment. In Anthony EJ, Chiland C (eds): The Child in His Family: Preventive Child Psychiatry in an Age of Transition. New York, John Wiley & Sons, 1980
32. Sullivan HS: The Interpersonal Theory of Psychiatry. New York, WW Norton, 1953
33. Sutton-Smith B: Play in cognitive development. In Schaefer C (ed): Therapeutic Use of Child's Play. New York, Jason Aronson, 1979
34. Vygotsky LS: Play and its role in the mental development of the child. In Bruner JS et al (eds): Play: Its role in development and evolution. New York, Basic Books, 1976
35. Winnicott DW: Playing and reality. New York, Basic Books, 1971
36. Winnicott DW: Therapeutic consultations in child psychiatry. New York, Basic Books, 1971

27

Group Therapy with Children

Nada Light

Introduction Social groups are a normal part of childhood. Children (5–12 years) separate from their families by forming peer groups. In groups, they play and talk freely, and motor and social skills are attempted, practiced, and refined. Individual therapy is sometimes difficult for a latency child because of strong defenses against dependent relationships with adults. Group therapy provides a format familiar to children.

Purpose[4]
1. To develop the capacity for healthier relationships
2. To develop defense mechanisms important for socialization: sublimation, reaction formation, identification with the aggressor
3. To strengthen ongoing development
4. To consolidate a conscience
5. To increase reality testing

Types A. **DIAGNOSTIC PLAY GROUPS**
1. A limited number of sessions is used, usually one or two.
2. The child's behavior, skills, and peer relationships are assessed.
3. An active leader designs situations to maximize periods of observation.

B. **ACTIVITY GROUP THERAPY**[5]
1. Activities are primary vehicles for children to discover their impact on others and to remedy individual problems.
2. The leader is a facilitator of activity and a helper with crafts, does not interpret behavior, and discourages transference.
3. The place and materials are predictable from session to session.

C. **PERMISSIVE PLAY THERAPY**[2]
1. The leader is nondirective, and behavior is not interpreted.
2. The place and materials are predictable from session to session.
3. This type of group is useful with withdrawn, phobic, immature children needing help in expressing aggressive and affective feelings, as well as in young latency children, when play and fantasy can be maximized.

D. **BEHAVIOR MODIFICATION**[3]
1. The leader is active and plans a token reward system, behavioral agreements, written contracts, and commitments with each child.
2. Specific behaviors are targeted for change, and recording methods are devised.
3. Group activities and discussion are used to help members evaluate necessary changes, progress, and successful mastery of behavior.
4. The group gradually simulates the outside world to transfer learned behaviors into home, school, and play relationships.

E. **GROUPS UNITED BY A COMMON EXPERIENCE** (partial list)
1. Examples
   a. Abused children
   b. Bereaved children (loss of parent or siblings)
   c. Diabetic children
2. Techniques of activity, discussion, and play are selected to work with specific problems.
3. The leadership and group's purpose determines the number and frequency of sessions and whether the membership is open or fixed.

Reasons for Group
Therapy with Children

1. The latency child uses activities to learn social skills.
2. Latency children can develop specific conflicts common at this time of development, for example, sibling rivalry, fear of hospitalization, and inappropriate classroom behavior. These can be explored in small groups of children within the hospital, school, or office setting.
3. Children are naturally dependent on adults in any social hierarchy: group treatment encourages child-to-child interaction and relationship problems can be explored productively with other children present.

Reasons for Play
Therapy Groups Rather
than Talking

1. Abstract thinking is not fully developed in the latency child; thus, the ability to learn through insight is limited.
2. Since mastery of small and large muscle skills dominate the developmental tasks of latency, crafts and activities capitalize on these needs.
3. Blending activities and discussion for the older latency child (ten to eleven years) becomes a leadership task handled best depending on group composition. Preadolescents are more capable of discussing issues, but not all may have the verbal interaction skills to do so.

Treatment Methods
Specific to Problems

Some methods of group therapy are more suitable for specific problems than are others. They are shown in Table 27–1.

Table 27–1
TREATMENT METHODS SPECIFIC TO PROBLEMS

Problem Behaviors	*Methods*	*Rationale*
A. Problems expressing feelings and conflicts: Phobias Repressed feelings Withdrawal Fears Feelings of powerlessness	The leader functions as a facilitator and designs an activity that encourages increased discussion time when the group becomes cohesive.	A phobic child can see others experiencing what is avoided; a fearful child observes the most feared behaviors tried by others; a child who feels powerless experiences mastery through activities and new friendships; a withdrawn child observes how relationships begin and develop.
B. Problems with behavior control: Conduct disorders with aggressive and socialization problems, and difficulty exerting self-control.	An active leader designs an activity group with behavior modification techniques. Before an activity begins, careful explanations of the group rules is essential. The rules are worded positively, that is, "children walk" rather than "no running," or "put equipment back in one piece" rather than "no breaking."	Members come with limit problems and require firm boundaries. The leader makes desirable behaviors explicit and encourages identification with the leader's methods of socialization, problem solving, and expressive behavior control.

Group Focus and Leader Behavior   Table 27–2 shows, for each age group, focus, rationale, and leader type and rationale.

Planning the Group   **A. WHOM TO INCLUDE**

A prospective group member is evaluated individually prior to beginning the group. When grouping children, the therapist considers positive behavioral characteristics, for example, assertiveness, craft-making abilities, aggressive expression, athletic abilities, and some appropriate school/study habits. Including two

Table 27–2
AGE, FOCUS OF GROUP, RATIONALE, LEADER TYPE, AND RATIONALE

Age	Focus of Group	Rationale	Leader Type and Rationale
5–7 years	A. Activity-oriented group— Vehicles include handcrafts, cooking, simple gardening, group trips, and simple sports.	At this age children have limited but developing skills in cooperation, competition, and compromise.	The activity leader is a facilitator and helper during the group session, letting interactions develop spontaneously. Children are struggling to function in any group and socialization deficits are explicit. These provide the leader with discussion ideas.
	B. Discussion-oriented group is limited to behaviors and relationships that grow out of related group activities: Planning and evaluation of activity are natural discussion times.	The discussion must be carefully led because children of this age lack the ability to be insightful and to reflect on their own problems or those of others.	The discussion leader is a model for language and behavior useful in planning, talking about, and evaluating problems or conflicts that evolve from the activity.
8–10 years[5]	A simple discussion format is possible. Activities may be used initially until the group is cohesive, and then fade as discussion–problem solving becomes the dominant focus, with activities secondary. For fun, or as a behavioral "reward," a trip, party, or special game can be provided.	The group becomes very important. Children at this age are more conscious of rules and competition, and there is a developmental leaning toward conformity, which can be used effectively to teach desirable behaviors. Positive media and sport heroes can be useful here.	The leader acts as a guide by delineating the purpose of the group, for example, "This group will help people learn how to get along better with others. We will do some projects together while we get to know each other, and talk about how we are working together." The leader must be active initially to encourage desirable behavior. Informal child leaders will emerge and encourage the peer identification process.
11–12 years	Discussion group and specialized techniques are used, for example, psychodrama, dance, or art therapies.	These children are capable of interacting on a verbal level. Social group identity is very strong, even in children with poor social skills, and the desire to belong is present. Specialized techniques capitalize on the preadolescent's increased ability to fantasize and to be more expressive.	An engaging adult provides clear, appropriate relationship behavior methods. The leader is an active facilitator and role model for developing more sensitive approaches to relationships. Limits are set clearly with a firm behavior code, for example, no physical violence, roughhousing or "horsing around." Preadolescence is a time when adults outside the home become significant for a deepening of the identification process; it is a fluid psychological state for therapeutic work to be successful.

children who share similar competence in one of these areas encourages support and beginning cohesiveness as each child's deficit areas are touched on and explored.

B. **WHOM TO EXCLUDE**

The following kinds of children need individual or family therapy to ready them for group therapy:

1. The child with intense sibling rivalry prevents a group's cohesiveness from jelling because of intense bullying, projecting, and destructive behaviors.
2. The child with impaired psychosexual development needs individual therapy. A sexually precocious child needs direct interpretations; a perversely abused child may find the group too stimulating, and group therapy may raise the child's anxiety too much, especially if the child, the abuser, and the group members are of the same gender.
3. The overly aggressive child needs too many verbal and physical restraints.
4. The child with reactive stress, for example, a death in the family or a traumatic event, can resolve anxiety more quickly with individual or family treatment.
5. The actively psychotic child is too frightening and confusing to other members. A child who has had psychotic periods but is reconstituted can be included.
6. The unsocialized child with poor social bonds needs individual treatment first.

C. **LENGTH OF TIME**

One and one half hours is adequate for most groups. Sessions begin and end on time because members pace their responses unconsciously. Also, boundaries must be predictable.

D. **FREQUENCY AND DURATION**

A child's growth and development continues despite problems. The leader may want to consider frequent sessions to capitalize on an age level that is fluid and responsive to treatment. For example, a group might meet twice weekly for 6 weeks or weekly for 12 weeks. A school-based group may begin on an intensive basis, meeting twice weekly. As behaviors resolve, the group would progress to a weekly and then biweekly session until termination were appropriate.

E. **OPEN-ENDED VERSUS CLOSED**

Closed groups, in which a number of children start together, have a certain number of sessions together, and end together, are best. The coming and going of children every so often is too disruptive. However, a well established, cohesive group can accommodate a new child occasionally.

F. **NUMBER**

The group begins with eight or nine members. Dropping out will occur as the group develops and inappropriate behavior patterns emerge, for example, excessive disruptiveness. The group should have at least three and no more than six members per leader. Fewer than three members does not provide enough interpersonal diversity; a large group presents management problems, with overly aggressive behavior and subdividing.

G. **ADDING AND DROPPING MEMBERS**

A group that is undergoing stabilization to a manageable and functional size creates anxiety in members. The leader offers simple statements about a child's entry or exit. "Mary is joining the group today," and avoids labeling any behaviors. If the child asks, "Does she see you too?" "Does she do bad in school?" the leader directs these questions child to child.

H. DEVELOPMENTAL LEVEL AND AGE SPREAD

The age spread should be 12 months at the most. Interests, level of sophistication, and emerging sexuality in preadolescents make closer age groupings generally more functional. Occasionally, developmental age or a behavioral problem may be best treated by mixing age levels, for example, placing a younger bully in an older group or an immature older child in a younger group. Both examples are not meant to intimidate or humiliate the children, but rather to expose the larger problem area to other children at a different age level who are working on similar behavioral issues. This kind of grouping is very difficult and can lead to an additional overlay of identification problems. It must only be used in selected children.

I. WHEN TO USE SAME SEX GROUPS

If the child's gender identification is weak, and self-concept and peer relations poor, a same-sex group is best. Also, preadolescents need same-sex groups because this is the period when sexual identification is being solidified. Members of the opposite sex create anxiety, which distracts from other problems. A heterosexual group can follow if further treatment is necessary.

J. WHEN TO USE MIXED-SEX GROUPS

Withdrawn and repressed, as well as preschool children can be treated in a mixed-sex group. This group can be modeled on Slavson's activity groups.[5] In our culture, boys and girls begin to play according to their gender in midlatency, that is, girls play in different ways than boys. When older latency children are in the same group, the girls see the boys as "too rough," and the boys see the girls' games as "silly." However, in younger latency, both boys and girls are still mastering large and small motor skills and can use a wider variety of activities, for example, doll play, cooking, and sports. The leader must keep in mind at all times that the activity is not as important as the behavioral and identity problems being worked out by each child.

K. WHEN TO MIX PROBLEMS

In general, a mixture of problems is best, however, the leader is careful to include only one of the following problems per group:
1. Stealing—If the stealing is confined to home and family members, the child is admitted to the group. If the child steals indiscriminately, the leader will have to spend valuable time and energy safeguarding equipment and the environment.
2. Young Undersocialized Conduct Disorders (under 8 years)—While these children are difficult to treat at any age, the younger child is not able to empathize with other children who are different. Also, because these children are so aggressive, it is best to keep them in small, homogeneous groups. The leader must observe problems carefully for behavioral changes.

L. PREPARATION OF MEMBERS

Children need preparation when entering a therapy group. The therapeutic process is a totally strange experience for a child "brought to treatment," and all the newness can be overwhelming. The leader explains the time the group starts and ends, the duration of the group, the place and general format, and specific therapeutic goals for that child. Concrete information in these areas includes the necessary boundaries, without preventing spontaneous behavior.

M. **RELATIONSHIP OF THE NURSE TO PARENTS**

The leader must have a strong alliance with the child's parents because once the immediate symptoms are relieved, the child's and parent's motivation to continue in treatment are greatly diminished. Regular conferences with the parents can help the leader assess if changes seen in the child's behavior in the group are also occurring in behavior at home and school.[4]

The Setting   Three dimensions influence the setting of the group:

A. **SIZE OF ROOM**

If the group is purely discussion, a comfortable room or part of a room with adequate privacy is sufficient. Very small spaces are more intimate, but they may cause high anxiety if the intimacy is forced and premature. Most latency groups combine both activities and discussion of the activities, that is, planning and outcome or impact on the members. Very large spaces can encourage random and wild running. A room that can be easily subdivided is best.

B. **PREDICTABILITY OF AVAILABILITY OF THE SPACE**

This may be an issue for some members. Treatment centers often switch groups, rooms, and so on. A leader must ascertain how important it is to the group to meet each time in the same location. Very disorganized children may need to explore each new area, interfering with the work of the group.

C. **THE ORIGIN OF THE GROUP**

This dictates where it can be held. If the group is from a school, a hospital outpatient or inpatient department, a mental health center, or a private office, these services are located in their own peculiar spaces. Nice weather may permit the use of outdoor neighborhood facilities. However, liability may be an issue and should be clarified by the leader. There may not be a good space choice. Too often, group therapy is an afterthought and no adequate space exists. A commitment to group work must be ascertained before a facility is designed or chosen.

Activities   A. **PLANNED BY THE LEADER**

A specific problem or conflict is chosen by the leader to be explored in the group, for example, hospitalization. The leader manipulates the equipment and themes to help members play through traumas and problems.

B. **PLANNED BY THE GROUP**

The leader offers guidance to the group during their planning sessions. This method offers members ''safer'' or ''controlled'' situations to experience problems with social participation, overcontrolling behaviors, frustration intolerance, shyness, and lack of self-confidence and self-worth.

Phases of Group   Since most latency groups have activities at some point in the group, these phases are
Development   obviously geared toward activity-oriented treatment. Pure discussion groups for older latency children or preadolescents follow the same stages of development as adult therapy groups. The activity group passes through the following phases:

A. BEGINNING

In early sessions, the least emotionally loaded situation is an individual project, for example, a craft or model. Children can initiate their choices, own styles, and abilities while adjusting to the group. This phase provides the leader with an immediate assessment of fine motor skills and social responses, for example, a child's ability to praise a friend, level of self-confidence, and need to criticize. Chart 27–1 shows typical behavior and nursing interventions in the orientation phase of any children's group.

B. MIDDLE

Once individual projects begin and the leader observes child-to-child interactions about projects, dyad experiences can be introduced. Board games, skill demonstrations, and group building activities encourage beginning group skills in taking turns, cooperation, and following rules. This phase outlines clearly the problem areas of most children. Patterns of isolation and alienation become apparent. However, opportunities for new friendships, support, and healthier patterns of interaction are the goals in this phase.

Chart 27–1
BEHAVIOR AND INTERVENTION IN THE BEGINNING

Behaviors	Nursing Interventions
1. Children may be silent and isolate themselves.	1. Tolerate initially; be alert to signs that the child is observing or listening and comment on these. "I noticed you watching Meg and Bonnie arguing. Would you like to be able to talk like that to your brother?" Another child's curiosity may be aroused, and he may talk about the sibling problem.
2. Children may become aggressive and test rules.	2. Set firm limits and their consequences at the outset; use verbal and physical limits if necessary.
3. Children may talk directly to the leader and ask personal questions.	3. Simple comments like, "It's easier to talk to me," state that you understand but that this type of question is not appropriate. Restate the purpose of the group and note that it is hard to get started with any new friendship. Give attention to the strongest dyad in the group.
4. Children may ignore other group members.	4. Observe those children a child ignores and those a child finds "comfortable." Use either as a stimulus for the more verbal child to respond to initially. Before and after group lingering adds to the withdrawn child's information about subgroups.
5. Children may misuse equipment or toys to attract attention.	5. Discourage this behavior. Call on members to help the noisy or disruptive child to censure this behavior. This helps the child verbalize needs, and control outbursts. "Okay, Bobby, we know you are here. What do you want to tell us?"
6. Children may bring in outside toys, friends, magazines, food, projects, pets.	6. The younger child needs props. Use them but discourage the child from bringing in any items in the future. Point out in a helpful way that there are two ways to get to know one another, sharing ideas and sharing special things.
7. Children may wander around and have difficulty sitting in a chair or on a mat.	7. Hyperactive children have a "driven" quality to their restlessness. Determine if the restlessness is anxiety or part of a hyperactive pattern. Hyperactivity can be helped through medication and firm limits.
8. Children develop cycles of play in groups. Destructive play is followed by quiet, constructive play. Switching back and forth occurs more frequently in this first phase.	8. Intervene if destructiveness occurs to others or materials. Otherwise observe for lengthening of constructive cycles as an indicator of beginning cohesiveness.

1. *Promoting Cohesiveness*—Treatment can occur when self-control, compromise, and mutual understanding lead to cohesiveness. If this has not occurred the nurse asks the following questions:
   a. Is there an unusually disruptive or scary child present?
   b. Is the leader too anxious?
   c. Are activities interfering with the discussion of problems?
   d. Is the leader overly optimistic about the members' ability to discuss, give feedback, and offer suggestions?
   e. Is the meeting place too large, too small, that is, too stimulating or too intimate, generating anxiety in some members?
2. *Characteristics of Cohesiveness*—Cohesiveness has begun when:
   a. Friendships form.
   b. Group rules are generally obeyed.
   c. Members are prompt or early.
   d. Members talk about their "group" or "us."
3. *Identification*—One of the important processes occurring in the middle phase of group development is identification. The number of sessions needed for this is dependent on the changing internal dynamics for each child and the external forces in each child's life (additional school and family stresses). Characteristics of this phase include the following:
   a. Members begin to focus on interactions in the group. Conversations are about what is happening in the group.
   b. Members model an active leader's style of question and answers.
   c. Parents and schools report some behavior improvement.
   d. Members gradually connect problem behaviors in group and the original referral problems. This particular area may take a long time to reach and then many sessions may be required to address each member's problem.

C. **LAST**

Group projects dominate this phase. The active leader first sets an example of appropriate group behavior and then fades as members work toward group goals. Evidence of healthy competition, cooperation, role taking, and expressive skills mark the beginning of termination planning.

Termination occurs when there is a time-limited group situation. Otherwise, each member will reach this point in treatment individually. Leader activities include

1. Making the group less attractive by giving less praise, less positive reinforcement, and less encouragement
2. Helping members explore joining social activity groups in the community (scouts, Y-groups, day camps, sports teams, church groups)
3. Readying those members who need further treatment for referral or as a nucleus for a new ongoing group

Use of Food   Any experience can be used to teach socialization skills. Feeding children and mealtime is a daily experience colored by parental emotions, culture, and style in relating to others. A leader must evaluate whether serving food presents more problems than it is worth or if it provides a good learning experience.

A. **ADVANTAGES**
1. The severely deprived child may be emotionally unavailable during the early stages of treatment; food literally fills the child who may be then able to

function on a more secure emotional level. The importance of the feeding process then fades as the members begin to function as a group.

2. The combination of discussion and food can be reminiscent of painful mealtime scenes that are important treatment issues to explore.

B. **DISADVANTAGES**

1. The main problem with serving food during treatment time is the distraction it can present. A clear message of therapeutic work must be conveyed by the leader from the outset.

2. New therapists may serve food as a friendly gesture or even a "bribe" to encourage attendance and may not be able to assess the confusion this creates for a troubled child who responds to the mixed message.

Ground Rules   Appropriate socialization with others is the primary aim of most groups. Expected behaviors must be explicit from the outset. Children are used to hearing this approach from their school teachers. However, some children may not be able to absorb abstract interpretations because of cognitive limitations. Using examples of *natural consequences* may be helpful, for example, broken equipment means a loss for all members, disruptive behavior brings an activity to a halt, and arriving late means no participation. It is useful to set rules, observe who breaks them, and help the child understand, with the group's assistance, "why" it happened.

Ground rules depend, in part, on the group's purpose. The following rules may be applicable to either verbal or activities groups:

1. One person speaks at a time.
2. No distractions like radios, food for self, noisy toys, animals
3. No physical violence
4. No wild running

Activities used in latency groups must be carefully planned. Stating general rules ahead of time provides structure for security and boundaries for those with control problems. In addition to the above rules these can be added for an activity:

1. No destruction of materials
2. No throwing of equipment
3. Cleanup is a part of every project.

Encouraging Interaction Among Members   The leader clarifies appropriate ways of behaving in the group and outside the group. Children will model a leader's behavior but will rely on the leader to ask and answer painful questions. Adults usually take a leadership role in directing children's behavior; however, the leader encourages a different style of interacting within the group, that is, child to child. For example, Joan and Susan were arguing and grabbing a particular piece of doll furniture. Each had intense sibling relationships that interfered with social friendships. The leader suggested, "You girls have the same sharing problems at home." Both girls stopped, but neither gave in. Joan punched Susan and grabbed the toy, all the while looking at the leader. Susan screamed so loud that the rest of the group censured her. "Just like home," the leader continued. Jill, a more easy-going child, suggested another way to arrange the doll furniture. Both girls liked Jill's suggestion, and Susan said to Joan, "It's okay now if you want the chair." Joan was reluctant to comply and said, "You can use it when my doll finishes." The give and take occurred after the explosion, but at least the possibility of taking turns may then occur to one or both girls in a future situation.

Types of Leaders   The group's purpose and composition shape the leader's role.

A. **THE ACTIVE LEADER**

The active leader deliberately becomes dominant.

1. Goal—Members incorporate methods used by the leader by the end of the group.
2. Leadership Methods
   a. Confronts unproductive patterns of behavior
   b. Reinforces positive behavior
   c. Sets limits both verbally and physically
   d. Encourages identification with the leader
3. Uses
   a. Children with control problems
   b. Children with weak or absent parental models
   c. Children with severely disorganized home environments

B. **THE PASSIVE LEADER**

The passive leader deliberately remains neutral.[5]

1. Goal—Members strengthen independent behavior and inner security.
2. Leadership Methods
   a. Is not active in interpersonal conflicts and relationships, but rather is supportive
   b. Helps with crafts and projects and matches members to be potentially supportive in behavioral areas
   c. Discourages transference to leader
3. Uses
   a. Children who have experienced adults as overprotective, coddling
   b. Children who have experienced adults as rejecting or depriving

Evaluation Expected outcomes of group psychotherapy with latency children include the following:

1. Less destructive behavior
2. Increased social acceptance by the child's peer group
3. Improved self-concept
4. Improved academic performance

These observations can be part of a general assessment. A behavioral chart recording specific changes, their frequency of occurrence, and related behavioral spin-offs is an additional method of evaluation. Comments from the family, school, and other groups that may involve the child are helpful in a general sense. However, the leader must see changes in the child within the group for more lasting treatment effects. A time-limited group can be followed by periodic reviews with the family or school system. A child may need to be seen by the leader or a therapist on an individual basis as a supportive postgroup experience until the child no longer wants the contact.

References 1. Epstein N, Altman S: Experiences in therapy with latency-age boys. In Schaefer C (ed): The Therapeutic Use of Child's Play. New York, Jason Aronson, 1976
2. Ginott HG: Group Psychotherapy with Children. New York, McGraw-Hill, 1961
3. Rose SD: Treating Children in Groups. San Francisco, Jossey-Bass, 1973
4. Sarnoff C: Latency. New York, Jason Aronson, 1976
5. Slavson SR: Play group therapy. In Schaefer C (ed): The Therapeutic Use of Children's Play. New York, Jason Aronson, 1976

28

Therapy with Adolescents

Candy Dato

Introduction   Adolescents present particular issues, concerns, and problems to nurses working with them in any setting. Therapeutic interventions with adolescents must take into consideration the developmental tasks of adolescence, the strong countertransference reactions encountered, and the difficulties of behavioral management. Adolescence, with its many changes, is a totally unique time of life. One enters it as a child and leaves it as an adult. The potential difficulties along the way are numerous for this relatively short time period.

The Impact of Puberty   Puberty is the start of adolescence, although adolescence is sometimes considered a response to puberty. At this time, increased hormonal secretions lead to increased sexual drives and impulses. These heightened feelings of sexuality can lead to anxiety about sexual adequacy. Because the age at which sexual development begins can vary greatly, adolescents sometimes suffer anxiety about premature or delayed development. An added dimension is added by rapid bodily changes, including the appearance of secondary sexual characteristics, which require a change in bodily self-image and public image.

A. **PHYSICAL MATURATION**

In adolescence there is increased awareness of one's body. Individual responses to bodily sensations and the seeking of familiarity in a "new" body becomes an initial step in forming a self-image. Growth is both individual and uneven in a single person. Still, adolescents tend to compare themselves to others, which also causes anxiety. Adolescents may be reluctant to have medical examinations that intensify masturbatory conflicts, sexual feelings, and guilt and arouse fear of finding abnormalities.[8]

B. **AFFECTIVE CHANGES**

There is an intensity of feelings that can be frightening in response to situations, events, and people, as well as mood swings. The adolescent often expresses feelings in actions instead of in words.

C. **CHANGES IN THINKING**

There is movement from the "concrete operations" of childhood to the period of "formal operations," including abstract thinking, more logical reasoning, and more effective evaluations.[11] In addition, there is a normal preoccupation with oneself and the need for self-expression, philosophical abstractions, social complexities, fantasies, theories and ideals, sexuality, hedonism, asceticism, and conformism.

D. **CHANGES IN RELATIONSHIPS**

There is an abrupt movement from the sheltered world of grammar school to busy junior high school, fraught with a multitude of fantasized opportunities and dangers. The need for adult life choices occurs very early, along with increased demands for self-sufficiency. Social changes such as getting jobs, traveling farther from home, attending high school, and meeting greater intellectual challenges present more fuel for the fires of introspection and self-absorption. Compatibility with peers becomes crucial; nonconformity and divergence can lead to ostracism. The importance of acceptance in a peer group leads to experimentation that may be growth producing or potentially destructive. Adolescents often have one very close friend whom they mimic as an aid in developing self-identity. Similarly, certain adults, such as celebrities or favorite teachers, can be idealized. Social situations are used to test out values. Relationships with the opposite sex often begin with a need for security and someone with whom to talk. They enhance self-esteem by demonstrating sexual attractiveness to oneself and the world, symbolizing acceptance, lovability, and value.

Tasks of Adolescence[4] These include
1. Consolidation of a sense of self-identity
2. Individuation from parents
3. Control of feelings
4. Learning to work and play with members of both sexes
5. Establishment of sexual relationships
6. Crystallization of values

Problems of Adolescence The common problems and psychological symptoms of adolescents can be viewed along a continuum from "normal" to psychotic. The differences are in the degree and persistence of symptomatology and the effect of the symptoms on the adolescent's life. These differences provide the basic criteria used to evaluate the need for treatment, to determine the best type of treatment, and to assist the adolescent toward growth. These differences, considered along a continuum from least to most serious, are
1. Family problems
2. Sexually related problems
3. Drug use
4. Poor social adjustment
5. School phobia
6. Violent acting out
7. Sexual acting out (promiscuity)
8. Hypochondriasis
9. Physically related problems such as anorexia nervosa, excessive overactivity, noncompliance with self-care, obesity, accident proneness
10. Juvenile delinquency
11. Running away
12. Psychosis
13. Depression
14. Suicide threats, gestures, attempts

Individual Therapy Individual psychotherapy with adolescents bears much resemblance to therapy with adults. As with adults, there are many possible approaches to treatment, depending on the goals of the adolescent, the therapist's theoretical orientation, and external realities that may impinge on the treatment. The focus here is on long-term, dynamically oriented outpatient treatment. Many of the principles also apply to other forms of individual treatment.

A. **REFERRAL**

Adolescents may be referred by parents, schools, or juvenile authorities. Often the adolescents themselves do not want to be in therapy and appear "unmotivated" to therapists who are accustomed to adults. These adolescents will probably have no understanding of the therapeutic process and, further, will be skeptical. There is a "culture" gap, since adolescents firmly believe adults cannot understand them.

B. **THE CONTRACT**

The nurse tells adolescents that they are free to leave therapy after discussing the reasons, unless they are required to remain in therapy because of an outside contract (usually juvenile authorities). This freedom decreases dependency fears and allows commitment to treatment. The adolescent often needs to stop treatment and then return to test or act out separation and reunion.

C. **ASSESSMENT**

The nurse sees the adolescent alone for the first contact if possible. This may help establish a relationship by reducing the adolescent's association of the nurse with parents. It aligns the nurse with the autonomous, mature, responsible part of the adolescent. Parents are then seen alone for a full developmental history to evaluate whether the adolescent is acting out some earlier relationship, deprivation, or conflict.

Family sessions are then used for diagnostic evaluation. Familial patterns, ways of relating and systems can be revealed, and necessary future support for the treatment can be elicited.

The first goal of therapy is evaluation of the likelihood of success in outpatient treatment. Out-patient therapy alone, at least initially, may not be enough, since it may offer nothing or only mild symptom relief. The danger lies in "losing" the client who may benefit from more extensive treatment. Individual outpatient therapy requires some ability to abstract, reason, judge, anticipate consequences, and delay gratification, albeit with some external help at times.

D. **CONFIDENTIALITY**

All issues regarding confidentiality are spelled out and agreed upon by therapist and client. Confidentiality is always an important issue in therapy. With adolescents, there is the particular sensitivity to information sharing with parents. The nurse tells the adolescent why, when, and what kind of information will be discussed with parents, for example, "Once a month, I will be meeting with your parents to let them know your general progress. I won't be discussing any specific details of our talks."

E. **THE TREATMENT**

Therapy with the adolescent requires alertness, flexibility, readiness to intervene, readiness not to intervene, objectivity, tolerance, and a capacity to invest in the therapy that no other age group demands.[6] This is necessary because of the frequency of "ego exhaustion" and the varying ego states seen in adolescence.[6] Chart 28–1 shows nursing interventions and the rationale for each in individual therapy with adolescents.

(Text continues on page 268)

Chart 28–1

NURSING INTERVENTIONS AND RATIONALE IN INDIVIDUAL THERAPY WITH ADOLESCENTS

Nursing Intervention	Rationale/Comments
The therapist is a "safe" adult, who listens carefully.	The adolescent wants and needs an objective adult with whom to talk. The listening is simultaneously an evaluation of what is said. Cathartic release of tension is one aspect of therapy.
The therapist forms a therapeutic alliance with the adolescent, although this is difficult.	The therapeutic alliance is the basis of any growth.
The therapist suggests environmental changes as indicated.	Needed changes can have a beneficial effect on both the adolescent and the therapy.[6]

(continued)

Chart 28–1
(continued)

Nursing Intervention	Rationale/Comments
The therapist does not force the adolescent to accept a label of being sick.	The adolescent is not a therapist's fantasy of a "good client." Adolescents often will not admit to hurting, or being "sick." They may be defending against any thoughts of having an identity that is seen as sick, incomplete, or inadequate (or whatever therapy may signify).
The therapist does not demand adult behavior, but reasonable behavior.	The adolescent is not an adult, and the therapist cannot expect adult behavior, ideas, or feelings.
The therapist is willing to shift focuses along with the adolescent.	The adolescent often changes mood, thoughts, and feelings. The therapist evaluates whether this is defensive or growth stimulating.
The therapist does not focus on the past but on connecting behaviors with their effect in the present.	Adolescents are often overwhelmed by the present and anxious about the future.[12]
Therapeutic regressions (and regressive transferences) are not encouraged as they might be with adults. When they occur, the therapist focuses on recovery.	"Regressions" appear spontaneously in adolescents as a beneficial movement toward growth. Adolescents' conflicts over dependency will cause them to run fearfully from regressive pulls in treatment.
The therapist fosters dependence initially with adolescents who act out.	This may produce a willingness to restrain some behavior in order to keep the relationship with the therapist.[9]
The therapist recognizes early defenses and interprets the propensity to act in order to avoid feelings.	The adolescent may feel impatient, frustrated, helpless, or embarrassed about needing therapy. Defenses against those feelings may include acting out, rebellion, disdain, condescension, or passive compliance. Adolescents are threatened by the thought of unconscious motivation. As part of separating from parents, they omnipotently view their actions as freedom rather than defenses against instincts and feelings.[12]
The therapist sets limits as necessary, with open discussion of all issues involved, including dependence versus independence.	Acting out can be harmful physically or psychologically, or it can interfere with therapy. With limit setting, adolescents' fears of losing control will be decreased, making them more accessible and free of the defenses that they employ to avoid losing control.
The therapist allies with the adolescent's ego, rather than imposing a superego.	Limit setting is done for protection, not to teach moral values. Adolescents are sensitive to manipulative control. All behaviors should be considered for understanding.
The therapist observes and points out adaptive behaviors and strengths as well as pathology.	This serves to strengthen the therapeutic alliance, with the therapist seen as neutral and friendly.
The therapist recognizes the defenses that the adolescent uses to avoid establishing a therapeutic alliance and points these out.	Adolescents defend against their dependency wishes by viewing the therapist negatively, inviting criticism, reducing the relationship to a peer or parent–child relationship, and by self-criticism.
The therapist avoids "unholy alliances"[10]: 1. With the id—by avoiding the temptation to be "hip," or to make premature interpretations of sexual or aggressive material.	An eager (sometimes young) therapist may try to appear more tolerant and accepting than any other adult. This approach causes adolescents to become very anxious because they need a firm sense of the therapist's position on talking, not acting.
2. With pathologic defenses (often intellectualization)—by a. Asking for definition of any jargon b. Avoiding use of any technical language	The adolescent must learn to experience and report feelings.

Chart 28–1
(continued)

Nursing Intervention	Rationale/Comments
3. With the *superego*—by limit setting in a careful, nonjudgmental way.	If used too early or harshly, it can reduce acting out without promoting any real maturation. The adolescent will attempt to recreate past dealings with adults, which can then be talked about.
The therapist recognizes when a therapeutic alliance has not occurred and discusses this with the adolescent. The therapist may consider referring the adolescent to another therapist.	Early interventions may have been incorrect, and a discussion may lead to an alliance. Both adolescent and therapist learn from the understanding of this response.
The therapist recognizes disruptions in the alliance and addresses it before anything else. The cause is identified, labeled, and interpreted (following the adolescent's cues).	All other work in therapy is dedependent upon the therapeutic alliance. Other inventions at this time could be ineffective or harmful. The most common cause for disruption in the alliance is anxiety. Other causes may be parental sabotage or other unfortunate events that draw the adolescent's attention for a period of time.
The therapist actively explores countertransference, using consultation or supervision as indicated.	Countertransferential responses to adolescents may be different from those encountered with adults. The aggression displayed by the adolescent makes special demands on the therapist, and there is often a relative lack of the positive reinforcement that is present in treating adults.[9]
The therapist guards against the possibility that the adolescent will act out the therapist's unconscious wishes and fantasies.	Problems arise when therapists have unresolved conflicts from their own adolescence, and countertransference feelings towards the adolescent's parents or any authority figures, or identify with rebellious behavior.
The therapist guards against punitive, impulsive, regressed, or retaliatory responses.	Adolescents will stop at nothing in putting the therapist on the "hot seat" as they attack all of the therapist's defenses. Retaliatory actions reduce feelings of trust.
The therapist identifies and explores the adolescent's relentless search for the fallibility of the therapist.	The therapist is human and will make errors that can be acknowledged, and then the therapy moves on. The adolescent often is looking for repetitions of prior experiences with adults.
The therapist avoids engaging in power struggles, corruption, or compromise.	Adolescents can be very seductive in tempting the therapist to leave the therapeutic role and engage in a peer–peer or adult–child competition. Adolescents respond to adults as if they were all parents or other authority figures and treat them as though they are wrong no matter what they do. Adult therapists are seen as adults who can be corrupted and compromised. Power struggles often arise in response to issues the adolescent is dealing with in therapy, such as independence and trust. When the therapist does not become seduced into living out the adolescent's fantasy, the adolescent is able to give up the fantasy, move on, and become separate from the parents.
The therapist is not unduly influenced by outside forces.	Parents, teachers, or others may pressure the therapist to get adolescents to stop certain behaviors. Unless a prearranged contract was established or the adolescents are placing themselves in great danger, these pressures should not influence the course of therapy, though they may be discussed. The therapist's resistance to this provides a role model.

(continued)

Chart 28–1
(continued)

Nursing Intervention	Rationale/Comments
The therapist may be a "special friend" or assist the adolescent in relating to one.[10]	This type of a relationship does not change the basic nature of a therapist–client relationship. Adolescents use a special, often older, friend to aid in developing an ego ideal, that is, a picture of the self that is perfect for the individual. Aspects of the friend, for example, the friend's values, are incorporated in the adolescent's own development.[10]
The therapist avoids prolonged therapy that is dependent in nature.	This can be a stumbling block to the adolescent's development.
Termination is discussed at a length appropriate to the length and work of the therapy and is not delayed.	Termination is always a difficult aspect of treatment. In adolescents, feelings about separation are easily aroused, since separation is the major task of adolescence.

Family Therapy Family therapy is a critical aspect of treatment with adolescents. A primary adolescent developmental issue is separation from the family; parents and adolescents may have resistances to this. Family therapy may be indicated in conjunction with individual therapy with an adolescent when there is an acute disruption in the family that affects the adolescent's behavior or development (for example, divorce, birth of a sibling, moves, death, illness). Chronically disturbed familial interactions and patterns affect an adolescent's behavior and may be another indication for family therapy. The choice of therapist(s) may be determined by the clinical situation and the therapist's preference, and it may be the adolescent's individual therapist, a different therapist, or a combination. Parents may be referred for couples therapy as an alternative. Sometimes the goal of treatment is to relieve adolescents of an impossible role in the family, thus freeing them for their own development. Adolescents are easily scapegoated or used to express unconscious desires of parents. Chart 28–2 shows nursing interventions and the theoretical rationale in family therapy with adolescents (see also Chap. 24).

Group Therapy Group therapy and group work have been particularly successful with adolescents. Group treatment uses the natural, developmentally appropriate tendency of adolescents to relate to peers. Group therapy can be a good catalyst for individual therapy.

A. **ADVANTAGES OF GROUP THERAPY**
   In group treatment peers may
   1. Assist in identity formation
   2. Help with learning age-appropriate behavior
   3. Provide opportunities for learning social skills
   4. Offer support, protection, and security
   5. Provide challenges and confrontation
   6. Be attentive to authority conflicts
   7. Be useful in conflict resolution through the testing out of ideas and thoughts
   8. Help dilute conflicts of independency–dependency with adults
   9. Assist in exploration of increased autonomy and skills of self-reliance
   10. Accept dependency upon each other more than they can upon adults because of their fears of regression
   11. Assist each other in ego development because of their varying abilities and uneven development

B. **COMMON PROBLEMS**
 1. Poor attendance
 2. High drop-out rate
 3. Antisocial behavior that interferes with group process
 4. Lack of cohesiveness
 5. Destructive sibling rivalry
 6. Defensive peer relationships
 7. Overuse of acting out instead of verbalization
 8. Resistances such as silence, passivity, disruptiveness, and intellectualization

C. **TYPES OF GROUPS USED WITH ADOLESCENTS**
 1. *Educational groups*—The primary task is to increase knowledge in a particular area that is appropriate and important in adolescent development. The advantages of adolescents working and learning together in groups are used in support of the primary task. These groups may take place in schools, community health or mental health centers, churches, mental hospitals, residential treatment centers, juvenile detention facilities, and community social organizations. Common topics include sex education, personal grooming and health, nutrition, drug use, pregnancy, career planning, assertiveness training, divorce, values clarification, and communications skills.
 2. *Activities groups*—Adolescent activities groups are similar to those used with latency-age children. They are useful with younger adolescents who are just

---

Chart 28–2
NURSING INTERVENTIONS AND RATIONALE IN FAMILY THERAPY WITH ADOLESCENTS

Nursing Intervention	Rationale
1. Assessment	
Treatment begins with a careful assessment of the familial interactions and the effect on the adolescent.	Adolescents remain the responsibility of their parents, who can exert tremendous influence on them.
The adolescent and parents are seen together.	The interactions between parents and the adolescent can be observed.
Siblings old enough to participate who are still involved in family life are included.	Young siblings may play an important role in the adolescent's life.
A history is obtained that includes the adolescent's developmental history and the family history. This can be done alone with the parents.	Basic data are necessary for an understanding of the adolescent's problems and the family's problems.
2. Treatment	
Parents are involved in the initial planning of goals and treatment.	Adolescents are not yet able to fully plan for themselves.
A safe, nonthreatening environment is established for the whole family.	This reduces anxiety and frees the family to act in a relatively usual manner.
Parents may need to be instructed about confidentiality (what they are and are not told about the adolescent's individual treatment), the meaning of behavior, and how to better supervise and protect the adolescent.	Changes effected in therapy should be reinforced at home.
An initial series of time-limited family sessions is set up.	There is observation and discussion of the family interactions and dynamics to determine better ways of interacting. This may aid the parents in supporting the individual treatment.

beginning to develop skill in verbal expression of feelings. The activities provide stimuli for age-appropriate behaviors and interests, and are used to stimulate verbal expression.

3. *Multiple family therapy groups*—Two to six families meet with one or more therapists in time-limited or open-ended groups. These groups are often used in hospitals and residential programs to provide an effective and efficient way of involving the families of clients in the understanding of hospital treatment and discharge planning. They may be particularly useful in the treatment of families who are socially isolated, have an absent parent, or operate in a rigid way that tends to continually reinforce pathology.

4. *Open-ended supportive groups*[10]—These groups are used with homogeneous groups of adolescents, often under some externally controlled situation (for example, in institutions or drug rehabilitation programs). There is a focus on changing self-destructive behavior and using peer pressure to change to more adaptive behaviors. Older group members influence newer group members by providing new superego models. Group leaders are inspirational, supportive, and directive, and do not place much emphasis on exploration. These groups are not indicated for adolescents who are very immature socially or severely neurotic because there is a risk of an antitherapeutic subgroup forming in response to the influence of a strong new member or a relapse of an older member.

5. *Transition groups*—These groups are for the purpose of easing important transitions, such as discharge groups in hospitals and placements in or out of foster care or institutions. They are both supportive and educational.

6. *Crisis intervention, drop-in, rap groups*—These groups may include adolescents alone or with their parents, may be diagnostic, or may provide a safe way to make an entry into a mental health care system.

7. *Homogeneous groups*—These groups make use of preexisting group formation, using common factors to positively influence cohesiveness. Some types of homogeneous groups include adolescents with drug abuse problems, legal problems, adjustment problems to new situations such as schools or emergency shelters, or as military dependents on a base.

D. **CONTRAINDICATIONS FOR GROUP THERAPY**[10]
   1. Adolescents with very poor coping skills, little ego strength, and tendencies toward severe disorganization may find the interpersonal stresses of a group detrimental.
   2. Adolescents who are fixated at early developmental levels require adult nurturance and cannot use peers for support.
   3. Some severely unsocialized, acting-out adolescents may be detrimental to a group, rather than the group being harmful to them. They have poor object relations and cannot respond to group pressures and expectations.

D. **NURSING INTERVENTIONS**
   Chart 28–3 shows appropriate nursing interventions and rationale in group therapy with adolescents.

Evaluation   The evaluation of an adolescent's treatment takes into consideration
   1. Outcome of the presenting problem
   2. Outcome of other problem areas that were identified during the assessment
   3. The adolescents' evaluation of their treatment and their own difficulties

Chart 28–3

NURSING INTERVENTIONS AND RATIONALE IN GROUP THERAPY WITH ADOLESCENTS

Nursing Interventions	Rationale
Groups are coeducational.	This decreases homosexual anxiety and anxious disruptiveness.
Group members are selected whose parents are supportive of group therapy.	Parents can easily influence the learning of healthier, adaptive behaviors. They can also support resistances such as flight from the anxiety generated in the group.
Members are selected who show motivation.	The motivation expected with adults is not seen in the same ways with adolescents. It is, nonetheless, necessary and may initially be only an interest in and willingness to try the group for a short time.
The age range of members is kept small (13–15, 15–17, 17–19).	The central issues in the younger group tend toward separation, sexual anxieties, and the movement out of childhood. Verbal abilities of self-expression are also more limited. Younger adolescents experience great anxiety about premature identification with the sexual behavior of older adolescents. The central issues in the older groups are the movement toward adulthood, identity, dating, vocation, drugs, and money. There is a tendency of older adolescents to regress in groups with younger adolescents. The oldest group will show more adultlike behavior and will be taking steps out of adolescence toward college and jobs.
The size of the group varies according to the ages of the members (younger adolescents, 5–6 members; older, 6–9 members).	A smaller group will allow younger adolescents the individual attention they need while keeping the group manageable. The larger number of members in an older group provides for more variety and expression and allows for potential low attendance.
Members are chosen who have social compatibility.	Adolescents can be both sensitive and judgmental about superficial characteristics.
There is a balance of personal styles and symptomatology.	The group functions more effectively when members have varied verbal abilities, tendencies to act out, degrees of withdrawal, and developmental social skills.
Group members are evaluated before the beginning and are given advance preparation.	A beginning of a therapeutic relationship can be established while simultaneously assessing the suitability of the adolescent for the group. Advance preparation decreases anxiety that might prevent the adolescent from attending.
Introduction of ground rules is dependent upon the population.	Adolescents vary in their ability to exercise internal controls and their concomitant need for expressed external limits.
The therapist does not overemphasize prohibition rules.	The therapist may have fears of potential problems of control in the group and thus heavily appeal to the superego of the adolescent. Some adolescents will react with meek, timid obedience. Others will see any rule as a potential target for rebellion and will quickly rebel.
Some rules for group behavior include No violence No hitting or fighting No drugs No sexual activity No leaving the room No interrupting when another person is speaking	More disturbed or younger adolescents may need the assurance of protection afforded by external controls on themselves and others. A safe atmosphere is a prerequisite for verbal expression. Major forms of acting out prohibit verbal work.

(continued)

Chart 28–3
(continued)

Nursing Interventions	Rationale
Members are told to inform the therapist if they cannot attend.	Regular attendance is expected because the group work requires members getting to know each other and relying on each other. Unexplained absences are an insult to other members.
The therapist comments on any absence.	Although absences are very common in adolescent groups, they should not go unnoticed. Therapists may elicit the underlying meaning of an absence by showing interest and concern as well as adherence to established norms.
Principles of confidentiality are described to the group with the expectation that they will be honored. Members' discussion outside the group should be limited to one's own feelings and thoughts, and reference to others should not be included.	Confidentiality is necessary for any amount of free and open discussion. Adolescents are generally very sensitive to exposure and may fear being excluded if "exposed."
The adolescent is told before the therapist contacts parents.	Parents may need to be informed of potential dangers (for example, a suicidal adolescent). Limited reports to parents may be appropriate.
With younger groups, refreshments may be served (soft drinks, candy, cookies), or members may bring their own snacks.	Adolescents are still close to the orality of childhood. Refreshments are discussed in terms of relationships, behavior, symbolic uses, and family styles.
With younger groups, an activity may be used to start the group.	This can have a stabilizing effect as well as offer stimuli for verbal expression.
There is one male and one female group therapist.	A solo therapist may evoke anxiety leading to fight or flight in members of the opposite sex. A male–female combination also offers easier recreation of the family and sets the stage for dealing with these current issues of adolescence.
Co-therapists handle disagreements openly.	It is helpful for adolescents to observe adults resolving a conflict in a healthy, constructive manner.
Duration of the group may be time limited.	Many groups are held in conjunction with a school calendar, since adolescents may be unavailable in the summer. Many adolescents will not attend a group regularly during the summer "holiday" unless they are required to, such as in an institutional setting. Some groups may develop a strong sense of cohesiveness and belonging and may continue all year.

4. The family's view of the adolescent
5. Reports from pertinent others (teachers, siblings, probation officers)
6. Progress toward developmental goals

References

1. Berkowitz I: Adolescents Grow in Groups. New York, Brunner-Mazel, 1972
2. Blos P: On Adolescence. New York, Free Press, 1962
3. Burns KJ: Adolescent adjustment reactions. In Haber J et al (eds): Comprehensive Psychiatric Nursing, 2nd ed. New York, McGraw-Hill, 1982
4. Erikson E: Childhood and Society. New York, WW Norton, 1963
5. Holmes M, Werner J: Psychiatric Nursing in a Therapeutic Community. New York, MacMillan, 1966
6. Josselyn I: Adolescence. New York, Harper & Row, 1971
7. Jurgenson K: Limit setting for hospitalized adolescent psychiatric patients. Perspect Psychiatr Care 9:173, 1971
8. Lidz T: The Person. New York, Basic Books, 1968

9. Malinquist C: Handbook of Adolescence. New York, Jason Aaranson, 1978
10. Meeks J: The Fragile Alliance. New York, Robert E Krieger, 1980
11. Piaget J, Inhelder B: The Growth of Logical Thinking. New York, Basic Books, 1958
12. Poll G: Psychophysiologic disorder in adolescents: Anorexia nervosa. In Heacock D (ed): Psychodynamic Approach to Adolescent Psychiatry. New York, M Dekker, 1980
13. Stuart G, Sundeen S: Principles and Practice of Psychiatric Nursing. St Louis, CV Mosby, 1979
14. Williams D: Substance use and abuse. In Howe J (ed): Nursing Care of Adolescents. New York, McGraw-Hill, 1980

Bibliography

Bragg TL: Teen-age alcohol abuse. J Psychiatr Nurs 14:10, 1976

Duffey M: Factors contributing to the development of a cohesive adolescent psychotherapy group. J Psychiatr Nurs 17:21, 1979

Fox K: Adolescent ambivalence: A therapeutic issue. J Psychiatr Nurs 18:29, 1980

Freeberg S: Anger in adolescence. J Psychosoc Nurs 20:29, 1982

Group for the Advancement of Psychiatry: Power and Authority in Adolescence: The Origins and Resolutions of Intergenerational Conflict, 1978

Hansborg HG: Adolescent Separation Anxiety, vol 1 and 2. Melbourne, FL, Robert E Krieger, 1980

Hart NA, Keidel GC: The Suicidal Adolescent. Am J Nurs 79:80, 1979

Henggeler SW: Delinquency and Adolescent Psychopathology. Littleton, MA, John Wright PSE, 1982

Lynch VJ: Narcissistic loss and depression in late adolescence. Perspect Psychiatr Care 15:133, 1976

Mellencamp A: Adolescent depression: A review of the literature with implications for nursing care. J Psychosoc Nurs 19:15, 1981

Parker G, Gibson C: Development of the hospitalized adolescent anxiety tool. J Psychiatr Nurs 15:21, 1977

Raubolt RR: Brief, problem-focused group psychotherapy with adolescents. Am J Orthopsychiatr 53:157, 1983

Sugar M (ed): Female Adolescent Development. New York, Brunner-Mazel, 1979

Walker P, Brook BD: Community homes as hospital alternatives for youth in crisis. J Psychiatr Nurs 19:17, 1981

29

Activities of Daily Living Groups

Rachel Parios

Introduction   Activities of daily living (ADL) groups are a part of inpatient therapeutic milieu programs as well as deinstitutionalization programs for psychiatric clients. Owing to the nature of their psychiatric illness and its resulting social deprivation, psychiatric clients often neglect or lack motivation to attend to their daily living needs. ADL groups offer psychiatric clients information, consideration, and the expectation that they are capable of learning or relearning how to live independently in the community.

Purpose   ADL groups help clients learn or relearn to
1. Maintain health and hygiene
2. Obtain housing
3. Plan and prepare meals
4. Manage money
5. Plan leisure time

Techniques   The components necessary for ADL groups include
1. The presentation of information through discussion and visual aids
2. A demonstration of learning by the client

Setting Up and Conducting Groups   Chart 29–1 shows how groups are conducted and the rationale for each nursing intervention.

Chart 29–1
CONDUCTING ADL GROUPS

Nursing Intervention	*Rationale*
1. Clients are expected to attend all groups.	1. a. Communicates the importance of the subject matter b. Allows for assessment of clients' understanding and application as they progress through various phases of ADL groups
2. Groups are composed of 4–8 clients having similar levels of functioning.	2. a. Allows for individualized attention b. Encourages peer interaction c. Is a manageable group size for field trips
3. Each topic is covered for 6–10 sessions, with review at the beginning and end of each session.	3. a. Allows time for individual advancement, learning, and comprehension b. Provides time for assessment and client/leader evaluation of the clients' capabilities c. Provides for repetition, enhancing learning d. Allows time limiting for each topic
4. Tasks are incorporated into each session for experiential learning.	4. a. Enhances the clients' ability to retain and recall information b. Allows for assessment of clients' learning
5. Group sessions are limited to 90 minutes (unless field trips require more time).	5. a. Allows adequate time for information sharing b. Provides adequate time for experiential learning c. Allows consideration for the clients' attention span
6. Group leader participates actively as a resource person and role model.	6. Provides for social learning through imitation
7. Progression is staged from simple to complex tasks.	7. a. Enhances clients' motivation toward independent living by offering reinforcement for early simple tasks b. Fosters development of new skills toward total independence
8. Clients' anxiety level is monitored.	8. a. Provides for assessment of issues that increase clients' anxiety level. b. Indicates areas that require individual attention.
9. Opportunity is provided for individual ADL guidance as needed.	9. Takes into account variations in individual learning abilities

Health and Personal Hygiene   The first step in learning to live in the community is learning personal hygiene. Clients who have been hospitalized for many years develop a "chronic look," which identifies them as "mental patients" to the community. This look consists of disheveled or dirty clothing and hair, poor posture and hygiene, and inappropriate makeup on women.

    Chart 29–2 shows nursing interventions and rationale in promoting health and personal hygiene.

Housing   Clients who have lived in hospitals or at home for many years need help to learn about arranging for their own housing. Chart 29–3 shows how to arrange sessions on this area of living.

Chart 29–2
HELPING WITH HEALTH AND PERSONAL HYGIENE

Nursing Intervention	Rationale
Sessions 1–4—Maintaining Health	
1. Conduct lecture and discussion groups using speakers from American Heart, Dental, Lung, and Cancer Associations.	1. Enhances understanding of optimum physical well-being
2. Incorporate audiovisual filmstrips on various health issues, that is, hypertension, smoking, obesity, and so forth.	2. Stimulates clients' thinking and discussion
3. Encourage yearly physical examination.	
Session 5—Medication Education (see Chap. 65)	
1. Identify clients' medication by name and action.	1. Fosters self-care
2. Discuss side effects.	2. Understanding of side effects may prevent them from becoming irreversible and may allay anxiety
3. Discuss compliance.	3. Prevents decompensation due to failure to take medication
4. Help clients indentifying symptoms and report them accurately.	4. Helps prevent decompensation
Session 6—First Aid	
1. Demonstrate use of a first aid kit.	1. Teaches client to respond appropriately to emergency situations
2. Discuss first aid treatment for minor injuries.	
3. Discuss emergency room use.	
Session 7—Sexuality (see Chap. 30)	
1. Provide guest speakers from planned parenthood, VD clinic.	1. Offers clients
2. Divide group into male and female. Discuss menstruation, menopause, masturbation, orgasm, and abortion.	a. Accurate information and understanding about sexuality
	b. Opportunity to ask questions and clarify misconceptions
Session 8—Personal Hygiene	
1. Direct discussions on the following aspects of grooming:	1. Provides clients with an understanding of areas important for functioning in society
a. Appearance	
b. Cleanliness—body and clothes	
c. Hair care	
d. Nails	
e. Skin	
f. Posture	
g. Clothing coordination	
h. Care of clothing	
2. Encourage peer participation.	

Chart 29–3
HELPING WITH HOUSING

Nursing Intervention	Rationale

Session 1—Types of Housing
(Supervised residential; temporary apartment; community apartment)

1. Discuss with client past living experiences.

2. Establish with client goals for future living situations.

3. Offer information about supervised residential living:
   a. Guidelines
   b. Duration of stay

4. Offer information about temporary apartment living (owned by institution for rehabilitation; time limited to 6 months).

5. Offer information about apartment living in the community:
   a. Vacancies
   b. Rental agencies

1. Establishes baseline from which to begin locating appropriate housing

2. Housing selection is based on client's skills for independent living.

3. Provides learning with supervision

4. a. Provides semi-independent housing
   b. Develops skills for independent apartment living

5. Provides information for client who has skills for independent apartment living

Session 2—Federal Government Housing Subsidies

1. Provide information about federal government housing subsidies.

2. Provide applications and assist client in applying for housing subsidy.

3. Explore housing possibilities where subsidies are accepted. (Not all landlords accept subsidies, and rents may be too high for subsidy consideration.)

1. Assists the client with rent while rehabilitating

2. Provides the client with guidance needed for application

3. Provides client with information needed to plan

Session 3—Housing Selection with Client

1. Introduce client to method of housing selection and application:
   a. May be done with one or two clients only
   b. Visit residence or apartment for client approval
   c. Make necessary application for living situation

1. Provides client with experience needed for future

Session 4—Living with Others

1. Discuss living with others:
   a. Responsibilities of household, that is, maintenance, cleaning, cooking, shopping
   b. Using electrical appliances
   c. Cooperation
   d. Respecting privacy
   e. Differences in interest
   f. Socializing, guests
   g. Verbalizing feelings, confrontation

1. a. Initiates understanding of and motivation to live with others
   b. Fosters less self-involvement on the part of clients

Session 5—Telephone Arrangements

1. Assist client with telephone purchase and installation.
2. Discuss fee and shared responsibility.

1. Fosters independence

Session 6—Landlord–Tenant Interaction

1. Discuss rent regulations:
   a. Date due
   b. Financial responsibility
   c. Consequences of not respecting this obligation

2. Discuss responsibilities of landlord:
   a. Repairs
   b. Heat
   c. Hot water
   d. Painting

1. Fosters knowledge and understanding of responsibility

2. Fosters awareness of tenants' expectations

(continued)

Chart 29–3
(continued)

Nursing Intervention	*Rationale*
3. Discuss establishing a tenant–landlord agreement about decorating an apartment, that is, nails in wall, paneling, and so forth.	3. Encourages client to understand boundaries with use of property
Session 7—Furniture and Necessities	
1. Take inventory of clients' possessions	1. Establishes items needed for apartment living
2. Assist client with obtaining donations from family or agency, that is, furniture, cooking utensils, curtains, towels, pictures, and so forth.	2. Enhances assertiveness
3. Introduce client to visiting "garage sales," warehouse sales, charity or nonprofit organizations that sell furniture or appliances.	3. Provides client with knowledge and understanding about bargain shopping
4. Introduce decorating ideas from magazines.	4. Encourages clients' creativity
Session 8—Independent Living	
1. Discuss benefits and problems:	1. Assists in exploration of motivation for independent living
a. Encourage clients to discuss fears and anxieties.	2. Assists client with working through unidentified feelings about new experiences
b. Confront dependency, social withdrawal, and resistance.	
Session 9—Laundry	
1. Discuss use of a washer/dryer.	
2. Discuss use of a laundromat.	

Chart 29–4
HELPING WITH MEAL PLANNING AND PREPARATION

Nursing Intervention	*Rationale*
Session 1—Nutrition	
1. Discuss nutrition and its importance, including food value, daily needs, and caloric value.	1. Provides clients with basic information about nutrition
2. Assess clients' eating habits:	2. Assists clients' awareness of their own eating patterns
a. Foods liked and disliked	
b. Quantities consumed	
3. Discuss effects of food on health, that is, malnutrition, obesity, and so forth.	3. Enhances clients' understanding of nutrition and health-related issues
Session 2—Dietary Adjustments	
1. Discuss dietary adjustments in conjunction with medical problems. Help client seek professional medical treatment.	1. Offers assistance and knowledge to keep client physically healthy and aware of when medical problems appear or worsen
2. Discuss:	2. Psychiatric hospitalized clients have acquired negative eating habits:
a. Self-controlled weight loss	a. Overeating for oral gratification
b. Metabolism of foods	b. "Starchy diets"
	c. Dependence on being served meals
Session 3—Food Processing	
1. Supply information about food processing:	1. Expands knowledge of food values and preparation
a. Fresh food	
b. Frozen food	
c. Canned food	
d. Fast food	
2. Take field trips to markets and food processing industrial corporations.	

Chart 29–4
(continued)

Nursing Intervention	*Rationale*
Session 4—Food Storage 1. Discuss food storage: a. Refrigeration b. Bacterial effects on foods c. Dry food storage	1. Helps clients learn importance of safe food storage
Session 5—Meal Planning 1. Discuss meal planning for one week, including breakfast, lunch, and dinner. (This may be done for residential setting and for apartment.) 2. Take into consideration the following: a. Food preferences b. Variety c. Using leftovers d. Cost containment e. Clients' level of functioning f. Food substitutes g. Sales h. Using coupons i. Quantitative shopping	1. a. Supplies clients with structure b. Offers information for food shopping c. Incorporates group or dual decision making.
Session 6—Purchasing Food 1. Have client prepare grocery list according to menu and personal needs. 2. Assist client with grocery shopping using sales and coupons. 3. Encourage client to do comparative shopping. 4. Encourage client to shop at large, national food centers because they stock more items, sell in volume, and offer larger choice. 5. Ensure that the client remains within budgeted limit. 6. Help client put away purchased groceries at home.	1. Allows client to apply previous discussions to actual experience 2. Allows opportunity for clients to ask questions 3. Helps client learn to budget responsibly 4. Helps client learn to set priorities in line with limited income 6. Helps client learn how and where to store food
Session 7—Preparation of Food 1. Assess clients' cooking skills, knowledge about using stove, kitchen utensils. 2. Provide information about food preparation, including method, measurements, and first aid for cuts and burns. 3. Observe (assist if necessary) as client prepares food. 4. Eat with clients. 5. Observe kitchen and dining area cleanup.	1. Helps in planning individualized program 4. Offers supportive encouragement 5. Promotes the inclusion of this task into meal preparation

Meal Planning and Preparation Institutionalized clients have had little experience with meal planning and preparation. Chart 29–4 shows nursing interventions and rationale in helping clients learn about meal planning and preparation.

Managing Money Clients who have been hospitalized for many years or who have lived in other protective environments often lack the ability to care for their finances. Chart 29–5 shows nursing interventions and rationale for helping clients learn this activity of daily living.

Leisure Time Planning One of the most difficult areas of daily living for chronic clients is planning satisfying leisure time. Chart 29–6 shows nursing interventions and rationale in helping clients do this. Chart 29–7 is a guide for choosing leisure time activities.

(Text continues on page 283)

Chart 29–5
HELPING THE CLIENT MANAGE MONEY

Nursing Intervention	*Rationale*
Session 1—Introduction	
1. Assess clients' knowledge and understanding of financial situation.	1. Formulates baseline from which to build knowledge and understanding about finances

2. Provide and assist with a questionnaire containing the following:
  a. Monthly income
  b. Source (SSI, welfare, family)
  c. Monthly expenses
      Rent/room and board
      Food
      Gas and electric
      Miscellaneous
	2. Provides information for nurse and client in planning budget

3. Encourage clients to participate verbally.	
Session 2—Budget Sampling	
1. Provide clients with three sample budgets within their income range, including varied expenditures.	1. Provides clients with direction and concrete data

2. Have clients explore all three:
  a. Identify differences
  b. Discuss each
  c. Identify budget closest to client's
	2. Stimulates thinking about designing budget

3. Discuss posting budget in visible area of room or apartment.	3. Fosters limit setting and enhances impulse control

4. Assign homework to document daily expenditures.	4. Assures reality testing
	  a. Establishes connection between sessions
	  b. Provides organization

Session 3—Creating a Personalized Budget	
1. Review material already covered.	1. Tests information learned

2. Have clients make out blank budget with
  a. Monthly income
  b. Monthly expenditures
	2. Provides personalized structure for budget; develops self-discipline, management

3. From balance, determine monthly savings and weekly spending money.	3. Fosters ego functioning

4. Provide information about individual restrictions and discipline of budgeting. Discuss:
  a. Consequences of overspending
  b. Process of making decisions
  c. Setting priorities
	4. Encourages self-determined limit setting

Session 4—Banking	

1. Discuss process of opening an account:
  a. Savings account
  b. Checking account
  c. Interest rates
	1. Motivates clients toward independent functioning

2. Discuss bank location within walking distance:
  a. Hours
  b. Walk-up windows	

3. Discuss banking responsibilities:
  a. Deposits
  b. Withdrawals
  c. Social Security Insurance (SSI) and Social Security Disability (SSD) check pickup
  d. Food stamps	

Chart 29–5
(continued)

Nursing Intervention	Rationale

Session 5—Field Trip to Bank
1. Assist with filling out:
   a. Application for checking and savings account
   b. Withdrawal slips
   c. Deposit slips
	1. Provides experiential learning

Session 6—Guest Lecturer-Investing
1. Discuss:
   a. Stocks and bonds
   b. Corporate sharing
	1. Broadens clients' perspective on finances

Chart 29–6
HELPING WITH LEISURE TIME PLANNING

Nursing Action	Rationale
1. Explore clients' present leisure pastimes and how they travel to activities.	1. Helps clients to plan activities and understand travel and transportation
2. Provide "Wondering What to Do?" questionnaire and list (Chart 29–7).	2. Provides clients with ideas about theatrical, cultural, educational, and recreational benefits of living in the community
3. Discuss passive versus active leisure time planning.	

4. Plan trips to
  a. Museums
  b. Arts and crafts shows
  c. Flea markets
  d. Theater
  e. Sports events
  f. Circus
  g. Animal shows	

5. Explore travel with public transportation and then plan overnight trips to
  a. Historical locations
  b. Camping sites at state parks	

6. Introduce handicraft activities.
  a. Woodworking
  b. Leather
  c. Sewing
	6. Completion of these projects increases satisfaction and self-esteem.

Chart 29–7
GUIDE FOR CHOOSING LEISURE TIME ACTIVITIES

Wondering What To Do?

To clarify your thinking about initiating and learning new activities, decide if you agree or disagree with the following statements.

_____ I feel I'm too old to start anything new.

_____ I'm not physically able.

_____ I don't have the skills.

_____ I won't succeed if I try anything new.

_____ It's almost impossible to make new friends.

(continued)

Chart 29–7
(continued)

_____ It's good for a person to break habits occasionally.
_____ An older person can learn new skills if he puts his mind to it.
_____ It is important to take risks in order to make changes.

Wondering What To Do?

Fond of sedentary games? Some of the most popular are

_____ chess
_____ bridge
_____ scrabble
_____ cards

_____ checkers
_____ Chinese checkers
_____ crossword or other puzzles
_____ adult games

_____ awareness games
_____ backgammon
_____ bingo

If you like to participate in sports, have you considered one of these?

_____ swimming
_____ boating
_____ shuffleboard
_____ horseshoes
_____ golf
_____ horseback riding
_____ bowling
_____ croquet
_____ table tennis
_____ baseball
_____ canoeing
_____ yoga
_____ gymnastics

_____ ice skating
_____ paddle tennis
_____ sailing
_____ track
_____ volleyball
_____ women's sports
_____ walking
_____ miniature golf
_____ fishing
_____ jogging
_____ exercise
_____ archery
_____ badminton

_____ bicycling
_____ boxing
_____ wrestling
_____ billiards/pool
_____ calisthenics
_____ football
_____ hiking
_____ judo–karate
_____ roller skating
_____ tennis
_____ skiing
_____ weight lifting
_____ water sports

Have you always liked pets? The following might be good pastimes.

_____ raising, training, or showing
      dogs or cats
_____ breeding tropical fish

_____ training parakeets or pigeons
_____ animal care, that is, dog
      sitting, and so forth

_____ working for the SPCA
_____ beekeeping
_____ keeping housepets (hamsters,
      turtles, birds)

Do you have a few items you've always thought might be the start of a good collection? Now's the time to find out about, or add to, those.

_____ antiques
_____ old coins
_____ stamps
_____ playing cards

_____ match covers
_____ buttons
_____ wildflowers
_____ seashells

_____ dolls
_____ prints and paintings
_____ other

Does nature and the outdoors appeal to you? Then consider whether to

_____ take a walking tour
_____ study landscape design
_____ join a bird-watching group

_____ go on picnics
_____ go mountain climbing; go
      camping

_____ garden in earnest
_____ learn about trees, wild
      flowers, rocks, minerals.

Have you often been told you have "a talent" for something? Perhaps you can polish up your skill in:

_____ cooking
_____ music
_____ acting
_____ hairdressing
_____ sewing

_____ entertaining
_____ dancing
_____ writing poetry
_____ oral interpretation of literature

_____ drawing, painting, modeling
_____ sculpture
_____ photography
_____ playing a musical instrument

Are you happiest when you're with a group of people? Then you can

_____ take up volunteer work
_____ join a church
_____ serve on committees for
      charity drives
_____ visit hospital patients

_____ organize a club for singles,
      retirees, drama, special
      interests, choral
_____ attend parties
_____ attend adult classes

_____ join a discussion and lecture
      group
_____ be active in your local
      government
_____ take part in cultural fairs,
      parades, festivals, ethnic
      activities

Chart 29–7
(continued)

Does working with your hands please you? Then you could consider

_____ making pottery	_____ paper mosaics	_____ puppet making
_____ photography	_____ crewel	_____ macramé
_____ quilting	_____ wire sculpture	_____ candle making
_____ upholstering furniture	_____ bottle lamps	_____ sewing
_____ painting	_____ découpage	_____ crocheting
_____ papercraft	_____ vegetable and sponge	_____ cooper tooling
_____ making toys	painting	_____ rug making
_____ making ships or airplane	_____ batik	_____ yarn pictures
models	_____ weaving	_____ papier-mâché
_____ leathercraft	_____ needlework	_____ pebble pictures
_____ mosaics	_____ refinishing	_____ spoon jewelry
_____ stained glass	_____ furniture woodworking	_____ god's eyes
_____ flower arranging	_____ metalwork	_____ clay modeling
_____ knitting	_____ printing and binding books	_____ tie-dyeing
_____ ceramics	_____ basket weaving	
_____ enameling	_____ jewelry making	

What subject would you like to learn more about? It's never too late to take an adult education or correspondence course in

_____ crafts	_____ current events	_____ creative writing
_____ languages	_____ history	_____ mathematics
_____ geology	_____ psychology	

Have you been wanting to do more reading? Ways to get started are

_____ read biographies of authors and their works	_____ gear your reading to your vacation: learn about spots of interest, ways to travel, etc.	_____ learn new hobbies and skills by reading
_____ pick an interesting subject and do research		_____ read to the blind
	_____ do book reviews for clubs or local papers	

Any other interests?

_____ CB radio	_____ theatre, ballet	_____ restaurants
_____ historical sites	_____ zoos, parks, museums	_____ electronics
_____ genealogy	_____ stereo	_____ tutoring
_____ television	_____ mechanics	_____ traveling
_____ shopping	_____ astrology	_____ book store browsing
_____ fixing things	_____ movies	_____ beaches, pools

(Designed by Sonia Zayas, OTR, and printed with her permission.)

Evaluation   The nurse is satisfied that the ADL group has been successful if the client shows an ability to
1. Maintain health and hygiene
2. Obtain housing
3. Plan and prepare meals
4. Manage money
5. Plan leisure time

Bibliography

Chaplin M: Indoor gardening for handicapped people. Comm Outlook 12:191, 1979

Currie-Gross V, Heimback J: The relationship between independent living skills attainment and client control orientation. J Rehabil 46:20, 1980

Dejong G, Wenker T: Attendant care as a prototype independent living service. Arch Phys Med Rehabil 60:477, 1979

Foster Z, Mendel S: Mutual help group for patients: Taking steps toward change. Health Soc Work 4:82, 1979

Haworth RJ, Hollings EM: Are hospital assessments of daily living activities valid? Int Rehabil Med 1:59, 1979

Hochbaum GM: Patient counseling vs patient teaching. Top Clin Nurs 2:1, 1980

Kartman LL: Therapeutic group activities in nursing homes. Health Soc Work 4:135, 1979

Kirchman MM, Loomis B: A longitudinal study assessing the quality of occupational therapy. Am J Occup Ther 34:582, 1980

Laing MM et al: The planning and implementation of a psychiatric self care unit. J Psychiatr Nurs 15:30, 1977

Landisman-Dwyer S, Sachett GP, Kleinman JS: Relationship of size to resident and staff behavior in small community residences. Am J Ment Defic 85:6, 1980

Levin LS: Self care—New challenges to individual health. J Am Coll Health Assoc 28:17, 1979

McMordie WR: Helping patients control their own money. Perspect Psychiatr Care 20:33, 1982

Meissner JE: Evaluate your patient's level of independence. Nursing 80, 10:72, 1980

Mocellin G: Occupational therapy and psychiatry. Int J Soc Psychiatry 25:29, 1979

Nelson GL, Cone JD: Multiple-baseline analysis of a token economy for psychiatric inpatients. J Appl Behav Anal 12:255, 1979

Neville A: Temporal adaptation–application with short-term psychiatric patients. Am J Occup Ther 34:328, 1980

O'Brien J: Teaching psychiatric inpatients about their medications. J Psychiatr Nurs 17:30, 1979

Rigger TF: Stages in the rehabilitation of the developmentally disabled. Rehabil Lit 40:305, 1979

Sheikh K et al: Repeatability and validity of a modified activities of daily living (ADL) index in studies of chronic disability. Int Rehabil Med 1:51, 1979

Smith VS: A new option: A day activity therapy center for the frail elderly. Oklahoma Nurse 25:15, 1980

Staff PH: ADL assessment. Scand J Rehabil Med (suppl) 7:153, 1980

Turner SL: Disability among schizophrenics in a rural community: Services and social supports. Resident Nurs Health 2:151, 1979

30

Women's Awareness Groups for Chronic Psychiatric Clients

Eleanor Rodio Furlong

OVERVIEW

Description
Qualifications of Nurse Facilitator
   Basic Requirements
   Development of Professional Skills
Criteria for Selection of Participants
Personal Interview
Program Design
Topics for Discussion
Sample Session
Pretest and Posttest
Additional Suggestions for Topics

Description   In women's awareness groups, nurses use group dynamics to help clients develop and increase understanding of their own biology, sexuality, and role as women in today's world. The principles addressed are drawn from current issues and trends in the women's health movement. Sessions are designed to increase understanding of body processes as well as political and social issues. The central objective of women's awareness groups is for the woman to achieve optimal self-realization of her female being.

Qualifications of Nurse Facilitator

A. **BASIC REQUIREMENTS**
1. Professional nursing license
2. Understanding of group dynamics
3. Understanding of the women's health movement and social/political issues pertinent to women
4. Self-awareness
   a. Rationale—By understanding their own values, prejudices, assets, and deficiencies, nurses can better provide the following:
      • Climate of acceptance of others' views and life-styles
      • Understanding of client difficulties
      • Appropriate objective responses to clients
      • Referral to appropriate resources
   b. Self-review—The following questions may serve as a guide for the nurse who seeks to further understand herself:
      • Am I educationally prepared to be a group leader?
      • How do I feel about my own sexuality?
      • What are my feelings about masturbation?
      • What are my feelings about people who have chosen alternate life-styles, for example, homosexuals, celibates?
      • What is my stand on birth control?
      • What is my stand on abortion?
      • Am I prepared to refer clients to appropriate therapists or other health services?
      • Am I cognizant of the social and political trends affecting women and their legal ramifications?
      • What are my feelings about the roles of women in today's society?

B. **DEVELOPMENT OF PROFESSIONAL SKILLS**
Nurses who lead women's awareness groups can increase their professional competence through
1. Readings
2. Workshops, seminars, conferences
3. Collaboration with colleagues
4. Community resources, for example, American Cancer Society, Mental Health Associations
5. Formal education

Criteria for Selection of Participants

A. **GENDER**
Participants should be limited to females.

B. **NUMBER**

The number of participants should be seven for optimal interaction; maximum number is 12.

C. **MENTAL STATUS**

Participants should be verbal, in relative contact with reality, and in reasonable control of anxiety.

D. **AGE**

Participants should be from 18 to 55. A mixture of ages provides the potential for participants to share more varied life experiences

E. **NEEDS ASSESSMENT**

Each client is evaluated prior to the first session using
1. Observation of general appearance
2. Review of clinical data
3. Personal interview (see Chart 30–1)
4. Conference with primary team members

F. **PRIORITY**

Preference is given to clients with
1. Promiscuous behavior
2. Poor personal hygiene
3. History of unwanted pregnancies
4. High risk for major health problems
5. History of abuse
   a. Rape
   b. Incest
   c. Wife-beating

(Text continues on page 292)

Table 30–1
TOPICS, OBJECTIVES, ACTIVITIES, AND RESOURCES IN WOMEN'S AWARENESS GROUPS

Topic	Objectives	Activity	Resources/Materials
1. Getting in Touch with Ourselves	The client will: Develop an awareness of female sexual identity and associated cultural roles.	Help client to prepare a collage to reflect thoughts, feelings, and values of womanhood. Encourage client to create title and captions for the collage. Provide time for each client to display and share significance and meaning of collage with other group members.	An array of current woman-oriented magazines Collage materials—construction paper, scissors, glue, tape, and magic markers *(continued)*

Table 30–1
(continued)

Topic	Objectives	Activity	Resources/Materials
2. How Are We Made?	The client will: Increase understanding of the general anatomy and physiology of the human body. Distinguish between truths and myths concerning the human body.	Explain and discuss normal body structure and functions. Discuss and dispel myths of body functions.	Diagrams and illustrations Models of skeletal system and other body structures when available (usually available on loan from hospital nursing education department)
3. Female Sexuality	The client will: Demonstrate an understanding of the basic anatomy and physiology of the female reproductive system. Develop an awareness of the physical and emotional female responses. Relate perceptions of women's role in society. Question known truths and myths of women's roles in today's society.	Illustrate and explain the structure and functions of the female reproductive system. Facilitate discussion of sex hormones, menses, and menopause. Facilitate discussion of female sexual responses. Encourage clients to discuss their beliefs about roles of women in today's society. Discuss and dispel myths about the roles of women in today's society.	Illustrations provided by Educational Department, Tampax Incorporated, Lake Success, NY 11042 The Boston Women's Health Book Collective: Our Bodies, Ourselves, pp 24–37[4] Bardwick JM: Psychology of Women, pp 22–29[2] Sherfey MJ: The Nature and Evolution of Female Sexuality, pp 66–110[11] Gornick V, Moran BK (eds): Women in Sexist Society[7]
4. Preventive Health Care of the Female Reproductive System	The client will: Develop an understanding of terminology related to gynecological care.

Develop an awareness of major health problems. State the importance of periodic physical and pelvic examinations. | Facilitate discussion of terminology and major health problems.

Orient the client to gynecological equipment and examinations (pelvic and breast). See sample session for a detailed outline of nursing actions and theoretical rationale. | US Department of Health and Human Services, Public Health Service, Health Service Administration, Bureau of Community Health Services, Rockville, MD 20857 Female Physical Examination for Contraception. Publication No. (HSA) 80-5609; an excellent self-instructional booklet to aid clients in the understanding of an interview, laboratory tests, and breast and pelvic examinations OMNI Education, Division of Ortho Pharmaceutical Corporation, Box 220, Somerville, NJ 08876 a. Teaching Breast Self-Examination. 16 mm color film, 10 min |

Table 30–1
(continued)

Topic	Objectives	Activity	Resources/Materials
			b. Breast Self-Examination. A self-instruction kit designed to help clients to learn about breast self-examination; an excellent source; three-dimensional illustrations c. Betsi. Breast Teaching Model. Designed to teach clients what a lump might feel like American Cancer Society. National Office, 219 East 42 Street, New York, NY 11017. Check telephone directory for listing of local office. Guest speakers, films, and literature available upon request. OMNI educational materials sometimes available from American Cancer Society.[1]
5. Understanding Sexually Transmitted Diseases (STD)	The client will: Develop knowledge and understanding of sexually transmitted diseases. Learn methods of prevention, contraception, and treatment of sexually transmitted diseases.	Facilitate discussion following film presentation. Encourage discussion of knowledge of STD. Discuss and dispel myths concerning STD.	V.D.: The Hidden Epidemic. Encyclopedia Britannica, 425 N. Michigan Avenue, Chicago, IL 60611; 16 mm film, color, 23 min; sometimes available through local Planned Parenthood Association About V.D. A Scriptographic Booklet by Channing L. Bete Co., Inc., Greenfield, MA, 1979 edition, 1116JJ-78
6. Family Planning	The client will: Discuss and recognize preparation necessary for parenthood. Compare and contrast the various available contraceptive devices. Demonstrate the ability to choose a personal method for family planning.	Assist client to determine ability to parent. Demonstrate contraceptive measures providing an opportunity for clients to examine devices. Discuss advantages and disadvantages of available control measures. Assist client to execute choices.	Planned Parenthood Federation of America, Inc., 810 Seventh Avenue, New York, NY 10019. See telephone directory for listing of local office. Guest speakers, films, and literature are available upon request. Two very good booklets are Basics of Birth Control, No. 1253, and To

(continued)

Table 30–1
(continued)

Topic	Objectives	Activity	Resources/Materials
			Be a Mother, To Be a Father, No. 590. G.D. Searle and Company, Medical Communications Department, Box 5110, Chicago, IL 60680. The Female Reproductive System, Illustrations for Patient Counseling. Copyright October 1976
7. How to Handle the Hard Times	The client will: Describe situations and experiences that have caused discomfort. Recognize and discuss early signs of anxiety. Develop awareness of precipitating factors. Demonstrate coping mechanisms for handling stress.	Encourage discussion of uncomfortable experiences. Help clients to understand their role in conflicts. Provide opportunity for client to consider alternative actions. Encourage role playing for reality testing. Facilitate relaxation exercises.	Everly GS, Rosenfeld R: The Nature and Treatment of the Stress Response. New York, Plenum Press, 1981[6] McKay M, Davis M, Fanning P: Thoughts and Feelings, The Art of Cognitive Stress Intervention. Richmond, CA, New Harbinger Press[10] Davis M, McKay M, Eshelman E: The Relaxation and Stress Reduction Workbook. Richmond, CA, New Harbinger Press, 1980[5]
8. Women Abuse	The client will: Discuss self-inflicted abuse. Recognize and discuss effects of abuse on body physiology. Relate abuse inflicted by others. Demonstrate knowledge of community resources for assistance.	Facilitate discussion of self-inflicted abuse situations, that is, Overeating Smoking Alcohol Drugs Provide information of effects on body physiology. Facilitate discussion of abuse inflicted by others: Rape Incest Wife-beating Provide information about community resources serving abused clients.	Women Against Rape, Box 02084, Columbus, OH 43202 National Clearinghouse for Mental Health, Rockville, MD 20852. Educational materials related to mental health are available upon request.
9. Personal Hygiene	The client will: Identify current hygiene habits.	Help client to log and discuss current hygienic habits.	That Certain Look. A booklet provided by the

Table 30–1
(*continued*)

Topic	Objectives	Activity	Resources/Materials
	Increase knowledge and skills for care of skin, hair, and nails. Demonstrate changes in hygiene habits.	Provide demonstration for skin and nail care. Assist client to arrange for beauty salon appointment.	Educational Services from Avon, 30 Rockefeller Plaza, New York, NY 10020 Total Beauty Care. A booklet provided by Noxell Corporation, 11050 York Road, Baltimore, MD 21204 Solicit local cosmetologists as guest speakers when available. Provide materials necessary for skin care and hair care.
10. You Are What You Eat	The client will: Identify current dietary habits. Gain knowledge of nutritional values of food elements. Develop awareness of various means of weight control. Participate in planning a nutritionally balanced meal.	Help client to log a 24-hour dietary recall. Discuss the basic four food groups and nutritional values of food elements. Discuss safe and sensible weight-control measures. Help clients to plan, shop, and prepare a nutritionally balanced meal.	National Dairy Council, Rosemont, IL 60018. Pamphlets are available upon request. Guide to Good Eating (available in Spanish). Choose Your Calories by the Company You Keep. The Basic Four. Use local dietitian as guest speaker.
11. Exercise for Physical and Mental Health.	The client will: Identify current level of physical activity. Develop awareness of the importance of physical exercise for maintaining health. Participate in a fitness program suitable to health needs.	Help client to log and discuss current physical activity. Discuss relationship of exercise and health. Obtain medical clearance when indicated. Design individualized physical fitness program for client.	Consultation with local school physical education department; in hospital, consultation with recreational department
12. Fashion/Styles of Dress	The client will: Decide on appropriate attire for work and play. Become familiar with current cost factors and budgetary techniques. Demonstrate skills as a consumer of clothing apparel and grooming supplies.	Provide materials for client to create a collage on fashion and styles. Help client order mail order catalogues to become acquainted with current cost factors. Plan shopping trips to local store.	Current fashion magazines, current mail order catalogues Collage materials— construction paper, scissors, glue, tape, and magic markers

Personal Interview	Chart 30–1 shows nursing interventions and theoretical rationale in conducting the initial interview with prospective group members.
Program Design	Chart 30–2 shows nursing interventions and theoretical rationale in designing the program.
Topics for Discussion	Table 30–1 is a list of topics, objectives, activities, and resources appropriate for group discussion. Topics are selected from a needs assessment. For example, if promiscuity is a problem, the topics venereal disease and contraception are included. The number of sessions needed to complete each topic is dependent upon the learning level of participants.
Sample Session	Chart 30–3 shows the way in which one session might be conducted. The session chosen as an example is Preventive Health Care of the Female Reproductive System.

Chart 30–1
GUIDELINES FOR PERSONAL INTERVIEW AND THEORETICAL RATIONALE

Nursing Action	*Theoretical Rationale*
A. Climate	
1. Provide privacy.	1. Subject matter is frequently sensitive to both client and nurse.
2. Allow sufficient time for discussion.	2. Client who is rushed will refrain from mentioning important details.
3. Assure confidentiality.	3. Confidentiality promotes trust.
4. Be nonjudgmental.	4. Objective attitude encourages honesty.
B. Content	
1. Begin with subjects that are easy to talk about and progress to the more anxiety-provoking areas, for example: a. When was your last period? b. How long are your periods? c. Do you have any bleeding between periods? d. Do you have pain during intercourse?	1. This order promotes ease and comfort for both client and nurse.
2. Use explicit, clear words, for example: Penis Vagina Orgasm	2. The nurse's comfort promotes client comfort, which enhances communication.
3. Seek clarification of client's terminology.	3. Validation of terms is necessary to correct misunderstandings.
4. Determine areas for evaluations: a. Personal hygiene b. Reproductive system c. Sexual patterns d. Social values e. Support system—family, friends, and so forth	4. Knowledge of each client's unique situation is used to help her later in group discussions.

Chart 30-2
NURSING INTERVENTIONS AND THEORETICAL RATIONALE IN PROGRAM DESIGN

Nursing Intervention	Theoretical Rationale
A. Prepare resources in advance.	

1. Arrange for audio and visual aids:
     Films   Posters
     Models   Diagrams
	1. Promotes efficiency and lessens clients' anxiety

2. Arrange for guest speakers, for example, representative of American Cancer Society.	
3. Prepare handouts.	
B. Prepare topics consistent with needs assessment, including behavioral objectives.	B. Subjects that are mutually interesting to members tend to solicit participation. Behavioral objectives provide direction and clarity.
C. Set climate conducive to group participation. Physical surrounding:	C. Learning is stimulated by a climate that promotes comfort.[9]

1. Sensory accommodations
     Lighting   Ventilation
     Acoustics	

2. Spatial arrangements—Arrange seats in a circle without obstructions.	2. Members of a group interact more effectively with direct eye contact.
D. First Session	
1. Welcome/introductions—Address clients by last name.	1. Indicates respect for the client as an adult woman.
2. Discuss mutual expectations.	2. Reduces anxiety and enhances learning
3. Establish meeting day(s). It is preferable to meet two to three times weekly.	3. Behavior that is reinforced tends to persist.[8]
4. Schedule meeting times for 1 to 1½ hours.	4. Sessions of less than 1 hour do not allow sufficient time for discussions. Sessions in excess of 1½ hours decrease tolerance level for both clients and nurses.
E. Reassessment of needs and evaluation	E. This is essential to determine effectiveness of program and degree of learning.

Chart 30-3
SAMPLE SESSION—PREVENTIVE HEALTH CARE OF THE FEMALE REPRODUCTIVE SYSTEM

Nursing Intervention	Theoretical Rationale
1. Administer pretest (see Chart 30-4).	1. Determine clients' knowledge upon which discussion is based.
2. Explain objectives for session.	2. Understanding of expectations reduces anxiety and enhances learning.
3. Distribute and discuss a list of commonly used gynecological terms (see Chart 30-5).	3. Understanding terminology enhances effective communication.

4. Facilitate discussion of major health problems such as
   • Anemia
   • Hypertension
   • Cancer (breast and uterine)
   • Pelvic inflammatory disease (PID)
	4. Increased knowledge promotes prevention and early detection of disease processes.

5. Arrange a visit to a gynecological examination room. Demonstrate table, positions, instruments, and so forth.	5. Knowledge that replaces misinformation relieves anxiety.[3]
6. In coordination with treatment team, assist client to arrange for physical, pelvic or other health service needs.	6. Providing these for all members promotes discussion of problems and mutual concerns.
7. Using Betsi, Breast Teaching Model, demonstrate techniques of breast self-examination.	7. Promotes discussion and learning
8. Provide privacy for a return self-demonstration.	8. Return demonstration measures learning level.
9. Administer posttest (see Chart 30-4).	9. A posttest indicates the degree of learning.

A pretest is given to determine the extent of clients' knowledge before the session begins. Clients are told not to worry about wrong answers, and that this test is to help the nurses know what material to include. The same test is given at the end of the session to determine what has been learned. See Chart 30–4 for a sample pretest and posttest. Chart 30–5 is a glossary to be used with the sample topic.

Additional Suggestions
for Topics

1. Childbearing
2. Parenting
3. The working mother
4. Abortion
5. Equal Rights Amendment (ERA)
6. Assertiveness training
7. Legal aspects

Chart 30–4
PRETEST AND POSTTEST*—PREVENTIVE HEALTH CARE, FEMALE REPRODUCTIVE SYSTEM

Circle Appropriate Answers

True False	1.	A speculum is a metal or plastic instrument that is used to open the vagina during a pelvic examination.
True False	2.	A Pap smear is a test that studies cervical and vaginal tissue for cancer.
True False	3.	Breasts are examined for lumps that may or may not be cancerous.
True False	4.	A complete physical and pelvic exam is not very important.
True False	5.	Iron deficiency anemia is a health problem for women who menstruate.
True False	6.	Swelling and tenderness of the breast often precede a period.
True False	7.	Hysterectomy is the removal of the breast by surgery.
True False	8.	Itching, discharge, and burning upon urination may be signs of a vaginal infection.
True False	9.	Frequent bleeding between periods is unimportant.
True False	10.	It helps to talk with your doctor or nurse when you feel upset.

*When clients give incorrect responses on the posttest, they may need further individual health counseling.

Chart 30–5
GYNECOLOGICAL TERMS

benign—noncancerous.
biopsy—the removal of tissue or fluid from the body for laboratory examination.
carcinoma—a malignant growth of cancer cells capable of spreading (metastasis) to other parts of the body.
CBC—complete blood count.
cyst—a sac in part of the body, usually filled with fluid (most often benign).
D & C—(dilation and curettage) a procedure to open the cervix and scrape the lining of the uterus.
fibroid—a benign tumor of the uterine muscles.
hysterectomy—removal of the uterus by surgery.

infection—an invasion by bacteria or other organism.
malignant—cancerous.
mastectomy—removal of one or both breasts by surgery.
oophorectomy—removal of one or both ovaries by surgery.
Pap smear—(named after Dr. George Papanicolaou who developed it) a method for early detection of cancer cells.
pus—an accumulation of white blood cells.
salpingectomy—removal of one or both fallopian tubes.
speculum—a metal or plastic instrument inserted into the vagina during a pelvic examination to provide visibility for the physician.

References

1. American Cancer Society. National Office: 219 E. 42nd Street, New York, NY 10017; telephone (212) 867-3700. Guest speakers, films, literature and Betsi, The Breast are available upon request.
2. Bardwick JM: Psychology of Women. New York, Harper & Row, 1971
3. Bellak L, Small L: Brief Therapies. New York, Behavioral Publications, 1971
4. The Boston Women's Health Book Collective. Our Bodies, Ourselves. New York, Simon & Schuster, 1979
5. Davis M et al: The Relaxation and Stress Reduction Workbook. Richmond, CA, New Harbinger Press, 1980
6. Everly GS, Rosenfeld R: The Nature and Treatment of the Stress Response. New York, Plenum Press, 1981
7. Gornick V, Moran BK (eds): Woman in Sexist Society. New York, Basic Books, 1971
8. Kidd JR: How Adults Learn. New York, Associated Press, 1976
9. Knowles MS: The Modern Practice of Adult Education. New York, Associated Press, 1976
10. McKay M et al: Thoughts and Feelings, The Art of Cognitive Stress Intervention. Richmond, CA, New Harbinger Press, 1981
11. Sherfey MJ: The Nature and Evolution of Female Sexuality. New York, Random House, 1972

Bibliography

Marieskind H: The Women's Health Movement: Women's Health Care. Nurs Dimen 1:64, 1979
Mindek L: Inpatient psychiatric womens groups: The concept of sexuality. J Psychiatr Nurs 17:36, 1979
Redman BK: The Process of Patient Teaching in Nursing. St Louis, CV Mosby, 1976
Smith ED: Women's Health Care: A Guide for Patient Education. New York, Appleton-Century-Crofts, 1981
Watts RJ: Dimensions of Sexual Health. Am J Nurs 9:1568, 1979

31

Therapeutic Community Meetings

Sharon Ward Miller

OVERVIEW

Introduction   The ANA Standards of Psychiatric and Mental Health Nursing Practice state that it is the task of the nurse to create and manage a therapeutic milieu or community. Central to this task is the leadership of therapeutic community meetings.

Therapeutic Community   A. **DEFINITION**

The therapeutic community is a complex social organization. The method of treatment lies in the experience, and in the understanding of the process by which people live together. This is arrived at through the participation of staff and clients in a series of social gatherings. Every social gathering is viewed as potentially therapeutic. The aim of treatment is to facilitate social learning by encouraging staff and clients to confront one another about their behavior. It is believed that, over time, this process of confrontation will increase one's awareness and lead to more socially acceptable behavior and eventual personality reorganization. The benefits of living and working in a therapeutic community are not limited to the client. It is likely to be a growth-producing experience for staff as well.

B. **BASIC BELIEFS**

The therapeutic community is built on four basic beliefs[4]:
1. Democratization
2. Permissiveness
3. Communalism
4. Reality confrontation

    See Table 31–1 for a description of each, with the purpose and rationale.

Table 31–1
THERAPEUTIC COMMUNITY IDEOLOGY—FOUR BASIC BELIEFS

Definition	*Purpose*	*Rationale*
I. Democratization— participation of all members of the unit in the exercise of power and decision making	1. To change basic orientation toward authority figures	1. Diffuses the focus of authority. Many clients have negative views of staff as authority figures, based on early unsatisfactory experiences with parents. The source of the difficulty can be refocused to within the individual rather than the environment. Improved communication confirms social norms through legitimization of client participation. 2. Increases clients' positive influence of each other through staff role modeling 3. Promotes development of strengths among clients so that they may begin to help each other 4. Increases individual client's self-respect

(continued)

Table 31–1
(continued)

Definition	Purpose	Rationale
II. Permissiveness—facilitation of emotional expression. Acting-out behavior is understood rather than sanctioned.	1. To teach clients tolerance of others through control of their own reactions. (Clients develop the habit of thinking before reacting, leading to eventual improvement in adjustment to social situations/interactions.) 2. To produce personality change 3. To facilitate rehabilitation	1. Facilitates expression of ordinarily repressed ideas and behaviors 2. Serves a cathartic function 3. Long-term results are analogous to analysis and insight—clients become aware of existence and causes of ideas and behavior via interpretations made about their original source. 4. Recognition of intolerance of others' behavior leads to new insight into own problems.
III. Communalism—general sharing in activities of daily living	1. To develop increased capacity to endure "real-life" situations 2. To improve social skills 3. To increase social interactions	1. Provides clients the opportunity to contribute relevant information about decision making that will affect them 2. Provides a "corrective emotional experience" for those clients suffering from chaotic family situations, which have led to feelings of isolation and social alienation 3. Clarifies social consequences of behavior 4. Highlights the wider range of a client's difficulties and leads to more specific modes of treatment or rehabilitation through total participation in all aspects of community life
IV. Reality confrontation— confrontations about behavior as observed by those in the environment	1. To counteract the clients' tendency to use defense mechanisms (denial, displacement, withdrawal) 2. To assist clients to develop more realistic perceptions of home and family	1. Increases the development of relationships with those in the real world 2. Leads to a more satisfactory posthospital adjustment

C. **ESSENTIAL ELEMENTS**[11]
   1. Everything is treatment
   2. All treatment is rehabilitative
   3. All clients should receive the same treatment

D. **ESSENTIAL ATTITUDES**[9]
   1. People have a potential for helping one another because of and despite their own problems.
   2. Within the proper atmosphere and environment, this potential can be maximized and the potential harm minimized.
   3. Openmindedness toward problems and solutions rather than application of ready-made solutions prevails.
   4. The process of attacking a problem can itself be of value, whether or not a solution is found.

5. The opportunity to experience achievement may also result in the opportunity for failure.

Therapeutic Community Meetings (Also known as client–staff meetings, ward meetings)

A. **DEFINITION**

All members of the unit, clients, nursing staff, therapy staff, and activities staff, gather together to discuss the day-to-day issues of living together.

B. **FREQUENCY**

Frequency varies, depending on the philosophy of the unit. It can be daily, three times a week, or once a week.

C. **DURATION**

Sessions last between 30 minutes and 60 minutes, most commonly 45 minutes.

D. **PURPOSE**

The purposes of therapeutic community meetings are
1. To facilitate open communication between all members of the community
2. To demonstrate all aspects of behavior in a setting in which it can be discussed, reacted to, and understood
3. To allow for "on-the-spot" discussion of the effects of such behavior, disturbed or otherwise, on the community
4. To encourage clients to develop ways of dealing with such behavior and preventing it in the future
5. To provide a "corrective emotional experience" (for clients who tend to be passively dependent) through active participation
6. To use staff as role models of rational thinking and socially appropriate behavior
7. To introduce new members to the community
8. To say good-bye to departing members
9. To make announcements about administrative issues, patient government, new admissions, or discharges

E. **TECHNIQUES**

Chart 31–1 shows nursing actions and rationale in conducting therapeutic community meetings.

The Staff Premeeting A. **DEFINITION**

The premeeting is a gathering of all staff immediately preceding the community meeting.

B. **FREQUENCY**

It occurs before every community meeting.

C. **DURATION**

It lasts 10 to 15 minutes.

D. **PURPOSE**
1. To inform staff of events within the community in the previous 24 to 48 hours
2. To foster cohesiveness among the staff as a group

Chart 31–1
NURSING ACTIONS AND RATIONALE IN CONDUCTING COMMUNITY MEETINGS

Nursing Action	*Rationale*
1. Begin and end the meeting on time.	1. A consistent structure is important. It allows clients to gauge the timing of their comments and defines the limits. Usually, most emotionally laden topics are raised during the last 15 minutes.
2. Arrange chairs in a circle.	2. Allows for all members to have a clear view of each other.
3. Encourage maximum attendance of clients and staff.	3. Whenever possible, a consistent core group of staff should be present. Continuity of attendance will eventually lead to more open discussion.
4. Instruct staff to scatter themselves within the room of each meeting, preventing clients from developing comfortable "niches."	4. While continuity and consistency are always important, clients should not be allowed to become too comfortable.
5. The same person(s) always lead(s) the meetings.	5. Changing leaders disrupts the sense of continuity and consistency. Having co-leaders, male and female, duplicates the parental configuration and may stimulate transference reactions. (Often the medical chief and head nurse co-lead the meetings.)
6. Instruct staff to sit next to a particularly disturbed client.	6. Staff can provide support and security needed for this client to remain in the meeting. Staff lends the client external control, which may be lacking internally.
7. Comment on unusual behavior.	7. It is likely that others have noticed the behavior and may need "permission" to comment. As the group becomes more cohesive, it is expected that clients will freely comment on each other's behavior.
8. Listen for themes that are relevant to current events on the unit.	8. Emotionally charged unit issues, if not discussed openly, often become acted out.
9. Make comments connecting these events and ideas being expressed.	9. Clients can benefit from open discussions of difficult issues by practicing verbal skills and thereby decreasing the need for acting them out behaviorally.
10. Be aware of the emotional tone of the meeting.	10. Tuning into the emotional tone will give clues to the nonverbal themes.
11. Comment on the tone of the meeting.	11. This facilitates the overt expression of covert feelings.
12. Comment on the unexpected absence of any client if it is not raised by the clients themselves.	12. Fantasies about the condition or whereabouts of the absent member may lead to more open discussion of fears and anxieties within the members.
13. Instruct staff to announce vacations or other departures well in advance (several weeks if possible).	13. Many clients are struggling with issues of separation and attachment. This allows for a thorough discussion of feelings related to the loss.
14. Announce the arrival of new members (staff, students, clients, and so forth).	14. Clients have difficulty dealing with change. This allows for open discussion of feelings and reactions.

The Staff Postmeeting A. **DEFINITION**

The postmeeting is a gathering of all staff members immediately following the community meeting.

B. **FREQUENCY**

It follows every community meeting.

C. **DURATION**

It lasts 10 to 15 minutes.

D. **PURPOSE**
1. To review events of the meeting
2. To do "on-the-spot" supervision of staff regarding its participation
3. To provide for teaching about dynamics of group behavior. The following are examples of problems and solutions which might come up in postmeetings:

Problems

As clients become more active and assume more responsibility, staff members may view this as a loss of their control.

Communication breakdowns within the system can easily occur.

Solutions

Encourage a positive attitude among staff members. The ultimate goal is the *sharing* of responsibility.

Assure that the system provides for all staff to give and receive information. This is especially important for evening and night staff who might be unable to attend community meetings.

Patient Government (Patient Council)

A. **DEFINITION**
The patient government meeting is a highly structured meeting in which clients have the delegated authority to make decisions, solve problems, and make recommendations related to their environment. The clients elect a leader in an organized fashion and may choose to elect other officers such as a secretary and a treasurer. A constitution is developed and unit policies written.

B. **FREQUENCY**
It occurs once each week.

C. **DURATION**
It usually lasts 45 minutes.

D. **PURPOSE**
1. To allow for personal authority
2. To allow the client group to make decisions and recommendations about their environment that meet the group's needs
3. To assign routine unit tasks
4. To develop unit rules and policies about client behavior and to recommend changes in existing rules
5. To channel complaints and suggestions through the administrative network
6. To plan and carry out any social activities either on the unit or within the outside community
7. To elect new officers

E. **TECHNIQUES**
Chart 31–2 shows the techniques used by the nurse to help clients with patient government, including nursing actions and rationale.

F. **EXAMPLES OF PATIENT GOVERNMENT ISSUES**
1. Rules and Regulations. Establishing and enforcing
   a. Television and stereo hours
   b. Smoking and nonsmoking areas
   c. Hours that all lights must be out

2. Activities planning
    a. Trips to museums, plays, concerts, and so forth
    b. Unit parties
    c. Fund-raising activities such as bake sales, quilt making, car wash, and so forth
    d. Use of money raised
    e. Unit decorations and furnishings
3. Tasks
    a. Assigning routine daily tasks such as keeping the patient kitchen tidy
    b. Choosing subcommittees to organize parties, trips

Staff Meetings A. **DEFINITION**
As many staff as possible meet on a regular basis, separate and apart from the client group.

B. **FREQUENCY**
The staff meets weekly.

C. **DURATION**
The meeting usually lasts 60 minutes.

D. **PURPOSE**
1. To discuss difficulties within the work environment and between staff
2. To enhance staff members' interpersonal skills
3. To discuss feelings generated as a result of treatment philosophy and modality
4. To facilitate problem solving
5. To facilitate the development of a viable peer support system, which permits free expression of doubt and concern about the work
6. To allow staff to assist each other to recognize therapeutic and nontherapeutic techniques of intervention with clients
7. To foster group cohesion

Chart 31–2
NURSING ACTIONS AND RATIONALE ASSOCIATED WITH PATIENT GOVERNMENT

Nursing Actions	*Rationale*
1. Provide support for development of patient government structure.	1. Fosters independent action through the assumption of responsibility
2. Provide consultation in the organizing and establishing of the structure of meetings.	2. Demonstrates support; provides a forum for client teaching
3. Provide resources for the development of a constitution and unit rules. Make hospital policies available as needed.	3. Provides an established set of guidelines and boundaries for clients
4. Hold regular meetings with patient government representatives.	4. Keeps channels of communication open, to both give and receive information
5. Avoid making any decisions about the environment that can best be handled by the patient government.	5. Fosters autonomy and group cohesion
6. Support any and all patient government decisions within allowable administrative limits.	6. Provides clients with evidence that their ideas and recommendations are listened to and respected; increases self-esteem and boosts morale
7. Assure staff support through ongoing supervision and education.	7. Alleviates members' feelings of loss of control as patient government becomes more effective. Prevents staff from unconsciously "punishing" clients for becoming independent.

Living–Learning Situation

A. **DEFINITION**

The living–learning situation is a face-to-face confrontation between individuals (staff or clients) who are emotionally involved in some crisis situation. The meeting deals with conscious material. A neutral person(s) acts as the facilitator or mediator.[8]

B. **FREQUENCY**

This happens whenever a crisis situation occurs.

C. **DURATION**

It is recommended that it last 60 minutes.

D. **PURPOSE**

1. To open up channels of communication so that learning can take place
2. To increase individual awareness
3. To assist those involved to become more aware of the thoughts and feelings of the other
4. To allow for a holistic view of the situation
5. To provide in-service training for staff
6. To promote maturity and personality growth
7. To lessen tension
8. To allow venting of feelings in a safe manner

E. **PROBLEMS AND SOLUTIONS**

Staff at all levels must be willing to participate in such meetings. Failure to allow one's own behavior to be examined can lead to a decrease in morale among community members and can lessen the effectiveness of the treatment modality as a whole.

Formal in-service workshops where role-playing techniques can be used may increase comfort with this type of intervention. Staff meetings can provide supplemental support and review of each situation.

Recommended Staff Attributes

All staff members in a therapeutic community

1. Must be willing to support the philosophy of the unit, its goals, and structure
2. Must have a high tolerance level for deviant social behavior
3. Must be committed to being honest with clients and staff
4. Must be willing to look at their own interpersonal problems and make efforts to change when necessary
5. Must be open to being confronted about their own behavior either by clients or staff
6. Must be able to react flexibly in the face of high levels of anxiety and frustration
7. Must be willing to accept and use supervision on an ongoing basis
8. Must have good interpersonal skills
9. Must be willing to initiate and sustain contact with clients and be aware of the inherent importance of this

Guidelines When Hiring Staff

1. Prospective staff members receive a detailed description, either verbally or in writing, of the philosophy of the unit and of the nursing department.
2. They are encouraged to ask questions and to react to the information. The role of staff in a therapeutic community is, at times, in contrast to traditional care-giver roles.

3. They are given examples of situations that might arise on a typical day and asked how each could best be handled.
4. They are asked their own philosophy of nursing.
5. They are asked to return for a second interview, which includes spending several hours on the unit attending meetings, and talking with staff and clients.

References

1. Almond R: The therapeutic community. Scientific American, March, 1971
2. Barnes E: Psychosocial Nursing. London, Tavistock, 1968
3. Burkitt P: The concept of a therapeutic community. Nurs Times 71:75, 1975
4. Campbell W: The therapeutic community: A history. Nurs Times 75:1985, 1979
5. Campbell W: The therapeutic community: Problems encountered by nurses. Nurs Times 75:2038, 1979
6. Holmes M, Werner J: Psychiatric Nursing in a Therapeutic Community. New York, Macmillan, 1966
7. Jones M: Therapeutic community practice. Am J Psychiatry 122:1275, 1966
8. Jones M: Maturation of the Therapeutic Community. New York, Human Sciences Press, 1976
9. Kennard D: Bulletin of the Association of Therapeutic Communities. London, January 1978
10. Margolis P: Patient Power. Springfield, IL, Charles C Thomas, 1973
11. Rappoport R: Community As Doctor, London, Tavistock, 1960
12. Skinner K: The therapeutic milieu: Making it work. J Psychiatr Nurs 17:38, 1979

32

Transactional Analysis

Janet Craig / Terrie Kirkpatrick

Definition   As a theory, transactional analysis is defined as a unified, systematic, and observable theory of personality and social dynamics that incorporates concepts from orthodox Freudian psychoanalysis and ego psychology. It makes possible the definition and observable description of psychopathology common to large categories of psychiatric disorders.[3] As a phase of treatment, transactional analysis refers specifically to the analysis of interpersonal "transactions" between two or more people.

As a therapeutic approach, in its contemporary application, the therapist facilitates integration of the cognitive, affective, and behavioral capacities of the client, generally in a group setting, and may use the specific experiential techniques of behavioral modification, gestalt therapy, and psychodrama, as well as didactic methods and the more traditional verbal interventions of confrontation, clarification, confirmation, interpretation, and so forth.[4] The objective may be limited to social control, that is, altering some aspect of behavior or thinking causing difficulty, or may extend to the actual resolution of internal archaic conflict(s) and distortions, thus freeing the individual for autonomous living. The goals and techniques of the therapist are specifically selected and determined by the client's defined, negotiated contract for change.

Settings   Nurses practice therapy using the transactional analysis framework in
1. Inpatient units
2. Outpatient clinics
3. Day hospitals
4. Private practice
5. Other settings, with special groups of clients

Qualifications   The nurse who practices transactional analysis
1. Is approved by the examining board of the International Transactional Analysis Association (ITAA) as a full clinical member whose requirements include
   a. Two groups with 50 hours' supervision
   b. Personal treatment within the transactional analysis framework
   c. Oral and written examination
2. Has completed an NLN-approved nursing program; has a license to practice nursing according to local standards

Role of the Therapist   The role of the therapist is to facilitate clients' attainment and maintenance of their goals while moving toward autonomous living.

Goals   A. THERAPIST'S GOALS
   The therapist's goals include [10]
   1. To foster a nurturing environment in which learning and changing is *fun*
   2. To model in actions and words the philosophy and values of the theoretical model
   3. To help individuals claim power and take responsibility for their choices

B. CLIENT'S GOALS
   The client's goals, in general, may include one or more of the following
   1. To relieve symptoms, for example, headache, depression, anxiety
   2. To change a particular attitude or behavior, for example, to stop drinking, overeating, smoking
   3. To make a decision, for example, to divorce or change jobs
   4. To resolve conflict with a significant other, for example a spouse, child, parent

Ego states. Transactional analysis takes into account the three ego states or parts of the personality identified by consistent feeling and behavior patterns. These are the Parent, the Child, and the Adult; they are observable in demeanor, gestures, voice, and vocabulary and are experienced subjectively as states of mind. Psychic energy shifts between ego states from moment to moment, depending on past experiences and on stimuli in the present. In *structural analysis,* the client is helped to identify each of the three ego states and to operate in the *Adult* ego state at will.[3] Table 32–1 shows each ego state, its definition, functions, decisions, and statements.

Transactions. Transactions are the smallest units of communication between two people; they consist of a stimulus and a response between ego states, for example:

$$\text{Child} \rightarrow \text{Parent} \quad \text{Parent} \rightarrow \text{Child}$$
$$\text{Child} \rightarrow \text{Adult}$$

In *transactional analysis* proper (as opposed to structural analysis), the clients are helped to identify transactions between themselves and others, and to use the *Adult* to monitor and evaluate.[3] Table 32–2 shows types of transactions (complementary, crossed, and ulterior), a definition of each, and outcome for each.

Strokes. People hunger for others to recognize them either through physical touch or verbalizations, to validate their human existence. We structure our lives to give and receive as many strokes as needed to prevent sensory or emotional deprivation. A person may do this through withdrawal, rituals, activities, pastiming, games, or intimacy. The order of these behaviors indicates increasing interpersonal involvement and, therefore, an increase in the stroke value.[2] Types of strokes are as follows:
1. Positive—Complimentary, direct, alive, significant; producing good feelings
2. Negative—Uncomplimentary; producing the feeling of being put down, discounted, slapped, or scowled at
3. Conditional—Received for *doing* something
4. Unconditional—Received for simply *being*

Games. Games are a series of repetitive complementary, ulterior transactions with a hidden message directed to a particular role (Position), which hooks the opponent's weakness (Racket) and results in a negative stroke for the player (Payoff).

Table 32–1
EGO STATES—DEFINITION, FUNCTIONS, KINDS OF DECISIONS, AND TYPICAL STATEMENTS

States	*Parent*	*Adult*	*Child*
Definition	Attitudes, beliefs, behaviors learned as a child from parents, or parental messages continuing in the client's mind	Objective, rational, realistic behaviors that deal with facts	Impulses, basic needs, desires, and feelings learned as a child and acted out in the here-and-now
Functions	Sets limits, preaches, teaches, protects, supports, reassures self and others. May be: NURTURING OR CRITICAL	Solves problems, weighs possibilities and probabilities, based on past and present experiences. Is always: RATIONAL	Acts intuitively, experiences intimacy, pleasure, pain, and other feelings. May be: NATURAL OR ADAPTED
Decisions	Imitative	Informed	Impulsive
Statements	"You should"; "I'll never"	"I think"; "I will figure"	"I want"; "I can't"

Table 32–2
TRANSACTIONS—COMPLEMENTARY, CROSSED, AND ULTERIOR

Types	Definitions	Outcomes
COMPLEMENTARY	Stimulus and response complement one another, that is, *Stimulus:* Child (self) to Parent (other) *Response:* Parent (other) to Child (self)	Mutually satisfying communication proceeds indefinitely.
CROSSED	Stimulus and response are dissonant, that is, *Stimulus:* Adult (self) to Adult (other) *Response:* Child (other) to Parent (self)	Misunderstanding, communication interrupted or stops
ULTERIOR	Hidden, complex involving more than one ego state in each person (social and psychological levels). *Stimulus:* Adult (self) to Adult (other) Parent (self) to Child (other) *Response:* Adult (other) to Adult (self) Child (other) to Adult (self)	Negative feelings, dishonest communication

In *game analysis,* clients are helped to identify games when they occur by recognizing certain sequences of maneuvers, to identify motives for the games, and to monitor their tendency to play games, that is, to manipulate and be manipulated.[2] For example, a client in a *Child* ego state may manipulate others to treat him like a victim, and then feel powerless as his payoff.

Scripts. Scripts are ways of living that were prescribed by early parental influences and messages of "how not to be" (injunction) or "how to be" (counterinjunction) which results in the feeling of being "OK" or "Not OK" (Life Positions).[7]

In *life script analysis* clients are helped to identify and rework their life plans by facilitating the re-enactment of the "early scene," identifying the early decisions, and redeciding the future course of their lives.[5]

Table 32–3 shows injunctions, counter-injunctions, and life positions.

Phases **Introductory phase.** In the introductory or initial phase of treatment, clients are seen individually for one or more sessions for the purpose of exploring and clarifying the nature of their difficulties and motives for seeking treatment, and providing information about what the therapist has to offer, including the therapist's beliefs about therapy and the techniques or procedures used.

If a mutual decision to work together is reached, a contract or clear statement outlining the client's difficulties and goals is formulated. As therapeutic development progresses, the initial contract may be amended to include other interpersonal or intrapsychic problems that emerge. However, clients generally work on only one contract at a time. Chart 32–1 provides an example of client behaviors, nursing interventions, and theoretical rationale relevant to client contracts.

Table 32–3
INJUNCTIONS, COUNTER-INJUNCTIONS, AND LIFE POSITION

	Definition	*Examples*
INJUNCTIONS	Indirect nonverbal "Don't" commands from the parent's *Child* ego state (parent's feelings of unhappiness, anger, anxieties)	"Don't be you." "Don't feel." "Don't grow up." "Don't be important." "Don't be."[7]
COUNTER-INJUNCTIONS	Direct, restrictive "Driver" messages from the parent's *Parent* ego state, which could stunt the child's growth and adaptability	"Be perfect." "Be strong." "Hurry up." "Try hard." "Please me."[7]
LIFE POSITION	An interpersonal style of being that is assumed at the time of the early decision by the child	"I'm OK, You're OK." "I'm OK, You're not OK." "I'm not OK, You're OK." "I'm not OK, You're not OK."[5]

Chart 32–1
POSSIBLE CLIENT BEHAVIORS, NURSING INTERVENTIONS, AND THEORETICAL RATIONALE

Client Behaviors	*Nursing Interventions*	*Theoretical Rationale*
1. The client presents herself for help focusing on negative feeling or thought. She describes feelings of hopelessness, talking in a childlike voice and rigidly sitting in chair, wringing her hands, "I'm nervous and tense all the time."	1. The nurse asks questions, and explores and clarifies the specific nature of the difficulties, "When is the last time you felt nervous and tense? . . . Where were you? . . . Was there anyone there with you? . . . What were you discussing (or thinking)? . . . How did it end?"	1. The exaggeration exhibited, ("all of the time") and the sense of helplessness in voice tone suggests cathexis of the *Child* ego state. Clarifying questions are aimed at the *Adult*.
2. In elaborating on her discomfort, the client reveals overtly or covertly: a. How she wishes people in her past or present life were different, or b. How others in her life want her to change, or c. How she "should" be different, for example, stop drinking, and stop losing her temper, or d. How she thinks the therapist thinks she could or should change As the client talks, her ego states, rackets, games, and life position are revealed in the style of presentation, for example, how she wishes people were different. Her *Child* ego state suggests a favorite game, "Ain't it awful," and a life position of "I'm OK, You're not OK," or "I'm not OK, You're not OK."	2. The nurse focuses, clarifies, and elicits an exact description of how she wants to be different, asking "If you were given wishes, what or how would you change? . . . How will you be different when you do the work you've come here to do?" Motives for treatment are confronted and clarified: "I'm aware of what you wish your husband would do. What do you intend to do for yourself?" Or, "I'm aware of what others in your life want for you. . . . I'm not clear on what it is you want for yourself."	2. Questions are aimed at cathecting the *Adult* and reinforcing responsibility.

(continued)

Chart 32–1
(continued)

Client Behaviors	Nursing Interventions	Theoretical Rationale
3. The client may persist in evading responsibility for specifying what she will do in treatment. This is usually verbalized or enacted via her discounting of: a. The nature, significance and solvability of her problem, or b. Her own or another's ability to influence her situation: "Nothing I try makes any difference. . . . I still feel nervous all the time. . . . I can't change."	3. The nurse listens for, observes, and confronts discrepancies in words and actions, thoughts and feelings, and discounting behaviors: "Will you say 'I won't do anything to relax me' and share your feeling?" She is asked to imagine the consequences of persisting in her present ways—"Suppose you choose not to make any changes, how will life be a year from now?"	3. Discounts, such as "I try" and "I can't" maintain dependency and are often the first move in a game. In this case, the implied message "Do me something" frequently hooks the "Why don't you" response, to which the client responds "Yes, but." Reassurance is obtained in the process at the cost of maintaining helplessness. Clarifications and confrontations are designed to bring into *Adult* awareness her self-sabotaging behaviors.
4. The client makes a clear, concise, simple, positive statement of exactly how she intends to change: "Instead of feeling tense and anxious, I will learn to do things to relax me."	4. The nurse asks the client to put her desired change in a simple sentence in words of two syllables or less. The therapist acknowledges a positive, clear contract asking when the client will start and how both client and therapist will know when the work is accomplished: "Now I know exactly what you want me to assist you with. . . . When will you begin and how will I know you are doing these good things for yourself?"	4. The contract is an agreement the therapist makes with the client to work on the client's goals. The initial contract generally: a. Is short-termed and open to redefinition and extension as work progresses b. Gives the therapist permission, direction, and a time frame within which to work. c. Provides criteria by which both can measure change. d. Is syntonic with both the *Child* and *Adult* ego states of the client and the *Adult* ego state of the therapist (an example of a complementary transaction) e. Has reasonable probability of fulfillment

A variety of tools has been developed to assist the therapist and client in this phase to assemble significant historical data, operationally describe the desired change, and familiarize the client with the conceptual framework and language of transactional analysis. All are generally considered preparatory to the client's entering the group treatment setting.[1,9,11]

Other issues pertinent to the contractual relationship are made explicit during this phase, including

Meeting schedule, attendance, and fees

Expected time frame and how termination will occur

Rules, though few, for behavior in the group[8]

Working phase. Theoretically, the working phase of treatment proceeds through four successive stages in individual or group work.[3] In contemporary application, however, once the client has completed the introductory didactic materials, with a trained and skillful therapist, it is possible to *simultaneously* work through the four stages as meaningful opportunities in the here-and-now experience arise. The four stages mentioned earlier are

1. Structural analysis
2. Transactional analysis
3. Game analysis
4. Script analysis

In the working phase of treatment, usually accomplished in an open-ended group of eight to ten members, the therapist observes samples of behavior exhibited by the clients and works directly with behavior and transactions in the context of the established individual contracts. Clients are asked to introduce themselves, share anything about themselves that they would like the group to know, and specifically to restate their contract. Statements that include discounts of themselves or others, often the first move in a game, are interrupted. Clients are asked to restate the comment and reflect acceptance of responsibility for thoughts, feelings, behavior, and choices, and to report internal responses (feeling or thinking). Focus is maintained on individual choice, responsibility, and obtaining strokes without exploitation of self or others.

When the clients bring examples to group of difficulties with others in past or present life outside the group, they are asked to re-enact the scene in the present tense, rather than tell about it, so that ego states, actual transactions, rackets, and games can be detected and new behaviors practiced.

Clients are actively encouraged to use all of their abilities to identify and monitor their active ego states, transactions, rackets, and games. They learn to cathect, or invest energy in, *Adult* ego states and evaluate the probable consequences in terms of desired outcomes for themselves. They learn when and how to shift ego states, when to engage in rackets and games, and what other choices they have to obtain recognition.

The essential task in working through *Child* ego state distortions is to facilitate clients' re-enactment of the traumatic "early scene" in which they made significant early decisions about themselves and their lives in response to parental messages (injunctions) in order to adapt, survive, and get strokes. Through the selected use of transactional techniques, the *Child* ego state of the client is experienced and with the assistance of the therapist, the childhood experience is understood and old conflicts resolved, so that emotional change can occur. The *Child* in the client is thus provided an opportunity to make a new decision, give up rackets, games, and a destructive life plan, and redecide the course of life.[8]

Group members in this setting are used to provide opportunities for mutual confrontation, practice of new behaviors, and positive stroking and recognition for authentic change. Group dynamics and process are not the focus and are not specifically promoted.

Though therapists differ in method, each is committed in the working phase to supplying clients with the cognitive framework, keeping clients informed of what is happening as they go along, and reinforcing affective work with cognitive information, verbally, and through visual imagery. Clients are encouraged to use their intelligence, "stop experiencing themselves as powerless, and take responsibility for their lives."[10] See Chart 32–2 for a working phase example of possible client behaviors, interventions, theoretical rationale, and key concepts with a potentially suicidal client.

Termination phase. Termination occurs when clients have made the change they want to make. When this happens, clients are encouraged to terminate, because termination is seen positively and as a beginning. Dependency is minimized from the outset. Anticipatory planning is facilitated at times by the use of imaginal techniques. Difficulties that emerge are discussed and possibly rehearsed. When further oppor-

Chart 32–2
POSSIBLE CLIENT BEHAVIORS, NURSING INTERVENTIONS, AND THEORETICAL RATIONALE WITH A SUICIDAL CLIENT[3,6]

Client Behaviors	Nursing Interventions	Theoretical Rationale
1. Verbal and nonverbal expressions indicative of depression: "I'm a bad wife and a bad mother. My family would be better off without me." Other observable behaviors include strained voice, tight body, slow movement as if weighted down, and expressions of worthlessness, guilt, or fear.	1. Ask for facts of current life situation. Summarize and reflect content and process: "So you feel your situation is hopeless?" Explore self-destructive or suicidal fantasies implied by the statement, "My family would be better off without me." Ask client to take responsibility and own her own feelings—"Would you be willing to say 'I make me guilty, worthless, afraid'?"	1. Symptoms are interpreted as exhibitions of a definite ego state. The first step is to diagnose which one. The body posture and statements suggest *Adapted Child* under heavy influence of the *Critical Parent*. The feeling rackets are guilt, inadequacy, or fear. Games might be "Kick Me," "Poor Me," or "Ain't it Awful?" Data suggest a "Don't Be" script injunction with an "early" decision, for example, "If things get too bad, I'll kill myself."
2. Awareness increases. May still resist taking responsibility for thoughts and feelings preferring to externalize or project blame on circumstances or significant others, seeing herself as a victim of impulses.	2. Ask directly about past or present thoughts of hurting self or wishing for death to happen either accidentally or on purpose: "At what age did you think you would die and how would death occur?" . . . "When did you last think about suicide?" . . . "And the time before that?" In the presence of past attempts or near attempts, also explore what she did to keep herself alive. Ask client to state, "No matter what happens, I will not kill myself, accidentally or on purpose, at any time now or in the future," and to report responses (feelings or thoughts) to the statement.	2. Unsolved problems are used as justifications by the *Child* to kill self. Informed decision from *Adult* ego state will facilitate getting past external sources of trouble, close "escape hatch," and allow reinvestment of psychic energy into solving the problems after the decision is made to live. Internal response provides clues to conflicts.
3. May repeat statement assertively without hesitation, without change in words. May report relief.	3. Test strength to maintain course: "You've said you'd stay alive . . . is there anything which could happen that you'd use as an excuse?" May use imaginal techniques to reinforce decision if there is a likelihood of situational crisis occurring. Elicit how client will use energy now: "What will you do instead of thinking about killing yourself? . . . Who will you use for support?"	3. Intention is for a rational *Adult* commitment. Interventions strengthen boundaries of *Adult* ego state via anticipatory problem-solving. Later in therapy when the *Child* is deconfused, a new decision to live made in the *Child* will affirm emotional change consistent with the *Adult* decision.
4. Instead of above, may verbally comply, or do one of the following: a. Change words or phrases—"I promise not to . . ." "I'll try not to . . ." b. Omit words or phrases—"I will not kill myself on purpose." c. Qualify the statement "unless or if my husband, child, and so forth . . ." "Until . . ." d. Exhibit inconsistent verbal and nonverbal voice tone, body	4. Point out hedging or overt compliance as resistance: "I'm aware you are saying the words . . . what other thoughts or feelings are you experiencing?" a. Counter with "But will you?" b. Ask client to assume responsibility for the "accidents" she might have . . . poor health habits, drinking and then driving, and so forth. c. Reflect her ambivalence back so	4. The client is in charge of what options she will allow herself. a. A "promise" is a *Child* response intended to get the perceived *Parent* to stop asking. b. Omissions are dealt with as direct risks. c. Qualifiers frequently shift the responsibility outside the self. d. Therapist strokes and acknowledges the *Child* investment in the feeling.

Chart 32–2
(continued)

Client Behaviors	Nursing Interventions	Theoretical Rationale
movements, agitation, or other negative feeling escalations, especially with repeated refocusing of responsibility for thoughts, feelings, and impulses. e. Refuse directly, "I won't," or indirectly, "I can't," or use silence and other mechanism of interpersonal withdrawal to avoid.	she can hear how other situations and people are used to keep herself at risk. d. May comment, "It sure seems important for you to be guilty (worthless, fearful)." Reiterate importance of staying alive so the work necessary to make life better can be done. e. Assume the risk of suicide is high whether or not a definite plan exists. Advise client of her choice to make a contract to stay alive for whatever length of time she wishes—72 hours, 1 week, 1 month, and so forth, *or* that arrangements for her security will be made (hospitalization).	e. Refusal to make a contract indicates an impasse with additional work necessary. In destructive scripts where the payoff or the "escape hatch" is suicide, it is ultimately important for the client to get in touch with the early decision and to redecide to live, that is, to kick the "Don't be" injunction. Ensures regular therapeutic contact for renewal of client decision before expiration date, or until redecision work completed.

(Bozeman W: Transactional Analysis 202 Course lectures and personal supervision, 1973)

tunities for practicing new behaviors in a controlled setting would be potentially beneficial, or specific skill deficits exist, referral may be made to classes or groups to meet the specific need.[7]

Evaluation The effectiveness of the therapy and the therapist is measured and evaluated by clients' attainment of their goals. Clients in a group are able to "stroke" one another for taking responsibility and initiating changes rather than inadvertently nurturing one another for helplessness, hopelessness, and passivity. Energy levels are high, laughter is frequent, and learning is maximized.

References

1. Barnes G: Steps for Developing and Implementing Problem-Solving Contracts. Chapel Hill, NC, Southeast Institute, 1974
2. Berne E: Games People Play. New York, Grove Press, 1964
3. Berne E: Transactional Analysis in Psychotherapy. New York Grove Press, 1961
4. Berne E: Principles of Group Treatment. New York, Oxford University Press, 1966
5. Berne E: What Do You Say After You Say Hello? New York, Grove Press, 1972
6. Drye R, Goulding RL, Goulding MM: No suicide decisions: Patient monitoring of suicidal risk. Amer J Psychiatry 130:2, 1973
7. Goulding MM, Goulding RL: Changing Lives Through Redecision Therapy. New York, Brunner/Mazel, 1979
8. Goulding RL, Goulding MM: The Power is in the Patient. San Francisco, TA Press, 1978
9. Holloway WH: Clinical Transactional Analysis with Use of the Life Script Questionaire. Akron Ohio, Midwest Institute for Human Understanding, 1973
10. McNeel J: Seven components of redecision therapy. In Barnes G (ed): Transactional Analysis After Eric Berne. New York, Harper's College Press, 1977
11. Steiner C: Transactional Analysis Made Simple. San Francisco, Transactional Pubs, 1971

Bibliography

Berne E: The Structure and Dynamics of Organizations and Groups. New York, Grove Press, 1963

Corey G: Theory and Practice of Counseling and Psychotherapy. Belmont, CA, Wadsworth, 1977

Harris TA: I'm OK—You're OK. New York, Avon Books, 1969

James M: Marriage is for Loving. Reading, MA, Addison-Wesley, 1979

James M: Breaking Free. Reading, MA, Addison-Wesley, 1981

James M, Jongeward D: Born To Win. Reading, MA, Addison-Wesley, 1971

James M, Savary L: A New Self. Reading, MA, Addison-Wesley, 1977

Jongeward D, James M: Winning With People. Reading, MA, Addison-Wesley, 1973

Jongeward D, James M: Winning Ways in Health Care. Reading, MA, Addison-Wesley, 1981

Jongeward D, Scott D: Women As Winners. Reading, MA, Addison-Wesley, 1976

McCormick P: Guide for Use of a Life-Script Questionnaire in Transactional Analysis. Berkeley, CA, Transactional Pubs, 1971

Novey T: TA For Management. Sacramento, CA, Jalmar Press, 1976

33

Primal Scream Therapy

Norine J. Kerr

Description	Primal therapy is a process that allows an individual to re-experience early, core pains from infancy and childhood. As these pains are relived, they become integrated into the personality structure in such a way that longstanding physical and psychological symptoms may be significantly diminished or totally eliminated.
Primal Pain and Primal Needs	Primal pain refers to the early catastrophic hurts that the child experiences from before birth throughout childhood. Catastrophic physical pain results from the birth process itself, as well as factors such as intrauterine hypoxia, childhood illness, and injuries. Primal pain that is psychological results from the fundamental rejection of the child as a lovable human being. A sense of rejection forms the mainspring from which all primal pain arises. Because they are unable to love, some parents are unable to meet the infant or child's most basic needs. Basic or primal needs arise internally and are a natural expression of the organism's tendency towards growth and expansion. A loved child is one whose natural needs are fulfilled. An unloved child has not had his needs met and consequently feels empty, cheated, and angry. Because primal needs become so painful when unattended, it is necessary to block awareness of the need in order to suppress the pain. The cost of such suppression is neurosis, the deadening of the real self and the creation of a pseudo, unreal self that does not "need." Thus, it is the suppression of pain, the suppression of basic primal needs, that is at the core of every neurosis.
Primal Scene	There is a theoretical point in time when these children realize that they are not loved and that they are totally alone. A young child cannot integrate the terror of this realization and so suppresses conscious awareness of it. It is this point of conceptual understanding that Janov terms the *Primal Scene*. He describes it as the "single most shattering event" of the child's life—that moment of "icy, cosmic loneliness" when he begins to discover he is not loved for what he is and never will be.[1]
Primals	Painful memories from the past are brought forth to awareness through an orderly dismantling of the defenses that have acted heretofore to keep the pain repressed. As defenses are countered, the pain is mobilized in such a way that the individual is transported back into his past. This journey into one's past, in which a segment of that past is relived, is what is known as a *primal*. A primal is an intense feeling–thought–body experience in which an individual relives specific childhood events that, owing to the great overload of painful affect, have been repressed and not accessible to consciousness. A primal is usually accompanied by such basic feelings as need, frustration, fear, anger, sadness, helplessness, and aloneness.
The Primal Scream	The primal scream itself is simply one expression of the pain being experienced during a primal. This pain has been likened to the feelings of someone who is about to be murdered. The scream that the ill child left stranded in the hospital without his mother emits when he comprehends that his mother is going to leave him there alone and helpless, is one that is similar to a primal scream.
Goal of Primal Therapy	The goal of primal therapy is to cure neurosis, and it is purported by followers to be the only cure.[3] Cure, in the primal context, does not refer to the traditional concepts of cure such as remission of symptoms, improved social adjustment, or enhanced ego integration. It simply means the absence of defenses that block feelings. Specifically, the following goals are accomplished when cure is considered to have occurred: 1. There is significant dissolution of the unreal self and emergence of the real self.

2. Inappropriate reactions in the present, compulsive behavior, neurotic symptoms, and destructive acting out are minimized.
3. Historical "real" feelings are no longer displaced onto "unreal" symbolic content.
4. Spontaneous choices are made in the present.
5. The neurotic struggle for parental love is abandoned so that more satisfying relationships can be formed.
6. The entire range of human emotion is experienced consciously.

Preparation for Therapy

To accomplish these goals, the therapy is structured in such a way as to allow individuals access to the very deepest core of pain residing in their own particular lives. Prospective clients are required to submit lengthy and detailed psychological biographies, undergo a medical examination, and in some cases, submit to an extended personal interview. Those who are selected for therapy are mailed explicit instructions informing them that for the first three weeks they will be unable to work or attend school and must devote themselves entirely to therapy. Mailed instructions inform the clients that for 48 hours prior to the therapy they must "give up all smoking and drinking . . . stop all pills four to five days before therapy . . . give up compulsive eating and smoking, biting nails, keeping busy and on the run, or oversleeping." Twenty-four hours prior to the first appointment, clients check into a hotel room located close to the therapist's office. They are not allowed to sleep, see friends, watch television, make phone calls or leave the hotel room until it is time for the initial visit. The aim of the isolation is to deprive clients of all usual outlets for tension, while the sleeplessness tends to weaken remaining defenses.[1]

Technique

The aim of all intervention is to uncover early pain through an orderly dismantling of the defenses that have kept the feelings repressed. The therapeutic techniques are powerful tools in accomplishing this end and represent a synthesis of approaches used in other therapies, including bioenergetic, gestalt, and psychodrama. During the initial three weeks, the client is seen daily on an individual basis in open-ended sessions. In the first session, the client is asked to talk freely about his early life. When areas of pain are encountered, the therapist attempts to help intensify the feeling and to assist the client to overcome resistance to feeling.

The therapist continually directs all conversation to the client's past in order to help relive childhood pains. The client is directed to speak with parents and loved ones as though they were actually present. "Tell Daddy not to hurt you," the therapist may encourage. As clients begin to evidence deep emotion, they are encouraged to breathe deeply and fully, since holding one's breath is a defense against feelings. As feelings intensify, a sensation within the abdomen or chest is often experienced. Clients are encouraged to "hook into this sensation" and let it overcome them. Finally, there is an intensive outpouring of emotion, usually accompanied by a deep piercing scream, which is "felt all over the body." Afterwards there is a sense of release and well-being.

Connection

At this point in a primal it becomes possible to compensate for the "split" that has occurred in neurotic development. It is proposed that this split takes place between the right and left hemispheres of the brain. The brain is composed of a dominant side, usually the left hemisphere of a right-handed person, and a minor side, the right hemisphere. The dominant side is the rational, intellectual side, while the minor side is the feeling, emotional side. To protect against primal pain, an actual split between the connection of these two sides occurs. This split consequently causes inappropriate connections between thoughts and affect, and leads to neurotic behavior patterns or physical manifestations that the person cannot comprehend with the rational mind. Only during a primal can the client reestablish the connection. Connection is the key in primal therapy because it provides the precise link between a particular past event and the affect being experienced in a primal. The client feels the connection between an old, early painful event and the present neurotic behavior and gains insight by virtue of "feeling the feeling" that was once unconscious.

Post-Primal Groups After the initial 3-week period, clients are assigned to postprimal groups composed of others who have completed the initial 3 weeks of therapy. The group sessions continue until the treatment is terminated, typically after 6 to 8 months. In the group sessions, the therapist moves from client to client, going through the procedures described to assist the client into a deep, emotional feeling experience. Baby bottles, cribs, teddy bears, and other infant/child paraphernalia provide useful psychodrama props to propel clients into the past.

References 1. Janov A: The Primal Scream. New York, Dell, 1970
2. Janov A: Anatomy of Mental Illness. New York, GP Putnam Sons, 1971
3. Janov A: The Primal Revolution. New York, Simon and Schuster, 1972

34

Hypnosis

Maureen Shawn Kennedy

Description	Hypnosis is an altered state of consciousness. It is a withdrawing of awareness of inconsequential data and environmental stimuli and a shift in concentration towards a focal goal, event, or person. Incidental facts, events, and people diminish in the hypnotized person's perception of reality, and the client becomes uncritical, accepting the reality that the hypnotist offers. Susceptibility to hypnosis is thought to be an inborn trait or tendency whose potential for use can be affected by environmental factors.

Hypnotherapy is the therapeutic use of the hypnotic phenomena, whereby the hypnotherapist assists clients to use their own hypnotic ability toward achievement of specific goals.

Types of Hypnosis

A. **INDUCED OR FORMAL HYPNOSIS**

A skilled hypnotherapist guides the client in achieving the hypnotic trance-state through methodologic instruction.

B. **SELF-HYPNOSIS OR AUTOHYPNOSIS**

The client consciously and knowingly enters into the hypnotic trance-state through a prelearned method.

C. **SPONTANEOUS HYPNOSIS**

Without the aid of a trained hypnotherapist or prelearned techniques for autohypnosis, an individual unknowingly enters into a hypnotic trance-state. This can happen frequently to those in the high hypnotizability range, especially when the individual is under duress or when a monotonous activity is being practiced, as with ''highway hypnosis.''

Therapeutic Uses of Hypnosis

1. Pain relief, from selective analgesia to complete anesthesia during surgery
2. Anxiety and stress reduction
3. Removal of undesired behavior or habits (smoking, eating to excess, phobias)
4. Removal of symptoms as part of therapy (hallucinations, motor disturbances such as tics, paralysis, amnesia, blindness)
5. Changes in physiological mechanisms (blood pressure and blood flow, heart rate)
6. Increased recall of events
7. Age regression for eliciting additional information and history for treatment purposes (in a limited population)

Myths Versus Facts About Hypnosis

Table 34–1 shows myths and facts about hypnosis.

Client Demographics

1. Seventy-five percent of the population is capable of achieving some degree of hypnosis.
2. Ten percent of this population is in the highly hypnotizable category.[4]
3. Gender has not been determined to be a significant factor.
4. Age is not a significant factor, although a child would have to have reached a developmental age that would allow for understanding and compliance with directions and the ability to sustain a short period of concentration (usually thought to be around 6 or 7).
5. Clients with psychopathology that results in significant disturbances in their ability to concentrate (for example, schizophrenics) seem to have little success in being hypnotized.
6. Heavy sedation, drug use, or alcohol all seem to decrease one's ability to be hypnotized, probably from their depressive effects on the cerebral cortex.

Table 34–1
MYTHS VERSUS FACTS ABOUT HYPNOSIS

Myth	Fact
Hypnosis is a sign of mental weakness.	Research has shown the contrary: pathology disturbs concentration and prevents hypnosis.
Hypnotists project their ability and skill onto the client.	The hypnotist merely guides clients in using their own inherent abilities
Anyone can be hypnotized.	About 25% to 30% of the population is lacking the ability (postulated to be a neurophysiological mechanism), and of those possessing the innate ability, problems in concentration or trust might interfere with their making use of hypnosis.
Hypnosis occurs only when clients allow themselves to be hypnotized.	Spontaneous hypnosis occurs frequently, especially in the highly hypnotizable.
Hypnosis is therapeutic by itself.	It is a useful tool that can enhance therapy.
A hypnotist must possess a certain charisma or mystique.	The personality and even the presence of the hypnotist has little to do with one's hypnotizability.
People will not do under hypnosis that which they would not do normally.	It is possible, especially in the highly hypnotizable, to have a client act out a posthypnotic suggestion that is foreign to normal behavior or beliefs, though this is controversial.

Client Screening The Hypnotic Induction Profile (HIP),[4] devised by Herbert Spiegel, provides the clinician with a rapid (5–10 minutes) assessment of the client's ability to use hypnosis in a therapeutic way. The HIP combines three components—eye-roll (Fig. 34–1), arm levitation, and a control differential—to arrive at a final "grade" of hypnotizability:

0–1 = Low
2–3 = Middle
4–5 = High

Research with over 4000 cases has demonstrated a 79% corollation between hypnotizability and one's eye-roll: the higher the eye-roll (the amount of sclera visible between the cornea and lower eyelid as one looks upward while closing the eyes), the greater the hypnotizability.[3] Since the eyeroll grade and the HIP score have a direct corollation, and both are graded on the continuum from grade 0 (nonhypnotizable) to grade 4–5 (very highly hypnotizable) the eye-roll grade itself is a good indicator of what the HIP score will be.[4]

Clinical Use 1. The HIP is administered to determine the client's ability to make use of hypnosis. The higher the score, the greater the ability to use hypnotherapy successfully, although a well-motivated client with a grade 2 score might be very successful.

2. While in the hypnotic state, clients are usually taught to hypnotize themselves for purposes of reinforcing therapeutic goals.

3. Based upon the HIP score and the hypnotherapist's knowledge of them and their problems, clients are given a strategy or suggestion.

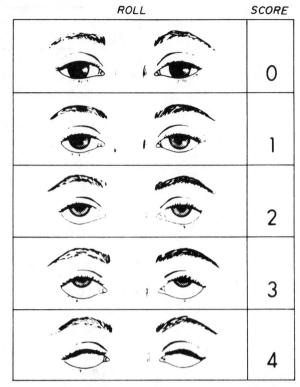

FIG. 34–1 Eye-roll test for hypnotizability. (From TRANCE AND TREATMENT: Clinical Uses of Hypnosis by Herbert Spiegel, M.D. and David Spiegel, M.D. Copyright © 1978 by Herbert Spiegel, M.D. and David Spiegel, M.D. By permission of Basic Books, Inc., Publishers, New York)

Inducing the Hypnotic Trance

1. The client is instructed to get as comfortable as possible, usually by sitting in a comfortable reclining chair. The environment should be quiet and neither warm nor cool. The atmosphere should promote quiet concentration, though highly hypnotizable individuals can be hypnotized virtually anywhere.
2. The following instructions should be given to the client in a moderately quiet tone (the phrase ''breathe deeply and comfortably'' can be repeated in tune with the client's inspiration and expiration):
   a. ''Looking at me (or straight ahead), roll your eyes up to the top of your head.
   b. Keeping your eyes up, take a deep breath.
   c. Holding your breath, slowly bring your eyelids down over your eyes. Keep looking upward. Let your eyes close.
   d. Now let your breath out as you slowly let your eyes relax.
   e. Take some deep breaths, breathing deeply and comfortably. Now imagine your body is floating, very light, buoyant, and restful. You feel very relaxed now, and the feeling is very pleasant.
   f. As you begin to feel light and relaxed, you can feel all the parts of your body relax. Your head and neck and face feel loose and relaxed, your arms hang limply, your back muscles are relaxed, and your legs are completely relaxed and restful.''

At this point, if you believe that the client is relaxed and receptive and concentrating on your voice and his internal feelings, proceed. If you believe that the client is not sufficiently relaxed, continue talking in soft tones, repeating steps e and f.

    g. "While you are feeling relaxed and concentrating on feeling light and buoyant and restful, it is also a good time to concentrate and think about: . . ."

At this point, you would instruct the client in a therapeutic manner, that is, you explore the topic in a nonthreatening, positive manner, one that will allow the client to formulate an approach that will help with the particular problem that is causing distress.

Strategies and Interventions

A. **RELAXATION TECHNIQUE**

Simply talk with clients about the pleasant feeling that they are experiencing, how this is beneficial for well-being, and how it often helps with problem solving. Clients can remain relaxed and buoyant for 30 seconds to 5 minutes and then return to work feeling relaxed, refreshed, and energized (see Chap. 35).

B. **PAIN RELIEF STRATEGIES**

It is of vital importance that the hypnotherapist have a thorough and complete knowledge of the client's pain before intervening with hypnosis. Pain is a symptom, and standard testing and evaluation should occur before *any* intervention, be it hypnosis, drugs, or so forth. When hypnosis is used to treat pain, all pain should not be relieved indiscriminately. See section on cautions. When the client seems relaxed and receptive, as much as possible given the pain, suggest that the pain feels very hot, as if there were a hot coal touching the skin at the site of the pain. Then suggest that there is a block of ice (or sheet or towel) placed at the site. Suggest that the client concentrate on the feeling of coolness. The coolness becomes colder and colder, and the "hot coal" is melting and is not so bothersome. The cold has now turned into a numbness, and there is no pain, just a small tingling sensation, which is not very bothersome. In fact, the client feels so much better now, that the tingling sensation would not even prevent sleep.

C. **HABIT CONTROL** (smoking, nail biting, overeating)

Suggest to the clients when they are relaxed and receptive that they are caring, trustworthy persons. You would not hesitate to have them take care of a pet or even a child. They would, of course, protect the child from harm and guide the child properly. "Just as we care for other living things, so too should we care for ourselves. Smoking (or whatever the habit may be) is harmful to us, and as caring, trustworthy individuals, we owe it to ourselves to care for ourselves and protect our body. Now think about this, knowing you have the power to protect yourself." After a few seconds of quiet reflection, count the clients out of trance.

D. **PHOBIA RELEASE**

Hypnosis can be used to help the client "experience" the phobia in a safe, supportive environment. Imagery can be used to desensitize the object by slow, progressive "exposure" in which the client imagines a phobic episode.

    Once a relaxed and receptive state has been achieved, remind the clients that you will constantly be with them and will let no harm come to them. Remind them that any distress or anxiety during this exercise will not harm them, and that should they become unduly distressed, you will help them to relax once again.

    At this point, have the clients imagine the phobic object. Remind them that they are relaxed, and merely watching the object from a distance and in a very detached manner. Depending upon the severity of the phobia, continue the exercise until the clients begin to be anxious. Then, remind them that no harm will come to them and end the trance and exercise. The goal is desensitization through gradual, progressive exposure. If clients are polyphobic (for example, fear of flying might also include elevators), progress might be slower.

From imagined experiences using hypnosis, the progression might then continue with films, then watching a significant other encounter the phobic object, encountering the object with a supportive "buddy," and, finally, a "solo" encounter. Hypnosis can be used throughout all stages of the desensitization to reinforce relaxation and already achieved mastery.

In the initial assessment of the client with a phobia, it is important that one rule out the presence of a thought disorder entailing a whole paranoid system, in which the presenting phobia is one small part.

Ending the Hypnotic Trance

Once the treatment strategy has been completed, clients may be returned to a normal state of awareness in the following way: "Now I will count backward. At two, you will again roll your eyes upward towards the top of your head with your eyelids closed. At one, you will take a deep breath, and then open your eyes and exhale. Ready? Three, two—with your eyes closed, roll your eyes up—and one, take a deep breath, open your eyes, and exhale." Allow clients a few minutes to collect themselves before continuing with any instructions or additional information.

The Hypnotherapist

Hypnosis should not be taken lightly. Nurses should use hypnosis only with a complete and thorough knowledge of both the process and the client. It is recommended that nurses who use hypnosis as a therapeutic skill

1. Have a graduate degree that includes study of personality assessment and dysfunctions
2. Be experientially skilled at the postgraduate level in their field (for example, medical or oncology nursing)
3. Have completed an approved program of study in hypnosis in an accredited university, college, or other educational institution

Cautions in the Use of Hypnosis

1. Hypnotized individuals can be induced to perform or take part in acts and events foreign to their normal ethics and beliefs. In addition, there is some data that improperly used hypnosis can precipitate serious psychological problems. It is for this reason that "parlor hypnosis" and stage hypnosis have been severely discouraged by both the American Psychiatric Association and the American Medical Association, and limited by an Act of the British Parliament.
2. There is much controversy surrounding the efficacy of symptom removal. Some contend that symptom removal can give rise to another, perhaps more dangerous or disabling symptom. Others charge that this presupposes that humans are closed energy systems incapable of change. While there is no conclusive data supporting either argument, hypnosis should not be used until and unless a complete assessment of the client and the importance of the symptom to the client has been made. Then hypnosis could be used with appropriate clinical follow-up to assist the client to dispense with the particular symptom.[3]
3. It cannot be overemphasized that hypnosis for pain relief should only occur when the following conditions have been met:
   a. A standard assessment and evaluation has been done to determine the source and pathology of the pain
   b. Standard therapeutics, if they are indeed indicated (such as surgery might be

for a progressing cancerous bone tumor), have been explained to the client and employed or rejected by the client with a full understanding of the risks

c. Analgesia has been limited to the specific area

d. Sufficient perception of the character and intensity of the pain has been left so that changes in the course of the illness or the onset of a new illness can be detected[1]

References

1. Crasilneck H, Hall J: Clinical hypnosis in problems of pain. In Jacox A (ed): Pain: A Source Book for Nurses and Other Health Professionals. Boston, Little, Brown & Co, 1977
2. Spiegel H: Is symptom removal dangerous? Am J Psychiat 123:1279, 1967
3. Spiegel H: An eyeroll test for hypnotizability. Am J Hypn 15:25, 1972
4. Spiegel H: Part III. Standardization and Theoretical Basis of the HIP in Hypnotic Induction Profile Manual. Revised prepublication draft, 1976
5. Spiegel H, Spiegel D: Trance and Treatment: Clinical Uses of Hypnosis. New York, Basic Books, 1978

Bibliography

Arnoz DL: Hypnosis and Sex Therapy. New York, Brunner/Mazel, 1982

Hilgard E: Hypnosis and Consciousness. Human Nature, January 1978

Kennedy MS: Integrating mind–body controls for the promotion of health. In Kennedy MS, Pfeifer GM (eds): Current Practice in Nursing Care of the Adult. St Louis, CV Mosby, 1979

Lankton SR, Lankton CH: The Answer Within: A Clinical Framework of Ericksonian Hypnotherapy. New York, Brunner/Mazel, 1983

Wein H: Hypnosis on a consultation–liaison service. Psychosomatics 20:678, 1979

Zahourek R: Hypnosis in nursing practice—emphasis on the 'problem patient' who has pain—Part I. J Psychosoc Nurs 20:13, 1982

Zahourek R: Hypnosis in nursing practice—emphasis on the 'problem patient' who has pain—Part II. J Psychosoc Nurs 20:21, 1982

35

Relaxation

Elizabeth Merrill Varcarolis

> If we look deeply into such ways of life as Buddhism or Taoism or Bendanta or Yoga, we do not find either philosophy or religion as these are understood in the East. We find something much more nearly resembling Psychotherapy.
>
> Alan Watts[11]

Introduction

It is well established that the body's emotional and physical health are interwoven. In the 1940s Hans Selye identified a reaction to stress in which the body prepared to handle any physical insult. He called this the *general adaptation syndrome* (GAS). This response is parallel to the *fight or flight* response of the sympathetic branch of the autonomic nervous system.[12] It has since been established that the body reacts physiologically in the same manner, whether the stressor (real or perceived) is of a physical, psychological, or social nature.[6] In the early 1970s, research demonstrated that clusters of certain life events (that is, death of spouse, marriage, job promotion, and so forth) can be, in themselves, stressful and can render one susceptible to illness.[9,21] Whereas the *fight or flight* sympathetic response can be useful in emergency situations, when this response is sustained and becomes chronic, it may lead to permanent pathophysiologic changes, such as high blood pressure, cancer, ulcers, and other diseases.[12,21,23]

Reducing Stress Responses

Recently it has been demonstrated that reducing the chronic sympathetic response to stress can

1. Alter the course of certain medical conditions such as high blood pressure, arrhythmias, arthritis, cancer, peptic ulcer[12,21]
2. Decrease the need for medications such as insulin, analgesics, antihypertensives[13,17]
3. Diminish or eliminate the need for unhealthy and destructive behaviors such as smoking, addictions to drugs, insomnia, overeating, and others[1,18]
4. Increase cognitive functions such as learning ability, concentration, and study habits[16,18]
5. Facilitate the Lamaze method of childbirth[20]
6. Enhance the effectiveness of therapeutic touch[8]

If nurses can help clients consciously to alter the body's inappropriate uses of the *fight or flight* sympathetic nervous system response, these clients can enjoy increased physical and emotional health.

Stress and the Relaxation Response

The autonomic nervous system consists of sympathetic and parasympathetic branches. These branches influence

1. Visceral targets—stomach, intestines
2. Somatic functions—gastric secretions, vasoconstriction
3. Skeletal muscles
4. Cerebral cortex—concentration and perception[7]

In the early 1970s, it was proposed that one could consciously alter the body's *fight or flight* sympathetic stress response to what was termed the relaxation response. This response is synonymous with the functioning parasympathetic nervous system.[7,12] Table 35–1 contrasts the psychophysiologic responses of the sympathetic and parasympathetic branches of the autonomic nervous system.[1,2,7,23,24]

The relaxation response seems to lead to more stability of the sympathetic nervous system and increased integration of the nervous system in general, directly opposite to the disordering effects of stress.[1]

The relaxation response has been identified in many forms throughout history; mysticism, Zen, yoga, t'ai chi, power of prayer, and Buddhism are but a sampling.

Table 35–1

SYMPATHETIC AND PARASYMPATHETIC RESPONSES OF THE AUTONOMIC NERVOUS SYSTEM[1,2,7,23,24]

Sympathetic *Fight or Flight Response* *(Epinephrine/Norepinephrine)*	*Parasympathetic* *Relaxation Response* *(Acetylcholine)*
Objective Findings	
1. Increase in heart rate	1. Decrease in heart rate
2. Increase in blood pressure	2. Decrease in blood pressure
3. Increase in O_2 consumption	3. Decrease in O_2 consumption
4. Peripheral vasoconstriction	4. Peripheral vasodilation
5. Decrease in digestion	5. Increase in digestion
6. Increase in blood lactate levels (associated with high anxiety)	6. Decrease in blood lactate levels (associated with lowered anxiety)
7. Increase in blood glucose, free fatty acid, and cholesterol levels	7. Amount of blood glucose, free fatty acid, and cholesterol needed for normal body functioning present
8. Minimal or absent slow alpha waves on EEG; no theta waves	8. Increase in slow alpha and theta waves on EEG (associated with subjective feelings of calm and well-being)
9. No release of endorphins	9. May be a release of endorphins (body's natural opiates)
Some Subjective States	
Tense, fearful, frustrated, difficulty concentrating, "pressured," shaky, jittery, confused	Increased sense of well-being, greater ability to cope with stress, refreshed, more energy, increased concentration

Today we are more familiar with the terms transcendental meditation (TM), progressive relaxation, autogenic training, and relaxation hypnosis (see Chap. 34). These techniques help to achieve the relaxation response.[2] The important components are

1. Physiologic relaxation
1. ↓ BP, ↓ respirations, ↓ O_2 consumption, ↓ blood lactate levels, and ↑ in alpha and theta waves on EEG

2. Altered state of consciousness
2. This varies subjectively from extreme calm to ecstasy. The crucial factor is the inherent possibility of breaking up static thinking and making fresh ways of perceiving things possible.[11]

Important Considerations

1. The relaxation response is a learned response and can be elicited in almost anyone. However
   a. It should not be used with people who are psychotic and who, therefore, have weak ego boundaries. Symptoms may intensify, for example, delusions and hallucinations.[25]
   b. For those who are unable to use relaxation techniques, biofeedback can obtain the same results.
2. There are many avenues for achieving the relaxation response, and these are adapted to each client according to individual preference.
3. These techniques are not a panacea. They are tools to help develop alternative responses to stress.
4. Clients have control over their actions and levels of relaxation.
5. Although deeply relaxed, the mind is alert and can respond to any sudden emergency in the environment.

Preparing the Client Before teaching clients the relaxation response, the nurse tells them that[2,11,17]

1. Motivation and receptiveness greatly enhance the process of learning relaxation techniques.
2. Relaxation is a skill. Learning it requires practice and work.
3. Once learned, relaxation techniques are simple to employ.
4. Some days it will be easier to practice than others.
5. Fifteen to twenty minutes, once or twice a day should bring desired results.
6. It may take weeks or months for results to appear.
7. Morning, midday, or evening are all good times to practice. Daily consistency is important.
8. Practicing at night might cause sleep. If that is not the desired goal, choose a time when concentration is facilitated.
9. The goal is improvement and not perfection.

Stages of the Relaxation Response

A. **INITIAL STAGE**

In this stage, concentration is usually extremely difficult. There are a number of resistances that are common and expected.[11,15] These resistances and ways to combat them are shown in Chart 35–1.

B. **RELAXATION STAGE**

Eventually another phase begins in which concentration is accompanied by a sense of calm stillness, a sense of energy and vitality, and letting go of old frameworks of static thinking.

Necessary Criteria to Elicit the Relaxation Response[2]

Four essential criteria have been identified for eliciting the *relaxation response*.[2] Whichever relaxation technique one chooses to employ, these four criteria will apply.

A. **A QUIET ENVIRONMENT**

Choose a calm, quiet environment with as few distractions as possible.

Chart 35–1
RESISTANCES TO RELAXATION AND NURSING ACTIONS[11,15]

Resistance to Relaxation	Action
	The client is urged to:
1. Mind wandering	1. Calmly and repeatedly bring self back to area of concentration.
2. Need to solve problems that have been a concern for weeks or months	2. Understand this as a resistance. Bring self back to area of concentration.
3. Feelings of boredom and unproductivity	3. Recognize this as an expected part of the process. Stay with it and work harder, and it will eventually go away.
4. Need to change position, scratch, sneeze, etc.	4. Change position, scratch, sneeze, etc., and then continue to focus on relaxation technique.
5. Immediate urgency to carry out some task, such as cleaning the stove, going through bills, or calling a friend	5. Calmly observe this manner of resistance and bring self back to the practice.

Toward the end of the initial stage, there is usually a feeling of pleasant "self-immersion," increased feelings of well-being, and greater ease with concentration. It is often at this time that another form of resistance may arise.

6. Interest in existing and dramatic phenomena, such as colors, images, and so forth. This experience may be met with anxiety or exhilaration.	6. Discontinue practice at this moment if it is uncomfortable; return later or observe what is happening until it passes. Do not get caught up in this phenomenon for it *is* a form of resistance and will hamper the arrival of the second stage. That is, the client may focus on these phenomena to avoid "giving in" to relaxation.

B. **A MENTAL DEVICE**

There are a variety of mental devices including visual, auditory or bodily sensations. The purpose of the device is to shift the mind from logical, externally oriented thought. There should be a constant stimulus, for example, a word repeated over and over.

C. **A PASSIVE ATTITUDE**

This is the most important aspect of the relaxation techniques and the most difficult to accomplish. When distracting thoughts interfere, as they will initially, the client acknowledges them and turns back to the mental device. Clients should not worry about how well they are doing. There is no good or bad way to relax.

D. **A COMFORTABLE POSITION**

A position best suited to minimize muscular tension is sitting in a chair with the head and shoulders supported, both feet on the ground and hands comfortably resting in the lap. Clothing should be nonrestrictive. Lying down may lead to sleep.

Techniques   **Benson's relaxation response.** This is a simple procedure for eliciting relaxation and very basic to most other meditative styles, but without the mystical or religious overtones. The nurse instructs the client as follows[2]:

1. Sit quietly in a comfortable position.
2. Close your eyes.
3. Deeply relax all your muscles, beginning at your feet and progressing up to your face. Keep them relaxed.
4. Breathe through your nose. Become aware of your breathing. As you breathe out, say the word "ONE" silently to yourself. For example, breathe IN . . . OUT, "ONE"; IN . . . OUT, "ONE"; etc. Breathe easily and naturally.
5. Continue for 10 or 20 minutes. You may open your eyes and check the time, but do not use an alarm. When you finish, sit quietly for several minutes, at first with your eyes closed then with your eyes open. Do not stand up for a few minutes.
6. Do not worry about whether you are successful in achieving a deep level of relaxation. Maintain a passive attitude and permit relaxation to occur at its own pace. When distracting thoughts occur, try to ignore them by not dwelling on them and return to repeating "ONE." With practice, the response should come with little effort. Practice the technique once or twice daily, but not within 2 hours after any meal, since the digestive process seems to interfere with the elicitation of the relaxation response.

Meditation. Meditations follow the basic guidelines described for the relaxation response. Other mental devices are available that might be better suited to individual needs and responses. They are all aimed at increasing awareness of what is happening inside while deeply relaxing the body. Mental devices that the nurse might suggest to the client are

A. **VISUAL**

This can be a candle, flower, vase, seashell, spot on the wall, etc. The purpose is to learn to concentrate. Neither analyze the object, think a series of thoughts about the object, nor associate thoughts about the object, but rather see the object as it exists in itself, without any connection to other things. Allow the perception of the object to fill all your awareness.[5]

B. AUDITORY

This refers to the repetition of a word or group of words that may or may not have a special meaning. Those who practice transcendental meditation use a special secret word or *mantra*, but any word used repetitiously will do just as well. *AUM* and *RAM* are popular mantras. Others frequently used are *PEACE*, *SERENITY*, and *SUPREME*. The constant repetition aloud or to the self allows the mind to focus inside and drown out external stimuli.[11]

C. BODILY SENSATIONS

This includes concentrating on breathing, the heartbeat, or muscle groups. For example, if one is using breathing as the mental device, one would let the breathing become natural and set its own pace. Concentrate on the breathing going in and out. Feel the chest expanding and count as you inhale and then exhale. Do not allow extraneous thoughts to pull your attention away from your concentration on breathing. Accept whatever thoughts or sensations arise, and then redirect your attention back to your breathing.[16]

Visualization. Visualization is a very effective means of deepening relaxation and desensitizing a real-life situation that is ordinarily met with undo stress and tension (for example, test taking). The important components are experiencing the projected image with all the senses (sight, sound, taste, smell, touch) and at the same time experiencing deep relaxation. For visualization, the client is instructed as follows:[3,11]

1. Relax yourself in your own usual way.
2. Take several deep breaths, slowly feeling your whole body becoming more and more relaxed.
3. See the tension drain from your feet, feel your calf muscles relaxing. Experience the tension leaving your thighs and your stomach becoming loose and comfortable. Feel your chest relax as you take a deep breath and feel all the tension drain from your shoulder, and out your head.
4. Spend some time feeling the warm, tingling sensation of being so very relaxed. It is nice to feel relaxed. Being relaxed feels good.
5. Now picture yourself in your favorite place, one in which you find joy and peace. If you do not know of a place, then imagine your own personal haven. For example, if you choose the seashore, *see* the waves with their frothy whitecaps, *smell* the tang in the air, *feel* the sea breeze on your arms and the warm sand under your feet. *Hear* the roaring of the waves and the cry of the gulls. *Taste* the salty spray on your lips. Let the feeling of quiet joy and peace embrace your whole being. Experience the beauty of the scene with all of your senses. Spend 3 to 5 minutes feeling more and more relaxed and refreshed by the experience.

Meditation and visualization with cancer patients. Meditation with visualization is currently being used for treatment of cancer patients in conjunction with medical treatment. Patients visualize the disease, the treatment, and the body's immune systems. They then picture the cancer being torn apart, erased, devoured, or in some form rendered ineffective at the same time experiencing the immune system becoming strong and dominant. A positive and optimistic attitude is encouraged while the client begins visually fighting the cancer, for the client's attitude seems to play a significant role in the course of the disease. There have been many encouraging results with this approach. Current research will be helpful in further evaluating the effectiveness of this method.[21,22]

Desensitization. Meditation can be used with visualization to desensitize a situation that causes stress. The following illustration applies to test-taking anxiety. The nurse would suggest that the client

1. Isolate the irrational thoughts that surround the situation. Irrational thoughts or goals set up conflicts that are experienced as anxiety. Rewrite the irrational thoughts into rational thoughts in which the goals or results implied can be met comfortably by the individual. Table 35–2 shows how this is done.
2. Write down two or three rational thoughts and commit them to memory. These thoughts should be clear and the goals comfortably obtainable, for example, "If I choose to study, I can increase my chances of passing the exam."
3. Follow the steps used for visualization.
4. In this relaxed state visualize going through your usual routine the morning of an exam. Experience the scene with all five senses, feeling peaceful and optimistic. Calmly repeat your rational thoughts.
5. Experience the incidents that usually cause you tension, for example missing the train or being spoken to rudely. See yourself meeting these situations with calm acceptance. Focus on your feelings of relaxation and the knowledge that you will be doing your best on the exam.
6. Continue to visualize going into the exam: Feel yourself sitting down and feel the pencil in your hand. Experience yourself relaxed and mentally alert. You see the first question and you read it. Give yourself time to read question #1. Look now at the distractors, feeling calm and confident, you make a choice. You are con-

Table 35–2
CONVERSION OF IRRATIONAL THOUGHTS TO RATIONAL THOUGHTS IN DESENSITIZATION WITH TEST ANXIETY

Irrational Thought	Discussion	Rational Thought
1. I have to study.	1. No one *has* to study. No one is forcing you to study. You have chosen this course of study to meet your own goal. In order to be successful, it is in your best interest to study.	1. Since I have chosen nursing as my career, I choose to do what is necessary to achieve my goal.
2. I have to get a 90 to pass this course.	2. You have no control over the numerical grade, but you do have control over how to prepare for the exam and to do your best.	2. I chose the time and amount that I studied. Now I will do my best.
3. This exam is going to be tricky. They want you to fail.	3. "They" most likely do not care one way or the other. This thinking puts the focus on something you cannot control, which will only raise anxiety. You have no control over how the exam will be written. You do have control over the answers you choose.	3. I cannot control the exam. I can control the answers I choose.
4. I am going to fail this test.	4. This is a very clear negative message. You have no way of seeing into the future. If you choose not to study, you may reduce your chances of passing.	4. If I choose to study, I can increase my chances of passing the exam.
5. I will never find time to study.	5. This is true. There is no time to find. Nowhere will you "find" an extra hour. You will have to make time to study. We make time for those things that have the highest priority for us.	5. If it is important for me to be successful, I will give myself every opportunity to understand the material.

centrating totally on the exam. Read question #2. You see the distractors, but at this time you do not find an answer. Calmly make a mark and go on to question #3. Come back to #2 when you have finished. Continue the exam in this manner, feeling relaxed and confident that you have done the best you could do.

7. Practice this daily after eliciting the relaxation response. It is helpful to tape record the scenario or to have someone run through it with you. Eventually it will come easily, and the anxiety will be reduced. The client may use this technique with almost any tense situation.

Progressive relaxation. Progressive muscle relaxation is based on systematically tensing and relaxing various muscle groups as a way of combating tension and anxiety. This method of relaxation is based on the idea that anxiety and muscle relaxation produce opposite physiologic states and cannot exist together[10] and that progressive relaxation reduces both physical arousal and psychological distress.[26] Initially, 39 muscle groups were used, but the method is effective when using 4 to 16.[26] The basic procedure is as follows:

1. Elicit the relaxation response.
2. Tighten each muscle group for a period of 5 to 7 seconds, but not to the point of discomfort (see Chart 35–2 for muscle group and suggestions). Abruptly release and relax that muscle group for about 20 seconds, concentrating on the feeling of relaxation and warmth.
3. During the tensing 5- to 7-second focus on the tension, study it and be very much aware of it. During the approximately 20-second relaxing period, tell yourself how relaxed and pleasant these sensations are and how enjoyable it is to feel so relaxed. From time to time, take slow, deep breaths, letting yourself feel more and more relaxed and peaceful.
4. At the end of the exercise, which will take from 20 to 30 minutes, let yourself relax for a short while and feel the pleasantness of such a relaxed state of mind and body.

Chart 35–2
MUSCLE GROUPS AND SUGGESTIONS FOR PROGRESSIVE RELAXATION[26]

1. *Right/left hand and forearm*—(Begin with your dominant side.) Make a very tight fist.
2. *Right/left upper arm*—Press your elbow down into the armrest. While pressing down, try to move your upper arm toward your rib cage.
3. *Left/right hand and forearm*—Same as 1.
4. *Left/right upper arm*—Same as 2.
5. *Forehead*—Raise your eyebrows as high as you can. If this does not cause tension, make a deep frown.
6. *Middle face*—Wrinkle your nose and shut your eyelids tightly together.
7. *Jaws*—Clench your teeth and pull back the corners of your mouth. At the same time, press your tongue against the roof of your mouth.
8. *Neck*—Pull your chin toward your chest with the muscles in the front of your neck while simultaneously pulling your head back with the muscles in the rear of your neck.
9. *Shoulders and upper back*—Pull your shoulders back as though you were trying to touch your shoulder blades together. An alternative movement is to shrug your shoulders. Raise your shoulders as though you were trying to touch your ears with the tops of your shoulders.
10. *Stomach*—Pull the muscles of your stomach inward while at the same time pressing them downward. This makes your stomach hard, as you would if you were preparing to be hit in the stomach.
11. *Right/left thigh*—Try to bend your knee forward with the muscles of the back of your thigh while at the same time bending in the opposite direction with the muscles on the top of your thigh.
12. *Right/left calf*—Bend your foot toward your shin as though you were trying to touch your shin with your toes. (This is the opposite movement from pointing your toes.)
13. *Left/right thigh*—Same as 11.
14. *Left/right calf*—Same as 12.

It is helpful for the nurse to verbally take the client through this process. If this is not possible, the client tape records the whole session, starting with the steps in relaxation through the muscle tensing, giving each muscle group the proper timing and instruction.

Autogenic training.[4] In this technique, autosuggestion is taught, and the main focus is passive attention to the body. Autogenic training requires that the nurse be trained in this technique before leading the client through the training. It may take from 4 to 10 months before optimal benefits are realized. The process of learning goes through six steps[12]:

1. Inducing sensations of heaviness of limbs: "My right arm is heavy, my left arm is heavy," and so forth
2. Inducing sensations of warmth in the limbs: "My right arm is warm, my left arm is warm"
3. Cardiac regulation: "My heartbeat is calm and regular"
4. Respiratory regulation: "My body breathes itself, my body breathes itself"
5. Induction of sense of upper abdominal warmth: "My solar plexus is warm"
6. Induction of sense of coolness in the forehead: "My forehead is cool"

As the individual gains control over the various musculature and internal functioning, suggested fantasy is introduced. These then progress to focusing on problems of living, and psychological conflicts.[3]

References

1. Aron A, Aron E: The transcendental meditation program's effect on addictive behavior. Addict Behav 5:5, 1980
2. Benson H: The Relaxation Response. New York, William Morrow and Co, 1975
3. Coe W: Expectation, hypnosis, and suggestion. In Kanfer F, Goldstein A (eds): Behavior Change: Helping People Change, 2nd ed. New York, Pergamon Press, 1980
4. Davidson RJ, Schwartz GE: Matching relaxation therapies and types of anxiety: A patterning approach. In White J, Fadiman J (eds): Relax: How You Can Feel Better, Reduce Stress and Overcome Tension. New York, The Confucian Press, 1976
5. Deikman A: Experimental meditation. In Tart C (ed): Altered States of Consciousness. Garden City, NY, Doubleday and Co, 1972
6. Engel GL: A unified concept of health and disease. Perspect Biol Med 3:459, 1960
7. Gellhorn E, Kiely W: Mystical states of consciousness: Neurophysiological and clinical aspects. J Nerv Ment Dis 154:399, 1972
8. Heidt P: Effects of therapeutic touch on anxiety level of hospitalized patients. Nurs Res 30:32, 1981
9. Holmes TH, Rahe RH: The social readjustment rating scale. J Psychosom Med 14:121, 1970
10. Jacobson E: Progressive Relaxation, 3rd ed. Chicago, University Press, 1974
11. LeShan L: How to Meditate. Boston, Little, Brown & Co, 1974
12. Luckman J, Sorenson K: Medical–Surgical Nursing: A Psychophysiologic Approach, 2nd ed. Philadelphia, WB Saunders, 1980
13. McCaffery M: Relieving pain with noninvasive techniques. Nurs 80, 10:57, 1980
14. Maxie Maultzy: Adapted from a tape recording on Test Taking Anxiety using Rational Behavioral Techniques
15. Maupin E: Individual differences in response to a Zen meditation exercise. In Tart C (ed): Altered States of Consciousness. Garden City, NY, Doubleday and Co, 1972
16. Maupin E: On meditation. In Tart C (ed): Altered States of Consciousness. Garden City, NY, Doubleday and Co, 1972
17. Morris C: Relaxation therapy in a clinic. Am J Nurs 79:1958, 1979
18. Morse D et al: A physiological and subjective evaluation of meditation, hypnosis, and relaxation. Psychosom Med 39:305, 1977
19. Peter L: The Peter Prescription. New York, William Morrow and Co, 1972
20. Pilletteri A: Maternal–Newborn Nursing, 2nd ed. Boston, Little, Brown & Co, 1981

21. Riley V: Stress and host resistance. In Achterberg J et al (eds): Stress, Psychological Factors and Cancer. Ft Worth, New Medicine Press, 1976
22. Scarf M: Images that heal. Psychol Today 4:33, 1980
23. Smith M, Selye H: Reducing the negative effects of stress. Am J Nurs 79:1953, 1979
24. Snyder SH: Opiate receptors and internal opiates. Scientific American 236:44, 1977
25. Spiegel H, Spiegel D: Trance and Treatment. New York, Basic Books, 1978
26. Woolfolk R, Richardson F: Stress, Sanity and Survival. New York, Sovereign Books, 1978

Bibliography

Garrison J, Scott PA: A group self-care approach to stress management. J Psychiatr Nurs 17:9, 1979

36

Behavior

Modification*

Maxine E. Loomis

OVERVIEW

*Material in this chapter is extracted from Loomis ME, Horsley JA: Interpersonal Change: A Behavioral Approach to Nursing Practice. New York, McGraw-Hill, 1974.

Introduction　Psychiatric nursing can be viewed as a process of altering the behaviors of clients, their families, and their environments. This alteration should provide for an increasingly more rewarding living situation for the clients and their families. Nurses perform four functions in the process of altering behavior:

1. Increasing the strength of clients' adaptive behaviors
2. Decreasing the strength of clients' maladaptive behaviors
3. Teaching clients new behaviors for living with themselves, their families, and their environments
4. Teaching clients new ways of adjusting to their environments

Basic Principles

Operant Behavior　**A. DEFINITION**

Operant behavior is behavior that operates on the environment in such a way as to produce a change in that environment. (For example, a client, Don, randomly hits clients whom he sees in the dayroom.)

B. OPERANT RESPONSES

Operant responses are individual units of operant behavior that are objectively defined and can be measured along some dimension such as frequency, duration, or intensity. (The frequency, duration, and intensity of Don's hitting behavior can be measured.)

C. RESPONSE CLASS

Response class is a grouping of operant responses according to some common characteristic (*e.g.*, social interaction). A response class may be broken down into many specific behavioral components. (Don's behavior could be classified as "social interaction," hitting, or making contact.)

Stimuli　**A. DEFINITION**

Stimuli are environmental events that interact with and influence a person's behavior.

B. DISCRIMINATIVE STIMULI

Discriminative stimuli precede a response and influence it by signaling, or setting the stage for the response to occur. (Don's hitting occurs when other clients are laughing together.)

C. REINFORCERS OR PUNISHERS

Reinforcers or punishers follow or provide the consequences for a response and thereby influence the future rate of occurrence of that response. (Don is either scolded or secluded when he hits clients.)

Operant Conditioning　**A. DEFINITION**

Operant conditioning is the learning process by which discriminative stimuli, operant responses, and environmental consequences become linked together in an orderly way.

B. CONTINGENCY SYSTEM

A contingency system is represented in the following manner:

Discriminative stimulus	$\rightarrow$	Operant response	$\rightarrow$	Environmental consequences
(other clients laugh)		(Don hits them)		(He is scolded or secluded)

What this model indicates is that certain discriminative stimuli set the stage for the occurrence of a behavior response, which is followed by environmental consequences that either increase or decrease the future probability that the response will occur. Nurses must identify and manipulate the discriminative stimuli, the responses (or human behavior), and resulting consequences to achieve the goal of change in client behavior.

Reinforcing Stimuli

A. POSITIVE REINFORCEMENT

Positively reinforcing stimuli are those consequences that increase or maintain the behaviors that they follow. Thus, a reinforcer is any event that increases the probability of the response that immediately precedes it. Reinforcement is one of the most direct ways of increasing behavior. Positive reinforcement is the presentation of desirable consequences following a behavior.

B. NEGATIVE REINFORCEMENT

Negative reinforcement is the removal of an aversive condition (such as alleviating pain) in order to strengthen behavior. This is classified as reinforcement because it increases the future probability of the response it follows.

C. LEARNING

Learning can occur whether we plan for it or let it take place accidentally. Much of the bizarre behavior demonstrated by psychiatric clients has been learned accidentally and is reinforced by attention. (Don's hitting other clients was followed by being placed in seclusion. For Don, seclusion was the reinforcer that maintained hitting behavior. That is, he hit clients in order to get into seclusion where he felt more in control.)

D. SPECIFICITY OF REINFORCERS

Reinforcers are individually specific, that is, an event that will serve as a reinforcer for one person may not do so for another person. (For some clients, seclusion is punishment; for others, like Don, it is a relief to have his behavior controlled.)

E. PREMACK PRINCIPLE

The Premack principle states that a more frequently occurring behavior can be used to increase the probability of a less frequently occurring behavior. (In Don's case, being in seclusion occurred more frequently than being with the other clients, so the former could be used to reinforce the latter.) The assumption underlying this principle is that activities in which people spend most of their time have some reinforcing properties. In other words, people choose activities that they like. These activities can be used as reinforcers.

F. **CONDITIONS INFLUENCING REINFORCER EFFECTIVENESS**
  1. Deprivation will increase the potency of a reinforcer (*e.g.,* thirst or hunger). (Don is more likely to control the hitting if he is hungry, and is promised dinner if he controls his behavior).
  2. Satiation will decrease the potency of a reinforcer, *e.g.,* food loses its reinforcing power following a big meal. (After dinner, Don is less likely to conform.)
  3. Primary reinforcers, which fulfill biological needs, (*e.g.,* food, sex, sleep, warmth), are more or less effective at predictable intervals. (Don gets hungry or sleepy at predictable times.)
  4. Conditioned, or secondary, reinforcers (*e.g.,* money, grades, praise) acquire their reinforcing value as a result of experience and are harder to satiate. (Once Don learns to accept praise for talking with other clients instead of hitting them, he can accept this secondary reinforcer at any time.)
  5. Immediacy of reinforcement is required to increase the strength of behavior; therefore, a token or praise given immediately following a behavior is a potent reinforcer. (Praise of Don's control upon seeing clients laugh must be given at once.)

Extinction A. **DEFINITION**
Extinction is the withholding of positive reinforcers following a response, which eventually decreases the response rate. (Theoretically, if Don's hitting behavior could be ignored, it would decrease and finally stop.)

B. **PROBLEMATIC SIDE EFFECTS OF EXTINCTION** (or ignoring behavior)
  1. The rate or intensity of the response subject to extinction may increase before it decreases. This is especially dangerous with self-destructive behavior. (If it were ignored, Don's hitting would initially increase, endangering him and others, before it began to decrease.)
  2. There may be an increased variability in clients' behavior as they randomly search to produce the desired reinforcement. Emotional (crying or yelling) escalations are not uncommon. (Don could become more and more verbally abusive.)
  3. Staff may engage in a process of *differential reinforcement* as the client does more and more extreme behaviors to get attention. (The staff may ignore less intense behaviors, for example, asking for medication, but be forced to respond to more upsetting behaviors, for example, hysterical crying or thrashing around.)

Aversive Stimuli A. **DEFINITION**
Aversive stimuli are stimuli that follow a response and result in a decrease of the future probability of that response. These aversive stimuli are commonly called *punishers*. When an aversive stimulus is used to decrease the future probability of the response that it follows, the operation is called punishment.

B. **PRIMARY AVERSIVE STIMULI**
Primary aversive stimuli directly threaten biological needs or existence (*e.g.,* extremes of heat or cold, physical blows).

C. **CONDITIONED OR SECONDARY AVERSIVE STIMULI**

Conditioned aversive stimuli acquire their punishing potential as a result of experience (*e.g.,* frowns or bad grades).

D. **PUNISHMENT**

Punishment can be delivered by the presentation of an aversive stimulus immediately following a response or by the withdrawal of an ongoing positive reinforcer immediately following a response. The use of punishment requires ongoing, accurate assessment of the consequences. When the response is not rapidly suppressed, the punishment should be stopped, or if safe, the magnitude of the aversive stimulus should be increased enough to produce rapid suppression.

E. **CONDITIONS INFLUENCING EFFECTIVENESS**

Effective punishment results in a suppression of the target response.
1. Punishment is less effective if the person is used to a high level of this punishment. Examples:
   a. Football players are gradually trained to tolerate increasing amounts of physical abuse. This is thought of as "conditioning."
   b. Abused children often become habituated to lower levels of punishment so that it takes increasingly severe abuse to get them to respond.
2. Punishment is less effective when positive reinforcers are mixed in with the aversive stimuli in an unplanned manner.
3. Punishment is more effective when aversive stimuli for specific responses are clearly combined with positive reinforcement for other specific responses.

F. **DISADVANTAGES OF PUNISHMENT**

1. The effects of punishment tend to be situationally specific, that is, associated with a place as the discriminative stimulus. (If Don were punished repeatedly by scolding in the dayroom, he might avoid the dayroom.)
2. Punishment tends to serve as the discriminative stimulus for escape responses. (If Don were scolded by the nurses frequently, he would avoid them.)
3. The use of punishment may sometimes result in the client's exhibiting aggressive responses. (Don could become assaultive to staff who scold him.)
4. The aversive properties of the punishment may be generalized to the person delivering the punishment. (If the same nurse scolded Don each time, he might become unable to relate to this nurse in a positive way at other times.)
5. Punishment has little holding power in relation to long-term behavior change unless the response has been totally suppressed. (As long as Don continues to hit clients even though scolding follows, the punishment has not been successful and will not be.)
6. While punishment can be an effective technique for changing behavior, few professionals are prepared to use it safely and ethically. Staff members would most likely not call the scolding "punishment" but rather refer to it euphemistically as "presenting reality through confrontation."

Issues of Control

Whether a person's behavior is considered appropriate or inappropriate depends upon whether that behavior has a high or low probability of being well received (reinforced) by others in the environment. Thus, the ability to discriminate when reinforcement is forthcoming is a basic function in successful interpersonal behavior.

Responding in
Appropriate
Environmental
Conditions

A. **DISCRIMINATIVE STIMULI**

Discriminative stimuli are stimuli that precede the emission of responses and serve to "set the occasion" for a particular response to occur. Discriminative stimuli do not cause a response to occur; instead they indicate when a response has a high probability of being reinforced. (When the nursing staff has helped Don change, he enters the dayroom, sees clients laughing and talking, and joins them, "knowing" that this response will be reinforced by staff members.)

B. **STIMULUS CONTROL**

Stimulus control exists when a given response is more likely to occur under the desired stimulus conditions than when these conditions are not present. (Don is more likely to respond appropriately when staff who tend to reinforce this behavior are present.) When a person's behavior is controlled by the situation in which he finds himself, the person is said to be able to *discriminate*.

C. **STIMULUS GENERALIZATION**

Stimulus generalization occurs when an environmental situation similar to, yet different from, the situation in which the response was originally reinforced acquires the capacity to set the stage for the occurrence of that response. (Once Don has learned that socially appropriate [nonhitting] behavior will be reinforced in the dayroom, he generalizes this response to the dining room as well.)

D. **RESPONSE GENERALIZATION**

Response generalization is a process whereby there is an increase in the reinforced response as well as in responses that are members of the same response class. (Once Don has learned that nonhitting behavior is reinforced, he generalizes to other socially appropriate behavior such as eating and dressing properly.)

Responding Without
Immediate
Reinforcement

People frequently respond without reinforcement. This is essential because the environment is not always capable of producing reinforcement every time a response occurs.

Reinforcement Schedules

A. **CONTINUOUS REINFORCEMENT**

The continuous reinforcement schedule is a special case in which every occurrence of the target response is followed by reinforcement. Continuous reinforcement is used primarily in the initial phases of generating new responses.

B. **PROBLEMS**

1. The person delivering the reinforcement must be continuously present to monitor the occurrence of the target response.
2. Because of the possibility of satiation, generalized secondary reinforcers (*e.g.*, money, points, tokens) must be selected that will maintain their reinforcing potential over time.
3. When continuous reinforcement is withdrawn, extinction occurs quickly.

C. **INTERMITTENT REINFORCEMENT**

Intermittent reinforcement schedules are used to combat the above problems. There are four types of intermittent reinforcement:

1. A *fixed ratio schedule* is a method of delivering reinforcement following a set

number of responses. (Don is given a token every time he eats a meal in the dining room without hitting anyone.)

2. A *variable ratio schedule* is a method of delivering reinforcement in which the number of responses required varies from reinforcement to reinforcement. (Don is given a token after some meals when he has not hit anyone, but not every meal.)

3. A *fixed interval schedule* is a method of delivering reinforcement for behavior following a set period of time. (Don is given a token at the end of every hour during which he has hit no one.)

4. A *variable interval schedule* is a method of delivering reinforcement in which the time interval varies from reinforcement to reinforcement. (Don is given a token at various times during the day when he is observed talking to clients without hitting them but not every time he spends time without hitting anyone.)

D. **CLINICAL APPLICATION**
1. A continuous schedule of reinforcement is necessary for the initial strengthening of weak responses.

2. *Ratio schedules* are more useful when a transition step is necessary to move from a continuous reinforcement schedule to a more real-life schedule, or when the target response occurs in well-specified and infrequently occurring situations (*e.g.,* preparing meals, washing the car, or doing the laundry). Ratio schedules are often impractical and inefficient in clinical situations because they require that the person delivering the reinforcement keep the client under constant observation in order to know when to deliver the reinforcement.

3. *Interval schedules* are practical in a clinical setting because the staff does not have to stay with the client between reinforcement intervals. Most everyday behavior is reinforced on an interval schedule. The variable interval schedule is the most resistant to extinction and can therefore be used to maintain behaviors that are not likely to be naturally reinforced every time they occur. For example, the instructor who wants her nursing students to be informed at all times about the conditions of their clients will spot check her students at randomly selected times. The student must then remain informed at all times, because she never knows when she will be questioned.

Response Chains   Normal behavior consists of numerous *response chains* with multiple links made up of discriminative stimuli, discrete responses, and conditioned reinforcers. At the end of this series of links is a very potent reinforcer. For example, a nurse may go to work every day and enjoy the daily reinforcement of a job well done, or of at least being able to go home at the end of the shift. Occasionally she receives a compliment from a supervisor (variable interval schedule), and every other week she receives a paycheck (fixed interval schedule). After a longer chain of working responses, she may receive an annual raise (fixed interval schedule) or a promotion (variable ratio schedule).

Response chains are learned in the reverse order from that in which they are eventually performed when they become a complex behavior. That is, the last behavior is taught first and reinforced, then preceding behaviors are added to the chain. For example, in toilet training, going in the toilet is reinforced first and then all of the behaviors for getting to the toilet in time are added in stages.

Modification Techniques

In order to apply the principles of behavior modification (operant conditioning) the nurse must consider these basic questions:

1. What is the target behavior, and how will all staff members recognize it when it occurs?
2. In what setting does the target behavior occur?
3. What are potent reinforcers or punishers for this client?
4. Can staff members control the reinforcers? the punishers?
5. What schedule of reinforcement or punishment should be used?

Table 36–1 can be used as a guide for the selection of appropriate behavior modification techniques.

Behavioral Nursing Process

Chart 36–1 shows a complete and individualized way to treat specific clients using the principles and techniques of operant conditioning and applying a problem–solving process.

(Text continues on page 347)

Table 36–1

PROBLEMS, GOALS, TECHNIQUES, AND TECHNICAL CONSIDERATIONS IN BEHAVIORAL MODIFICATION

Behavioral Problem	Goal	Techniques	Technical Considerations
Response too infrequent (for example, client will not leave his room to socialize with others)	Increase frequency of ongoing response	1. Positive reinforcement	1. Response definition, reinforcer identification, reinforcer control
		2. Negative reinforcement	2. What is the aversive stimulus? Who will initiate it? What client response will result in the termination of the aversive stimulus?
Response too frequent (for example, client constantly washes her hands)	Decrease frequency of ongoing response	1. Punishment	1. Response definition, definition of consequence, presentation of an aversive or removal of a positive stimulus? Delivered by whom? Strength of the punisher? Emotional side effects and generalization—how wil they be prevented or dealt with? With which other modification techniques will punishment be combined?

(continued)

Table 36–1
(continued)

Behavioral Problem	Goal	Techniques	Technical Considerations
		2. Extinction	2. Response definition, definition of consequences, reinforcer control. What other responses will be reinforced?
		3. Reinforce incompatible responses	3. Response definition of incompatible response, reinforcer quantity and quality.
		4. Satiation	4. By what means will the client be satiated? Is this practical?
		5. Time-out from positive reinforcement	5. Definition of responses (a) being punished, (b) being extinguished, and (c) being negatively reinforced. Definition of consequences for (a), (b), and (c) above.
		6. Response cost	6. Definition of response, determination of cost, potential for desirable responses to occur
Response never occurs (includes never did or used to occur) (for example, client is mute except for primitive sounds)	Teach or retrain response	1. Shaping	1. Target response definition, identify prerequisite response currently in client's repertoire. Define sequential response steps of successive approximation. Reinforcer identification, differentially reinforce each successive step until target response reached
		2. Chaining	2. Response definition, analyze response in relation to its temporal sequence, define backward or forward chain. Teach response at end of chain that results in reinforcement, and then add on the next step.

Table 36–1
(continued)

Behavioral Problem	Goal	Techniques	Technical Considerations
		3. Imitation	3. Does the client imitate? Response definition, reinforcer identification, generalization of imitative responding
		4. Behavioral rehearsal	4. How, where, and by whom will the behavioral rehearsal be conducted? How closely does rehearsal situation simulate real world situation?
Response occurs but inappropriately: 1. Occurs when it should not occur (for example, bed-wetting)	Stimulus discrimination	1. Discrimination training	1. What is the stimulus setting in which the response is desired? What will be used to reinforce the response when it occurs in that setting? What will happen when the response occurs in an inappropriate setting?
2. Occurs in some but not all instances when it should	Generalization of response to all appropriate situations	2. Generalization training	2. Define current stimulus situation in which response is emitted. Define other situations in which response should occur and identify any aspects that are similar to situations where response already occurs. Identify reinforcers for use in new situations.

(Adapted from Loomis M, Horsely JA: Interpersonal Change: A Behavioral Approach to Nursing Practice, New York, McGraw-Hill, © 1974. Reproduced with permission.)

Chart 36–1
NURSING PROCESS OUTLINE FOR BEHAVIOR MODIFICATION

1. *Statement of behavioral problem*
   a. What is the problem?
   b. Who defined the problem?
      1) The identified patient?
      2) An external agent? (for example, the patient's mother)
      3) Society?
2. *Behavioral history*
   a. Responses
      1) What are the appropriate responses present within the patient's behavioral repertoire?
      2) What are the inappropriate responses present within the patient's behavioral repertoire?
      3) What are the age-appropriate responses absent from the patient's behavioral repertoire?
   b. Consequences
      1) What are reinforcers for this patient?
      2) What are punishers for this patient?
      3) What are potential mediators for this patient?
   c. Discriminative stimuli
      1) Under what conditions do appropriate responses occur?
      2) Under what conditions do "inappropriate responses" occur?
      3) Under what conditions is it hoped that the response will occur?
   d. Control
      1) Can the nurse control the stimulus to the patient's response?
      2) Can the nurse control the reinforcers?
3. *Baseline*
   a. Select problem response(s) and stimulus condition(s)
      1) Define objectively. (When Don sees patients laughing together in the dayroom, he hits a patient.)
      2) Quantify response(s). (This happens about once an hour.)
   b. Empirically validate potential reinforcers
      1) Apply Premack principle. (Note how Don spends most of his time.)
      2) Manipulate reinforcers under consideration. (Reward Don with what he likes best.)

4. *Assessment*
   a. Are the empirical baseline data different from the "armchair" behavioral history information?
      1) Are there newly identified problems?
      2) Are the originally defined problems substantiated by the data?
   b. Can the problem be redefined and therefore eliminated?
   c. What type of learning problem is involved?
      1) Response too frequent?
      2) Response too infrequent?
      3) Response never occurs?
         a) Never did occur?
         b) Used to occur but does not currently?
      4) Response occurs but in inappropriate stimulus situations?
         a) Discrimination problem—response occurs when it should not occur?
         b) Generalization problem—response occurs only in some of the instances when it should occur?
5. *Intervention*
   a. What is the behavioral goal?
   b. What behavioral technique can be used to accomplish this goal?
   c. How can the technique be operationalized?
6. *Evaluation*
   a. Was the goal reached?
      1) Yes
         a) Plan for maintenance of the change.
         b) Is there another behavior that requires modification?
      2) No
         a) Is more time required?
         b) Is the plan in need of alteration? If so, return to assessment step and continue.

(Adapted from Loomis M, Horsley JA: Interpersonal Change: A Behavioral Approach to Nursing Practice. New York, McGraw-Hill, © 1974. Reproduced with permission.)

Bibliography

Agras WS: Behavior Modification: Principles and Clinical Applications. Boston, Little, Brown & Co, 1978

Atthowe JM Jr, Krasner L: Preliminary report on the application of contingent reinforcement procedures. Token economy on a 'chronic' psychiatric ward. J Abnorm Psychol 73:37, 1968

Ayllon T, Azrin N: Reinforcer sampling: A technique for increasing the behavior of mental patients. J Appl Behav Anal 1:13, 1968

Ayllon T, Azrin N: The Token Economy. New York, Appleton-Century-Crofts, 1968

Ayllon T, Michael J: The psychiatric nurse as a behavioral engineer. J Exp Anal Behav 2:323, 1959

Baer DM et al: The development of imitation by reinforcing behavioral similarity to a model. J Exp Anal Behav 10:405, 1967

Baer DM, Sherman JA: Reinforcement control of generalized imitation in young children. J Exp Child Psychol 1:37, 1964

Bandura A: Principles of Behavior Modification. New York, Holt, Rinehart & Winston, 1969

Birnhauer JS: Generalization of punishment effects—A case study. J Appl Behav Anal 1:201, 1968

Bostow DE, Barley JB: Modification of several disruptive and aggressive behaviors using brief time-out and reinforcement procedures. J Appl Behav Anal 2:31, 1969

Buehler RE et al: The reinforcement of behavior in institutional settings. Behav Res Ther 4:157, 1966

Burchard J, Barrera F: An analysis of timeout and response cost in a programmed environment. J Appl Behav Anal 5:271, 1972

Carigan ST: Self-motivation and self-control in operant conditioning. Perspect Psychiatr Care 12:36, 1974

Closurdo JS: Behavior modification and the nursing process. Perspect Psychiatr Care 13:25, 1975

Davis J: Treatment of a medical phobia including desensitization administered by a significant other. J Psychosoc Nurs 20:6, 1982

Ferster CB, Perrott MC: Behavior Principles. New York, Meredith Corporation, 1969

Fife BL: The use of operant conditioning to increase the frequency of a child's verbal responses of questions. J Psychiatr Nurs 15:31, 1977

Freitas L, Johnson L: Behavior modification approach in a partial day treatment center. J Psychiatr Nurs 13:14, 1975

Gelfand DN et al: Unprogrammed reinforcement of patients' behavior in a mental hospital. Behav Res Ther 5:201, 1967

Graziano AM (ed): Behavior Therapy with Children. New York, Aldine-Atherton, 1971

Haus B, Thompson S: The effect of nursing intervention on a program of behavior modification by parents in the home. J Psychiatr Nurs 14:9, 1976

Hauser MJ: Nurses and behavior modification: Resistance, ignorance, or both. J Psychiatr Nurs 16:17, 1978

Kelleher RT: Chaining and conditioned reinforcement. In Honig W (ed): Operant Behavior: Areas of Research and Application. New York, Appleton-Century-Crofts, 1966

Kelleher RT, Gollub LR: A review of positive conditioned reinforcement. J Exp Anal Behav 5:543, 1962

Loomis ME, Horsley JA: Interpersonal Change: A Behavioral Approach to Nursing Practice. New York, McGraw-Hill, 1974

Lovaas OI, Simmons JQ: Manipulation of self-destruction in three retarded children. J Appl Behav Anal 2:143, 1969

Matheson WE et al: Control of screaming behavior using aversive conditioning and time-out. J Psychiatr Nurs 14:27, 1976

Matheson WE et al: Control of food aversion using a reward model. J Psychiatr Nurs 14:35, 1976

McMorrow MJ, Epstein MH: The use of the premack principle to motivate patient activity attendance. Perspect Psychiatr Care 16:14, 1978

Nakanishi DA, Anderson DR: Behavioral treatment of psychogenic vomiting among children—A review and case example. J Psychosoc Nurs 20:17, 1982

Niemeier DF, Allison TS: Nurses can be effective behavior modifiers. J Psychiatr Nurs 14:18, 1976

Peterson KA, Errickson E: Use of reinforcement principles to reinstate self-care activities in a deaf and blind psychiatric patient. J Psychiatr Nurs 15:15, 1977

Pratt SJ, Fischer J: Behavior modification: Changing hyperactive behavior in a children's group. Perspect Psychiatr Care 13:37, 1975

Premack D: Toward empirical behavior laws: I. Positive Reinforcement. Psychol Rev 66:219, 1959

Provost J: Intervention in a schizoaffective depressive behavior pattern: A behavioral approach. Perspect Psychiatr Care 11:126, 1973

Redmond GT: A study of modification of socially acceptable eating behavior. Perspect Psychiatr Care 11:126, 1973

Reynolds GS: A Primer of Operant Conditioning. Glenview, IL, Scott, Foresman & Co, 1968

Rumpler CH, Seigerman C: A behavioral modification approach to dealing with violent behavior in an intensive care unit. Perspect Psychiatr Care 16:206, 1977

Sidman M: Tactics of Scientific Research. New York, Basic Books, 1960

Skinner BF: Science and Human Behavior. New York, Macmillan, 1953

Skinner BF: Cumulative Record. New York, Appleton-Century-Crofts, 1961

Staats AW, Staats CK: Complex Human Behavior. New York, Holt, Rinehart & Winston, 1963

Ullmann LP, Krasner L: Case Studies in Behavior Modification. New York, Holt, Rinehart & Winston, 1966

Whaley DL, Malott RW: Elementary Principles of Behavior. New York, Appleton-Century-Crofts, 1971

Wike, EL: Secondary Reinforcement. New York, Harper & Row, 1966

Wolpe J, Lazarus A: Behavior Therapy Techniques. New York, Pergamon Press, 1966

37

Assertiveness

Training

Kathleen McQuade

Description   Assertiveness training, a component of behavior therapy, is the process through which the client learns to communicate both positive and negative feelings in an open, honest, direct, and appropriate way.[4] Assertive actions result in a feeling of respect for oneself because integrity has been upheld by standing up for one's own rights without abusing the rights of others.[6] There are three elements involved in any assertive behavior: thinking rationally about a situation and the options, making a conscious choice of behavior based on one's goal(s), and then performing the action(s).

Acquiescent, Aggressive, and Assertive Behavior   It is important to be able to distinguish between acquiescent, aggressive, and assertive behavior so that one can make an informed choice about the appropriate action to take. Table 37–1 shows these differences and examples of each.

Setting Goals[2,4]   Some clients have difficulty acting assertively because they are unsure of their goals. It is important to know and clarify what one wants and whether it is feasible. Long-term and short-term goals give the client a sense of direction, and the attainment of goals increases feelings of self-esteem. Goal-directed behavior is more likely to continue if one begins with something that can be achieved within a relatively short time. Goals should be realistic, reflecting an awareness of both the client's real talents and limitations.

A client can more effectively set appropriate goals by answering the following questions:

1. What would the "ideal me" be like? Think or fantasize about this in detail, such as what one would do or say in various situations, how one would dress, etc.
2. What assets do I possess?
3. What behaviors would I like to change?
4. What activities do I like most?
5. What activities do I like least?

Table 37–1
ACQUIESCENT, AGGRESSIVE, AND ASSERTIVE BEHAVIOR

Behavior	Description	Example
Acquiescent	Does not stand up for rights; speaks placatingly; equivocates; avoids situations; performs unwanted tasks; feels and acts like a powerless victim	A client tries to avoid her supervisor, who wants someone to work a double shift. When the supervisor asks the client to do this, she says "yes" even though she does not want to work overtime.
Aggressive	Stands up for own rights but abuses those of others; speaks in an attacking and/or derogatory way; does not monitor words and/or actions; often feels powerless because of seeming inability to control own behavior	A client is asked by the supervisor to work a double shift. She replies: "Are you crazy? You have some nerve!"
Assertive	Stands up for own rights and respects those of others; speaks in a nonthreatening but firm way; chooses appropriate words and actions; feels power over *own* behavior	A client is asked by the supervisor to work a double shift. She says: "No. I am already tired from working one shift."

6. A goal I would like to achieve in 6 months is . . . . In order to do this, I need to . . . .

7. A goal I would like to achieve in one year is . . . . In order to do this, I need to . . . .

8. A goal I would like to achieve in 5 years is . . . . In order to do this, I need to . . . .

Inhibitors of Assertive Behavior

It is necessary to know what makes it difficult for the client to act assertively in order to be able to institute an effective plan for change. Typical inhibitors are skill deficits and anxiety.

One example of a skill deficit occurs when a client does not know what words to use when making a request. Sometimes clients know the words but are so anxious that they are unable to utter them.

Constructing an Assertive Plan for Change

Assertiveness training is based on the principle that clients act in certain ways because that is what they have learned. It follows, then, that they can learn new behaviors. It is not necessary to change one's feelings before altering one's actions. Self-respecting behaviors can cause an increase in an individual's actual feelings of self-respect. Chart 37–1 shows the steps in construction of a plan and theoretical rationale.

Positive Reinforcement[5]

One form of positive reinforcement occurs when pleasurable feelings, happenings or concrete rewards result from an assertive behavior. The reinforcement may come from the self or peers.

Self-reinforcement may come from

1. Commenting positively to one's self: "How great that I made an assertive response to that request!"
2. Rewarding oneself tangibly for acting assertively: Taking time for a hot bath or buying oneself a present.
3. Counting specific assertive responses: Keeping a record of responses.

Chart 37–1
AN ASSERTIVE PLAN FOR CHANGE AND THEORETICAL RATIONALE

Action	*Theoretical Rationale*
1. Target the behavior that one wishes to change. For example, a client finds it difficult to say "no" when he wants to and decides to work on saying "no."	1. Working on one behavior at a time makes it easier to set up and effect a focused, systematic plan for change and to achieve success, which reinforces assertive actions.
2. Set up a plan of action. For example, the client makes a list of approximately 20 situations in which he has difficulty saying "no." He rank orders them so that #1 is the least difficult situation and #20 is the most difficult. He then decides (based on his anxiety level) which practice method to begin with. The ways to practice the behavior, in order of increasing difficulty, are imagery, tape recorder feedback, role playing, and practice in the real-life situation.	2. Change is more likely to occur if one begins with situations in which there is a higher probability of success. The increased self-respect and self-esteem that result from successful performance reinforce the behavior and make it easier to progress through the hierarchy.
3. Institute the plan. One may begin with any of the practice modes, depending upon one's anxiety level. For example, the client begins with #1 to practice the guidelines for saying "no" (described later) and works his way through the hierarchy to #20. An individual should feel competent and reasonably comfortable performing the behavior by the time he has completed item #20 of the hierarchy in the real-life situation.	3. One becomes more assertive only through taking action.

Peer reinforcement may occur through

1. Talking at regular intervals with someone else who is working at being more assertive and who will be supportive.
2. Forming a group of colleagues or friends who meet once a week to share assertive experiences and support one another's assertiveness.
3. Attending workshops and seminars on assertiveness.

Behavioral Guidelines When the client has set up an assertive, goal-directed plan of action and decreased the effectiveness of inhibitors, there are behavioral guidelines to follow. It is a good idea to observe them strictly in the beginning phase of change, since they are designed to guard against common pitfalls. When the assertive behavior has become more spontaneous, the guidelines need not be adhered to as closely or, perhaps, at all. Chart 37–2 shows the desired behavior, guidelines for action, and theoretical rationale.

Chart 37–2
DESIRED BEHAVIOR, GUIDELINES FOR ACTION, AND THEORETICAL RATIONALE

Desired Behavior for Clients	*Guidelines for Clients*	*Theoretical Rationale*
Saying "no"[4]	1. Say "no" as the first word. 2. Follow this with a simple, declarative, explanatory sentence or two. For example, "No, I will not change my day off. I am looking forward to it."	The answer and the reason are clear without confusing the issue or apologizing for exercising the right to say "no." When the client begins to apologize, there is a regression to helpless or powerless feelings, which inhibit assertive behavior.
Making a request	1. If you want something, ask for it. 2. Use the pronouns "I" or "me" with a requesting verb such as want or give. You may follow this with the reasons why you think that the request should be granted. For example, "I would like the next holiday off, please. I have worked on the last two and believe it is my turn to be off."	One has the right to make a request. Since others cannot be expected to read minds, there is a greater probability that one will get what one wants by asking for it. Direct language conveys responsibility for wants, which, in turn, increases self-respect. Directness also makes it hard for others to ignore requests. The presentation of logical reasons may influence the person to grant the request, reinforcing assertive behavior.
Asking for a change in behavior[1]	1. Describe the behavior in descriptive terms. For example, "I have noticed that you often do not clean up and replace the equipment after you have completed a procedure." 2. Let the other person know the feelings that the behavior engenders. For example, "I feel resentful when you do this." 3. Request a specific behavioral change. For example, "I would like you to clean up after yourself." 4. a. Point out the positive consequences. For example, "When you clean up after yourself, it is a pleasure to work with you." b. If no indication is given that the behavior will change, or the behavior continues, point out the negative consequences. For example, "If you do not clean up after yourself, I will not do it and I will let others know who left the area in a mess."	1. One has the right to request a change. This lets the person know that it is one behavior or set of behaviors that is focused on rather than the total person. This increases the probability of a positive response. 2. One has the right to express one's feelings. People are often unaware of an individual's feelings unless told them. They will sometimes change because they do not wish to generate ill will. 3. This clarifies one's expectations, leading to a greater chance of change. 4. People are often willing to change because of positive consequences; some change because they do not wish to pay the price of the negative consequences. It is helpful for people to know that their behavior has consequences.

Chart 37–2
(continued)

Desired Behavior for Clients	Guidelines for Clients	Theoretical Rationale
Handling disrespectful, derogatory comments[4]	1. If you feel put down, plan a response. 2. Think before speaking. Don't say the first reply that comes to mind. 3. Do not use "I," "me," or "because" in the first sentence. 4. Say something that indicates that you do not accept being spoken to in a derogatory way. For example, "That was not necessary"; "What's with you?"	1. One has the right to respectful treatment. One decreases the chance of leaving the situation with negative feelings about oneself and the other person if one makes a response. 2. A fast response tends to be either passive or aggressive. It is important to *choose* a response. 3. Initial use of these can tend to make the response defensive. 4. Individuals increase self-respect if they deserve and expect to be treated with respect. An assertive response also gives people a chance to apologize or explain (they may not have meant to be hurtful).
Expressing anger[1*]	1. Use the pronoun "I" with a feeling verb and a behaviorally specific description about why you are angry. For example, "I am angry because you have been late all week and it delays the change of shift report." 2. If you do not get a positive response, tell the person what you specifically want. For example, "I would like you to be on time for report." 3. a. If you do not get a positive response, point out the positive consequences. For example, "When you arrive on time, I feel as if we are a smoothly functioning team." b. If there is still no positive response, point out the negative consequences. For example, "If you continue to arrive late, I will start report without you." 4. If there is no positive response at this point, call it to a halt. For example, "Well, there is no point in discussing this further at this time."	1. One has the right to express anger. One claims responsibility for and power over the anger by using "I." The person is less apt to be defensive than if one said: "You make me angry." A specific description criticizes one behavior or set of behaviors rather than the whole person and increases the probability of a positive response. 2. This clarifies expectations and again makes clear that one is not "attacking" the other person. 3. People are often willing to change because of positive consequences. Some change because they do not want to pay the price of the negative consequences. It is important for people to know that their behavior has consequences. 4. The assertive goal is to express honestly one's feelings and to exercise the right to ask for what one wants. It is important to remember that there is great value in an honest expression of feelings and that one will not always get what one wants. To engage in endless discussion is to risk a power struggle, which is self-defeating.
Handling negative responses to one's assertion	1. Remember that others also have the right to express themselves. 2. Do not become intimidated by another's displeasure. Remember that you can survive without continuous approval from others. 3. Remember that one does not *make* another unhappy or angry. Individuals are responsible for their own feelings and behaviors. 4. Remind yourself that a negative response does not necessarily mean that you are wrong. 5. Be direct with the other person. For example, "I know that you don't like it, but the answer is 'no.'"	1–4. Assertiveness means standing up for one's own rights while at the same time respecting the rights of others. One has the right to express anger, to say "no," and so forth, and others have the right to not like it. It is important to realize that others may not always like or agree with one. There are times when one must choose between having the approval of others or feeling respect for oneself. 5. This lets the person know that one respects both one's own rights and those of others.

(continued)

Chart 37–2
(continued)

Desired Behavior for Clients	Guidelines for Clients	Theoretical Rationale
	6. If you feel empathy, you may express it. For example, "I can appreciate your feelings, but my answer is still 'no.'"	6. One does not have to apologize for exercising her/his rights, but it is not usually necessary (or advantageous) to be arbitrary either.
	7. Use relaxation techniques if needed (see Chap. 35).	7. This decreases anxiety engendered by another's response.
Expressing feelings	1. Be specific. For example, "I like the way you summarized what that man said."	1. Specific comments are more meaningful and interesting than general ones.
	2. Use "I" followed by a verb that expresses feeling. For example, "I admire how you handled that distraught customer."	2. One claims responsibility for the feeling; this indicates to the listener that a feeling rather than a thought will be expressed.
	3. Be simple. For example, "I would like to be off the first week in June."	3. Long, qualifying sentences confuse and blur the expression of feeling for both the sender and the receiver.
	4. Be honest. For example, "I admire the way you stood up to Dr. Smith"; or "I am angry that you would speak to me so abusively."	4. One can become real and genuine to oneself and others only through honest acceptance and communication of feeling.
	5. Be appropriate. For example, "I feel sad (but not despairing) that your wife has been readmitted to the hospital."	5. One does not have to dramatize or exaggerate in order to fully express feeling. Some people can confuse feeling talk with emotional outbursts. (In general, the use of feeling talk promotes openness and closeness.)
Giving and receiving positive comments	1. To self: a. Make a list of twenty or more assets or strengths that you possess (e.g. compassion, ability to take risks, etc.). b. Make a positive comment about yourself to a partner. For example, "One thing that I like about myself is that I am dependable; if I say I'll do something, I get it done." c. Think self-affirming thoughts. For example, "I just made a very insightful interpretation of that person's behavior." d. Receive positive comments affirmatively. For example, "Thank you, that makes me feel very good!"; "You've made my day!"	1. Assertiveness includes the ability to appropriately express the range of human emotions. It is just as important and often as difficult to feel and to communicate genuine positive feelings as it is to experience and express negative ones. One maintains and increases feelings of self-esteem and self-respect by affirming oneself and by accepting the affirmation of others. By reinforcing the positive comments of others, one also increases the probability of their recurrence.
	2. To others: Communicate clearly that you like or appreciate something. For example, "I really value your contributions at case conferences."	2. The more honest feelings that one can express, the more alive and exciting one makes oneself and one's relationships.
Nonverbal assertive skills[5]	Look directly at the other person.	This helps one to maintain contact and shows interest in the other person. It also conveys self-confidence.
Facial expression	Assume a facial expression that is congruent with what is felt or said. For example, If you feel angry, rather than pleasant, assume an angry expression.	A congruent facial expression adds fullness and validity to what one says. A disparate facial expression belies and distracts from one's verbal content. For example, if one says something serious and smiles or laughs, the other person may not take the verbal message seriously.
Posture	Stand and walk in an erect, straight position.	This conveys confidence in oneself and communicates that one "stands up" for oneself.

Chart 37–2
(continued)

Desired Behavior for Clients	Guidelines for Clients	Theoretical Rationale
Gestures	Use movements that enhance and emphasize what is said. Avoid gestures that distract from the message, such as playing with your hair.	Gestures help to focus an individual's attention, and thus have the potential either to add or detract from the verbal message.
Physical distance	Stand at a distance that is comfortable for both you and the other person. People indicate that they are uncomfortable by moving backward or forward.	For both cultures and individuals, there is a physical distance that is comfortable and acceptable. One indicates sensitivity and interest by maintaining an appropriate physical distance.
Tone of voice	Use a firm, suitably loud tone of voice.	This connotes confidence and assurance. The tone of voice conveys whether a message is assertive, acquiescent, or aggressive.

*NOTE: It is not always appropriate to express anger directly. It may sometimes, for example, endanger an individual's job to directly express anger to the boss. One may choose not to take the risk but to express the anger indirectly by fantasy or talking with friends. The key element in all assertive behaviors is *choice*.

Important Considerations

1. When clients begin to work on becoming more assertive, there can be a tendency to behave aggressively. The nurse helps clients to note this and to monitor behavior appropriately. It is helpful to remember that others also have rights. For example, the client has the right to make a request; others have the right to refuse to grant it.

2. Rights have accompanying responsibilities. For example, the client has the right to make a mistake but is then responsible for the consequences.

3. When the client has doubts about whether or not to take an action, two questions can be most helpful in decision-making:[4] "Do I have the right to . . . ?" and "Will I respect myself more or less if I . . . ?"

4. Statements that begin with "I," as a general rule, are most assertive.

5. In many situations, it is advantageous to use a combination of assertive behaviors. This is illustrated in the section on expressing anger, where one may use an "I" statement, make a request, point out consequences, and set limits (calling it to a halt).

6. Negotiation skills are important. The client cannot always get exactly what is desired and may choose to "trade-off" with another. For example, one nurse may say to another: "I will work this Saturday for you if you will work next Saturday for me." The key point is that the clients choose freely what each will do.

7. Even when clients do not get what they want, self-respect is increased by making the effort.

8. Clients cannot change others but can change their own behaviors to achieve increased feelings of self-esteem and self-respect.

References

1. Bower SA, Bower CH: Asserting Yourself: Practical Guide for Practical Change. Reading, MA, Addison-Wesley, 1976
2. Clark CC: Assertive Skills for Nurses. Wakefield, MA, Contemporary Publishing, 1978
3. Ellis A, Harper R: A New Guide to Rational Living. Englewood Cliffs, NJ, Prentice-Hall, 1975
4. Fensterheim H, Baer J: Don't Say Yes When You Want to Say No. New York, Dell, 1975
5. Herman S: Becoming Assertive, A Guide for Nurses. New York, Van Nostrand Reinhold, 1978
6. McQuade K: Leadership styles, The calendar. NY Counties Registered Nurses Assoc 41:1, 1981

Bibliography

Cohen S, McQuade K: Programmed instruction. Assertiveness in nursing, Part I. Am J Nurs 83:417, 1983

Cohen S, McQuade K: Programmed instruction. Assertiveness in nursing, Part II. Am J Nurs 83:911, 1983

Cotter SB, Guerra JJ: Assertion Training. Champaign, IL, Research Press, 1976

Edmunds M: Non-clinical problems: Assertiveness skills. Nurs Pract 6:27, 1981

Eisler R et al: Components of assertive behavior. J Clin Psychol 29:295, 1973

Eisler R et al: Situational determinants of assertive behaviors. J Consult Clin Psychol 43:330, 1975

Gareri EA: Assertiveness training for alcoholics. J Psychiatr Nurs 17:31, 1974

Hauser MJ: Assertiveness techniques: Origins and uses. J Psychiatr Nurs 17:15, 1979

Hersen M et al: Development of assertive responses: Clinical measurement and research considerations. Behav Res Ther 11:505, 1973

Jakubowski P: Assertive behavior and clinical problems of women. In Carter D, Rawlings E (eds): Psychotherapy for Women: Treatment Towards Equality. Springfield, IL, Charles C Thomas, 1980

Jakubowski P, Lachs P: Assessment procedures in assertion training. Counsel Psychol 5:84, 1975

Jakubowski P, Spector P: An Introduction to Assertive Training Procedures for Women. Washington, DC, American Personnel Guidance Association, 1973

Lange A et al: Cognitive behavioral assertion training procedures. Consult Psychol 5:37, 1975

Lange A, Jakubowski P: Responsible Assertive Behavior: Cognitive/Behavioral Procedures for Trainers. Champaign, IL, Research Press, 1976

Numerof RE: Assertiveness training. Am J Nurs 80:1796, 1980

Rathus S: A thirty item schedule for assessing assertive behavior. Behav Ther 4:398, 1973

Rathus S: Principles and practices of assertive training: An eclectic overview. Counsel Psychol 5:4, 1975

Rimm DC et al: Group assertive training in the treatment of inappropriate anger expression. Psychol Rep 34:791, 1974

Wood D et al: The nurse as therapist: Assertion training to rehabilitate the chronic mental patient. J Psychiatr Nurs 13:41, 1975

38

Gerontological
Counseling

Joyce J. Fitzpatrick

Introduction A wide range of physical, social, emotional, and mental problems can occur among the aged. These problems are often related to the multiple losses that occur for the elderly, including, for example, loss of health and loss of significant others. Certain intervention techniques have been targeted for use with the elderly to meet the specialized needs of these individuals.

Psychodynamics of Aging Erikson[3] has described the last stage of psychological development as ego integrity versus despair. During the aging process, the individual is faced with the inevitability of death, the final loss. A number of other losses may occur during this period, for example, loss of family members and friends through death, and loss of physical and mental functioning. Those who are not satisfied with their life accomplishments often feel despair and may fear death or deny death. Those with ego integrity appear more other-directed, expressing concern for the future in a broad perspective, that is, in terms of family, culture, or world order.

The psychiatric nurse should be prepared to address issues of loss and grieving, understandings and fears of death, despair, and depression. The elderly have a range of resources available to them to cope successfully with the losses and challenges they experience. Psychiatric nursing interventions often are focused on helping the elderly person mobilize both internal and external resources.

Settings Settings in which the psychiatric nurse might work with aged clients include

A. **GENERAL HEALTH CARE FACILITIES**
   1. Acute care facilities (hospitals)
   2. Community mental health centers
   3. State and county mental hospitals
   4. Visiting nurses associations
   5. Veterans administration hospitals
   6. Alcohol treatment programs

B. **SPECIALIZED AGENCIES FOR THE ELDERLY**
   1. Nursing homes or health-related facilities
   2. Geriatric day-care centers
   3. Senior citizens programs

Assessment Chart 38–1 presents a comprehensive plan for holistic assessment of the aged, which includes demographic data, health–illness data, psychological health data, economic resource data, and cultural and social data. The nurse uses this guide while interviewing the client, taking care to use language that is familiar to the client.[9]

Life Review Therapy A. **DEFINITION**
   Life review therapy is a mental process through which past experiences are progressively returned to consciousness for review, assessment, and resolution. It is often initiated by the realization of approaching death.

B. **GOALS**
   The goals of life review therapy are to
   1. Review unresolved conflicts
   2. Increase hopefulness about the rest of life
   3. Increase flexibility in meeting current or future conflicts and frustrations

4. Enhance purpose in life by providing meaningful activity
5. Enhance personal integrity and life satisfaction through a review of past accomplishments and satisfactions
6. Provide opportunity to make amends and restore harmony with friends and relatives
7. Gain self-understanding

Chart 38–1
NURSING ASSESSMENT GUIDE FOR THE AGED

Demographic Data

Name, age, sex, marital status, address, telephone number, occupation, name(s) of primary health care provider(s)

Health-Illness Data

1. Belief—Define health; define illness
2. Own physical health status—Description of current, recent changes in
3. Compare own health status with that of others in age group
4. Health practices—Rest, activity, nutrition, drugs, immunizations, habits
5. Specific health problems (past and present)
   • Allergies—Food and drugs
   • Integumentary
   • Sensory—Touch, vision, hearing, smelling, tasting
   • Gastrointestinal—Dental health, ingestion, digestion, and elimination
   • Cardiopulmonary—Diseases, symptoms (shortness of breath, pain, cough), activity change (ordered by physician or self-imposed)
   • Breasts—Changes, practice of self-examination
   • Musculoskeletal—Pain, weakness, swelling, cramps, fractures, stiffness
   • Neurologic—Tremors, dizziness, depression
   • Genitourinary—Pain, frequency, difficulty starting stream, bleeding, incontinence

Psychological Health Data

1. Ego differentiation
   • Do you enjoy life now?
   • Does life seem to get better or worse for you?
   • How did you adjust to retirement?
   • What creative activities do you participate in?
2. Body transcendence
   • How do you feel when you notice that your body is getting older?
   • What do you do to cope with the aging process?
   • Does physical activity influence your self-concept? How?
3. Ego transcendence
   • How satisfied are you with your accomplishments in life?
   • How is your belief system a resource to you?
   • Have most of your goals been achieved in the past?

• What are some of your goals for the future?
• What do you see as your role in relation to younger people?
• How have you dealt with death of people you care about?
4. In general terms, how would you describe your personality?

Economic Resource Data

1. Income
   • Change in past 5 years
   • Adequacy to meet basic needs—food, shelter, clothing
   • Adequacy for desired goals—"splurge," trips, recreation, entertaining, donations
2. Resources shared by others with client
3. Housing
   • Quality—space, heat, security, etc.
   • Privacy
   • Client satisfaction with housing
   • Proximity to activities of choice
4. Neighborhood
   • Client satisfaction
   • Security
   • Is it a good place for older people?

Cultural and Social Data

1. Client perception of own status and respect within own social network
2. Who is in client's social network? family, neighbors, friends?
   • To whom would client go for affective or instrumental assistance?
   • Frequency of interaction with persons in network (daily, weekly, monthly—with number of persons)
3. Reciprocity of relationships
   • For whom is client an affective or instrumental resource?
   • Does client have at least one confidant?
4. Participation in groups/organizations, organized and casual
   • Frequency
   • Adequacy

(Adapted from Schrock MM: Holistic Assessment of the Healthy Aged. New York, John Wiley & Sons, 1980)

C. **PURPOSE OF NURSING INTERVENTION**
The nurse enhances the process by helping clients to review their lives consciously, deliberately, efficiently, thoughtfully, and emotionally. The therapist may work with individuals or groups.

D. **METHODS OF INTERVENTION**
The nurse
1. Encourages
    a. Written or taped autobiographies, diaries, journals
    b. Attending reunions
    c. Tracing genealogy
    d. Visiting hometown
    e. Visiting relatives
    f. Preserving/exploring ethnic identity
    g. Reading literature (*e.g.,* novels, poetry) evocative of the client's life or being (for example, the journals of May Sarton)[8]
2. Reviews and discusses scrapbooks and photographs with the client
3. Reviews work accomplishments
4. Enhances and encourages
    a. Creativity
    b. Sharing favorite foods
    c. Discussion of family traditions
    d. Intergenerational groups
    e. Groups with contemporaries
    f. Oral histories
    g. Visits to museums
5. Emphasizes the quality of the present life rather than quantity
6. Discusses fears, answers questions about death
7. Helps client deal with present conflicts, in light of past accomplishments
8. Listens actively and sensitively

Reminiscence A. **DEFINITION**
Reminiscence is the therapeutic process of sharing memories of past experiences and events (especially those considered personally significant), conscious recall of these experiences, and purposeful seeking of memories.

B. **GOALS**
The goals of reminiscence are to
1. Maintain a sense of familiarity about life and the world
2. Develop increasing understanding and integration of life experiences
3. Increase self-esteem
4. Enhance interpersonal relations
5. Improve cognitive activity
6. Exercise memory
7. Maintain a unique identity
8. Bridge the generation gap through memories of past events similar to current activities of young people
9. Entertain others

C. **PURPOSE OF NURSING INTERVENTION**
The nurse encourages and enhances the process by structuring the environment so as to facilitate the process either with individuals or groups.

D. **METHODS OF INTERVENTION**
   It is the same as for life review process.

Reality Orientation A. **DEFINITION**
   Reality orientation is a specific remotivation process that trains individuals to recall recent and remote memory (experiences, ideas, facts, and general information such as time and place).

B. **GOALS**
   The goals of reality orientation are to
   1. Evaluate contact with the environment
   2. Increase contact with the environment
   3. Improve social and cognitive functioning
   4. Increase self-esteem

C. **PURPOSE OF NURSING INTERVENTION**
   The nurse helps the client to reverse or halt confusion, disorientation, social withdrawal, and apathy in a group setting.

D. **METHODS OF INTERVENTION**
   The nurse
   1. Questions reality contact: "Can you tell us what day today is?"
   2. Rewards positive behavior: "Good! Your memory is improving."
   3. Focuses on behaviors: "Show us how you use your comb."
   4. Confirms what clients see and hear: "Yes, there is a lot of noise on the unit today."
   5. Does not give false reassurance
   6. Uses touch

Grief Work A. **DEFINITION**
   Grief work is an acute state of despair and anguish caused by the loss of a person or object.

B. **GOALS**
   The goals of grief work are to
   1. Express grief with a view toward resolution and acceptance
   2. Prevent social isolation and withdrawal
   3. Prevent physical illnesses
   4. Prevent depression and suicide

C. **PURPOSE OF NURSING INTERVENTION**
   The nurse assists the client to accept the loss, express feelings, and learn and grow from the experience. Usually the nurse intervenes with individuals, but may lead a group of clients who have suffered recent loss.

D. **METHODS OF INTERVENTION**
   1. Assist person in working through grief: "Tell me what you're feeling today."
   2. Accept ambivalence: "Sometimes we feel angry at people who die and leave us."
   3. Anticipate somatic complaints: "Do you sometimes feel like not even eating?"
   4. Prevent isolation and loneliness: "Why not join the others for lunch today?"
   5. Prevent self-destruction: "Please call me when you feel really down."

6. Involve peers: "Are you playing cards with the other women today?"
7. Increase morale and self-esteem: "You've been through a lot lately, and handled it fine. As time goes on, you'll feel better."

Touch   A. **DEFINITION**
Touch is the process of tactile human contact.

B. **GOALS**
The goals of touch are to
1. Decrease stress and anxiety
2. Increase communication
3. Enhance relationships

C. **PURPOSE OF NURSING INTERVENTION**
The nurse provides touch as a means of communication when words seem insufficient, or when the client seems to prefer touch to words. The nurse may hold the patient's hand, pat her arm, etc.

D. **USES OF TOUCH**
Touch is used to
1. Assist in ambulation
2. Assist with physical care
3. Communicate support
4. Decrease stress and anxiety
5. Increase reality orientation
6. Decrease pain experience

Activity Therapy   A. **DEFINITION**
Activity therapy is a method to increase the quality and quantity of physical movement and social interaction (extent to which the client relates to others in the environment and more generally the total environment).

B. **GOALS**
The goals of activity therapy are to
1. Avoid withdrawal
2. Maintain social contact
3. Enhance self-esteem
4. Increase morale
5. Maintain health
6. Develop body awareness

C. **PURPOSE OF NURSING INTERVENTION**
The nurse attempts to facilitate and enhance movement and interaction and to provide goal-directed activities. This is usually done with groups.

D. **METHODS OF INTERVENTION**
The nurse intervenes by
1. Acting as a role model
2. Using art forms such as dance, music
3. Promoting rhythmic movements
4. Using touch
5. Promoting the value of exercise

6. Encouraging verbalization and socialization
7. Introducing spontaneity
8. Teaching the need for physical safety

Movement Therapy   A. **DEFINITION**
Movement therapy is the use of body motion and language in a dynamic process to meet therapeutic goals.

B. **GOALS**
The goals of movement therapy are to
1. Increase body awareness
2. Increase relaxation
3. Increase stimulation
4. Increase attentiveness
5. Increase physical mobility
6. Increase flexibility
7. Increase socialization
8. Increase self-esteem
9. Decrease anxiety

C. **PURPOSE OF NURSING INTERVENTION**
The nurse provides a group situation with focus on movement as primary means for intervention.

D. **METHODS OF INTERVENTION**
The movement therapist
1. Initiates and directs the movement
2. Interprets the client's movement
3. Supports group process
4. Monitors physical and emotional states and paces activity
5. Offers alternative movements
6. Encourages creativity and spontaneity
7. Maintains rhythmic flow

E. **OTHER SIMILAR APPROACHES**
1. Dance therapy
2. Exercise programs

Evaluation   Goals for each individual or group are determined prior to initiation of any intervention. It is expected that outcomes of the intervention will be evaluated against the preintervention assessment. Success in the work with the elderly clients would be demonstrated by a heightened sense of self-worth, overall improvement in morale, and a sense of the contribution they could make to others based on their life experience.

Some studies of outcomes of nursing interventions with the elderly have been published.[1,2,4-7,10] Clearly, there is a need for more of these studies.

References

1. Dennis H: Remotivation therapy for the elderly: A surprising outcome. J Gerontol Nurs 2:28, 1976
2. Dominick JR: Nursing care factors in psychotic depressive reactions in elderly patients. Perspect Psychiatr Care 6:28, 1968
3. Erikson EH: Childhood and Society, 2nd ed. New York, WW Norton, 1963
4. Goldberg WG, Fitzpatrick JJ: Movement therapy with the aged. Nurs Res 29:339, 1980

5. Gray P, Stevenson JS: Changes in verbal interaction among members of resocialization groups. J Gerontol Nurs 6:86, 1980
6. Hogstel MO: Use of reality orientation with aged confused patients. Nurs Res 28:161, 1979
7. Langland RM, Panicucci CL: Effects of touch on communication with elderly, confused patients. J Gerontol Nurs 8:152, 1982
8. Sarton M: The House by the Sea. New York, WW Norton, 1977
9. Schrock MM: Holistic Assessment of the Healthy Aged. New York, John Wiley & Sons, 1980
10. Voekel D: A study of reality orientation and socialization of confused elderly. J Gerontol Nurs 4:13, 1978

Bibliography

Beaton SR: Reminiscence in old age. Nurs Forum 19:270, 1980

Birren JE, Sloane RB: Handbook of Mental Health and Aging. Englewood Cliffs, NJ, Prentice Hall, 1980

Brink TL: Is TLC contraindicated for geriatric patients? Perspect Psychiatr Care 15:129, 1977

Burnside IM: Psychosocial Nursing Care of the Aged. New York, McGraw-Hill, 1980

Butler RN, Lewis MI: Aging and Mental Health: Positive Psychosocial Approaches, 3rd ed. St Louis, CV Mosby, 1982

Chenitz C: Primary depression in older women: Are current theories and treatment of depression relevant to this age group? J Psychiatr Nurs 17:20, 1979

Copp LA: Care of the Aging. Edinburgh, Churchill Livingstone, 1981

Doona ME: The process of psychiatric nursing. In Travelbee J (ed): Intervention in Psychiatric Nursing, 2nd ed. Philadelphia, FE Davis, 1979

Ebersole P, Hess P: Toward Healthy Aging: Human Needs and Nursing Response. St Louis, CV Mosby, 1981

Epstein C: Learning to Care for the Aged. Englewood Cliffs, NJ, Prentice Hall, 1977

Freideman JS: Factors influencing sexual expression in aging persons: A review of the literature. J Psychiatr Nurs 16:34, 1978

Isaacs AD, Post F: Studies in Geriatric Psychiatry. New York, John Wiley & Sons, 1978

Jackson BS: The role of the psychiatric nurse specialist in caring for the institutionalized aged. J Psychiatr Nurs 17:20, 1979

King KS: Reminiscing therapy with aging people. J Psychosoc Nurs 20:21, 1982

McMordie WR, Blom S: Life review therapy: Psychotherapy for the elderly. Perspect Psychiatr Care 17:162, 1979

Mental Status Assessment: A Programmed Unit. Am J Nurs 81:1493, 1981

Murray R, Huelskoetter MM, O'Driscoll D: The Nursing Process in Later Maturity. Englewood Cliffs, NJ, Prentice Hall, 1980

Pfeiffer E: The psychosocial evaluation of the elderly patient. In Busse E, Blazer D (eds): Handbook of Geriatric Psychiatry. New York, Van Nostrand Reinhold, 1980

Sarton M: As We Are Now. New York, WW Norton, 1973

Velardo CC: Geriatric Psychosocial History Outline. J Am Geriatrics Soc 24:470, 1976

Weiner B et al: Working with the Aged: Practical Approaches in the Institution and Community. Englewood Cliffs, NJ, Prentice Hall, 1978

Wells TJ: Problems in Geriatric Nursing Care. Edinburgh, Churchill Livingston, 1980

Wolanin MO, Phillips LR: Confusion: Prevention and Care. St Louis, CV Mosby, 1981

39

Thanatological Counseling of Adults and Their Families

Thomas F. Nolan

Introduction The clinical nurse specialist is often called upon either formally or informally to help a family who has a member with a chronic, life-threatening illness such as cancer, or a family who has lost a member through sudden and unexpected death.

The family is defined as a set of people who are connected to each other by a relationship system formed by blood, marriage, adoption, or another strong bond. A person's family includes at least three generations, regardless of whether all members are alive, whether all relationships are legally intact, or whether members live in proximity to one another.

Often, nurses first come in contact with the family members of someone who is dying only after they have already formed a relationship with the dying person. Nevertheless, it is important for nurses to focus on the entire family because all members of the family participate in the process of losing a member through death. Treating the family as a client is in contrast to the traditional primary focus on the dying member, with only secondary concern for family members. If families are understood to be systems of interacting members, the peaceful dying of one member is contingent upon the successful resolution of the loss of that member by other family members, and vice versa.

The Family with a Dying Member When a family member is dying, there is a shift in the roles of all the family members resulting in system imbalance and widespread anxiety. Helping the whole family to use this anxiety to complete necessary tasks is the central challenge facing families with a member who is dying. Each family member, including the dying one, has specific tasks to accomplish, some in relation to self and some in relation to each other, as the entire system changes in response to losing a member. Role tasks must be divided up, reassigned, and accepted before the family can move through the painful transition to a new stage of development. These tasks may include functions such as breadwinning, parenting, caretaking, protecting, and listening. The family as a whole also must complete the critical tasks of bereavement step by step as it moves through the "before death" phase to the "terminal" phase to the "after death" phase.

"Before Death" Phase **Stages of normal grief.** Just as the dying person's family members influence the person's response to the illness and the dying process, so also does the dying person influence the family's responses to the impending loss. All persons, whether dying themselves or losing a family member through death, go through a series of well-identified stages of grieving, that is, denial, anger, bargaining, depression, and acceptance.[3] In fact, it is important for each of the family members to go through all the steps of grieving, whether or not in sequence, in order to resolve the loss and advance to the next phase of development in the life cycle. Table 39–1 shows the stages of normal grief and clinical examples.

The nurse's role with the dying person. Chart 39–1 shows the role of the nurse in helping the dying person move through the stages of normal grief.[1]

The nurse's role with the family of a dying person. During the time they have to prepare for the loss of a member, family members can be helped to identify whatever issues of "unfinished business" each may have to resolve with the dying person before death occurs. For example, a son may want to say, "I love you" to his dying father, or a dying daughter might have to ask forgiveness of her mother for some years' old transgression about which she still feels guilty. It is much easier for everyone in the family if such mutual reconciliations can occur before the death takes place. There is power in the absolution one family member can give another, especially at the time of death. The goal is for each member of the family to be able to feel at the

Table 39–1
STAGES OF NORMAL GRIEF AND EXAMPLES

Stages	Description	Clinical Examples
Denial	The unconscious avoidance of being aware of the seriousness of impending death, or of death having occurred	Two days after her mother's death, Marge was back in the store with a cheery "business as usual" look.
Anger	Open or subtle hostility, manifested in affect, speech, and behavior	35-year-old John, who was dying of complications associated with his juvenile onset diabetes, threw his insulin syringe on the floor and screamed that it wasn't fair that he should be dying.
Bargaining	Engaging in behavior designed to change the reality of the illness or death	Peg promised herself that she would attend church weekly if only her mother would live to see Peg's baby born.
Depression	Feelings of sadness and, sometimes, despair	After hearing of the diagnosis of his son, who had cancer, Mr. Jones was unable to accomplish much at work and said that he just didn't have energy or interest in anything anymore.
Acceptance	Resolution of feelings about death	Mrs. Henry, though dying with cancer, had finally come to terms with her illness and told her family that she didn't need to live forever and that she would like to spend the time left with them at home.

time of death that nothing more must be said or done. A nurse can be helpful to the family either by calling the family together for a formal session to discuss how things are going for them, or by informally talking to family members when they are visiting.

Chart 39–2 shows nursing actions and the rationale when working with a family about to lose a member.

Fears of the dying person.[6] Dying persons experience special fears, which the nurse can help to allay:

A. **FEAR OF PAIN**[6]

Most dying persons fear pain and assume that death is painful. Although there is little if any pain as one passes from life to death, there are realistic fears about pain associated with the disease process and its treatment. The nurse can assure dying people that they will be kept as comfortable as possible and that supportive people will be nearby.

B. **FEAR OF LONELINESS**[6]

An even greater fear than that of pain is the dread of loneliness. The nurse must be especially sensitive to the pleas of dying persons who do not want to be left alone. The nurse can encourage family members and friends to be physically present to a dying loved one by reassuring them that their mere presence brings comfort and that they need not be talking to the client to be helpful.

(Text continues on page 372)

Chart 39–1

THE NURSE'S ROLE WITH THE DYING PERSON[1]

Major goal—To facilitate the dying person's living as fully as possible by helping the person maintain dignity and self-respect as a human being.

Nursing Intervention	Rationale
1. Develop self-awareness.	What nurses find in themselves can make their interaction with the dying person more effective and satisfying. For example, the nurse who recognizes the tendency to keep at a distance from the dying person can make a conscious effort to change that behavior in order to be more effective in providing care for the dying.
2. Think about your own death.	Despite the difficulty healthy people have in thinking about their own deaths, it is important for nurses to come to terms with their feelings about their own death. If nurses run from their own feelings about death, they will run in fear from the dying and their feelings.
3. Assess how you feel about the person who is dying.	Honestly facing one's feelings is useful for both the nurse and the client. If, for example, nurses are fearful about being with the dying, or feel inadequate or insecure, these feelings will become apparent to the dying observer despite efforts to hide them.
4. Distinguish between the client's need for denial and your own need to deny.	By accepting the client's denial and maintaining a reality reference for themselves, nurses can provide experiences to help relieve feelings of panic and reduce feelings of stress. However, if nurses have a personal need to deny the reality of dying, it may be more difficult for the dying person to give up the denial and move to a more realistic stance.
5. Support the client in dealing with the denial of family and friends.	If clients are unable to talk to family and friends about what is uppermost in their minds, they will be forced to pretend interest in other matters or keep silent. Nurses can let clients practice with them what might be said to family members. Or a nurse might act as a temporary liaison to the family by carrying the message to them that the client realizes the fact of dying and that their continual denial only serves to keep the client isolated from them.
6. Respond to the denial.	For example, if the client says, "I can't believe it! It's not possible!" the nurse might respond with "I suppose it does feel a bit unreal." In this way the nurse neither reinforces nor rejects the client's denial, but implies acceptance of the need for it. This is a better response than to say, "I'm sorry, but it's true. There's no doubt about it. As the doctor said, you have cancer." If nurses insist that clients believe before they are ready, chances are they will either close themselves off to further communication by withdrawing or take a firm stand in rejecting the validity of the information.
7. Encourage clients to freely express feelings without fear of censure.	Anger is not a socially approved feeling. Thus, the nurse who says to a man, "How happy you must be to have a family who rally around you when you need them!" may merely force the client to keep quiet about how *un*happy that "rallying around" is making him. Conversely, the nurse who says, "Mary, you seem to be uncomfortable when your mother comes to visit," and then just waits, may encourage the client to express feelings without fear of censure.

Chart 39–1
(continued)

Nursing Intervention	Rationale
8. Give clear messages that you are ready to listen to whatever the client wants to say without making any kind of judgment.	For example, if the nurse says to a middle-aged female married client, "Wouldn't you like me to help you get out of that hospital gown and put on your pretty nightgown?" The nurse is offering help, but may also be saying, "I think it's only natural that you should want to look attractive for your husband." If the client feels differently, the nurse may be adding to her fears that she is "unnatural" and to her feelings of guilt.
9. Learn to accept the anger of clients by looking behind it, without reacting personally or defensively.	Sometimes anger is a function of the panic clients feel when they believe no one will respond quickly enough should they need someone desperately. At other times, clients may be angry at the moment and furious at the knowledge that they are dying, while still being frightened underneath. It is important for nurses to look behind the client's anger even though it may appear to be directed at them.
10. Find resources within yourself for appreciating the unfulfilled wishes and yearnings of others.	There are no set answers for helping clients who are bargaining for a little more life or a little less pain. A sensitive, accepting nurse may be of direct assistance in providing an individual with the time and opportunity to make amends for past failures or grievances.
11. Identify the stages of grieving as part of the dying process.	Grieving is a stage of the dying process. As people die, they grieve for the ultimate loss, the loss of themselves. Although the family of the client is generally thought of as grieving, the dying person certainly also has a basis for grief.
12. Allow people their right to grieve the loss of themselves.	Many people associate the grieving behavior of a dying person with self-pity. People have the right to cry for themselves when faced with the loss of everything known and loved. Not only is this a right, it is reasonable behavior. If a person keeps grief hidden, it is important to conjecture about the reason for hiding the grief. It may be that the person pretends not to grieve to present to others an image of an "acceptable" person.
13. Assist family members to identify stages of dying as experienced or expressed by their dying member.	Family members may be shocked to see their loved one accepting death without fear, and they may need reassurance by identifying this as a stage of dying. They may also need an opportunity to explore more fully their feelings about the client's acceptance of death, especially if they are unable to accept it yet and if they experiece it as rejection of them.
14. Try to determine the needs of the client.	If nurses completely identify with a client, they may be less likely to test the accuracy of their perceptions about the client's needs. Because both the nurse and the client have a separate self, it is important that the nurse very carefully ascertain what the client needs.
15. Recognize unverbalized needs of the client.	People who are aware of their own death may have needs and wants that they cannot put into words. They may be so overwhelmed by the knowledge of their dying that their feelings are confused. The nurse can help them sort through their feelings in order to express their wants.
16. Learn to read the client's cues.	The nurse must become sensitive to the cues clients give about their needs. When a young woman says, "Come tomorrow," instead of "Don't bother me," she may be implying *(continued)*

Chart 39–1
(continued)

Nursing Intervention	Rationale
	that tomorrow she may need help, that she will no longer be able to maintain her denial of death. When a wife says, "How terrible I am; I wish my husband wouldn't visit me so often," she may be asking for help in making a decision about whether or not to discuss her feelings honestly with her husband.
17. Clarify communication.	For example, to discover the real meaning of the angry behavior a nurse may be witnessing, the nurse first identifies the behavior and then feeds back to the client a brief description of the behavior observed: "You seem so angry." Then the nurse waits for the client to respond. The nurse has recognized the client's anger without judging it or the client. The client is free to continue the tirade, give some further explanation of feelings, or say nothing at all. It is important for the nurse to listen, to understand, and to care.
18. Help clients discover their own answers.	What works for one person does not necessarily work for another person who brings to the situation different experiences, feelings, and perceptions. It is important for the nurse to help people explore their problems, try out alternative solutions, and find the solution that best suits the individual person, rather than to offer solutions based on the nurse's own background and experience.
19. Provide opportunities for clients to change their level of awareness about dying.	It is part of the nurse's responsibility to assess how aware clients are of impending death. Then the nurse can provide a window through which the client may see an alternative to the present behavior. However, the choice of whether or not to change is left to each client. For the nurse to try to force awareness or push clients to behave differently is an unwarranted interference with their freedom, no matter how well intentioned the interference may be.
20. Recognize that nurses who care for the dying need help too.	Just as family and friends of the client suffer from loss and the feelings surrounding loss, so also does the nurse experience bereavement. It is important in order for the nurse to be effective and to avoid professional burnout to be able to share feelings of bereavement and resolve them with professional colleagues.

Chart 39–2
THE NURSE'S ROLE WITH THE FAMILY

Nursing Intervention	Rationale
1. Assess the degree of potential disruption the death will have on the family.	Any death of a family member leads to disruption in the balance of family energy. The significant factors affecting the degree of disruption are 1) the timing of the death or serious illness in the life cycle; 2) the nature of the death or serious illness; 3) the openness of the family system; and 4) the family position of the seriously ill, dying, or dead family member.[2]
a. The timing of death and serious illness in the life cycle	Understanding the life cycle tasks and issues for the family is crucial to understanding the effect of death on that family.

Chart 39–2
(continued)

Nursing Intervention	Rationale
	These tasks vary, depending on whether the dying person is an elderly grandparent, a middle-aged parent, a newly married young adult, an adolescent, or a child.[2]
b. The nature of death	Death can be expected or unexpected and may or may not involve long periods of caretaking. Each type of death has implications for the family's reaction and adjustment.[2]
c. The openness of the family system	Many reactions and long-term adjustment difficulties arising from death originate in the lack of openness in the system. Openness is the ability of family members to remain calm despite the emotional intensity in the system and to communicate their thoughts and feelings to others without expecting others to act on them.[2]
d. The family position of the dying or dead family member	Not all deaths have equal importance in the family system. In general, the more emotionally significant the dying or dead family member is to the family, the more likely it is that the death will be followed by an emotional shock wave or ripple effect up and down the generations.[2]
2. Use open and factual terminology and information.	It is important for nurses to avoid using expressions such as "deceased," "passed away," or "passed on." Using direct words such as "death" and "dying" suggests to the family that the nurse is able to be open and relatively comfortable with such a discussion. It is important for the nurse to be a model by presenting information in a factual way to the family and by letting them make decisions about the use of this information. In this way, the nurse encourages the family and the dying person to take maximum responsibility for life decisions.[2]
3. Facilitate the establishment of at least one open relationship within the family system.	Since the discussion of death often provokes much tension in family members, it is not uncommon that as the tension increases between any two of the family members around the death issue, the most uncomfortable individual will draw in a third to relieve the tension.[2] The nurse, when recognizing this triangle, can help at least one of the three to separate from the other two and face the issue openly. One way is to identify the most uncomfortable person, who may be the most motivated to make a change in role in the process. By coaching these people to control their emotions enough and to plan a method to broach the death issue, the nurse is often successful in opening the family system to deal with death.[2]
4. Respect the hope for life and living.	No one knows exactly when someone will die, except perhaps the dying person, who often senses the time of death. Often clients outlast the predicted survival time; often they live a shorter time. Since families are constantly living on an emotional seesaw of uncertainty, it is very difficult for them to deal continuously with death. Some people will not deal with certain death-related issues during a remission from the effects of serious illness, but they can deal with these same issues during exacerbations. Each family develops a timing and style of accomplishing its work. Although the nurse may want the family to deal with the death issues at all times, it is necessary to develop a respect for the family's timing and need for hope.[2]

(continued)

Chart 39–2
(continued)

Nursing Intervention	Rationale
5. Remain calm or unreactive.	Families who are dealing with anticipated or actual death are not only coping with the normal life cycle stresses but also have the additional stress of living with dying. A nurse who is unable to remain calm with the family increases the family stress even further. Certainly the nurse may experience emotions, but actions should not be guided by emotions. The nurse for whom death is a toxic issue will often be reactive and will instinctively cut off discussion, collude with the family in not discussing the issue or, conversely, insist that the family deal with the death. Or nurses may even present the family with their own tears or upset emotions to deal with. Nurses who begin behaving in one of these ways need to examine why.[2]
6. Evaluate the progress of relationships and issues.	Since the stress level is so high in families with a dying member, it is not unusual for the nurse to see symptoms developing in some part of the system because tension is not being dealt with in another area. For example, the diabetic son of a woman with terminal cancer may experience an imbalance in his blood sugar for no apparent physiologic reason. Such a symptom is not to be ignored, since it is an indication of stress. However, it is important not to get lost in such a symptom, but rather to check on the family's progress in dealing with the major stress in the relationships. These symptoms are signals that the stress should be discussed.[2]
7. Use family rituals, customs, and styles.	All families have personal or religious rituals or customs for dealing with death. In obtaining a family history, it is useful for the nurse to ask how deaths have been handled in the extended families. Not only does one gain a picture of the rituals, but the nurse also gains information about the way families deal emotionally with death, whether it be angry fights over money, depression, or physical illness. Another area to be explored eventually with families is the dying person's plan for the death, funeral, and burial. That is, where does the person want to die, who does the person want to be present, where will burial take place, and what will the funeral be like? It is important for the nurse not to take a position on the "right" way or "best" way, since what is right or best is what the family members want and agree to.[2]

(Adapted from Herz F: The impact of death and serious illness on the family life cycle. In Carter E, McGoldrick M (eds): The Family Life Cycle: A Framework for Family Therapy. New York, Gardner Press, 1980, pp 223–240)

C. **FEAR OF MEANINGLESSNESS**[6]

Dying people need to believe that their lives have been meaningful and that they are leaving behind a part of themselves. The nurse helps the client and the family to recognize this and to talk about the meaning of the client's life.

"During Death" Phase It is helpful in eventual resolution of the grieving process for family members to take an active role in the final phase of a member's life, *to the extent that the dying person is agreeable*. Some clients prefer to die in a more private way, and this must be respected.[5] When the client wants involvement, the following ways may be provided:

1. Members, regardless of age, are allowed to be physically present to the dying person.
2. Opportunities are provided for members to assist with the care of the dying person, such as bathing, positioning, applying lotion, and so forth. It is at times comforting to family members to be able to touch and talk to the dying person. The senses of touch and of hearing are the two final senses lost while a person is dying. By encouraging family members to assist with these nursing actions of comfort, people are given an opportunity to touch or communicate in a purposeful way that might otherwise be awkward or frightening for them.
3. Each family member is given an opportunity for time alone with the dying person and encouraged to say any final messages. Nurses can be particularly useful to the family by keeping a sensitive, respectful distance from them, though not abandoning them, as they go through these final tasks together.
4. When imminent signs of death appear, all family members are encouraged to gather around the dying person's bed. Individuals may wish to whisper a final farewell in the dying person's ear, offer a kiss, or hold the person's hand. Someone may choose to sit on the bedside and hold the person. Sometimes families like to say aloud together a formal prayer that may possibly be heard by the dying person as the final breaths are taken. Once death has occurred, family members may want to spend some time alone in the room with the body before the nurses begin postmortem care.

"After Death" Phase   With the actual death of a family member, families move into another phase of the separation process. Regardless of how much time the family may have had to prepare for the death ahead of time, the fact of death brings with it a kind of finality that anticipation of the death can never achieve.

During the few days immediately following death, family members direct much of their energy to the tasks of the death announcement and the funeral ritual. Preparation in advance reduces some of the stress of this period. At the time of the burial ritual, families face a number of challenges:
1. Being in close proximity with family members and friends who may not be seen frequently under other circumstances
2. Coming into contact with family members who have become emotionally cut off or the family "black sheep," with whom old unresolved conflicts now surface
3. Presenting a "stiff upper lip" under scrutiny of the public eye
4. Doing what is perceived to be socially approved or acceptable

Families usually manage to make it through the funeral experience with the support of many people, including other family members, friends, neighbors, funeral directors, and clergy. It is only after the funeral celebrations are completed and out of towners have returned to their homes that the immediately bereaving family members begin to acutely experience their new loss. One of the painful tasks confronting them is to dispose of the dead member's clothes and belongings. Suddenly, those who were most responsible for taking care of and visiting the dying person in the weeks or months before the death now have much empty time on their hands.

Nurses' Feelings about Working with the Dying[4]   A. **ISSUES THAT BOTHER THE NURSE MOST WHEN WORKING WITH THE DYING[4]**
1. Anger and guilt toward clients because of their hopeless circumstances
2. Anxiety over seeing clients lose control of their lives
3. Lack of skills and power, created by not knowing how to be helpful, leading to feelings of frustration and confusion

4. Overidentification with and overinvolvement in the struggles of clients and families with life and death
5. Depression and sadness over pains and struggles of clients and families
6. Avoidance of clients and families so as not to be depressed or sad
7. Confusion over role expectations stemming from expectations for the nurse from clients and families, self, and the profession

B. **FEELINGS NURSES HAVE ABOUT THEIR OWN DEATH**[4]
1. Fear of pain
2. Fear of losing control
3. Regrets about leaving people behind in death

C. **ISSUES THAT INHIBIT NURSES FROM DISCUSSING EMOTIONAL CONCERNS WITH DYING CLIENTS AND THEIR FAMILIES**[4]
1. The withholding of information by physicians or family members
2. Wishing to be superhuman, or the inability to reach every client in one's care
3. Isolation because of lack of support and understanding from other health professionals, leading to feelings of failure

D. **WAYS NURSES COPE WITH THEIR OWN FEELINGS**[4]
1. Physical care is believed to be more essential than meeting emotional needs.
2. Humor is expressed, allowing the safe expression of feelings and opening up channels of communication.
3. Outside activities are sought so that the nurse's life does not revolve solely around care of the dying.
4. There is awareness and acceptance of one's own feelings, of the client's feelings and of one's relationship with the client and family.
5. Limitations are faced insofar as nurses are aware of their inability to meet all the needs of their clients at all times.
6. Some of the issues surrounding death are denied.
7. Thoughts, feelings, and concerns are shared with other nurses and health practitioners.

Evaluation   The nurse who works with dying clients and their families considers the following signs of success in the work:
1. The dying person and family members move through the normal stages of grief to acceptance.
2. The person dies with dignity and self-respect.
3. The family experiences the normal feelings of loss after the death and operates at the same or a higher level afterwards.

References

1. Epstein C: Nursing the Dying Patient. Reston, VA, Reston Publishing Co, 1975
2. Herz F: The impact of death and serious illness on the family life cycle. In Carter EA, McGoldrick M (eds): The Family Life Cycle: A Framework for Family Therapy. New York, Gardner Press, 1980
3. Kübler-Ross E: On Death and Dying. New York, Macmillan, 1969
4. Mandel HR: Nurses' feelings about working with the dying. Am J Nurs 81:1194, 1981
5. Sarton M: A Reckoning. New York, Norton Paperbacks, 1981
6. Williams JC: Allaying common fears. In Nursing Skillbook, Dealing with death and dying. Jenkintown, PA, Intermed Communications, 1977

Bibliography

Ames B: Art and a dying patient. Am J Nurs 80:1094, 1980

Barstow J: Stress levels of hospice nurses. Nurs Outlook 28:751, 1980

Beauchamp T, Perlin S: Ethical Issues in Death and Dying. Englewood Cliffs, NJ, Prentice-Hall, 1978

Bowen M: Family reaction to death. In Guerin PJ Jr (ed): Family Therapy: Theory and Practice. New York, Garden Press, 1976

Caughill RE: The Dying Patient: A Supportive Approach. Boston, Little, Brown & Co, 1976

DuBois PM: The Hospice Way of Death. New York, Human Services Press, 1980

Goldstein V, Regnery G, Wellin E: Caretakers and the role of fatigue. Nurs Outlook 29:24, 1981

Murphey JC: Communicating with the dying patient. Am J Nurs 79:1084, 1979

Nolan TF: The dying process. In Haber J et al (eds): Comprehensive Psychiatric Nursing, 2nd ed. New York, McGraw-Hill, 1982

Nursing Skillbook, Dealing with Death and Dying. Jenkintown, PA, Intermed Communications, 1977

Speer GM: Learning about death. Perspect Psychiatr Care 12:70, 1974

Winder AE, Elam JR: Therapist for the cancer patient's family: A new role for the nurse. J Psychiatr Nurs 16:22, 1978

40

Thanatological Counseling of Children and Their Families

Karen Davis Frank

Introduction	The nurse is often called upon to help the dying child and family in a variety of community settings as well as in the acute-care hospital. The nurse intervenes at all three levels of prevention: primary, secondary, and tertiary.
Levels of Prevention[6]	The levels of prevention and goals are as follows:

A. **PRIMARY PREVENTION**
The goal of primary prevention is to reduce the incidence (new cases) of mental illness in the populations at risk by finding families with dying children and intervening early.

B. **SECONDARY PREVENTION**
The goal of secondary prevention is to reduce the prevalence (new and old cases) of mental illness through early case finding and effective treatment in the populations at risk by treating families with dying children who are having problems.

C. **TERTIARY PREVENTION**
The goal of tertiary prevention is to reduce the disability associated with the mental illness through rehabilitation by treating families who are recovering from the death of a child.

Primary Prevention

Populations at Risk	The following are high-risk situations for the child and family. In these situations, neither the child nor the parents and siblings demonstrate symptomatology of mental illness. They are identified as part of a vulnerable population, however, and may profit from limited, supportive care.

1. The family coping with a miscarriage
2. The family coping with a neonatal death
3. The family coping with a seriously ill child or with the death of a child
4. The family coping with a seriously ill adult or with the death of an adult
5. The child coping with a seriously ill parent or with the death of a parent
6. The child coping with a seriously ill sibling or with the death of a sibling
7. The child coping with a seriously ill friend or with the death of a friend
8. The child coping with his or her own serious illness or possible death
9. The adolescent who is a passenger when there is an auto accident fatality
10. The adolescent who is a driver when there is an auto accident fatality
11. The child and family coping with suicide or suicide attempts
12. The child and family coping with multiple losses of loved ones

The Nurse's Role	Nurses can intervene in the community to prevent mental illness resulting from the death and dying of a child. They explore resources available:

1. From the speakers' bureau for the local mental health association
2. From the consultation and education department at the local community mental health center
3. At local schools by contacting the school health nurse and the child study team
4. At employment sites by contacting the local occupational health nurse at each company
5. In health care settings by contacting the local community nursing service and the directors of nursing at local hospitals, hospices, and clinics
6. From self-help support groups

7. From local social agencies, religious institutions, police departments, or correctional facilities

Once nurses have assessed the community for the availability of these programs they
1. Develop new programs
2. Participate in existing programs
3. Refer children and their families to these programs

Secondary Prevention

Assessment The nurse determines the seriously ill or dying child's need for services by assessing as follows:
1. What is the child's perception of his or her health status? Is this perception age appropriate? Has the child voiced fears of pain or fears of being separated from the parents? How have these fears been addressed? (See Table 40–1.)
2. What is the family's perception of the child's health status? What is the family's perception of the child's understanding of the situation? What is the family's belief system concerning death and dying?
3. What support systems are available to the child, including nuclear family, extended family, school friends, religious groups, or community services?
4. If the child is in the acute-care setting of a hospital, what are the feelings of the care-givers involved? How does the child get along with hospital roommates? What is their understanding of the child's health status?
5. If the child is at home, what are the feelings of the community nurses and volunteers involved in the child's care? How does the family feel about the sick child at home? How do the the child and family relate to the local hospice workers?

Feelings of the Dying Child's Siblings Each sibling living at home with the dying child will probably experience disturbing feelings. Since these feelings are considered negative or unacceptable by Western culture, the child may not even be aware that he or she is trying to defend against them. They are:
1. Happiness at the prospect of being rid of the sibling
2. Guilt stemming from death wishes toward the sick brother or sister[3]
3. Fear of also becoming ill[3]
4. Jealousy at the attention paid to the sibling[3]

Table 40–1
CHILDREN'S PERCEPTIONS OF DEATH AND DYING

Age	Perception
3–5 years	Death is reversible, not final.
5–9 years	Death is final, but not everyone dies. Death is personified, rather than viewed as an abstract concept. (For example, death is "old people.")
9–11 years	Death is final. Everyone dies.
11 and older	Fantasies of rebirth, reunion, and reincarnation develop.
All ages	The underlying fear is of separation and pain, rather than fear of death itself.

---

5. Rage at the leniency with which the sick child is treated at home during remissions[3]

Defenses of the Dying Child's Siblings

The following defense mechanisms can be expected to develop in the grieving child, although the child's behavior may not always reflect negative feelings.[2]
1. Denial—"It's just a dream. Danny will come back."
2. Bodily distress—"I have a tightness in my throat . . ."
3. Hostile reactions to the deceased—"How could Danny do this to me?"
4. Guilt—"He got sick because I was naughty. I killed him . . ."
5. Hostile reactions to others—"It's the doctor's fault. He didn't treat him right. It's God's fault . . ."
6. Replacement—"Uncle John, do you love me, really love me?"
7. Assumption of the mannerisms of the deceased—"Do I look like Danny?"
8. Idealization—"How dare you say anything against Danny! He was perfect . . ."
9. Anxiety—"I feel like Danny when he died. I have a pain in my chest."

Changes in the Parents

Behavior changes in the adult family members may provoke the further development of negative feelings in the siblings[2]:
1. Parents may become angry more often than before.
2. Parents may leave siblings in the care of surrogates more often. For children under 3 years, these separations can be particularly difficult.
3. Siblings with preexisting emotional problems may have trouble mastering normal developmental tasks in the face of increased stress.
4. Siblings may develop psychosomatic problems, school difficulties, and interpersonal problems with friends.
5. Parents may develop overindulgent or overprotective attitudes toward the surviving siblings.

The Parents' Feelings

Parents of dying children experience anxiety, depression, guilt, hostility, worry, and negative self-image. These occur in the following areas[5]:

A. **VOCATIONAL ENVIRONMENT**
The child's illness affects such things as how parents evaluate their present job performance, time lost on the job, changes in their vocational investment and the goals they have set for themselves, and interpersonal conflicts that they have been experiencing within their work situation.

B. **DOMESTIC ENVIRONMENT**
The child's illness affects the quality of the relationship with others living in the home, communication patterns and styles, changes in the dependency relationship that they have with others outside the family, potential physical disability, and the family's financial resources.

The Nurse as Counselor—Nursing Interventions

The nurse in both inpatient and outpatient settings has opportunities to develop ongoing relationships with dying children and their families. Nursing interventions are outlined below*:

---

*The following section (A–H) is adapted from Frank K: Dying children. In Haber J et al (eds): Comprehensive Psychiatric Nursing. New York, McGraw-Hill, © 1982

A. **BE SURE THE CHILD HAS A PRIMARY NURSE**
The primary nurse should be able to develop a close relationship during periods of hospitalization. Establish lines of communication with other nurses who serve the child when the child is an outpatient or a hospice client. Notify these nurses when the child is hospitalized and encourage visits. Being involved in such an intense relationship is stressful, so be sure to take time off from the case occasionally. Communicate your feelings openly to other staff members.

B. **OBSERVE CHANGES IN CHILD'S AND PARENTS' BEHAVIOR**
Interpret changes in relation to the child's age level and perception of body image. Body-image distortion can be magnified by fantasy. Projective play techniques such as drawing, storytelling, or play with puppets can elicit the child's current feelings. Provide support for the child who returns to the community after therapy has produced observable side effects. Consult together with the child and school health nurse to plan how the child can cope with loss of hair, loss of weight, or even loss of a limb. Establish lines of communication with teachers and fellow students to prevent the development of ostracism, oversolicitude, and other destructive behaviors.

C. **EXPRESS YOUR CONTINUING AVAILABILITY**
"I know this must be a horrible experience for you. No one likes to endure so much pain and uncertainty. If you'd like to talk about it with me, perhaps you won't feel so alone."

Provide support for the family as they ride an emotional roller coaster through the child's exacerbations and remissions, trying to establish a normal rhythm of living in a constantly changing situation. This support is crucial when the child is ill for a period of years.

D. **TRY TO ANTICIPATE THE CHILD'S RESPONSES**
1. "Sometimes kids think it's their fault when they get so sick."
2. "It must be hard for you to understand how you can be sick when your body looks fine outside. Maybe I can help explain it to you. Shall I draw a picture?"
3. "You seemed to have so much pain and be so scared during your liver biopsy this morning. Let's talk about it." Or, "Why don't you draw us a picture of what it felt like?"
4. "Have you ever seen a television program about a person with the same illness you have? Tell me about it."
5. "Do you ever feel that your parents have been treating you differently since you were hospitalized? What do you think about that?"
6. "Since it is your body that is sick, we would like to help you understand what is wrong and why certain diagnostic tests and treatments are necessary. We will always tell you in advance what test you will have, when you will have it, what it is for, and how you can help us. Whenever possible, we will try to talk to you to find out when you would prefer to have the tests done, and maybe you can pick your own premedications."

E. **TRY TO ANTICIPATE THE PARENTS' RESPONSES**
1. "It seems your child became sick so suddenly. Perhaps you've been wondering if he was sick earlier, and you and your physician hadn't noticed it."
2. "How much do you think your child knows about her illness? How do you think we can best help her through this?"

3. "You must be exhausted. Life has changed so much in such a short time. Has it changed for the whole family?"
4. "Mrs. G is sitting in the next room with her son who has also been very sick. Would you like to speak with her? She has been very interested in meeting you."
5. "Your child seems to be suffering so these past few weeks. Perhaps sometimes you think it would be kinder if her suffering were all over."
6. "With Johnny so sick between remissions, it must be hard to treat him as normally as possible. Do you find this difficult?"
7. "Johnny has a younger brother and sister. Have they been asking a lot of questions about Johnny's hospitalization? Has their behavior changed? Perhaps they are more reluctant than usual to let you leave, or perhaps they have been 'too good'?"

F. **GIVE OTHER CHILDREN ON THE UNIT A CHANCE TO WORK THROUGH THEIR FEELINGS ABOUT THE DEATH AND DYING OF THEIR FRIENDS**
This can be done by means of projective play techniques or verbally. "I'm sure you noticed that Johnny's bed is empty this morning. Let's talk about it. You were such good friends, weren't you?"

G. **HELP THE CHILD AND FAMILY TO MAKE USE OF ALL AVAILABLE RESOURCES**
Resources include extended family members, the clergy, and family service agencies. Help parents determine who can most appropriately serve as the surrogate parent for siblings who are unattended during recurring periods of hospitalization.[2]

H. **BE ESPECIALLY SENSITIVE TO THE FAMILY'S NEEDS IN SITUATIONS OF SUDDEN DEATH OR INJURY**
1. Suggest that they contact a relative or close friend to come to the hospital for immediate support.
2. Avoid needless delay in conveying bad news.
3. Arrange for a private area for conferring. If possible, have nurse and physician both present with the family.
4. Arrange for the family to view the body of the deceased and to have time in private to say good-bye, if desired.
5. Use touch, eye contact, and creative listening as appropriate.

Evaluation of Secondary Prevention
Treatment of the grieving family has been successful if the child and his family[2]
1. Complete the stages of normal growth and development, as appropriate, within the limitations of the illness
2. Maintain healthy self-esteem, in spite of the poor body image that the illness may produce in the sick child or parent
3. Continue to play an active role in the community, in the home, in the school, and at work, within the limitations of the illness
4. Continuously participate in health teaching programs concerning the nature of the child's disease
5. Are active participants, as appropriate, in planning care with the health team
6. Are consulted by the hospital health team, the community nursing service, and the hospice home-care program as the child's health status changes and new needs emerge
7. Are able to express their angry, despairing, and tender feelings

8. Participate, if desired, in a group forum to share feelings with others in similar circumstances
9. Develop and maintain support systems that continue to be in effect after the child's death

Tertiary Prevention

Assessment Although many children and their families appear to adjust well to the death of a loved one, appearances can be deceiving. Failing grades, poor job performance, running away, and even separation or divorce may be related to unresolved conflicts concerning the death.

Table 40–2
COMMUNITY SELF-HELP GROUPS[2]

Name and Function	Address
1. *The Compassionate Friends, Inc.*, is a self-help organization "offering friendship and understanding to bereaved parents." The organization provides sharing groups that meet monthly, provides "telephone friends" who may be called, and offers information about the grieving process through lecture programs and a library.	The Compassionate Friends, Inc. National Headquarters PO Box 1347 Oak Brook IL 60521 Telephone (312) 323-5010
2. *The Candlelighters Foundation* is an organization that coordinates and maintains communications among parents and parent groups, developed to meet the needs of families who have children with cancer. One such group is Impact, Inc., which developed in New Jersey. Impact provides ongoing family-to-family support from the moment of diagnosis and assists families to obtain needed services.	The Candlelighters Foundation 123 "C" Street SE Washington, DC 20003
3. *The Jamie Schuman Center* is an organization that offers family support groups, which meet for weekly 2-hour sessions, counseling services upon request, a speaker's bureau, workshops, and education and training for interested community professionals.	The Jamie Shuman Center 600 Blue Hill Road River Vale, NJ 07675 Telephone (201) 391-4473
4. *The Center for Attitudinal Healing* is a self-help group for children, which offers weekly sharing groups for children only, plus "telephone friends" whom the children can call. Children need to have the opportunity to share their feelings openly in a receptive group environment, if desired. This organization believes that these children have a better chance for healthy personality development in spite of their illnesses than children who are forced to suppress their feelings to meet the needs of others.	The Center for Attitudinal Healing Dr. Gerald Jampolsky, Director 19 Main Street Tiburon, CA 94920

When death comes suddenly, the mourners have no opportunities to right old wrongs. Guilt arises inevitably in situations of death due to trauma, as the mourners seek to find a cause and often blame themselves. Families who have nursed a sick child through a lengthy illness may experience hostility toward the deceased, which they internalize as guilt for such unacceptable feelings. Nurses, therefore, must assume that *all families who have experienced a death need tertiary prevention services* until they demonstrate otherwise.

Intervention   A. **COUNSELING THE FAMILY MEMBERS**

The nurse offers direct services to the family to help them rebuild their lives after the death of their child. This may be done in individual, group, or family therapy or in play therapy with the surviving child. This therapy is directed toward helping family members resolve any remaining guilt, anger, or sadness and toward helping them to withdraw emotional investment from the lost person, and redirect interest to their future lives. It is kept in mind that grief and mourning takes 1 to 2 years and that family members may all move at their own individual paces.

B. **REFERRAL TO SELF-HELP GROUPS**

The nurse coordinates client needs and community resources by becoming aware of available self-help groups, as well as by playing the role of consultant to parents who wish to initiate a new group. Table 40–2 provides examples of community self-help groups and their addresses.[2]

Evaluation   Coping with loss over the long-term cannot be easy, and it is work that each family must ultimately do for itself. Nurses can evaluate how well families and individuals, working in concert with other bereaved people, have learned to live again. The following objectives for behavior after the child's death are useful benchmarks.[1] The family members have completed

1. Full realization and acceptance of the loss
2. Resolution of anger and irrational guilt related to the loss
3. Significant withdrawal of emotional investment from the lost person
4. Redirection of interest and involvement with life

References

1. Cain A, Cain BS: On replacing a child. J Am Acad Child Psychiatry 3:443, 1964
2. Frank K: Dying children. In Haber J et al (eds): Comprehensive Psychiatric Nursing. New York, McGraw-Hill, 1982
3. Gourevitch M: A survey of family reactions to disease and death in a family member. In Anthony DJ, Koupernik C (eds): The Child in His Family: The Impact of Disease and Death. New York, John Wiley & Sons, 1973
4. Grollman EA (ed): Explaining Death to Children. Boston, Beacon Press, 1967
5. Morrow G: Parental interrelationships in living with pediatric cancer. Proceedings of the First National Conference for Parents of Children with Cancer, National Cancer Institute, Bethesda, Maryland. NIH Pbulication No. 80–2176, June 1980
6. Ramshorn MT: Mental health services. In Haber J et al (eds): Comprehensive Psychiatric Nursing. New York, McGraw-Hill, 1978

Bibliography

Fife BL: Childhood cancer as a family crisis: A review. J Psychiatr Nurs 18:29, 1980
Lonetto R: Children's Conceptions of Death. New York, Springer-Verlag, 1980

Part IV

Counseling

Specific

Clients

41

The Client
Who Is Anxious

Marie C. Smith

OVERVIEW

Description
Definition
Relief Behaviors
Levels of Anxiety
Nursing Interventions

Description   Anxiety is experienced by everyone at one time or another. Extreme forms of anxiety early in life lead to the development of defense mechanisms, personality traits and interpersonal behaviors intended to make the person feel relatively secure. When these overall defense mechanisms fail, the client can suffer intense emotional and physical discomfort. Chart 41–1 lists the subjective and objective (physiologic) symptoms of anxiety.[1]

Definition   Anxiety occurs when a severe, unexpected threat to one's feeling of self-esteem or well-being occurs. It has been noted that anxiety often takes place when a person expects one thing, and is suddenly confronted with something quite different. This process has been operationalized as follows[2]:
1. Client has expectations related to need for prestige or status.
2. Expectations are not met.
3. Unexpected powerlessness or extreme discomfort is felt.
4. Power is mobilized through some automatic relief behavior (for example, anger, withdrawal, somatization) to relieve the feeling of powerlessness.
5. There is justification of the relief behavior.

Relief Behaviors   Anxiety may be directly felt or, more characteristically, may not be felt at all. That is, as soon as the client senses a threat, a relief behavior occurs automatically. Over

---

Chart 41–1
SYMPTOMS OF ANXIETY

Subjective *(Reported by Clients)*	*Objective* *(Observed by the Nurse)*
Intense apprehension	Increased heart rate
Fear, terror	Increased rate and depth of respiration
Feelings of impending doom	Shifts in body temperature
Dyspnea	Alternating blood pressure from norm
Palpitations	Abnormal or absent menstrual flow
Chest pain or discomfort	Urinary urgency or retention
Choking, smothering sensations	Dryness of the mouth
Dizziness	Loss or increase in appetite
Vertigo	Cold, clammy skin
Unsteady feelings	Dilation of pupils
Numbness and tingling of fingers/toes	Release of sugar by the liver
Hot and cold flashes	Retention of sodium (aldosteronism)
Sweating, particularly in the palms	In extreme cases, there can be enlargement of adrenal and
Faintness	pituitary glands with overworking of organ systems to the
Trembling or shaking	state of exhaustion and death.[3]
Fear of dying	
Fear of going crazy	
Fear of doing something uncontrolled	
Apprehensive expectation	
Motor tension with hyperactivity	
Vigilance and scanning	
Phobias	
Hallucinations	
Delusions	
Ringing in the ears	
Visual disturbances	
Anger or hostility	
Increased irritability	

---

time, the individual develops a characteristic pattern of relief behaviors intended to provide comfort and protection in the face of anxiety. Four major conversion patterns for anxiety have been identified[3]:

A. **ACTING-OUT BEHAVIOR**

There may be overt expressions of anger and aggression, or covert expressions of resentment.

B. **SOMATIZING**

Somatizing includes a number of "psychosomatic" disorders. The autonomic nervous system quickly converts anxiety to an organ function. Rather than the client having the felt experience of anxiety, the organ takes the stress and strain.

C. **FREEZING-TO-THE-SPOT BEHAVIOR**

Withdrawal into depression or schizophrenia may be seen.

D. **USING THE ANXIETY IN THE SERVICE OF LEARNING**

The nurse encourages the client to tolerate the anxiety while assisting the client to figure out the cause of the anxiety.

Levels of Anxiety   Four levels of anxiety have been identified. It is important for the nurse to assess the client's anxiety level, since the intervention is based on the level. In mild (+) or moderate (+ +) anxiety, the nurse intervenes by helping the client to figure out what is causing the anxiety. In severe anxiety (+ + +) or panic (+ + + +), the nurse helps the client through nonverbal means (walking with the client, or just remaining quiet) or by offering sedation to reduce the anxiety. Chart 41–2 shows the effect of anxiety on the client's ability to observe, focus, and learn.[2]

Chart 41–2

LEVEL OF ANXIETY AND THE CLIENT'S ABILITY TO OBSERVE, FOCUS ATTENTION, AND LEARN

Level of Anxiety	Effects on Client
Mild (+)	Sensory perception and ability to focus are broad. The ability to observe oneself and what is going on is enhanced. Connections between events are made and verbalized. At this level, learning can take place. The individual who is at this level of anxiety is alert and able to function in emergencies.
Moderate (+ +)	Sensory perception is somewhat narrowed, but alertness continues to the extent that the individual is able to concentrate on a delineated focus. With some effort, concentration on relevant data is possible, and appropriate connections are made as long as the individual is able to "shut out" irrelevant data.
Severe (+ + +)	Sensory perception is greatly reduced. The person focuses on a small detail of an experience and is unable to make connections between scattered details. The individual is unable to get a total picture of an experience. Learning cannot take place.
Panic (+ + + +)	There is major dissociation of experience, and the person does not notice or remember major experiences. Details become enlarged and distorted. Communication is not understood by the listener, and personality disorganization is apparent. The individual is in a state of "terror". At this level of anxiety, learning cannot take place. The immediate goal is to get relief.

Nursing Interventions The nurse intervenes with anxious clients in the following way[2]:

1. The nurse observes that the client is exhibiting some relief behavior (for example, pacing in a circle).
2. The nurse approaches the client and attempts to assess the client's level of anxiety: "Hello, Mr. Smith, I see you are pacing. What are you feeling now?"
3. Depending on the level of anxiety, the nurse continues to intervene. If the anxiety is at the severe or panic level, the nurse remains with the client, speaks in a calm way and offers sedation if needed. If the anxiety is mild or moderate the nurse continues as follows:

a. Helps the client to name the feeling	"Are you feeling anxious?"
b. Helps the client to describe what was happening before the anxiety occurred	"What happened just before you became anxious and began to pace?"
c. Connects the anxiety to the unmet expectation and threat to self-esteem	"So, you expected your wife to visit, and she hasn't come. You feel helpless and anxious."
d. Connects the relief behavior to the anxiety	"The pacing makes you feel less anxious."

The mere process of walking and talking with the nurse alleviates anxiety. Clients often feel calmer when they feel understood by another person. In addition, the cognitive process of understanding *themselves,* the connection between their anxiety, and the occurrence that triggered it almost always brings relief.

References

1. Diagnostic and Statistical Manual of Mental Disorders, 3rd ed. American Psychiatric Association, 1980
2. Field WE (ed): The Psychotherapy of Hildegard E. Peplau. New Braunfels, TX, PSF Productions, 1979
3. Selye H: The Stress of Life. New York, McGraw-Hill, 1956

Bibliography

Kerr NJ: Anxiety: Theoretical considerations. Perspect Psychiatr Care 16:36, 1978
Mathew RJ: The Biology of Anxiety. New York, Brunner-Mazel, 1982

42

The Client
Who Is Depressed

Linda Barile

OVERVIEW

Conditions Associated with Depression
Endogenous and Exogenous Depression
Psychodynamics
Description
Nurses' Nonproductive Reactions
Nursing Interventions

Conditions Associated with Depression

Depression is a state associated with a number of accepted diagnostic categories. It is important that the nurse be able to identify the etiology or source of the client's depression, since treatment and knowledge of the course of illness follow from this assessment. Table 42–1 shows the DSM III categories that include depression and the theoretical description of the depression.[4]

Endogenous and Exogenous Depression[2]

The term depression refers to a mood state, a symptom, or a group of clinical syndromes. As a mood state, feelings of sadness, disappointment, and frustration are normal in all individuals. The syndrome of depression is distinguished from the symptom by the severity and duration of the depressed mood.

An early division of depression categorized this syndrome into endogenous depression and exogenous or reactive depression. In endogenous depression, a clear-cut identifiable precipitating factor is usually nonexistent. There is, however, a strong family history of depression, and the client has experienced a recurrent major episode of depression in the past, both of which suggest a hereditary, biologic, or hormonal component to this depression. The severity of symptoms sometimes experienced in endogenous depression, particularly psychotic symptoms of hallucinations and delusions, resulted in this depression being called ''psychotic depression.'' Endogenously depressed people respond less to environmental stimuli or psychotherapy and more to electroconvulsive treatment and administration of antidepressants. Examples of endogenous depressions include manic depressive psychosis, involutional melancholia, and some postpartum psychoses.

In exogenous depression, an identifiable situational event or stress exists as a precipitating factor. Examples of external stresses are loss of a significant other, loss of employment, and financial reverses. Exogenously depressed people usually respond to psychotherapy. The term neurotic depression is often used synonymously with exogenous depression.

There is considerable controversy over the separation of exogenous and endogenous depression, with some authors arguing that the distinction is artificial and that the differences are primarily quantitative.[2] In some settings, the Dexamethasone Suppression Test (DST) is being used to determine whether the depression is endogenous. However, this test is not conclusive.[6]

Psychodynamics

Exogenous depression occurs when clients experience a real or symbolic loss and come to believe that they will never be the same again. When any loss occurs, there is an interruption in one's goals or plans. This interruption causes a period of grief. When the grief feelings turn to hopelessness about ever achieving any goals again or ever feeling good again, depression is operating.

One prominent psychodynamic theory asserts that depression is a result of anger turned inward. The real or symbolic loss causes the client to experience anger, usually unconsciously. The client who becomes depressed is usually unable to accept being angry and has a history of[3]

1. A chronic hunger for affection
2. Chronic guilt
3. A need for control
4. Feelings of inadequacy and inferiority
5. Feelings of helplessness, powerlessness
6. Low self-esteem

In the depressive personality,[3] the anger toward the loss is turned toward the self.

Another theory poses that reactive depression is a belief in one's own helplessness and that depression results when rewards as well as punishments come independently of one's own efforts.[7]

Table 42–1
CONDITIONS ASSOCIATED WITH DEPRESSION AND DESCRIPTION[4]

Condition	Description
1. Major depressive episode	1. Depression caused by external factors such as identifiable situational or maturational events or losses in a person's life or by internal factors. Depressions caused by internal factors are thought to have some biologic, biochemical, or hereditary aspect. There is usually a good premorbid adjustment and a previous episode of affective disturbance from which there was complete recovery.
2. Bipolar disorder	2. Mood disturbance in which there is usually a family history and previous episodes of a manic attack that alternate or intermingle with a depressive mood
3. Cyclothymic disorder	3. Chronic mood disturbance of at least 2 years' duration, involving numerous periods of depression and hypomania, but not of sufficient severity and duration to meet the criteria for a major depressive or manic episode
4. Dysthymic disorder (depressive neurosis)	4. Chronic disturbance of mood involving depressed mood, but not of sufficient severity and duration to be a major depressive episode
5. Organic–affective syndrome with depression	5. Organic disturbance due to substances such as reserpine, to infectious diseases such as influenza, or to endocrine disorders such as hypothyroidism
6. Dementia	6. Organic disturbances caused by Alzheimer's disease, central nervous system infection, brain trauma, toxic or metabolic disturbances and neurologic disease
7. Psychological reaction to the functional impairment associated with physical illness	7. Temporary depression caused by a psychosocial stress such as the amputation of a leg or a life-threatening illness
8. Schizophrenia	8. In schizophrenia, there is usually considerable depressive symptomatology. An individual with a major depressive episode may also have psychotic symptoms; however, the diagnosis of schizophrenia is made only if the affective symptoms follow the psychotic symptoms or are brief.
9. Schizoaffective disorder	9. Schizophrenia and an affective disorder exist simultaneously.
10. Chronic mental disorders—obsessive compulsive disorder, alcohol dependence or addiction	10. Chronic mental disorders often have associated depression.
11. Separation anxiety disorder	11. Depression and excessive anxiety following separation from major attachment figures or from home or other familiar surroundings.
12. Uncomplicated bereavement	12. A full depressive syndrome is frequently a normal reaction to a major loss. However, if bereavement is unduly severe or prolonged, the diagnosis may be changed to major depression.

13. Personality disorder
    Borderline
    Histrionic
    Dependent
	13. Depressive features viewed as secondary to the underlying personality disorder

A third theory suggests that depressed or depression-prone persons have certain self-defeating, negative thoughts that become activated by specific stresses. These automatic self-statements pervade the individual's thinking and result in the feeling of depresion and behaviors associated with depression.[2]

Description   The client who is depressed suffers from a number of painful symptoms. These have been divided into emotional, cognitive, motivational, and physical categories as follows[2,4]:

A. **EMOTIONAL MANIFESTATIONS/AFFECT OR MOOD**
    1. Depression, sadness, hopelessness, discouragement, emptiness
    2. Lack of ability to experience pleasure
    3. Negative feelings about self, that is, worthlessness, shame, guilt, low self-esteem
    4. Anxiety or agitation, anger

B. **COGNITIVE MANIFESTATIONS/THOUGHT**
    1. Worries and preoccupations
    2. Slowed, impoverished thoughts; difficulty with thinking or memory; distractions; self-blaming, self-critical, self-devaluing thoughts
    3. Negative outlook or expectations
    4. Indecisiveness, ambivalence
    5. Exaggeration of problem—distortion in perception
    6. Distorted thoughts of body image or excessive concern with physical health, somatic delusions
    7. Self-devaluing hallucinations or delusions
    8. Thoughts of death or suicide

C. **MOTIVATIONAL MANIFESTATIONS/BEHAVIOR**
    1. Psychomotor retardation, that is, slowness of speech and lack of energy; fatigue; sad facial appearance; inattentiveness to personal hygiene
    2. Passivity and dependence
    3. Avoidance, escapism, withdrawal
    4. Psychomotor agitation, that is, inability to sit still; pacing; handwringing; pulling or rubbing hair, skin, clothing, or other objects; pressure of speech
    5. Panic attacks or phobias

D. **PHYSICAL MANIFESTATIONS/SYMPTOMS**
    1. Loss of appetite or increased appetite with accompanying weight loss or gain
    2. Insomnia, difficulty falling asleep, waking in the middle of the night, or early morning wakening
    3. Constipation
    4. Dry mouth
    5. Amenorrhea, impotence, or loss of sexual response

Nurses' Nonproductive   Working with a depressed client is often extremely difficult and challenging. The
Reactions   client's overwhelming, hopeless feelings and lack of response to environmental stimuli or to nurses' interventions often produce loss of objectivity, depression, hopelessness, helplessness, and a sense of failure in the nurse. In addition, the client's anxiety and depression are often communicated empathically. The nurse who feels the same painful feelings begins to use avoidance or withdrawal from the client as a means of coping.

The client's response of a childlike helplessness and dependency can often produce either anger and frustration or a reciprocal parental approach on the part of the nurse. The frustration experienced can result in inconsistent approaches on the part of the nursing staff.

Nursing Interventions   Chart 42–1 shows nursing interventions and theoretical rationale with depressed clients.

Chart 42–1
NURSING INTERVENTIONS AND THEORETICAL RATIONALE ASSOCIATED WITH DEPRESSED CLIENTS

Nursing Intervention	*Theoretical Rationale*
Assess suicide potential (see Chapter 3).	The most serious complication of depression is suicide.
Assess and observe for physical symptoms.	Physical symptoms can provide information about the type of depression.
1. Assess or observe and record sleep pattern. Investigate the reasons for sleeplessness. Implement appropriate relaxation techniques, sedation, and so forth. 2. Assess or observe eating pattern. Encourage and supervise proper nutrition. 3. Assess whether the client has difficulty in elimination. Tell the client to inform staff if there is difficulty in elimination. Take appropriate action. 4. Encourage exercise and recreation. 5. Encourage the client in personal hygiene and activities of daily living and give positive reinforcement.	1. The client who is exhausted from lack of sleep has little energy left to work on the reasons for the depression. A vicious cycle is set in motion. 2. The client who is undernourished lacks energy to work on and resolve the conflicts underlying the depression. 3. Constipation and urinary retention cause secondary problems, increasing the depression. 4. Exercise and social contact reduce depressive symptoms. 5. When clients neglect physical hygiene, their feelings of self-worth decrease and others avoid them.
Assess what change or changes have recently occurred: "What was happening in your life that made you seek help at this time?" "What problems or changes have you had at home? Work? School? With family?" and so forth.[1]	Sometimes the client does not recognize the significance of changes and events. Recognizing these as precipitating factors often brings relief.
Determine the meaning or the client's perception of the precipitating stress or change. "What is most upsetting about this situation?" "What is the meaning of this to you?"[1]	The number of life changes and the meaning of these changes are assessed to better understand what the client is experiencing. Depending upon the degree of depression, these events might be distorted, but it is the client's experience that matters. This assessment helps the nurse figure out why the client is angry.
When distortions are extreme such as "I'm dying," attempt to correct distorted perceptions by supplying accurate information, posing possible alternatives, or discussing different interpretations of the events. Try to find out why the client needs this distortion, that is, what is the symbolic meaning of the distortion?	Once the nurse understands the distortions and why they are needed, the client can be helped to understand the meaning of the depression.
Help the client gain an intellectual understanding of the situation. Help the person see the relationship between the depressive symptoms and the precipitating event.[1] For example, "Is it possible you believe you are dying because you're anxious about going off to school in the Fall?"	The person may not see the relationship between events and symptoms and is often relieved to see the connection.
Assist the person to recognize, accept, understand, and ventilate feelings, particularly anger. 1. Use an empathic approach to help the client identify feelings. Observe and comment on the verbal and nonverbal	1. The use of empathy, respect, genuineness, and concreteness establishes a helping relationship. The warmth and *(continued)*

Chart 42–1
(continued)

Nursing Intervention	Theoretical Rationale
expression of feelings: "You look angry. Are you?" "Right now, you feel hopeless about the situation." "How do you feel about what has happened?"	acceptance of the nurse encourages self-respect and self-acceptance in the client. The use of empathy allows the client to verbalize thoughts and feelings, discuss troublesome life events, and connect the feeling to the situation.
2. Connect the feeling to the content: "You feel angry because you have to leave people who are familiar and supportive to you."	2. Communicates that the feeling has some concrete as well as symbolic basis
3. Tell the client how others might feel in a similar situation: "Lots of people have trouble separating from their families and friends. It's one of the hardest things we all face."	3. Helps the client gain a more realistic perception of self and events
4. Encourage the client to identify feelings as they occur in talks with you, to accept and understand feelings, and to talk feelings over with you and with others in similar situations.	4. Helps the client to learn more direct, assertive ways to express feelings. The depressed person often has feelings of unconscious anger that do not get expressed, but are internalized to feelings of guilt and worthlessness.
5. Give positive reinforcement when the client expresses feelings appropriately, but do not push an artificial expression. If the client expresses anger before being ready, anxiety, guilt, and suicidal thoughts may result. If client is expressing anger at you, wait until later to provide praise.	5. Reinforces the direct expression of genuine feelings. Praise during an angry outburst will interrupt its expression.
6. Have the client attend to bodily responses that indicate feelings. When clients feel anxious or depressed and cannot express feelings, encourage them to write the feelings experienced, the circumstances and events, the reason, and action taken.	6. Helps establish a pattern of observing, describing, and analyzing behavior with a view toward testing, validating, and using new behaviors.[5]
7. Point out ways the client avoids expression of feelings.	7. Helps the client to observe avoidance behaviors, which may contribute to the internalization of anger
Use support systems[1]	
1. Assess support systems: "Who are the important people in your life?" "Who has helped you with difficult problems?" "Who are the people you believe you can go to for help or can be helpful to you?"	1–3. The depressed person is usually isolated and needs to reopen social contacts.[1] When clients spend time with others, depressive symptoms are usually less severe.
2. Encourage the client to contact others who are important.	
3. Plan ways of using community groups to establish support systems.	
Encourage discharge planning	
1. Ask the client to formulate problems, expectations, and standards. In the beginning, encourage clients to make simple decisions. Avoid dealing with difficult decisions when they are acutely depressed. When the client is able, encourage him to assume responsibility.	1. The more involved the client is in planning, the more likely the follow through.
2. Talk with the client and significant others about discharge plans, that is, living arrangements, work, school, and leisure time.	2. The more involved the family and client are in planning, the more likely the follow through.
3. Encourage the client to anticipate problems or areas of difficulty and discuss possible ways of coping and problem solving.	3. Avoids readmission
4. Educate the client and significant others about the client's illness, signs and symptoms that indicate a return of the depression, whom to contact in times of stress, follow-up treament, and effects of medication. For example, if the client is taking an MAO inhibitor, high tyramine-content foods such as aged cheese, yogurt, chicken liver, chocolate, beer and wine are contraindicated.	4. Same as #2.

References

1. Aguilera DC, Messick J: Crisis Intervention: Theory and Methodology. St Louis, CV Mosby, 1970
2. Beck A: Depression. Philadelphia, University of Pennsylvania Press, 1967
3. Bibring E: The mechanism of depression. In Greenacre P (ed): Affective Disorders. New York, International University Press, 1953
4. Diagnostic and Statistical Manual of Mental Disorders, 3rd ed. Washington, DC, American Psychiatric Association, 1980
5. Field WE (ed): The Psychotherapy of Hildegard E. Peplau. New Braunfels, TX. PSF Productions, 1979
6. Harris E: Dexamethasone Suppression Test. Am J Nurs 82:784, 1982
7. Seligman MEP: Learned helplessness. Annu Rev Med 23:407, 1972

Bibliography

Authier J, Authier K, Lutey B: Clinical management of the tearfully depressed patient: Communication skills for the nurse practitioner. J Psychiatr Nurs 17:37, 1979

Chenitz C: Primary depression in older women: Are current theories and treatment of depression relevant to this age group? J Psychiatr Nurs 17:20, 1979

Drake RE, Price JL: Depression: Adaptation to disruption and loss. Perspect Psychiatr Care 13:163, 1975

Jacobson A: Melancholy in the 20th century: Causes and prevention. J Psychiatr Nurs 18:11, 1980

Knowles RD: Dealing with feelings: Handling depression by identifying anger. Am J Nurs 81:968, 1981

Knowles RD: Handling depression through activity. Am J Nurs 81:1187, 1981

Provost J: Intervention in a schizoaffective depressive behavior pattern: A behavioral approach. Perspect Psychiatr Care 12:86, 1974

Rowe D: The Experience of Depression. New York, John Wiley & Sons, 1978

Shmagin BG, Pearlmutter DR: The pursuit of unhappiness: The secondary gains of depression. Perspect Psychiatr Care 15:63, 1977

Swanson AR: Communicating with depressed persons. Perspect Psychiatr Care 13:63, 1975

43

The Client
Who Is Suicidal

Linda Barile

OVERVIEW

Conditions Involving Suicide
Psychodynamics of Suicide
Warning Signs
Nurses' Nonproductive Reactions
Nursing Interventions

Conditions Involving Suicide Nurses care for suicidal clients in both inpatient and outpatient settings. Table 43–1 shows the conditions that may include suicidal behavior and a description of each.[2]

Psychodynamics of Suicide Suicide and suicide attempts have been examined from a number of different viewpoints. These include[5]

A. **SUICIDE ATTEMPTS AS A COMMUNICATION**
   Suicide has been widely viewed as a "cry for help," an attempt to call attention to the plight of the attempter.

B. **SUICIDE AS A MASTERY OVER FATE**
   Deeply depressed people often believe that they have no control over their fate. One way to gain control is to take their own lives.

C. **SUICIDE AS MURDER TURNED INWARD**
   When the person feels strong aggression toward another, suicide can serve to
   1. Control the aggression by turning it toward the self
   2. "Murder" the other person who has been incorporated by the suicidal individual

D. **SUICIDE AS AN ESCAPE FROM PAINFUL OR HUMILIATING SITUATIONS**
   Cultural or socially sanctioned suicides are sometimes carried out to spare the person's family or friends, as in the case of "rational suicide." Also, suicide may be seen as a way to drift into peaceful sleep or to reunite with dead relatives or friends.

(Text continues on page 402)

Table 43–1
CONDITIONS INVOLVING SUICIDE AND THEIR DESCRIPTIONS

Category	*Description*
1. Major affective disorders Bipolar disorder Major depressive episode	Suicide is always of major concern with depressed clients. If depressive symptoms are severe or if suicide assessment shows high lethality, there is reason for extreme concern. Manic depressive clients in the depressed phase are usually highly suicidal.
2. Schizophrenia	There is a high suicide risk if the client is experiencing hallucinations and delusions that are of a harmful nature.
3. Organic mental disorders	Suicide may be a risk in this disorder if the client is experiencing severe depressive symptoms, is impulsive, confused, hallucinating or delusional, or is using alcohol or drugs.
4. Substance use disorders	The combination of depression and impulsivity may account for the high incidence of suicide in this disorder.
5. Personality disorders • Histrionic • Antisocial • Borderline	The impulsive, demanding, and manipulative behavior coupled with depression may indicate suicidal risk.

Chart 43–1

NURSING INTERVENTIONS AND THEORETICAL RATIONALE WITH SUICIDAL CLIENTS

Nursing Intervention	*Theoretical Rationale*

If the client has attempted suicide, restore physical health.
1. Maintain life support.
   a. Institute CPR.
   b. Apply pressure if client is bleeding.
2. Assess vital signs and do a brief neurologic assessment.
3. Maintain an open airway.
4. Maintain fluids and electrolytes; start IV, monitor intake and output.
5. If client has overdosed, investigate name and amount of drug taken. Contact Poison Control Center.

1–5. Medical management of a suicide attempt requires immediate first aid and maintenance of life support. Nursing management depends upon the method used to attempt suicide.

Provide a warm, nurturant, and protective environment.
1. The client is placed on a special observational status or one-to-one supervision and restricted to certain observable areas.
2. Silverware and sharp objects are not allowed for the client's use or are counted daily.
3. The client sleeps in a room with others but spends a minimum amount of time in this room during the day
4. The client is accompanied to the bathroom.
5. Windows and screens are shatterproof or impenetrable, particularly if the unit is not on the first floor.
6. Utility and storage rooms are locked.
7. Electrical appliances and lamp cords are shortened to a minimum length. Light bulbs are counted daily.
8. The client's belongings are inspected upon admission, as are items from visitors.
9. Staffing is planned to ensure that the unit is covered, especially at change of shift, meal times, breaks, vacations, and weekends.[6]

1–9. There is controversy about the necessity of suicide-proofing the physical layout of the environment. Some feel that a restrictive environment is antitherapeutic and has not prevented suicides. Frequent methods of suicide in hospitals are hanging, jumping, cutting, and ingestion of toxic substances. Suicides often occur when there is a shortage of staff.

Establish a trusting relationship with the client by using empathy and respect.

This improves self-esteem and encourages the client to talk over feelings rather than act them out.

Help the client to recognize, ventilate, and accept feelings.
1. Feelings of guilt[1]
   a. Investigate what it is about the client or the situation that would be destroyed through suicide.
   b. Help clients see that there are positive things about themselves and their lives.[1]
   c. Investigate with the client ways that they can change the things they find intolerable.
   d. Attempt to relieve guilt. Investigate precipitating events and help clients gain a realistic perception of these events.
   e. Help clients to accept that they cannot change what happened in the past, and that they did the best they could at the time. Help them learn from the past and accept responsibility for doing something now.

1. The suicidal person usually wants the death of the whole self in order to get rid of the part of the self that is felt to be intolerable.[1] If the client can explore and understand both intellectually and emotionally the source of the guilt, the need for self-punishment is decreased.[1]

Chart 43–1
(continued)

Nursing Intervention	Theoretical Rationale

f. Discuss and work through unrealistic expectations that they have of themselves and others.[1]

g. Avoid comments that add to clients' guilt, such as "What about your children? husband? family?"

2. Feelings of ambivalence. Talk about ambivalence and point out clients' ambivalence. Discuss and reinforce thoughts, feelings, or actions indicating a will to live. "In each of us there is a will to live and a will to die. It's like a seesaw in balance. Right now, your will to die is overbalancing the will to live. But we are all here to be on the side of life and help you find your reasons to live."

2. All suicidal persons are ambivalent, and the will to live should be capitalized upon. Usually if the person did not have a will to live, suicide would have been successfully completed.

3. Feelings of hopelessness. Discuss with clients ways that they can be different and things can be different.

3. If hope can be increased without giving false reassurance, suicidal wishes will decrease

a. "With therapy, you can work on some of your problems, change some of the things you would like changed, and feel different about yourself and your current situation."

b. "Together we can find your reasons to live."

c. "Though you feel terrible now, you won't always feel this way. Sometime in the future, you'll feel like your old self again."

c. Depression is always time limited. This information can reassure clients.

d. "With time and working on your problems in therapy you could solve some of those problems and get more pleasure out of life."

e. "There are probably many solutions that you have tried and some that you might not have thought of. With time and therapy, you may find a satisfying approach to your problems."

f. "Right now you're feeling miserable and hopeless and believe you have little to live for, but I have seen others who felt similar to you and were helped by medication and treatment. You have nothing to lose by giving yourself a chance to get well."

4. Feelings of low self-esteem.
   a. Encourage the client to perform responsible acts, and provide positive reinforcement.
   b. Help the client achieve a more realistic, positive self-concept and sense of worth.

4. The suicidal person needs increased self-esteem, self-respect, acceptance, and belongingness. A helping relationship of empathy, respect, and genuineness fosters self-respect and acceptance in the suicidal person. Behavioral techniques are also useful in achieving this goal.

5. Feelings of anger
   a. Help the client to recognize and express anger directly.
   b. Teach assertiveness training.

5. Depressed and suicidal people often have anger turned inward and must learn how to recognize and express anger. As clients become more assertive, they are less likely to be exploited and, in turn, feel angry.

Discharge planning

1. Educate the client and family about the signs and symptoms of depression and the warning signs of suicidal thoughts.
2. Inform the client and family of suicide prevention centers and other places for help.
3. Arrange for referral and follow-up treatment.
4. Educate the client and family about the effects of medication and special precautions.

1–4. Depression can be treated early and suicide avoided.

The method used to attempt suicide is a clue to the dynamics of the suicide. For example, the person who takes an overdose of sleeping pills may be equating death with a prolonged sleep, and the use of firearms often suggests violent rage.[5]

Warning Signs   Nurses who care for suicidal clients must be aware of the behaviors that indicate that the client will attempt suicide. They are as follows:[3,4,6]:

1. Depression[4]
2. Hopelessness and helplessness[4]
3. Anger or hostility[4]
4. Anhedonia—absence of any pleasure or satisfaction
5. Guilt leading to a wish for punishment
6. Isolation or withdrawal[4]
7. Insomnia
8. Impulsiveness
9. Ambivalence
10. Preoccupation with death[3] or suicide
11. Thoughts, words, and actions that are "end-centered"[3]
12. Givng things away, making a will, checking on life insurance[6]
13. Termination of significant relationships or commitments
14. A sudden uplift in mood, or serenity, when the client was previously deeply depressed

Nurses' Nonproductive Reactions   The suicidal client presents a psychiatric emergency. Nearly always, nurses feel anxious that the client may attempt suicide or commit suicide. They often feel powerless to effect a change in the client's depressed feelings or suicidal behavior and become frustrated by the client's dependency and manipulation. Nurses cope with their own anxiety by the use of denial or by feeling anger, frustration, indifference, and avoidance.

Nurses naturally have attitudes and feelings about the meaning of life and the right to death, which are formed by personal experience, cultural beliefs, and moral or societal views. These attitudes influence the nurse's response to the client.

Feelings and reactions of shock, omnipotence, responsibility, and guilt are particularly common if the client has committed suicide, in which case, nurses go through the stages of grief and mourning.

Nursing Interventions   Working with suicidal clients requires that the nurse be patient, alert, and empathetic. Chart 43–1 outlines applicable nursing interventions and theoretical rationale.

References

1. Berger MM: Working with People Called Patients. New York, Brunner-Mazel, 1977
2. Diagnostic and Statistical Manual of Mental Disorders, 3rd ed. American Psychiatric Association, 1980
3. Grosicki JP: Nursing Action Guide. Washington, DC, Veterans Administration, Committee on Research in Clinical Nursing, 1970
4. Hatton C et al: Suicide Assessment and Intervention. New York, Appleton-Century-Crofts, 1977
5. MacKinnon R, Michels R: The Psychiatric Interview in Clinical Practice. Philadelphia, WB Saunders, 1971
6. Neal MC, Cohen PF: Nursing Care Plan Guide, The Patient Who is Suicidal. NURSECO 3:38, 1977

Bibliography

Atkinson JM: Discovering Suicide: Studies in the Social Organization of Sudden Death. Pittsburgh, University of Pittsburgh Press, 1978
Evans DL: Explaining suicide among the young: An analytical review of the literature. J Psychosoc Nurs 20:9, 1982

Farberow NL (ed): The Many Faces of Suicide. New York, McGraw-Hill, 1980

Floyd GJ: Nursing management of the suicidal patient. J Psychiatr Nurs 13:23, 1975

Hart NA, Keidel GC: The suicidal adolescent. Am J Nurs 79:80, 1979

Leonard CV: Treating the suicidal patient: A communication approach, J Psychiatr Nurs 13:19, 1975

Loughlin Sr N: Suicide: A case for investigation. J Psychiatr Nurs 18:8, 1980

Miller M: Suicide After Sixty: The Final Alternative. New York, Springer-Verlag, 1979

Stafford L: Depression and self-destructive behavior. J Psychiatr Nurs 14:37, 1976

Vollen KH, Watson CG: Suicide in relation to time of day and day of week. Am J Nurs 75:263, 1975

Wekstein L: Handbook of Suicidology: Principles, Problems, Practice. New York, Brunner-Mazel, 1979

44

The Client
Who Is
Passive–Aggressive

Marie C. Smith

OVERVIEW   *Description*
Etiology
Psychodynamics
Characteristic Behaviors
Nurses' Nonproductive Reactions
Nursing Interventions

Description   Passive–aggressive behavior may be seen as an isolated personality trait disturbance or it may occur in conjunction with more severe psychopathologic conditions such as depression, alcoholism, obsessive–compulsive personality, borderline personality, psychosomatic disorder, and many others.[1]

   Passive–aggressive behavior is defined as behavior intended to mask anger and anxiety from the self and significant others.[4] It is shown in subtle resistance to demands for adequate performance in both work and social environments.[1] The person with this disorder sidetracks or channels anger into passive measures, which consciously and more frequently unconsciously obstruct growth in love and work relationships. Typically, resentment is expressed through procrastination, dawdling, stubbornness, intentional inefficiency, and forgetfulness.[1]

Etiology   Early experiences in the child who is to become passive–aggressive as an adult include dependency on adults who are hypercritical, demanding, unloving, and sometimes punitive. Punishment may have been physically violent or psychologically threatening, causing fears of abandonment and rejection.[5] The early gratification of needs for nurturance and physical protection are essential to the growing child. The threat of loss of gratification is constantly feared by the child. As the child grows, anxiety and helplessness become masked by anger. Anger in the child becomes as frightening as the initial anxiety and is seen by the child's mind as all destructive. The perception of destruction of those upon whom one is dependent is equal to self-destruction, a predicament unacceptable to the child's growing ego. The compromise that is struck by the growing ego is to unconsciously channel anger and aggression very quietly, into passive–resistive and passive–aggressive behaviors.[3]

Psychodynamics   The adult or child who is passive–aggressive has difficulty trusting normal dependency on others; he may become overdependent and compliant and will not tolerate normal anger or anxiety in the self or others without intense discomfort. Failure to express anger constructively, over time, causes its covert or passive expression in a manner that causes the least discomfort to the client. Most passive–aggressive behaviors are unconscious to the client but have a demoralizing effect on others. The behavior of significant others toward the client becomes more and more unrewarding, the very response the client feared most in childhood. Withdrawal of affection and attention of loved ones stimulates the passive–aggressive mode of relating, and the client is stuck in a pathologic trap originally designed to provide relative comfort in a threatening environment.

Characteristic Behaviors   The following behaviors have been identified as hallmarks of the passive–aggressive style[2,5-7]
1. Procrastination and failure to meet deadlines
2. Stubbornness, especially refusal to compromise with loved ones and co-workers
3. Sullen, moody attitudes
4. Intentional inefficiency or chronic failure to do what is expected
5. Whining and chronic complaining, pessimism
6. Pseudo-compliance without follow through
7. Subtle antagonism, verbal and nonverbal oppositional behavior
8. Externalization of responsibility through blaming the establishment
9. Resentment of those who do not meet the client's needs
10. Fearfulness of authority figures
11. Failure to reach a consensus with others after lengthy group discussion, or sabotage of social and work group goals *after* verbal agreement

12. Failure to remember an assignment or social commitment
13. Avoidance of open hostility in self or others
14. Unconscious enjoyment of victimization
15. Helplessness when action is called for
16. Self-defeating behavior
17. Chronic lateness
18. Falling asleep at inappropriate times and places (for example, after client or someone else has started a heated discussion)
19. Socially annoying behavior such as putting on lipstick or filing nails during group therapy, spitting on others in conversation, driving an automobile below the speed limit in the fast lane of a commuter highway, excessive flatulence in groups, and other seemingly ''minor'' violations of etiquette

Nurses' Nonproductive
Reactions

Initially, the well-meaning nurse may not notice the passive–aggressive behavior as abnormal or provocative in view of the client's good reality testing. Nurses may even support it through their own passivity and mistakenly think that the client's complaints are valid, that this point of view warrants consideration, and that this behavior is ''seminormal.'' Sooner or later, depending upon the degree of the client's pathology, nurses catch on to the pattern of passive–aggressiveness, feel angry or resentful themselves, and defend against it as the client does. Initially, oversolicitousness of the client may be seen with well-meaning efforts at being empathic to cover up the direct expression of exasperation and hopelessness. Genuine empathy for the client's anger is lacking. As time goes on, it becomes clear to the nurse that these clients really do not know why or how they are so ''obnoxious'' to others. It is indeed difficult to believe that the client's behavior is not deliberate or intentional. As the pathology

---

Chart 44–1
NURSING INTERVENTIONS AND THEORETICAL RATIONALE WITH THE PASSIVE–AGGRESSIVE CLIENT

Nursing Intervention	*Theoretical Rationale*
1. Define responsibilities of both parties and avoid authoritarian attitudes.	1. Discourages artificially compliant behavior and resentment and guards against duplication of early pathologic relationships in which excessive demands were made with critical attitudes.
2. Provide a spontaneous, flexible attitude with a sense of humor.	2. Encourages genuineness in the client, who will be more likely to give up passive–aggressive behavior when the atmosphere is open and the nurse is not sitting in judgment.
3. Present active, directive approaches, rather than passive listening and nondirective approaches.	3. Encourages clients to be curious about themselves and diminishes indecisiveness and passivity.
4. Assist the client to identify and clarify feelings of irritation and resentment.	4. Unacknowledged and unexpressed anger is at the root of the client's difficulties in living.
5. Assist the client to express hostility openly when it is being shown passively.	5. Hostility that arises naturally in the relationship reduces the need for passive–aggressive responses over time, and more appropriate expressions of anger can be applied to the client's life. Artificially induced hostility will cause too much anxiety and may drive the client away.
6. Avoid arguments and driving interpretations when the client offers excuses for passive–aggressive behavior. Instead, explore feelings.	6. Arguments that force the client to ''see the light'' induce stubbornness, passive resistance and more passive–aggressive behavior.

becomes clearer, there is an emergence of new rules and regulations aimed at stopping the "slippery" passive–aggressive client. Typically, nurses themselves experience passive–aggressive, passive–dependent and aggressive–aggressive responses to the client, including

1. Moodiness and feelings of demoralization
2. Ambivalence toward the client
3. Feelings of discouragement and helplessness
4. Avoidance and withdrawal (may "work *around*" the client)
5. Excessive sympathy and "understanding"
6. Compliance to client's suggestions

Over time, anger, frustration, and ultimate exasperation may lead to acting out through

1. Argumentativeness
2. Excessive rules and regulations, which tend to be punitive
3. Severe confrontations of the behavior without exploration of its meaning (to make the client see the "light")
4. Care plans designed to artificially induce open anger and hostility in the client
5. Excessive labeling with psychiatric nomenclature
6. Assertiveness training for staff and client
7. Sadistic joking and humoring of the client
8. Threats of discharge from treatment or the less direct quiet transfer of the client

Nursing Interventions   Chart 44–1 shows the nursing interventions and theoretical rationale in work with passive–aggressive clients.

References

1. Diagnostic and Statistic Manual of Mental Disorders, 3rd ed. Washington, DC, American Psychiatric Association, 1980
2. Giovacchini P: Treatment of Primitive Mental States. New York, Aronson, 1979
3. Mahler MS et al: The Psychological Birth of the Human Infant. New York, Basic Books, 1975
4. Mullahy P: Psychoanalysis and Interpersonal Psychiatry: The Contributions of Harry Stack Sullivan. New York, Science House, 1970
5. Noyes AP, Kolb LC: Modern Clinical Psychiatry. Philadelphia, WB Saunders, 1961
6. Salzman L: The Obsessive Personality. New York, Aronson, 1973
7. Shapiro D: Neurotic Styles. New York, Basic Books, 1965
8. Zamora LC: The client who generates anger. In Haber J et al (eds): Comprehensive Psychiatric Nursing. New York, McGraw-Hill, 1978

45

The Client ─────────────
Who Is Anorexic ──────────

Marie C. Smith

OVERVIEW

Description
   Appearance
   Physiology
   Mood
   Behavior
Etiology
   Developmental Issues
   Premorbid Personality
   Dynamics
   Family Patterns
Nurses' Nonproductive Reactions
Interventions

*Description**   Anorexia nervosa was until recently considered a rare disease. The appearance of hospital treatment units that specialize in the care of these persons is one of many indications of the increased incidence of this life-threatening disorder.

Anorexia nervosa has been defined as a conscious and stubborn determination to emaciate the self despite the presence of an intense interest in food[5] and as a relentless pursuit of thinness.[1] Anorexia nervosa appears most frequently in prepubertal girls but may occur in late adolescence up to the early thirties.[4] Diagnostic criteria for anorexia nervosa are as follows[4]:

1. Intense fear of becoming obese, which does not diminish as weight loss progresses
2. Disturbance of body image, for example, claiming to ''feel fat'' even when emaciated
3. Weight loss of at least 25% of original body weight
4. Refusal to maintain body weight over a minimal normal weight for age and height
5. No known physical illness that would account for the weight loss

Clinical research conducted in the United States and Italy reveals international concern over the prevalence of the disorder as well as uniformity of symptoms and characteristic behaviors of these clients.[3,5] Some of the common symptoms of anorexia follow[1,5]:

A. APPEARANCE
　　1. Emaciation
　　2. Hollow face with sunken eyes
　　3. Lanugo on skin
　　4. Yellow tinge to skin
　　5. Dry hair, which may fall out

B. PHYSIOLOGY
　　1. Amenorrhea
　　2. Slow pulse
　　3. Decrease in body temperature
　　4. Constipation
　　5. Loss of appetite late in the disease
　　6. Death due to starvation or alteration in body chemistry

C. MOOD
　　1. Hyperactivity
　　2. Depersonalization
　　3. Inability to recognize feelings
　　4. Fear of becoming fat, but desire for food
　　5. Guilt after having eaten
　　6. View of life as a constant struggle with weight
　　7. Depression and suicidal thoughts
　　8. Separation anxiety

D. BEHAVIOR
　　1. Denial of hunger, thinness, or need for treatment
　　2. Calorie counting and preoccupation with recipes and exercise
　　3. Cooking for others, forcing family to eat
　　4. Overeating followed by vomiting

*The female pronouns will be used throughout, since most anorexics are female.

5. Stealing of food and money
6. Hoarding of food
7. Phobias about the scale
8. Use of laxatives, enemas, and diuretics
9. Refusal of food as a threat
10. Bizarre eating habits
11. Excessive dawdling over food
12. Lying, teasing, deceitfulness
13. Inability to separate from parents
14. Delusional denial of thinness
15. Pride in self denial
16. Striving for perfection
17. Demanding and bargaining behavior
18. Irritability and arrogance
19. Need to be special
20. Exhibitionism of thin figure
21. Private ecstatic experiences
22. Denial of ill health
23. Chronic devaluation of treatment team
24. Playing off dieticians, nurses, and physicians
25. Suicide attempts following forced weight gain

Etiology   The causes of this disorder and subsequent symptoms are complex and include developmental precursors, the parent–child relationship, the meaning of the symptoms for the client, and interactional patterns within the family. These are as follows:

A. DEVELOPMENTAL ISSUES[2,3,5]
1. Early feeding experiences were mechanical and rigid, and the mother usually did not enjoy feeding times.
2. Feeding schedules were superimposed by a dominant mother without an accurate estimate of the child's need for feeding, holding, and so forth.
3. Responses to the child's expressions of joy and physical tenderness were ignored and offered by the mother when *she* wished to express them.
4. Over time, control by the mother led to an inability in the child to recognize bodily sensations, or there was a mistrust of bodily sensations such as hunger, fatigue, body temperature, tactile pleasure, anxiety, bowel and bladder sensations, and sexual impulses and sensations.
5. The child did not learn to identify accurately, or to trust emotional states originating within herself nor to identify and differentiate between hunger and an empty stomach.
6. Initiative coming from the child in the growing years was overwhelmed by the parent and subject to correction and invalidation.
7. The child's experiences of the mother included the feelings of imperviousness, criticism, and overt and covert suggestions about "how one should feel."
8. Spontaneous and unique verbal expressions were questioned and disqualified consistently.
9. The child never had a genuine experience that could be called her own, such as bodily internal physiological states or emotional reciprocity.
10. A sense of body image identity was poorly formed, and there was considerable personality identity diffusion.

B. **PREMORBID PERSONALITY**

These children usually demonstrate the following:

1. Compliance, obedience, passivity, perfectionism, dependence, and obsessive neatness, leading them to be considered "the pride and joy of the family"
2. Intelligence and high achievement in school
3. Above average athletic ability
4. Serious attitude toward responsibility
5. Lack of a sense of humor
6. Superficial friendships, with the client assuming the follower role
7. Preferred friendship with one person at a time
8. Need to please others, especially parents and teachers
9. Guilt when expressing a wish
10. Acceptance of gifts graciously, pretense at liking the gift to please the giver
11. Generally a "goodie-goodie" attitude in one who remains quiet for fear of drawing unnecessary attention to herself

C. **DYNAMICS**

1. It is thought that the child experiences her growing body as an extension of her mother.[5]
2. The body comes to represent the bad mother image.
3. Putting food into the body causes it to grow and become overpowering as was the early experience of the mother.[5]
4. Continued dependency leads to ambivalence toward the mother and body. The child must therefore keep the body in control. The intent is not to destroy it but to keep it in check.[5]
5. The onset of puberty and adolescence, with bodily growth and psychological requirements, calls for strengths that are lacking. A search for an independent and separate identity is desperate and leads to a disidentification with the mother, and concretely, the body, which represents the mother.
6. The child feels incompetent, helpless, and ineffective in dealing with a new body and new social and emotional requirements.
7. Eating and not eating represent a struggle for control, which is seen as her only alternative in a search for identity and effectiveness—the opposite of previous robotlike childhood behavior.
8. Giving up food serves the singular goal of achieving autonomy and effectiveness through bizarre control of the body and its functions.
9. There is perpetual conflict between the dread of overweight and the greed for food.
10. There is a gross inability to understand or tolerate interpersonal difficulties as well as considerable feelings of incompetence when dealing with others. Interpersonal difficulties are dealt with by excessive starvation or binge eating and vomiting, deception, manipulation and secretiveness.

D. **FAMILY PATTERNS**[3]

1. The parents of anorexics are rarely divorced.
2. Anorexic clients usually come from middle class, upper class, and wealthy families.
3. Mothers have had careers and have given birth in their middle thirties.
4. The average number of children is 2.8, predominantly girls.
5. The anorexic child is overvalued by both parents.

Chart 45–1
PROBLEMS, INTERVENTIONS, AND RATIONALE WITH ANOREXIC CLIENTS

Problem	Intervention	Rationale
Malnutrition Dehydration Electrolyte imbalance	Provide nutritional restitution that is compatible with life.	One needs to eat to live. Starvation impairs psychological functioning, and learning cannot take place.
	a. Offer a choice of food from a hospital menu, or	a. The client experiences more control when given a choice of nutritious foods.
	b. Provide liquid diets, by mouth (1400–1800 calories), or	b. Some clients have a morbid fear of solid food.
	c. Provide tube feeding of liquid diet, or	c. This is used when the client has not been able to maintain or increase weight.
	d. Provide intravenous hyperalimentation	d. Restores electrolyte and fluid/nutritional balance with slow weight gain. Guilt for eating is minimized since client views this as "medication."
	Provide for weight gains of ¼–½ lb per day, or 3 lb per week.	Slow weight gains are less anxiety producing and more likely to be maintained. Weigh daily or weekly, depending on client's phobias regarding the scale.
	Maintain weight of at least 90–95 lb.	Client cannot tolerate normal weight without feeling "too fat." 90–95 pounds is considered to be the "out of danger" weight. This compromise is usually acceptable to clients after a brief period of therapy.
Client uses starvation to avoid facing deeper problems.	Provide exploratory and supportive interpersonal psychotherapy that uses a fact-finding approach as opposed to interpretive methods.[1,3]	This type of psychotherapy, over time, allows the client to discover impulses, feelings and needs that originate within her. It is thought that this learning about oneself helps repair cognitive and perceptual difficulties that started in childhood. Perceptions are examined to assist the client to discover differences in physiologic and emotional states. The interpretive analytic approach is not indicated because the lack of identity of these clients leads them to seek clues from the therapist about their identity, which they either take in and regurgitate or are suspicious of, since the interpretations come from outside of the self. The discovery of thoughts and impulses that originate within the self leads to autonomy, self assertion, and independence.[1]

Chart 45–1
(continued)

Problem	Intervention	Rationale
Family members harass client about eating.	Provide family therapy.	The family system of the anorexic is concerned with power and control of its members in addition to massive denial of parental conflicts. These conflicts are approached in family therapy, in which the parents are asked to focus on their problems and release the client from their persistent control.[1]

6. The child may have been given everything, including items not requested or desired.
7. Anorexic children tend to feel guilty about not being able to pay back the debt of the parents' generosity.
8. Intense involvement with the child's life comes from one or both parents who have great ambitions for the child.
9. Marital strife is seen but denied by parents.
10. Family members speak for one another as if they read each other's minds.
11. There is a lack of communicative matching and consensual validation between parent and child.
12. Closeness with the mother is symbiotic in families in which the father is passive.
13. Fathers express admiration and praise for the daughter's more masculine qualities, such as athletic abilities.
14. The child wants to live up to the family traditions and expectations.
15. Mothers are proud of the early care that they gave their infant daughters and tend to provide copious detailed reports of the child's growth and development.
16. Parents may be obsessed with the "body beautiful" image.
17. Corporal punishment is lacking, while strict eating patterns are enforced.
18. Refusal to eat becomes the focus of family conflict and a preoccupation for the entire family.
19. Power struggles are demonstrated at meal times.
20. The family actively deprives the child of the right to live and experience her own life.

Nurses' Nonproductive Reactions

The skin-clad skeleton appearance of the anorexic is terrifying and unforgettable. Nurses have marked emotional responses, based partly on the realistic fear that the client may die. Some of the responses which are understandable but not helpful include

1. Power struggles with the client over eating, which lead her and the staff to feel angry, frustrated, helpless, and ineffective. Power struggles reenact old familiar and pathologic family patterns.
2. Desperate need to rebuild the anorexic's body in a hurry. This approach may terrify the client, who will then lose more weight. Overzealous nutritional restitution may be interpreted as a "cure" without psychological change within the client. Some clients have attempted suicide after rapid weight gains.

3. Inconsistency in team approaches toward the client's deceitfulness about eating

4. Aggressive interpretation of the unconscious meaning of symptoms in order to make the client change. These interpretations are alien to the client, who feels intruded upon by the all-knowing therapist (mother).

5. Impatience at the client's dawdling over food.

6. Use of trickery, bribery, cajoling, force, and threats to get the client to eat, stimulating more deceitfulness and power struggles.

7. Anxiety in staff, leading to excessive vigilance toward the client, similar to the intrusive mother's vigilance.

8. Arguing and excessive limit setting in response to the client's devaluation of nurses.

9. Intimidation by the very fragile anorexic who seems to be "running the show," leading staff to support the pathology instead of change.

10. Splitting among staff, especially disciplines and nursing shifts, leading to chaos.

Interventions

Three main areas of intervention are necessary for the successful treatment of anorexia nervosa. They are nutritional restitution, psychological change in self-concept, and family intervention aimed at loosening pathologic interaction. Chart 45–1 outlines the problems, interventions, and rationale.

References

1. Bruch H: Eating disorders. New York, Basic Books, 1973
2. Bruch H: Obesity and anorexia nervosa. Psychosomatics 19:208, 1978
3. Bruch H: The Golden Cage. Cambridge, Harvard University Press, 1978
4. Diagnostic and Statistical Manual of Mental Disorders, 3rd ed. Washington, DC, American Psychiatric Association, 1980
5. Selvini-Palazzoli M: Anorexia nervosa. In Arieti S (ed): The World Biennial of Psychiatry and Psychotherapy, vol 1. New York, Basic Books, 1971

Bibliography

Ciseaux A: Anorexia nervosa: a view from the mirror. Am J Nurs 80:1468, 1980
Claggett MS: Anorexia nervosa: A behavioral approach. Am J Nurs 80:1471, 1980
Garfinkel PE, Garner DM: Anorexia Nervosa: A Multidimensional Perspective. New York, Brunner-Mazel, 1982
Goodstein RK: Eating and Weight Disorders: Advances in Treatment and Research. New York, Springer-Verlag, 1982
Grossniklaus DM: Nursing interventions in anorexia nervosa. Perspect Psychiatr Care 18:11, 1980
Richardson TF: Anorexia nervosa: An overview. Am J Nurs 80:1470, 1980

46

The Client
Who Has a Borderline
Personality Disorder

Marie C. Smith / Suzanne Lego

The behaviors that accompany anger, acting-out, self-destruction, and mutilation are seen in a number of clients, including those who are psychotic, neurotic, addicted, depressed, antisocial, and organically impaired, as well as in children, adolescents, adults, and the aged. However, when these behaviors are seen in combination and occur consistently in one client, the nurse is alerted to the possibility that the client has a borderline personality disorder.

Definition   This disorder has been defined as a specific and stable form of personality organization that lies between the neurosis and psychosis.[5] In other words, the client may at times look normal or neurotic but has had transient psychotic episodes. The client maintains reality testing when not under stress, but involvements with others are marked by a long history of difficult interpersonal relationships.

Etiology   Theoretical explanations about the early experiences of the client who is borderline are numerous, complex, and well documented.[4,7,8] In general, it is thought that the client's behavior and personality warp are in part caused by early difficulty separating emotionally from a significant parental figure (the mother or surrogate). While the tendency in a developing child is to grow and to develop an independent identity, there is an accompanying fear of "freedom" and a desire to remain with the mother. The mother in this case rewards the child's clinging behavior and withholds emotional support as the toddler begins to explore the immediate environment. The child learns to abandon the tendency to grow apart from the mother, and instead quickly returns to the mother with frightened, clingy behavior. The mother consistently responds positively to this clinging and negatively to independent behavior. The child develops a fear of moving away, and internal, unconscious rage.

In adulthood, reenactment of the separation–individuation conflict is seen in the form of clinging behavior; anger, rage, discomfort, and acting out when the urge to separate occurs; and depressive episodes, self-mutilation, and substance abuse when separation has occurred, either symbolically or by actual physical separation from a parent. The extreme discomfort of personality growth and change in positive directions is accompanied by "abandonment depression." It is believed that mourning of the loss of the mother must occur before one can become an adult and that acting out and defiance are defenses against the painful depression that must emerge.[8]

Description   Recent research has led to the following comprehensive description of the borderline client[9]:

A. **APPEARANCE AND BEHAVIOR**
    1. Appears less attractive than those of other diagnostic categories
    2. Behavior is not adaptive to interview
    3. Expresses angry feelings at variety of targets
    4. Is argumentative
    5. Devalues others
    6. Is overtly manipulative
    7. Is demanding
    8. Acts entitled
    9. Acts special
    10. Does inappropriate things
    11. Is irritable
    12. Is sarcastic

B. **MOOD**
   1. Reports feeling angry
   2. Reports feeling lonely
   3. Reports anhedonia

C. **SPEECH CONTENT**
   1. Lacks anxiety tolerance
   2. Has episodic depersonalization (feels strange or unreal)
   3. Has episodic derealization (the environment seems strange or unreal)
   4. Has chronic feelings of emptiness

D. **COGNITIVE PROCESSES**
   1. Reality testing is intact
   2. Seems bright, intelligent
   3. Demonstrates poor judgment
   4. Makes arbitrary or doubtful inferences from one thing to another

E. **PERSONAL HISTORY**
   1. Has had limited, transient psychotic episodes, which sometimes developed during psychotherapy or following intoxication
   2. Is generally impulsive and displays highly unpredictable behavior
   3. Has slashed wrists or mutilated self in other ways
   4. Abuses alcohol habitually or is addicted
   5. Reports unusual sexual behavior
   6. Lacks creative achievement, given ability
   7. Lacks creative enjoyment or recreation
   8. Has good scholastic abilities or potential, whether used or not
   9. Has one or several repetitive impulses that periodically erupt
   10. Has made suicide attempts which were deemed manipulative
   11. Displays a regressed behavior during hospitalization
   12. Has a history of discrete depressive episodes, hypomanic episodes, or undue elations
   13. Has been destructive to property or things

F. **INTERPERSONAL RELATIONSHIPS**
   1. Is manipulative, clinging, demanding, hostile, angry, ambivalent, controlling, exploitative, intense, unstable, sadistic, or masochistic in close relationships
   2. Seeks out others to *avoid* being alone rather than to *be* with the other
   3. Shows a lack of real concern or regard for others
   4. Has little capacity to evaluate others realistically
   5. Close relationships are typically transient and brief
   6. Has promiscuous sexual relationships

G. **DEFENSE MECHANISMS**
   1. Externalizes and acts out anger
   2. Acts impulsively when tensions from any source build up
   3. Sees others as hostile and dangerous
   4. When feeling hostile, accuses others of hostile feelings (projection)
   5. Expresses contradictory and unreconciled ideas of others, talking about them as all good or bad (splitting)

6. Uses bland denial when faced with contradictions in feelings or actions
7. Denies relevance of past feelings when opposite to current ones
8. Denies relevance of a sector of life that is obviously important
9. Talks as if omnipotent
10. Seems gratified by talking of alleged relationships with idealized people
11. Has distorted ideas and perceptions of others

H. **OTHER ASPECTS OF PERSONALITY**
1. Is emotionally shallow
2. Lacks a sense of own identity
3. Is not usually psychotic
4. Suggests grossly inappropriate treatment for self
5. Overreacts to minor external stressors
6. Is narcissistic, preoccupied with self
7. Is deficient in empathy for others
8. Has underlying feelings of inferiority and insecurity

Primitive Defenses and Clinical Examples

The anger, acting out, and self-destructive behavior seen in borderline clients is caused by primitive defenses. Table 46–1 shows these defenses and gives clinical examples of each.

Nurses' Nonproductive Reactions

A. **INDIVIDUAL REACTIONS**
The emotional intensity of the borderline client as well as the ability to intuitively strike at each staff member's "weak spots" have a profound effect on the nurse's treatment of the client. Some of the reactions of the nurse include[2,3]:
1. Feelings of massive responsibility for the client's welfare
2. Feelings of guilt because of failure to help the client
3. Omnipotent urges to rescue the client from the mishandling of others
4. Feelings of intense love and attachment to the client
5. Promises to keep secrets for the client as a token of trust and esteem
6. Feeling honored that the client "finally opened up"
7. Feeling highly confirmed in professional identity
8. Feeling highly repudiated in professional identity
9. Experiencing a need for excessively firm limits on the amount and quality of attention given to the client
10. Guilt by association with some value or person viewed as hostile by the client
11. Feelings of disappointment in one's work
12. Feelings of being emotionally drained to the extent that one's personal relationships suffer
13. Manifestations of the nurse's latent personality difficulties
14. Hostile acting out toward the clients by discharging them or resigning from the setting
15. Contempt, jealousy, and envy of the seeming "normal" client who manages to get considerable attention
16. Feelings of general paranoia and fear of the client's "next" projection
17. Feeling emotionally exposed and vulnerable because of the client's "part-true" projections
18. Defensiveness, counterattacking, rejection, and appeasement of the client
    In addition to setting off irrational reactions in individual nurses, these clients often set in motion group dynamics that are unusual and potentially destructive. The staff members may find that they begin to idealize the head nurse or clinical

Table 46–1
PRIMITIVE DEFENSES AND CLINICAL EXAMPLES

Defense	Definition	Clinical Example
Splitting	Active separation of affects of opposite quality so that one does not contaminate the other. Is differentiated from repression, ambivalence, and reaction formation, in which one affect is kept unconscious. In splitting, opposite affects remain conscious but separate.[5]	The client displays a clinging attitude toward one nurse and stormy, aggressive behavior with another. The client may plead to talk to only one person: "You're much nicer than those people on nights," or "You're the only nurse who really understands." Nurses are seen as all good or all bad. The same nurse may be seen alternately as good or bad.
Projective identification.	Primitive form of projection used to externalize aggressive feelings. Once projection has occurred, fear of the person is coupled with a desire to control the person.[5]	The client accuses the nurse of the strong aggressive feelings the client experiences: "You hate me just because I don't adore you like all the other patients do!"
Primitive idealization	Archaic form of intense idealization to protect the client from recognizing strong aggressive, angry tendencies toward one on whom the client is dependent	The client expresses strong, exaggerated positive feelings toward the nurse. "You're a wonderful person. Your children are sure lucky."
Omnipotence	Fantasies of greatness, which lead these clients to believe they need not adhere to the conventions others follow, and that they cannot be touched by illness, death, or the passing of time	When the client is confronted with impulsive or unconventional behavior just displayed he replies, "That's ridiculous! You don't know what you're talking about!" These clients often abuse drugs or make suicide attempts.
Devaluation	Consistent, exaggerated criticism designed to deflect the client and others from the client's strong feelings of inadequacy and insecurity	"You've made me much worse since I came here. Does anybody ever get well here?"
Denial	Unconscious shutting out of aspects of an experience, particularly feelings	"I was bored so I took a bottle of valium, drank some whiskey, and cut my wrists." Feelings that preceded the self-destructive behavior are not consciously available to the client.

coordinator, become dependent, compete with one another, develop coalitions and even sexual involvements with one another. This is because the daily intense bombardment of primitive material and behavior leads to regression and the eruption of primitive feelings in the staff.

Chart 46–1
PROBLEMS, INTERVENTIONS, AND RATIONALE WITH BORDERLINE CLIENTS

Problem	Intervention	Rationale
Splitting	1. The nurse recognizes the behavior as defensive, rather than feeling flattered by the positive feelings or destroyed by the negative, and remains neutral. The nurse does not attempt to stop the behavior outright, but rather explores the underlying feelings. *Client:* I'm so glad you're here today! or God, not you today! *Nurse:* You feel like you need a 'friend' today?	1. Splitting is a major defense against the client's intense aggressive and needy feelings. Prevention of the use of the defense would make the underlying feelings less available for exploration. When nurses become aware of the process and understand the meaning of splitting, the client becomes more comfortable with the intense underlying feelings.
	2. The nurse or therapist assigned to the client should not be changed according to the client's whim.	2. Firm limits are set so that the client is forced to face the feelings rather than run from them.
	3. Regularly scheduled staff meetings are held.	3. Each member brings a different experience of the client to the attention of the total group. When combined, these pieces of information help provide a total picture of the client that is more comprehensive than a picture given by a single staff member. The nurse's sense of having private knowledge and responsibility for the client is lessened so that individual nurses are relieved of the burden of being the "only" viable helper. The need to "rescue" the client from the other staff is diminished, as well as guilt resulting from not meeting the client's insatiable demands. Blaming of colleagues is diminished, and increased tolerance of the opinions of others emerges. Comprehensive treatment approaches are developed, individual members having full knowledge of their roles in the care of the client. Administrators and clinicians are less likely to work at cross-purposes. A split staff is detrimental to clients who have part identity and splitting problems.[2]
Projection	1. The nurse recognizes the part of the client's accusation that is a projection, notes the underlying feeling, and questions that: *Client:* You certainly are an angry person. How'd they ever let you into the nursing profession? *Nurse:* How come you're so mad at me today?	1. Rather than engage the client in a power struggle over who was angry first, the nurse moves straight to the client's feeling. Over time, as the nurse readily accepts the client's anger, the client is able to do the same and to explore it further.
	2. The nurse recognizes the part of the accusation that is a half-truth and acknowledges it: *Client:* You treat me differently from the others: You're more strict with me and you get mad. *Nurse:* You're right. I think you need to know exactly what we expect of you. Sometimes your behavior does make me mad.	2. As the nurse is able to acknowledge and accept responsibility for her own behavior and feelings, the client will do the same. The client can see anger communicated in a nondestructive way, rather than acted out destructively.
	3. The nurse encourages the client to explore feelings and experiences instead of making interpretations of the client's behavior.	3. Correct interpretations tend to create a feeling of distance, inferiority, and unconscious envy of the nurse.[3]
Anger and acting out	1. In a nonpunitive way, the nurse a. Tells the client to stop the behavior and to talk about the feeling b. Offers empathic statements c. Clarifies what has happened d. Provides safety for all clients	1. Provides temporary ego boundaries, assists with impulse control, helps client delay gratification, inhibits self-destruction and violence, helps client to talk about feelings, helps client to work cooperatively and to gain self-understanding[1]

Chart 46–1
(continued)

Problem	Intervention	Rationale
	2. If these measures fail, the nurse provides medication, restraint, or seclusion. Once these measures are started, they are followed to completion.	2. Assists the client to regain control, prevents violence, provides safety. Premature release from restraint or seclusion causes anxiety and may lead to a sudden escalation of violent behavior. The implicit message of ambivalent use of restraint or seclusion is that the nurse is insecure and not in control. This terrifies the client.
	3. Secluded or restrained clients are observed at all times.	3. The client often suffers remorse and humiliation over having lost control. The incidence of suicide is great following a violent act.
Self-mutilation	1. The nurse provides first aid.	1. Prevents further loss of function and treats the injury
	2. The nurse encourages discussion of thoughts and feelings that preceded the act.	2. Most self-destructive behavior follows a real or fantasied disappointment. All disappointments must be discussed because these clients are chronically disappointed with life.
	3. The nurse avoids elaborate focusing on the injury itself.	3. Once the injury is treated, avoidance of discussing it prevents unnecessary development of secondary gains. When self-mutilation is deemed manipulative, healthier ways of getting attention are encouraged. Discussion and oversolicitous care of the wound serve as a defense against what the client was actually thinking and feeling.
Serious suicide attempts	Interventions are the same for all suicidal clients (see Chap. 43).	

B. **GROUP REACTIONS**

Specifically, the splitting and massive projections from clients may lead to the following group behaviors[2,6]:

1. Diagnostic uncertainty with contradictory evaluations of clients occurs.
2. Groups of staff members may feel emotionally isolated from one another.
3. Two or more staff members may become suspicious of the motives and behavior of other staff members toward the client.
4. Lunch-hour and coffee-break time may be dominated by discussion of specific clients.
5. The nucleus of an in-group may believe that they are the only ones who can help the client.
6. Loss of morale and confusion may be seen in the "out group."
7. Staff cleavage with excessive clash of opinions is seen by outside observers.
8. Blurring of staff–client role boundaries is seen in many forms (for example, client and staff discuss another staff member, or staff share personal information with the client).
9. Split in- and out-groups make the following accusations:
   a. "Ins" accuse "outs" of being cold and insensitive.
   b. "Outs" accuse "ins" of being too permissive and gullible and of spoiling the client.
10. Splits between departments in a hospital structure may be seen.
11. Administrative decisions to change the client's therapist occur when the therapist is part of the "bad" split.

| *Interventions* | Intervention with these clients involves concerted efforts to deal effectively with splitting and projection, to diminish the acting out of anger and self-destructive behavior, and to promote the beginning of new, more mature, and genuinely independent ways of relating with others. Chart 46–1 lists problems, interventions, and rationale. |

| *References* | 1. Adler G: Hospital treatment of borderline patients. Am J Psychiatry 130:1, 1973 |

2. Burnham DL: The special problem patient: Victim or agent of splitting? Psychiatry J Stud Interpers Proc 29:2, 1966
3. Epstein L: Countertransference with borderline patients. In Epstein L, Feiner AH (eds): Countertransference. New York, Aronson, 1979
4. Hartocollis P: Borderline Personality Disorders. New York, International Universities Press, 1977
5. Kernberg OF: Borderline Conditions and Pathological Narcissism. New York, Aronson, 1975
6. Kernberg OF: Leadership and organizational functioning: Organization regression. Int J Group Psychother 28:1, 1978.
7. Mahler MS: The Psychological Birth of the Human Infant. New York, Basic Books, 1975
8. Masterson JF: Intensive psychotherapy of the adolescent with a borderline syndrome. In Arieti S (ed): The American Handbook of Psychiatry. New York, Basic Books, 1974
9. Perry C, Klerman GL: Clinical features of the borderline personality disorder. Am J Psychiatry 137:2, 1980

Bibliography

Adler G, Buie DH: Aloneness and borderline psychopathology. Int J Psychoanal 60:83, 1979

Carser D: The defense mechanism of splitting: Developmental origins, effect on staff, recommendations for nursing care. J Psychiatr Nurs 17:21, 1979

Groves J: Borderline personality disorder. N Engl J Med 305:259, 1981

Herron WG: The borderline problem. Perspect Psychiatr Care 15:72, 1977

Hickey BA: Transitional relatedness and engaging the regressed, borderline client. J Psychosoc Nurs 21:26, 1983

Kerr N: The destruction of goodness in borderline character pathology. Perspect Psychiatr Care 17:40, 1979

Kerr N: Pathological narcissism. Perspect Psychiatr Care 18:29, 1980

LeBoit J, Capponi A: Advances in Psychotherapy of the Borderline Patient. New York, Aronson, 1979

Lego S: Treatment of the acting out borderline patient in private practice, clinical and scientific sessions, 1979. Kansas City, American Nurses Association, 1979

Lynch VJ, Lynch MT: Borderline personality. Perspect Psychiatr Care 15:72, 1977

MacVicar K: Splitting and identification with the aggressor in assaultive borderline patients. Am J Psychiatr 135:229, 1978

Mark B: Hospital treatment of borderline patients: Toward a better understanding of problematic issues. J Psychiatr Nurs 18:25, 1980

Masterson JF: The Narcissistic and Borderline Disorders: An Integrated Developmental Approach. New York, Brunner–Mazel, 1981

Maynard CK, Chitty KK: Dealing with anger: Guidelines for nursing intervention. J Psychiatr Nurs 17:36, 1979

Nadelson T: Borderline rage and the therapist's response. Am J Psychiatry 134:748, 1977

Platt-Koch LM: Borderline personality disorder: A therapeutic approach. Am J Nurs 83:1666, 1983

Searles H: Some aspects of separation and loss in psychoanalytic therapy with borderline patients. In Giovacchini P, Boyer LB (eds): Technical Factors in the Treatment of the Severely Disturbed Patient. New York, Aronson, 1982

47

The Client Who Is Addicted to Alcohol

Linda Barile

	The client is considered to be addicted to alcohol when there is either a pattern of

Introduction   The client is considered to be addicted to alcohol when there is either a pattern of pathologic use or impairment in social or occupational functioning due to alcohol and either tolerance or withdrawal.[2]

Although alcoholism is a disease in itself, it is often seen with other categories of mental illness. Borderline clients often abuse alcohol, as do schizophrenics, seeking quick relief from anxiety.

Etiology   Alcoholism is currently viewed as a multilevel problem with no single causative factor. The following factors, in concert, appear to contribute to alcoholism[1]:

A. **BIOLOGIC FACTORS**
   There is strong evidence that alcoholism is either inherited as a physical trait or as a predisposition.

B. **PSYCHOLOGICAL THEORIES[6]**
   Generally, it is believed that alcoholics experienced early childhood rejection, overprotection, and premature responsibility, resulting in excessive dependency. This dependency cannot be met in reality; consequently, the alcoholic feels rejection. This rejection leads to feelings of anxiety, which are dealt with by a number of defense mechanisms, particularly denial and grandiosity. The grandiosity causes the individual to try harder but this only results in inevitable failure and increases the anxiety, depression, anger, and guilt. Alcohol initially reduces these intolerable feelings and induces feelings of power and omnipotence, thus reinforcing the denial and grandiosity. Over time, the alcoholic behavior itself causes anxiety, guilt, shame, remorse, and self-hatred as the self-enhancing effects of alcohol lessen.[6]

C. **SOCIAL FORCES[1]**
   Alcoholism is higher among Catholics, and certain national groups, suggesting that cultural patterns are involved. For example, in France and the United States, drinking is considered ''macho'' behavior among men. In general, alcoholism is higher in societies that sanction the use of alcohol to feel better or in societies that have considerable ambivalence about the use of alcohol. Alcoholism among American women has increased considerably, and has been tied to stress, anxiety, and depression.

Description   Clients addicted to alcohol may display any of the following behaviors[2,3,5,6]:
   1. Physiological dependence evidenced by tolerance (increased amounts of substance needed to get the desired effect or decreased effect with the same amount of alcohol) or by withdrawal
   2. Impairment of physical and psychological functioning
   3. Decreased social or occupational functioning leading to a loss of friends, family, or job and criticism from significant others
   4. Obsession with alcohol[3]
   5. Sneaking of alcohol[3]
   6. Safeguarding the supply of alcohol[3]
   7. Nonintentional use[3]
   8. Use of alcohol to produce altered mood[3]
   9. Blackouts, that is, temporary amnesia or a permanent and complete loss of memory for a given time[3]
   10. Loss of control over alcohol use. The client must have alcohol after a period of nonuse

11. Use of defense mechanisms to justify alcohol use
12. Anxiety, fears, remorse
13. Resentments
14. Antisocial behavior, that is erratic, impulsive, aggressive, abusive behavior, sometimes leading to legal difficulties
15. Omnipotence, grandiosity, narcissism[5]
16. Poor frustration tolerance[5]
17. A tendency to do things in a hurry[5]

Chart 47–1

NURSING INTERVENTIONS AND THEORETICAL RATIONALE WITH THE CLIENT WHO HAS ACUTE ALCOHOL INTOXICATION[4]

Nursing Intervention	*Theoretical Rationale*
Physiological Stability	
1. Assess safety needs and provide for protection and necessary restrictions.[4]	1–2. Clients who are acutely intoxicated represent a real physical threat to themselves and sometimes others owing to unsteady motor behavior and impulsive behavior.
2. Assess degree of intoxication in client to determine safe and appropriate care.[4]	
3. Check vital signs at indicated intervals.[4]	3–5. Clients may go into shock, seizures, coma, and death due to alcohol withdrawal. Withdrawal can last from 6 hours to 7 days.
4. Administer medical orders for acute intoxication as prescribed.[4]	
5. Report any unusual findings and follow up. An increase in blood pressure, pulse over 100 beats per minute, and temperature above 100°F may indicate impending delerium tremens.[4]	
6. Ascertain duration of drinking episode, time, and amount of last drink, drinking pattern, and history, if possible.[4]	6. It is important to know the extent of alcohol use and physical effects (for example, to liver, esophagus, and stomach) to plan for care.
Treat the Delirium Tremens (DTs)	
1. Ascertain whether client has history of DTs.[4]	1–2. If client has had DTs before, steps can be taken to reduce discomfort by giving medication.
2. Observe for symptoms of impending or current DTs, such as increased pulse, blood pressure, and temperature, increased tremors, excitement, anxiety, increased disorientation, hallucinations, rigidity, and convulsions.[4]	
3. Administer medications as prescribed and observe response.[4]	3. Sedation reduces discomfort. Librium and other minor tranquilizers have been proven effective.
4. Provide oral fluids.	4. Clients often become dehydrated during DTs.
5. Reduce stimuli by placing client in a partially lighted room. Talk in a calming voice.	5. Clients are often very frightened.
6. Provide physical protection and restraint, as needed.[4]	6. Restraints will prevent client from harming self.
7. If necessary, transfer client to a more secure ward.[4]	7. Provides safety
Help Client to Become Aware of and Accept Alcoholism as a Disease	
1. Maintain nonjudgmental attitude. Avoid either negative or positive judgments.[4]	1. Negative judgments increase client's feelings of guilt and self-degradation, which are not productive. Positive judgments reinforce client's denial.
2. Provide for client contact at regular specified intervals.[4]	2. Avoidance of the client increases his negative self-appraisal and self-pity.
3. Help the client recognize how alcohol use has interfered with having a satisfying life.	3. Treatment cannot progress until the client recognizes and accepts that he has a disease.
4. Identify and point out defense mechanisms concerning the alcohol use.	4. Helps the client recognize and accept that he has a disease requiring treatment. Confronts the alcohol use early in treatment when the memory of the alcoholic episodes is alive and defenses have not rebuilt.
5. Help the client accept the fact that he cannot tolerate alcohol in any amount.	5. Total abstinence is the only way to control alcoholism. Belief in controlled use is a poor prognostic sign.[6]

Chart 47–2
NURSING INTERVENTIONS AND THEORETICAL RATIONALE WITH CHRONIC ALCOHOLIC CLIENTS

Nursing Intervention	*Theoretical Rationale*

Encourage Client to Make a Commitment to Treatment

1. Explain program and treatment plan and have client sign treatment contract upon admission.[4]
2. Use a concerned, nonjudgmental, matter-of-fact approach in exploring problems related to use of alcohol.[4]
3. Test for alcohol content with random urine samples.[4]
4. Provide professional instruction on physical, psychological, social, and economic effects of alcohol.[4]
5. Give client a written test before discharge.[4]

1. Commitment in writing increases chances of follow through.
2. The client is helped to see alcoholism in a practical, straightforward way rather than as a moral problem.
3. Ensures that staff know if client is not following treatment contract.
4. Helps client to make a decision about using alcohol.
5. Helps staff to know what information the client still lacks.

Help Client to Form Positive Relationships

1. Confront manipulative behavior; maintain frequent communication with staff to validate impressions of manipulative behavior.[4]
2. Assist in identifying and clarifying needs of self and others. Focus on here and now.[4]
3. Define staff expectations and consequences of noncompliance whenever client is manipulative.[4]

1. This helps clients to confront their own behavior and reduces staff frustration.
2. These clients are often self-involved. They are surprised to know that others have needs. Others respond positively when clients become more sensitive.
3. Same as #1

Help Client to Confront Frustration and Anxiety in Constructive Ways

1. Have clients attend group meetings twice weekly.[4]
2. Assist clients to identify ways of dealing with feelings, particularly anger, in ways other than by drinking. Schedule clients to participate in tension-relieving activities.[4]
3. Present lectures on alternatives for dealing with stress, including relaxation techniques.[4]

1. Provides an atmosphere for clients to discuss current feelings and maintain control under stress.
2. If clients learn to handle frustration more effectively, drinking will not be necessary.
3. If clients learn to prevent stress or handle it effectively when it occurs, they will be less likely to drink.

Prevent Depression and Suicide

1. Observe and protect as needed according to the severity of depression; consider move to locked ward.[4]
2. Help client to express anger openly, rather than turning it inward.
3. Encourage client to participate in social activities and daily exercise.

1. Chronic alcoholics are at high risk for suicide.
2. Open expression of anger obviates depression.
3. These reduce depression and raise self-esteem.

Help Client Solve Socioeconomic Problems

1. Assist client to identify problems related to family or significant others.[4]
2. Help client plan for alternative living arrangements if separation from family is imminent.
3. Help client learn to socialize and have fun without alcohol by attending social activities.
4. Explore options client has when offered a drink in social situations.
5. Refer client who is unemployed for vocational counseling.

1. When clients become aware of the effects of their drinking on others, they may be further motivated to stop drinking.
2. Otherwise, client may start drinking when discharged without a home.
3–4. Helps clients accept life without alcohol.
5. Work may provide satisfactions that replace alcohol.

Assist with Discharge Planning

1. Refer clients to Alcoholics Anonymous (AA). Have them begin to attend meetings before discharge.
2. Refer families of clients to Alanon and Alateen.
3. Involve the family and client actively in plans following discharge.

1. AA has proved to be very useful in continuous treatment of alcoholism.
2. These have proved helpful in providing support for families and, in turn, the alcoholic.
3. Full involvement in planning increases follow through.

18. Low self-esteem
19. Either a proneness to feel guilt or no guilt feelings at all[6]
20. Depression
21. Suicide attempts or completed suicide
22. Dependency and passivity
23. Passive, aggressive, or passive–aggressive behavior
24. Manipulative behavior
25. Demanding and critical behavior
26. Obsessive–compulsive behavior[6]
27. Perfectionism or rigidity[6]
28. A need to maintain control[6]
29. The inability to recognize, express, and accept feelings, particularly anger
30. Sexual problems

Nurses' Nonproductive Reactions

Some nurses find it very difficult to work with alcoholics. This is particularly true when the client displays provocative, manipulative, hostile, testing, or dependent behavior. It is also true when nurses view the drinking as "normal" owing to their own values regarding alcohol.

When the client is resistive to recovery and is repeatedly readmitted for detoxification, nurses respond with anxiety, frustration, anger, criticism, avoidance, rejection, moral judgments, guilt, or authoritative behavior. The nurse may feel unrewarded and hopeless about the client.

Nurses who have been raised in families with alcoholics or are married to alcoholics are particularly vulnerable to these feelings. The appearance of the alcoholic out of control may evoke painful early memories.

Nursing Interventions

Chart 47–1 shows nursing interventions and theoretical rationale in the care of clients with acute alcohol intoxication. Chart 47–2 shows interventions and rationale in the care of clients with chronic alcoholism.[4]

References

1. Chafetz ME et al: Alcoholism: A positive view. In Arieti S (ed): American Handbook of Psychiatry, vol 3, 2nd ed. New York, Basic Books, 1974
2. Diagnostic and Statistical Manual of Mental Disorders, 3rd ed. Washington, DC, American Psychiatric Association, 1980
3. Heilman R: Early Recognition of Alcoholism and Other Drug Dependence, Center City, MN, Hazelton Foundation, 1973
4. Kurose K et al: A standard care plan for alcoholism. Am J Nurs 81:1001, 1981
5. Tiebout H: The Act of Surrender in the Therapeutic Process. Q J Stud Alcohol 10:48, 1949
6. Zimberg S et al: Practical Approaches to Alcoholism Psychotherapy. New York, Plenum Press, 1978

Bibliography

Adams-Woodward C; Wernicke-Korsacoff syndrome: A case approach. J Psychiatr Nurs 16:38, 1978
Bakdash D: Essentials the nurse should know about chemical dependency. J Psychiatr Nurs 16:33, 1978
Bragg TL: Teen-age alcohol abuse. J Psychiatr Nurs 14:10, 1976
Carruth GR, Pugh JB: Grieving the loss of alcohol: A crisis in recovery. J Psychosoc Nurs 20:18, 1982
Cornish RD, Miller MV: Attitudes of registered nurses toward the alcoholic. J Psychiatr Nurs 14:19, 1976
Corrigan EM: Alcoholic Women in Treatment. Oxford, Oxford University Press, 1980
Davidhizor R, Gunden E: Recognizing and caring for the delirious patient. J Psychiatr Nurs 16:38, 1978
Gareri EA: Assertiveness training for alcoholics. J Psychiatr Nurs 17:31, 1979
Gibson DE: Reminiscence, self-esteem, and self–other satisfaction in adult male alcoholics. J Psychiatr Nurs 18:7, 1980
Janosik E: Reachable and teachable: Report on a prison alcoholism group. J Psychiatr Nurs 15:24, 1977
Kinney J: Loosening the Grip: A Handbook of Alcohol Information. St Louis, CV Mosby, 1978
McCabe TR: Victims No More. Center City, MN, Hazelden Books, 1978
Marks VL: Health teaching for recovering alcoholic patients. Am J Nurs 80:2058, 1980

Morton PC: Assessment and management of the self-destructive concept of alcoholism. J Psychiatr Nurs 17:8, 1979

Pugh JB: My love: The story of an addiction. J Psychosoc Nurs 20:22, 1982

Vaillant GE: The Natural History of Alcoholism. Causes, Patterns, and Paths to Recovery. Cambridge, MA, Harvard University Press, 1983

Valentine NM: Women and alcoholism: A bibliography. J Psychiatr Nurs 14:23, 1976

Van Gee SJ: Alcoholism and the family: A psychodrama approach. J Psychiatr Nurs 17:9, 1979

Zimberg S: The Clinical Management of Alcoholism. New York, Brunner/Mazel, 1982

48

The Client Who Is Abusing
Toxic Substances
Other than Alcohol

Marie C. Smith

OVERVIEW

Description
Symptoms of Intoxication and Withdrawal
Nurses' Nonproductive Reactions
Intervention

Description Substance abuse is determined by three major criteria: a pattern of pathologic use, impairment in social or occupational functioning caused by the pathologic use of the substance, and duration of use.[2] Each is considered separately:

A. **A PATTERN OF PATHOLOGIC USE**
    A pattern of pathologic use refers to continuous or frequent intoxication with the substance; an inability to reduce intake; efforts to control use to specified times; continuation of use despite known physical contraindications; the daily need for the substance in order to function, which is followed by intoxication.[2]

B. **IMPAIRMENT IN SOCIAL OR OCCUPATIONAL FUNCTIONING CAUSED BY THE PATHOLOGIC USE OF THE SUBSTANCE**
    Impairment in social or occupational functioning refers to any disturbance in family or social relationships and may include difficulty with the law. It also refers to any difficulties arising in work or school as a result of substance abuse.[2]

C. **DURATION**
    "Abuse" requires that the disturbance last at least *1 month*. Use does not have to be continuous throughout a given month but must be frequent enough within a month's time to cause noticeable difficulties in social and occupational functioning.[2]

(Text continues on page 434)

Table 48–1
SYMPTOMS OF INTOXICATION WITH AND WITHDRAWAL FROM TOXIC SUBSTANCES THAT ARE ABUSED[2]

Substance	*Intoxication*	*Withdrawal*
Barbiturates, tranquilizers, hypnotics	1. Mood lability 2. Disinhibition of sexual and aggressive impulses 3. Irritability 4. Loquacity 5. Slurred speech 6. Incoordination 7. Unsteady gait 8. Impairment of attention or memory 9. Impaired social judgment	Recent cessation of heavy use: 1. Nausea and vomiting 2. Autonomic hyperactivity (*e.g.*, tachycardia, sweating, elevated blood pressure) 3. Anxiety 4. Depressed mood or irritability 5. Orthostatic hypotension 6. Coarse tremor of hands, tongue, eyelids Delirium may occur within 1 week after cessation of heavy use.

Opioids
  Heroin
  Morphine
  Meperidine
  Methadone
	1. Pupillary constriction
	2. Pupillary dilation due to anoxia from severe overdose
	3. Euphoria
	4. Dysphoria
	5. Apathy
	6. Psychomotor retardation
	7. Drowsiness
	8. Slurred speech
	9. Impairment of attention or memory
	10. Impaired social judgment
		Recent cessation of heavy use or administration of a narcotic antagonist following a brief period of use:
		  1. Lacrimation
		  2. Rhinorrhea
		  3. Piloerection
		  4. Sweating
		  5. Diarrhea
		  6. Yawning
		  7. Mild hypertension
		  8. Tachycardia
		  9. Fever
		  10. Insomnia
		  11. Pupillary dilation

Table 48–1
(continued)

Substance	Intoxication	Withdrawal
Cocaine	Within 1 hour of use: 1. Psychomotor agitation 2. Elation 3. Grandiosity 4. Loquacity 5. Hypervigilance 6. Tachycardia 7. Pupillary dilation 8. Elevated blood pressure 9. Perspiration or chills 10. Nausea and vomiting Overdose: 1. Syncope 2. Chest pain 3. Seizures 4. Death may result from cardiac and respiratory failure.	None known Full recovery is seen within 24 hours of last dose

Amphetamine
Speed
Diet pills
	Within 1 hour of use:
	1. Psychomotor agitation
	2. Elation
	3. Grandiosity
	4. Loquacity
	5. Hypervigilance
	7. Tachycardia
	8. Pupillary dilation
	9. Elevated blood pressure
	10. Perspiration or chills
	11. Nausea and vomiting
		1. Long-term use of high doses yields a rapidly developing delusional syndrome following cessation, characterized by:
		  a. Persecutory delusions
		  b. Ideas of reference
		  c. Aggressiveness and hostility
		  d. Anxiety
		  e. Psychomotor agitation
		2. Prolonged heavy use yields a withdrawal syndrome following 2–4 days cessation with:
		  a. Depressed mood
		  b. Fatigue
		  c. Increased dreaming

Phencyclidine (PCP, "angel dust," "crystal"), Tetrahydrocannabinol (THC)	Within 1 hour of use: 1. Vertical or horizontal nystagmus 2. Increased blood pressure and heart rate 3. Numbness or diminished response to pain 4. Ataxia 5. Dysarthria 6. Euphoria 7. Psychomotor agitation 8. Marked anxiety 9. Emotional lability 10. Grandiosity 11. Sensation of slowed time 12. Synesthesias—seeing colors when a loud sound is heard. 13. Suicide has been reported.	None known
LSD, DMT, mescaline	Hallucinogen hallucinosis: 1. Perceptual changes occurring in a state of full wakefulness (*e.g.*, subjective intensification of perceptions,	None known

(continued)

Table 48–1
(continued)

Substance	Intoxication	Withdrawal
	depersonalization, derealization, illusions, hallucinations, synesthesias) 2. Pupillary dilation 3. Tachycardia 4. Sweating 5. Palpitations 6. Tremors 7. Uncoordination 8. Ideas of reference 9. Fear of losing one's mind 10. Impaired judgment	
Cannabis, marijuana, hashish, (THC)	1. Tachycardia 2. Euphoria 3. Subjective intensification of perceptions 4. Sensation of slowed time 5. Apathy 6. Conjunctival injection 7. Increased appetite 8. Dry mouth 9. Excessive anxiety 10. Impaired judgment	None known.
Tobacco	None known	When use of tobacco occurs for at least several weeks at a level of more than 10 cigarettes per day, containing at least 0.5 mg nicotine, cessation is followed within 24 hours by: a. Craving for tobacco b. Irritability c. Anxiety d. Difficulty concentrating e. Restlessness f. Headache g. Drowsiness h. Gastrointestinal disturbances
Caffeine	Consumption of caffeine in excess of 250 mg. (1 cup of coffee contains 100–150 mg caffeine): 1. Restlessness 2. Nervousness 3. Excitement 4. Insomnia 5. Flushed face 6. Diuresis 7. Gastrointestinal complaints 8. Muscle twitching 9. Rambling flow of thought and speech 10. Cardiac arrhythmia 11. Periods of inexhaustability 12. Psychomotor agitation	None known.

Chart 48–1
PRESENTING PROBLEMS, NURSING INTERVENTIONS, AND RATIONALE WITH CLIENTS WHO ABUSE DRUGS

Presenting Problem	Intervention	Rationale

1. Overdose:
Barbiturates
Heroin
Cocaine
Amphetamine
	1. Frequently observe and record vital signs (B/P, TPR, Neuro). Support breathing. Observe and record seizure activity. Physically support head and limbs during seizure, maintaining patent airway. Monitor urinary output and save specimens for drug screening.	1. Clients who are intoxicated or who have overdosed on these drugs have placed cardiopulmonary functions in jeopardy either by the direct effect of the drug or by its effect on the central nervous system. Cocaine has been known to cause seizures and sudden death. Amphetamine has been known to cause cerebral vascular accidents. Heroin has caused death from "wet lung syndrome".[3] The symptoms of pulmonary edema are
		    Anxiety and restlessness
		    Gray complexion
		    Cold, moist hands
		    Cyanotic nail beds
		    Incessant coughing
		    Noisy and moist breathing[3]

2. Intoxication in the ambulatory abuser who is Anxious Agitated Paranoid Having "out of body experiences" Synesthetic Hallucinating Fearful of losing his mind	2. Do not give psychotropic medication even if the client was taking it regularly. Sedation may be used once the abused substance is known. Reduce stimuli by placing client in a partially lighted room. Maintain one-to-one contact. Orient client to reality. Speak slowly, clearly, and in a low voice. Avoid loud noise.	2. The addition of psychotropic medication may further depress the central nervous system or cause paradoxical reactions when mixed with the abused substance. The major and minor tranquilizers have been used successfully for "bad trips" on LSD and PCP. Dimly lighted rooms have a calming effect, whereas fluorescent lighting increases agitation. Clients respond to reality orientation and become aware that the distress is due to the drug and not to psychosis. Noise produces color "rushes" in LSD users.

3. Nursing and medical intervention has restored the client's equilibrium, and the client is anxious to "get back on the street."	3. Educate clients about the hazards of drug abuse:
	    Use the client's past experiences with drugs.
	    Use the recent experience in the hospital.
	    Provide resource materials, names of agencies, and telephone numbers of locations where further assistance is available.
	    Do not threaten clients with police action.
		3. The best time to make the most of educational approaches is when the client's bad experiences are fresh in the mind.
		
		This approach will sabotage any educational efforts and will discourage the client from seeking treatment in the future.

4. A particular client is a chronic repeater and has not responded to educational approaches.	4. Assume that the client has serious psychological problems:
	    Provide psychological treatment,
	        or
	    Assist the client in locating a therapist or other community resources.
		4. The client's life depends upon willingness and ability to use psychotherapy.

Substance abuse is seen in the ''normal'' population, in which a variety of drugs are used for recreational purposes, as well as in persons suffering serious psychiatric difficulties. For example, persons with personality disorders and affective disorders are known to abuse substances to reduce anxiety and depression.

Symptoms of Intoxication and Withdrawal

Table 48–1 identifies the most frequently abused substances and the symptoms of intoxication and withdrawal.[2]

Nurses' Nonproductive Reactions

While nurses may identify with and have sympathy for the caffeine and tobacco addict, responses to hard-core drug abusers may not be as sympathetic. Substance abusers, and in particular repeat substance abusers, are subject to the disdain of many nurses. A client who has overdosed on heroin, LSD, or amphetamine is often viewed with disapproval, intolerance, moralistic condemnation, and a tendency to see the client as morally weak.[4] In addition, the manipulative behavior often seen in these clients leads nurses to feel angry and exploited.

In some cities, the recreational use of cocaine, cannabis, and speed is so common that the nurse may view the occurrence of intoxication or overdose as ''rather normal'' and may not have much emotional reaction. This attitude is as detrimental as strong disapproval because the nurse forgets the importance of supportive measures and client education and the need for follow-up psychotherapeutic intervention.

Intervention

Presenting problems, suggested nursing interventions, and their rationale appear in Chart 48–1.

References

1. Brunner LS et al: Textbook of Medical Surgical Nursing, 2nd ed. Philadelphia, JB Lippincott, 1970
2. Diagnostic and Statistical Manual of Mental Disorders, 3rd ed. Washington, DC, American Psychiatric Association, 1980
3. Wendkos MH: Sudden Death and Psychiatric Illness. New York, SP Medical and Scientific Books, 1979
4. Zamora LC: The client who generates anger. In Haber J et al (eds): Comprehensive Psychiatric Nursing. New York, McGraw-Hill, 1978

Bibliography

Bakdash D: Essentials the nurse should know about chemical dependency. J Psychiatr Nurs 16:33, 1978
Betemps E: Management of the withdrawal syndrome of barbiturates and other central nervous system depressants. J Psychosoc Nurs 19:31, 1981
Glatt MM: Drug Dependence: Current Problems and Issues. Baltimore, Baltimore University Press, 1977
Ray O: Drugs, Society, and Human Behavior. St Louis, CV Mosby, 1982
Vourakis C, Bennett G: Angel dust—Not heaven sent. Am J Nurs 79:649, 1979
Walker L: Coping with drug abuse by children of the wealthy: A new high-risk group. Perspect Psychiatr Care 20:65, 1982

49

The Client Who Is Organically Brain Damaged

Marie C. Smith

OVERVIEW

Description
Symptoms
Client's Emotional Responses to Deficits
Nurses' Nonproductive Reactions
Interventions

Description   Organic brain damage is diagnosed whenever there is psychological or behavioral abnormality associated with transient or permanent dysfunction of the brain.[1] Clients with organic mental disorders demonstrate a wide variety of symptoms with varying degrees of severity. The differences seen in the clinical picture reflect the cause of pathology. Traditionally, these disorders are related to

1. Aging of the brain
2. Ingestion of toxic substances
3. Any physiologic condition that inhibits adequate oxygenation of brain tissue

Organic brain damage can be classified as reversible or irreversible. Reversible types are those that respond to treatment of the underlying cause, such as restoration of nutritional and metabolic balance, correction of cardiac and circulatory disease, surgical removal of tumors, removal of toxic substances from the environment, and many others. The diagnosis of irreversible brain damage is reserved for conditions that cannot be corrected and that are usually due to long standing arteriosclerosis, the aging process, and permanent damage caused by trauma and volatile or toxic substances.

Symptoms   Regardless of the cause or progress of brain disease, any of the following symptoms may be seen, either in clusters or as isolated symptoms:

1. Clouding of consciousness
2. Reduced capacity for sustained attention
3. Perceptual disturbance
4. Incoherent speech
5. Disturbances of sleep–wakefulness patterns
6. Change in psychomotor activity
7. Disorientation
8. Loss of intellectual capacities
9. Impairment of abstract thinking
10. Impaired judgment
11. Aphasia—language disorder
12. Apraxia—motor disorder
13. Agnosia—failure to identify objects
14. Constructional difficulty—inability to copy three-dimensional figures
15. Short-term memory impairment—inability to learn new information
16. Long-term memory impairment—inability to remember information that was known in the past
17. Delusions and hallucinations caused by specific organic factors
18. Mood disturbance with alternating laughing, crying, temper outbursts
19. Poor impulse control
20. Poor social judgment, characterized by behavior such as sexual indiscretions and shoplifting
21. Marked apathy and indifference
22. Suspiciousness
23. Dementia with a uniformly progressive deteriorating course
24. Patchy distribution of intellectual deficits
25. Focal neurologic signs such as gait abnormalities, weakness of extremities, exaggeration of deep tendon reflexes
26. Repetitive questions

The existence of organic impairment and the degree of severity are determined by the mental status examination. It is essential that nurses assume responsibility for observing and recording the client's mental status on an ongoing, periodic basis. The collection of mental status data provides baseline and comparative data, which is used to determine the degree of reversibility of the organic syndrome following treatment (see Chap. 1).

Client's Emotional Response to Deficits Although psychiatric symptoms are seen in combination with organic symptoms, it is important to note that many psychiatric symptoms represent the client's emotional response or defense against the acknowledgment of intellectual deficits. The emotional responses may become pronounced whenever the client notices self-deficits or the deficits of other clients. Frequently, these reactions gain much attention from nurses without a full understanding that they are defenses against anxiety and loss and are to be dealt with as such. Some of these defenses are[2]

1. Anergia—lack of energy and passivity
2. Declining interest
3. Alterations of affect
4. Shallow affect
5. Impulsivity
6. Refusal to communicate
7. Confabulation
8. Rationalization
9. Sublimation and substitute tasks
10. Denial and repression
11. Negativism
12. Profound depression
13. Assaultive aggressiveness
14. Psychosis or neurosis
15. Disorganization of activity with agitation
16. Projection
17. Hallucinations and delusions
18. Illusions
19. Behavior representing an exaggeration of previous personality
20. Socially obnoxious behavior

Nurses' Nonproductive Reactions Nurses who work with the organically impaired client are frequently confronted with their own human limitations in effecting change in their clients, especially when deficits are irreversible and become progressively worse over time. Repeating oneself constantly, knowing that the client will soon forget is inherently frustrating. Attempts to control the inevitable deterioration of some clients and the subsequent failure causes a number of emotional reactions in the nurse. The responses of nurses are viewed as psychological processes that, when examined and resolved, can restore the nurse's functioning to a more realistic potential. Some of these responses are[2]

1. Overprotectiveness
2. Chronic helpfulness
3. Withdrawal, emotional and physical
4. Frustration
5. Disgust
6. Anger
7. Impatience
8. Avoidance of client
9. Coercive manipulation of client to behave
10. Impotence
11. Helplessness

12. Depression
13. Lack of caring, leading to mechanical, impersonal nursing care
14. Transfer to a different client care setting because of "burn-out"

Interventions Interventions should include clarification, empathy, and some problem solving. The client's ability to learn must be carefully assessed before the process of problem solving is employed. However, modifications in the problem-solving model may be adapted in the care of specific clients. See Chart 49–1 for problems and interventions.[2]

Chart 49–1

PROBLEMS AND NURSING INTERVENTIONS WITH THE ORGANICALLY IMPAIRED CLIENT

Client Problem	Nursing Intervention
Disorientation	1. Orient to time, place, and person with clocks, calendars, and visual aids. 2. Establish a set routine to be repeated daily. 3. Address by name and title ("Good morning, Mr. Smith"). 4. Repeat basic information frequently during the day. 5. Orient client when awake at night, especially to self and staff. 6. Do not agree, argue, or insist with a confused patient. 7. Gently correct the client. 8. Do not allow the client to ramble incoherently, clarify statements. 9. Respond openly and honestly. 10. Maintain a calm, quiet, and unhurried atmosphere. 11. Speak slowly and distinctly. 12. Avoid stressful situations to decrease stimuli. 13. Convey warmth and concern. 14. Respond patiently and consistently.
Impaired attention and concentration	1. Look directly at client during interaction. 2. Position self in client's line of vision. 3. Use clear, distinct, simple directions, step by step. 4. Direct conversation toward concrete, familiar subjects. 5. Provide simple activities that have a purpose. 6. Repeat messages slowly, calmly, and patiently until the client shows comprehension. 7. Vary media and words to fit client's comprehension; speak his social language. 8. Modify environmental stimuli that affect attention, when possible.
Social isolation	1. Support client's statements that describe his life with significant others (life review). 2. Convey concern and helpfulness. 3. Help client seek and accept reasons why significant other's behavior is not meeting client's expectations. 4. Encourage display of mementos. 5. Actively listen to the client's perceptions of the past and present (life review). 6. Help client maintain communication with significant others. 7. Help client select and accept alternate social networks.
Memory loss for recent, day-to-day information	1. Use simple, clear, step-by-step directions even for uncomplicated activities. 2. Interpret feigned deafness or refusal to perform as a defense against memory loss ("I guess it's hard to go to dinner when the location of the dining room slips your mind"). 3. Repeat ADL routines when the client's behavior suggests that he cannot remember this information. 4. Initiate assistance in the performance of a task that the client refuses to do, giving verbal reminders for each step. 5. Interpret fabricated stories or untruths as defenses against memory loss ("Sometimes when people forget where they put things, they think they've been stolen"). Do not directly confront the client about a lie or falsehood.

Chart 49–1
(continued)

Client Problem	Nursing Intervention
	6. Interpret irritability and/or anger as defenses against the client's realization that he cannot cope with demands of the situation ("I guess it's easier to get annoyed than it is to notice that you can't handle things the way you used to").
	7. Interpret difficulty in intellectual functions as a possible symptom of organic function ("Changes in circulation to the brain sometimes affect your ability to think straight").
	8. Recognize negativistic behavior and substitute activities as a defense. Do not interpret or confront here, as long as the substitute activities are not harmful. This fosters sublimation.
Catastrophic fear, profound depression, aggressive assaultiveness.	1. Since anxiety is great, do not use confrontation or probing for deep feelings.
	2. Support, temporarily, the client's efforts to deny or ignore intellectual impairment. However, do not be dishonest with client.
	3. Do not communicate in a way that increases client's awareness of his deficits. Allow use of coping defenses.
	4. Accompany client when he wanders, gently providing guidance back to the specified area. Do not force with physical contact. Offer your hand, but do not pull client along.
	5. Avoid restraints. They usually cause greater feelings of helplessness and inadequacy.
	6. Gently inquire about fears if client is suspicious.
	7. Do not leave client alone or unobserved. The possibility of harming self or others exists.
Loss of independent functioning	1. Avoid "doing for" the client. Give verbal step-by-step directions.
	2. Provide as much freedom as possible within safe limits.
	3. Accept and allow time for compulsive orderliness, since this allows client autonomy in structuring time and the environment.
	4. Maintain established daily living activities.
	5. Listen to somatic complaints but help client remain physically active within medically defined limits. Follow up somatic complaints with physical examination.
	6. Provide diversion activities for clients who cannot be physically active.
	7. Modify client's personal space in a way that facilitates independent functioning.
	8. Help the client only when there is data indicating sensorimotor impairment that would prevent him from functioning without help.
Misinterpretation, distortion of reality, false recognition of staff as significant others.	1. Reality-oriented feedback, in the "here-and-now."
	2. Use calming verbal reassurance for delusional fears.
	3. Support medical treatment for medical problems.
	4. Let the client know that he is safe.
	5. Protect client from excessive stimulation by restricting number of people in the environment, but *do not* leave client unobserved.
	6. Provide sufficient night light so that client can correctly identify surroundings.
	7. Staff should identify themselves whenever entering client's room.

(Adapted from Sideleau BF: Response to clients with organic brain syndrome. In Haber J et al [eds]. Comprehensive Psychiatric Nursing. New York, McGraw-Hill, 1978. Used with permission of McGraw-Hill.)

References   1. Diagnostic and Statistical Manual of Mental Disorders, 3rd ed. Washington, DC, American Psychiatric Association, 1980

2. Sideleau BF: Response to clients with organic brain syndromes. In Haber J et al (eds): Comprehensive Psychiatric Nursing. New York, McGraw-Hill, 1978

Bibliography

Burnside IM: Psychosocial Care of the Aged. New York, McGraw-Hill, 1980

Butler RN, Lewis MI: Aging and Mental Health: Positive Psychosocial Approaches, 3rd ed. St Louis, CV Mosby, 1982

Copp LA: Care of the Aging. Edinburgh, Churchill Livingston, 1981

Ebersole P, Hess P: Toward Healthy Aging: Human Needs and Nursing Response. St Louis, CV Mosby, 1981

Murray R, Huelskoetter MM, O'Driscoll D: The Nursing Process in Later Maturity. Englewood Cliffs, NJ, Prentice-Hall, 1980

Wolanin MO, Phillips LR: Confusion: Prevention and Care. St Louis, CV Mosby, 1981

50

The Client
Who Is Overactive

Linda Barile

OVERVIEW *Conditions Associated with Overactivity*
Description
Nurses' Nonproductive Reactions
Nursing Interventions

Conditions Associated with Overactivity

Overactive behavior is observed most often in the manic depressive, paranoid schizophrenic, or cyclothymic client. In these states, aggressive drives erupt because of the failure of repression. The behavior is often speeded up, and the client is loud, aggressive, and sometimes bizarre.

In the organic affective syndrome, aggressive behavior stems from organic changes in the brain. In some disorders, such as multiple sclerosis, the reason is unknown. Chemicals such as amphetamines and steroids may also cause overactive behavior.

Description

The overactive client displays the following symptoms[1–3,6]:

A. **EMOTIONAL MANIFESTATION (AFFECT OR MOOD)**
  1. Is elated, euphoric, irritable, distractible
  2. Mood swings, with shifts from euphoria to anger and depression; vacillates between being happy, amusing, irritable, negative, argumentative, angry, or hostile
  3. Is happy, playful, and humorous
  4. Acts on impulses and gratifies self
  5. Is grandiose and extravagant with time, money, opinions and advice; may give away money, lose money on business deals, or spend money extravagantly
  6. Gives the impression of a positive self-image
  7. Is outgoing and sociable, seeking others out

B. **COGNITIVE MANIFESTATIONS (THOUGHT PROCESSES)**
  1. Thoughts, speech, and behavior are rapid and pressured
  2. Verbalizes positive thoughts about self
  3. Seeks attention; has unrealistic, positive expectation of self and others
  4. Is hypercritical and blames others
  5. Denies problems
  6. Is authoritarian and decisive; shows impaired judgment
  7. Speech is loud, rapid, difficult to follow and interpret (shows flight of ideas and loose associations)
  8. Has ideas of reference
  9. Delusions are self-enhancing, grandiose, persecutory, or religious
  10. Makes insulting comments referring to others' physical defects, unusual name, or nationality

C. **MOTIVATIONAL MANIFESTATIONS (BEHAVIOR)**
  1. Is driven and impulsive—takes in and responds to massive amount of external stimuli
  2. Is domineering and prone to action
  3. Wants independence, dislikes restrictions or restraint of impulses
  4. Uses omnipotence and narcissism as a defense against a low self-esteem

D. **PHYSICAL MANIFESTATIONS**
  1. Is hyperactive
  2. Is not easily fatigued
  3. Appetite is variable—may eat voraciously or not at all
  4. Is hypersexual; may walk around naked or wear colorful garments; makes sexual references or uses obscenities
  5. Is insomniac
  6. Neglects personal hygiene, grooming, and health

When the client is playful, humorous, and witty, the nurse may be drawn into an "appreciation" of the client, which may escalate the behavior. When encouraged by staff, the client may perform more and more outlandish behavior, which will later lead to embarrassment and shame. Sometimes nurses encourage this behavior because of their unconscious anxiety about the regressed behavior, unconscious anger at the client, or even envy of the client's attention-getting behavior.

When the client is hostile, angry, critical, or manipulative, the nurse may respond by being angry in return. This may lead to excessive limit setting and other unconsciously retaliatory behavior.

Since these clients frequently do not respond readily to nursing intervention, frustration and confusion of the staff may lead to inconsistent approaches.

Nursing Intervention

Chart 50–1 shows nursing interventions and theoretical rationale used in work with the overactive client.[3–6]

Chart 50–1
NURSING INTERVENTIONS AND THEORETICAL RATIONALE WITH THE OVERACTIVE CLIENT[3–6]

Nursing Intervention	*Theoretical Rationale*
Establish and Maintain Physical Health and Safety.	
1. Provide for adequate nutrition; offer snacks and fluids between meals.	1–2. Hyperactivity may become a physical concern because the client who does not eat, drink, or sleep may suffer complete exhaustion.
2. Promote rest and sleep by removal from stimulating situations and administer sedatives as ordered.	
3. Remove to a quiet area (*i.e.*, quiet room or client's room) for periods of time during the day to prevent and reduce overactive behavior.	3. These clients are overstimulated and are processing massive stimulation from the environment; removal to a nonstimulating environment reduces overactivity.
4. Encourage personal hygiene.	4. Increases self-esteem and prevents the embarrassment client may suffer later.
5. Assess the client for suicidal, homicidal, or elopement behavior and intervene accordingly.	5. Overactive clients who become depressed are at high risk for suicide.
6. Observe for side effects of somatic therapies, that is, lithium carbonate, tranquilizers, sedatives, or electroconvulsive treatment (ECT). Lithium toxicity symptoms include abdominal cramps, vomiting, diarrhea, thirst, frequency of urination, drowsiness, and weakness. Encourage client to drink 6–8 glasses of fluid daily and to avoid excessive use of salt when on lithium.	6. Lithium is highly toxic when the dose is too high, so that clients must be observed closely. Side effects also occur with other drugs and ECT. These may be treated, or the somatic therapy may be discontinued. Sodium intake has an effect on the absorption of lithium and, therefore, must be carefully monitored.[4]
7. If the client is displaying acting-out behavior, physical restraint or sedation may be necessary. When the anxiety has lessened, the client is given an opportunity to express thoughts and feelings and to discuss the situation.	7. Moderate to severe anxiety may lead to threatening behavior or destructiveness of property or people. In this stage, physical control or restraints and chemical control may be necessary to protect the client and others.
Establish Safeguards Against Destructive Behavior.	
1. Observe for mood or behavioral change such as increasing irritability, demandingness, or increasing physical activity.	1–4. Acting-out behavior may be prevented by assessing the behavior and intervening early. In the early stages, expecting the client to control behavior, providing diversion, encouraging the release of anxiety with physical activity, or "talking it out" will de-escalate the behavior. If the anxiety or overactivity is moderate or severe (evidenced by negative response to rules and requests, provoking arguments, and so forth), then limit setting is essential.
2. Provide diversion and physical activities which expend energy and decrease anxiety.	
3. Assign one staff member to the client to assess and provide ego control.	
4. Give the client physical distance or space.	
5. Set limits on the client's escalating behavior.	5. Setting limits results in greater calmness, a sense of security, and lessening of activity.
6. Give the client the expectation that the behavior can be controlled.	*(continued)*

Chart 50–1
(continued)

Nursing Intervention	Theoretical Rationale
7. De-escalate client's behavior by using direct, simple, quiet comments and avoiding lengthy conversation.	
8. Remove client to a quiet area.	

Orient Client to Reality.

1. Orient client to reality in every contact, protect client from stressful situations, provide protective environment, and assure client of safety.	1. The client may experience flight of ideas, looseness of association, and unrealistic, grandiose ideas, which put the client in an unsafe position and provide distance from other clients.
2. Give positive reinforcement for rational thoughts and appropriate behavior.	2. Increases client's self-esteem and increases appropriate behavior.
3. Tell clients when their statements are difficult to understand.	3. Clients may not realize that they are not communicating appropriately.
4. Approach the client frequently but for short periods of time at first. Keep conversation simple, talk about the here-and-now, that is, ward life, eating, sleeping, and so forth.	4. This prevents overstimulation of the client.
5. Set limits when inappropriate comments and behavior are displayed.	5. The overactive client may be provocative or insulting and needs limits set on this behavior for protection and reality testing.

Help the Client to Recognize, Ventilate, and Cope with Painful Feelings.

1. Teach the client the appropriate expression of anger. Accept the client's angry feelings that are expressed appropriately.	1–3. If the client can recognize and accept these dissociated feelings, the need to act them out will be lessened. Talking about the feelings helps to bring them into awareness.
2. Recognize the client's feelings and reflect these back.	
3. Encourage expression of anger, depression, and guilt. Discuss situations that precipitate these feelings.	
4. Assess for signs that indicate that the client may be becoming depressed.	4. Depression often follows a hyperactive period and is devastating to the client.

Establish Discharge Planning with the Client.

1. Educate the client and significant others to early signs and symptoms of an overactive episode.	1–3. Overactive clients often have recurrent episodes because they like the feeling of euphoria and stop taking their medication, especially lithium. If the client is educated about the illness, the effects of medication, and the importance of regular testing for lithium blood levels, recurrences can be eliminated.
2. Establish follow-up treatment.	
3. Educate the client and family to the purpose, dosage, side effects and special instructions of medication.	
4. Discuss and formalize discharge plans with the client.	4. Active involvement in planning increases the client's chances for follow through.

References

1. Beck A: Depression Causes and Treatments. Philadelphia, University of Pennsylvania Press, 1967
2. Diagnostic and Statistical Manual of Mental Disorders, 3rd ed. Washington, DC, American Psychiatric Association, 1980
3. Grosicki JP: Committee on Research in Clinical Nursing, Nursing Action Guides. Washington, DC, Veterans Administration, 1970
4. Hunn S et al: Nursing care of patients on lithium. Perspect Psychiatr Care 18:214, 1980
5. Kalkman M, Davis AJ: New Dimensions in Mental Health–Psychiatric Nursing. New York, McGraw-Hill, 1974
6. Neal MC, Cohen PF: Nursing Care Planning Guides. The Patient with Manic–Depressive Psychosis. 3:36 California, NURSECO, 1977

Bibliography

Barile LA: A model for teaching management of disturbed behavior. J Psychosoc Nurs 20:9, 1982

Block B: Preparing students for physical restraint. J Psychiatr Nurs 14:9, 1976

DiFabio S, Ackerhalt EJ: Teaching the use of restraint through role play. Perspect Psychiatr Care 16:218, 1978

DiFabio S: Nurses' reactions to restraining patients. Am J Nurs 81:973, 1981

Fitzgerald RG, Long I: Seclusion in the treatment and management of severely disturbed manic and depressed patients. Perspect Psychiatr Care 11:59, 1973

Karshmer JF: The application of social learning theory to aggression. Perspect Psychiatr Care 16:223, 1978

Kilgalen R: The effective use of seclusion. J Psychiatr Nurs 15:22, 1977

Lathrop VG: Aggression as a response. Perspect Psychiatr Care 16:203, 1978

Lanefsty B, DePalma T, Locicero D: Management of violent behaviors. Perspect Psychiatr Care 16:212, 1978

Pilette PC: The tyranny of seclusion: A brief essay. J Psychiatr Nurs 16:19, 1978

Rouslin S: Developmental aggression and its consequences. Perspect Psychiatr Care 13:170, 1975

Stewart AT: Handling the aggressive patient. Perspect Psychiatr Care 16:228, 1978

Whaley MS, Ramirez LF: The use of seclusion rooms and physical restraints in the treatment of psychiatric patients. J Psychiatr Nurs 18:13, 1980

51

The Client
Who Is Hallucinating

Linda Barile

Conditions Associated with Hallucinations	Hallucinations are associated with organic and nonorganic disturbances. The organic causes are delirium and dementia, amnestic syndrome and organic hallucinosis, organic affective syndrome, organic delusional syndrome, intoxication and withdrawal, and atypical or mixed organic brain syndromes.

The nonorganic disturbances are schizophrenia, affective disorders, and the personality disorders, including borderline, schizoid, paranoid, and schizophreniform.

Psychodynamics[3]	Nonorganic hallucinations usually begin in a person who experiences stressful events resulting in moderate to severe anxiety and lacks supportive people with whom to talk, leading to intense loneliness. In auditory hallucinations, these clients recall a helping person and interact with this person to relieve the anxiety and loneliness. Initially, the voices are supportive, but over time the clients' past and present perceptions are projected on the voices, and they begin to contradict reasonable action. Clients retreat more and more into nonreality, invoking the original invented helper and interacting with this "person" rather than with real people. As anxiety increases, the ability for attention, focus, and self-control lessens.

Others observe the hallucinating experience and begin to comment on or criticize this behavior, further increasing clients' anxiety and withdrawal. Clients feel low self-worth, and their tendency toward self-criticism is reinforced by others' comments and criticism. These negative feelings become incorporated in the hallucinatory experience, and the voices become derogatory and accusatory, causing even greater anxiety. By this time, clients have made the abstract voices concrete and begin to believe that they are influencing their lives and changing their behavior. They try desperately to regain the "helping person" by bargaining, compromising, and promising not to reveal the presence or content of the voices. This painful cycle is interrupted over time when anxiety is reduced and interaction with supportive people (for example, nurses) in the real world is regained.

Description	The client who is hallucinating

1. Experiences sensory perceptions (auditory, gustatory, olfactory, somatic, tactile, or visual) without external stimuli[2]
2. Often has delusions that accompany the hallucinatory experience
3. May act on the hallucinatory experience, as with command hallucinations
4. Appears to be listening and watchful in the absence of environmental stimuli[2]
5. Appears preoccupied and unaware of surroundings
6. Is apprehensive; expression is fragmented
7. May not follow conversation
8. Talks to self[2]
9. Uses the pronouns "they," "them," "everybody"[2]
10. Demonstrates impaired reality testing
11. Tends to be concrete and literal and may misinterpret the words and actions of others[2]

Nurses' Nonproductive Reactions	Because they may not understand what the client is experiencing or because the client is impervious to their attempts to stop the hallucinations, nurses may become anxious or angry, avoid the client, experience feelings of helplessness, hopelessness, failure, and inadequacy, and may even laugh at the client. Often the laughter stems from anxiety at the exposure of repressed material not unlike the nurse's (or anyone's) own repressed feelings or thoughts.

Novice nurses may attempt to reason with the client, for example, "You could not possibly be smelling your own flesh rotting; I don't smell a thing.'' Frustration following this approach may lead to inconsistency of approaches, arguing, and challenging.

Nursing Interventions Chart 51–1 shows appropriate nursing interventions and the theoretical rationale for each.[2,3]

Chart 51–1
NURSING INTERVENTIONS AND THEORETICAL RATIONALE WITH CLIENTS WHO HALLUCINATE[2,3]

Nursing Intervention	*Theoretical Rationale*
1. Establish a trusting relationship with the client.	1. The client must trust the nurse before talking about the hallucinations.
2. Assure the client that the hospital is a safe place and that no harm will come.	2. Clients are often anxious and frightened and need to know that they are in a safe place in order to explore their feelings.
3. In organic states, use reality orientation and factual explanation, for example, "Mr. Jones, I am the nurse. You are at County Hospital. You are going through withdrawal, and there are no green and yellow men here. In time you'll feel better." Explain to the client that the experience is caused by organic changes, which will reverse.	3. This technique is useful *only* for hallucinations resulting from organic causes such as sensory deprivation or alcohol withdrawal. Knowing the cause of the hallucination and that it can be removed may decrease anxiety.
4. In nonorganic states, reasoning, arguing, or challenging the hallucinations is useless, and should not be attempted.	4. Attempts to deny, reason, or provide accurate information about hallucinations only increases anxiety and, in turn, the hallucinations.
5. Observe for behavior that suggests the client is hallucinating. Observe whether there is a precipitating stress that triggers the hallucinatory experience.	5. Hallucinations involve anxiety and, in turn, withdrawal from people to relieve this anxiety in nonorganic states. If the nurse can learn the cause of the anxiety, attempts can be made to explore the process with the client or to remove the anxiety.
6. Tell the client when you observe hallucinatory behavior. "You appear to be focusing on something other than our conversation," or "I noticed you began looking at the wall." "Is something distracting you?"[3]	6. Asking clients whether they hear voices or see things may produce a negative reply. Observing aloud the client's behavior usually elicits a response.
7. Refer to the client's underlying feelings rather than the content of the hallucinations, "Are you uncomfortable or anxious?" "Is something happening to make you uncomfortable?" "You appear frightened—are you?"[3]	7. Clients may hallucinate when they are in an anxiety-producing situation, but often the hallucinations themselves produce anxiety for the person. When anxiety is discussed and the reasons explored, it tends to decrease.
8. Help the client identify the cause of the anxiety. Connect this to the hallucinating behavior that relieves the anxiety.	8. Same as above
9. If the person talks about hallucinations, investigate the content: "What do the voices you say you hear tell you?" Find out if the client hears voices suggesting harm to the client or others.	9. Concern and intervention to prevent injury to the client or others may be necessary if the voices are saying to hurt someone. Auditory hallucinations may be of an accusatory, derogatory, or harmful nature.
10. Investigate the meaning of the hallucination, the purpose it serves, and the ways it interferes with the client's functioning.	10. Understanding may lessen the need for the hallucinations.
11. Do not imply belief in the voices. State that you do not hear the voices but would like to know the client's experience.	11. The client will be able to sense insincerity, which will increase paranoia.
12. Do not give the voices any status. Refer to them as the "so-called voices" or "voices you say you hear."[3]	12. This does not convey belief in the voices but respects the client's experience.
13. Help the client dismiss or devalue the voices: "Tell the voices that you say you hear to go away." Encourage the person to interact with real people in the environment. Provide competition for the voices by encouraging the client to talk with others, sing a song, or do something of interest.[3]	13. Telling the voices to go away helps the client have some control over these. All of these techniques create competition for the voices and distraction.

Chart 51–1
(continued)

Nursing Intervention	Theoretical Rationale
14. Meet the need that the hallucination fulfills. Approach the client frequently, interacting for short periods of time, and providing replacement for the hallucinatory experience.	14. Clients may feel anxious after dismissing voices. Voices have prevented loneliness, and clients need real people to fill this void. Clients will give up hallucinations when these are replaced with more satisfying situations.
15. Teach the client to relieve and cope with anxiety in an adaptive manner, that is, by talking to other people.	15. If the client learns to recognize anxiety and explore feelings with others, the hallucinations will not be needed.
16. Reinforce reality thinking and help the client cope with life events as they are in the here-and-now. Reinforce reality if the client starts to hallucinate. Give recognition and positive reinforcement to anything the client talks about that is real.	16. This is a behavioral technique and is based on the concept that reinforced behavior is repeated.
17. Provide a safe, healthy, structured environment. Use openness, honesty, and consistency in all interactions.	17. The use of a structured, safe milieu decreases anxiety and increases trust.
18. Observe for side effects of medication. Educate the client and family about the effects of medication and to signs and symptoms of the illness.[2,3]	18. These clients are usually taking major tranquilizers to relieve anxiety, enabling them to be amenable to psychotherapy.[2,3]

References

1. Diagnostic and Statistical Manual of Mental Disorders, 3rd ed. Washington, DC, American Psychiatric Association, 1980
2. Grosicki JP: Committee for Research in Clinical Nursing. Nursing Action Guide. Washington, DC, Veterans Administration, 1970
3. Field WE, Ruelke W: Hallucinations and how to deal with them. Am J Nurs 73:638, 1973

Bibliography

Arieti S: Interpretation of Schizophrenia. New York, Basic Books, 1955
Field WE (ed): The Psychotherapy of Hildegard E. Peplau. New Braunfels, TX, PSF Productions, 1979

52

The Client

Who Is Delusional

Linda Barile

OVERVIEW

Conditions Associated with Delusions[1]   Delusions are a common feature of the nonorganic psychotic disorders, including schizophrenia, paranoid disorders, and affective disorders. In addition, delusions may appear in organic illnesses caused by acute infective, metabolic disturbances, substance intoxications, and systemic illness. The organic disorders associated with delusions include[1]

A. **AMPHETAMINE OR SIMILARLY ACTING SYMPATHOMIMETIC DELUSIONAL DISORDER**
   Delusions, usually persecutory in nature, occur during the long-term use of moderate or high doses of amphetamines and other sympathomimetic drugs.

B. **HALLUCINOGEN DELUSIONAL DISORDER**
   Delusions may occur during and after hallucinogen use. This syndrome can persist beyond the period of direct effect of the hallucinogen, that is, for 24 hours after cessation.

C. **CANNABIS DELUSIONAL DISORDER**
   Persecutory delusions can occur immediately following cannabis use or during the course of use.

D. **OTHER OR UNSPECIFIED SUBSTANCE-INDUCED ORGANIC MENTAL DISORDERS**
   Delusions may occur in organic brain syndrome caused by levodopa or anticholinergic delirium, or after taking a bottle of unlabeled pills.

Description   Delusional behavior is occurring when the client displays[2]
   1. A false, fixed, personal belief that is not based on reality
   2. Thoughts, beliefs, or perceptions that are a misinterpretation and distortion of reality
   3. Exaggeration of facts
   4. Belief as an attempt to explain reality and reduce anxiety
   5. Inability to distinguish delusions from reality and action based on delusional beliefs
   6. Systems of belief that are either paranoid, grandiose, sexual, religious, hypochondriacal (somatic), or exaggerations of inferiority
   7. Concrete and literal thinking and misinterpretation of the words and actions of others
   8. Anxiety, loneliness, and avoidance of contact with others
   9. The defenses of projection, intellectualization, and omnipotence
   10. Incorporation of staff or other clients in the false beliefs

Psychodynamics   A psychodynamic view of delusions is that
   1. They result from overwhelming anxiety and are formed to give "logic" to existing fears and doubts, using the defenses of projection, intellectualization, and omnipotence.
   2. They protect the client from recognizing unconscious feelings that are often the opposite of those represented by the delusion.
   3. They represent an exaggerated picture of what the client truly believes.
   This is demonstrated as follows:

A. **PARANOID DELUSIONS**
   Paranoid delusions represent the client's own aggression, which is projected onto those outside who are "against" the client, for example the CIA or FBI. At the

same time, these delusions result from the client's low self-esteem, for attention from organizations such as the CIA would mean that the client is very important.

B. **GRANDIOSE DELUSIONS**
Grandiose delusions represent the client's low self-esteem and are the opposite of what the client really believes.

C. **SEXUAL DELUSIONS**
Sexual delusions represent the client's feelings of sexual inadequacy or guilt.

D. **RELIGIOUS DELUSIONS**
Religious delusions represent guilt or low self-esteem, like grandiose delusions.

E. **HYPOCHONDRIACAL OR SOMATIC DELUSIONS**
Hypochondriacal or somatic delusions represent low self-esteem and a need for punishment, for example, the delusion that the client is "rotting away" inside.

F. **INFERIORITY DELUSIONS**
Inferiority delusions represent low self-esteem or a fear of the opposite, being adult and successful.

Nurses' Nonproductive Reactions

Nurses sometimes respond to delusional clients by[2]

A. **BECOMING ANXIOUS AND AVOIDING THE CLIENT**
The anxiety may lead to annoyance, anger, a sense of hopelessness and failure, feelings of inadequacy, and laughing at the client. This anxiety is caused by the glimpse of the clients' deep repressed feelings (inferiority, fear, and anger), which touches off the same repressed feelings in the nurse. In addition, the clients' inadequate and exaggerated handling of the feelings generates anxiety that the nurse may not be able to successfully repress or disguise the same feelings.

B. **REINFORCING DELUSIONS**
This occasionally occurs because the nurse actually believes the delusion. More often it occurs when the nurse "goes along" with the delusion to get the client to cooperate, for example, "If the CIA is after you, you better eat a good supper to keep up your strength."

C. **ATTEMPTING TO PROVE THE CLIENT MISTAKEN**
The fledgling psychiatric nurse sometimes believes that if a logical argument is presented, the client will see that the delusion could not be true, for example, "How could you be Christ, when we know He died on the cross?" This approach diverts the nurse from the feelings underlying the delusion and in so doing, reduces the nurse's anxiety.

D. **SETTING UNREALISTIC GOALS**
Because the delusions are often so unbelievable, the nurse may expect that the client can put it aside and accomplish certain goals. The nurse then underestimates the power of the delusion, and the client's need for it, and sets unrealistic goals. This leads to disappointment, frustration, and sometimes anger.

Chart 52–1

NURSING INTERVENTIONS AND THEORETICAL RATIONALE WITH DELUSIONAL CLIENTS

Nursing Intervention	Theoretical Rationale
1. Establish a trusting relationship with the client through listening to and accepting feelings.	1. The client must trust the nurse before talking openly about delusions, describing underlying feelings, and giving up the delusions.
2. Assure the client that the hospital is a safe place and no harm will come.	2. Clients are often anxious and frightened and need to know that they are in a safe place before they can discuss feelings.
3. In organic delusions, investigate the cause and eliminate it, if possible. Explain to the client that the thinking is caused by temporary chemical changes.	3. This may lower the client's anxiety about what is happening.
4. In nonorganic delusions, reasoning, arguing, or challenging the delusion is useless. Attempting to disprove the delusion by tasting food or medicine or performing tests is nonproductive.[2]	4. Attempts to correct distortions or explain reality solidifies the symptoms more. When anxiety is increased in the client, the delusional material increases. The delusion meets an underlying need and thus decreases anxiety.
5. Investigate whether there is a precipitating stress that triggered the delusional material.[3]	5. This information may be important in understanding the client's delusions.
6. Investigate the meaning of the delusion, the purpose the delusion serves, and the concrete ways the delusion interferes with functioning. Inquire whether the client has taken action based on the delusion.[3]	6. When nurses investigate the delusional material without conveying belief, they can better understand the client and the purpose the delusion serves. It is important to know the secondary gains that clients get from the delusions if they are to give them up.
7. Without arguing or agreeing, question the client as to the logic or reasoning behind the delusion, for example, "Why are people against you?" or "What could you have done for others to be against you?"[3]	7. Understanding the delusion is necessary in helping the client eventually to give it up.
8. Offer concern and protective intervention to prevent injury to the client or others.	8. If the delusion involves harming others, they must be protected from the client.
9. Use the *process* of the client's conversation, rather than the *content,* for example, "It must be frightening for you to think that people are against you." Listen to the feeling and reflect this back to the client.	9. Using an empathic approach not only helps establish a relationship but helps clients focus on how the delusion interferes with their lives.
10. Acknowledge the plausible elements of the delusion, for example, "I have no doubt that you were driven to the hospital in a black car, however, I have no reason to believe that there were FBI men or that the FBI is interested in making your life uncomfortable."[3]	10. There is always a plausible element of a delusion, and if the nurse knows this element, it can be acknowledged. Delusions usually develop from some reality.[3]
11. If the client asks directly if you believe the delusion, respect that this is the client's experience: "I believe you are telling me this as you see it." "I believe that you think you have a serious illness."[3]	11. This respects clients' experiences and interpretations without arguing, challenging, attempting to prove them wrong, or conveying belief.
12. If the client persists in asking if *you* believe the delusion, simply state that you do not share the perception or delusional belief. The more bizarre the delusion, the more direct you can be with disbelief.[3]	12. Same as #11
13. Meet the needs that the delusion fulfills, for example, if the delusion fulfills dependency needs, attempt to meet these needs in everyday life.	13. The delusional material will usually decrease when the needs that the delusion fulfills are met in other ways.
14. Once the dynamics of the delusion are understood, repetitious talk of the delusion should be discouraged, and conversation should focus on the underlying feelings instead.	14. Once the underlying feelings have been resolved, the delusion will no longer be needed.
15. Decrease paranoia. Use openness and honesty in all situations.[3]	15. Delusions are usually paranoid in nature. If the nurse is open and consistent with the client, paranoia is decreased.
16. Involve the client and family in treatment. Encourage the client to make decisions when possible.	16. Follow through is more likely if the client and family are involved.
17. Observe for side effects of the medication. Educate the client and family about the signs and symptoms of illness and the effects of medication.	17. Clients are usually taking major tranquilizers to reduce anxiety and break through delusional material.

E. **INCONSISTENCY**

Because the delusional client's behavior is often confusing, nurses may "try anything," and approaches become inconsistent.

Nursing Intervention   Chart 52–1 presents nursing interventions and theoretical rationale in the work with delusional clients.[2,3]

References

1. Diagnostic and Statistical Manual of Mental Disorders, 3rd ed. Washington, DC, American Psychiatric Association, 1980
2. Grosicki JP: Committee on Research in Clinical Nursing Program Guide, Nursing Action Guide. Washington, DC, Veterans Administration, 1970
3. Mackinnon RA, Michels R: The Psychiatric Interview in Clinical Practice. Philadelphia, WB Saunders, 1971

Bibliography

Pasquali EA: Personification: Patient and nurse problem. Perspect Psychiatr Care 13:58, 1975
Wilson JS: Deciphering psychotic communication. Perspect Psychiatr Care 17:254, 1979
Wright LM: A symbolic tree, loneliness is the root; delusions are the leaves. J Psychiatr Nurs 13:30, 1975

53

The Client Who Is Experiencing Sleep Disorder

Ardis R. Swanson

Normal Sleep   Counseling clients for their problems of sleep requires a knowledge of normal sleep. With current knowledge about normal sleep and the disorders of sleep, the nurse selects practices and techniques appropriate to the client's problem and the nurse's expertise.

Sleep duration. Average sleep duration is 8.0 to 8.9 hours, but it is not well understood why duration of sleep varies among people. Among young adults, 7.0 to 7.9 hours of sleep a night is nearly as common. Differences between short sleepers and long sleepers has been explored and some evidence has been found that longer sleepers tend to worry more or are mildly depressed. Inconclusive by itself, this association suggests that the function of sleep is to work over material experienced in the waking state.

The sleep/wake cycle. Humans develop a sleep and wake rhythm, or wave, over each 24-hour period of day and night, such that adults generally do their sleeping at night and are awake and alert all the other hours in a day. The sleep/wake cycle is one of the most obvious and best known "circadian" rhythms, but there are shorter fluctuations of consciousness within sleep and wakefulness. Although philosophers, psychologists, and others for generations had spoken of varied levels of consciousness, it was not until the 1950s that the identification of rapid eye movements, or REM, occurred and three states of consciousness, namely, REM, nonREM, and wakefulness, were delineated. There followed a more refined delineation of recurring periods within each state, achieved by monitoring the experience of subjects throughout all states.

The stages of normal sleep. The following stages have been identified:

A. **STAGE 0**
   The person is relaxed, with eyes closed. High frequency alpha waves are predominant in the EEG. There may be eye movements. Muscle tension begins to decrease.

B. **STAGE 1**
   The person feels relaxed and dreamy. The EEG shows mixed frequency signals with high frequency waves predominating up to stage 2 sleep. Slower theta waves begin to appear. There is substantial muscle tone of the eyes and chin. Pulse and respirations slow down. There may be involuntary jerks of muscles. This stage lasts only about 5 minutes.

C. **STAGE 2**
   The theta wave background continues, with bursts of high frequency waves, called spindles, and high amplitude waves, called K complexes, lasting 0.5 seconds or more, imposed upon the theta background. About 50% of an adult's total sleep time is spent in stage 2 sleep.

D. **STAGE 3**
   When still slower delta waves predominate, the person is in stage 3 sleep.

E. **STAGE 4**
   When slow delta waves predominate, the person is in stage 4 sleep, known also as deep sleep. There is little body movement. Pulse, respirations, and blood pressure are at a low point. There is some muscle tonus of the face. Of all stages, arousal is most difficult from this stage.

Stage 4 sleep is believed to be necessary to restore one physically. When strenuous physical activity during the day is followed by deep sleep, the person awakens with the feeling of having slept long and soundly. After stages 1, 2, 3, and 4, the person comes up out of deep sleep not enough to awaken completely but enough to experience REM sleep. Normally, this occurs several times each night.

REM sleep. The EEG looks similar to EEGs in stage 1 sleep. There is rapid eye movement, and muscular twitching may be observed. Upon awakening, dreaming is reported. Blood pressure is variable and pulse irregular. Gastric secretions increase their flow. In men, penile erections occur (nocturnal penile tumescence).

REM sleep is believed to be necessary to restore one mentally and emotionally. It is theorized that the day's events are reviewed, problems solved, and perspective gained. After days of stress, there is more need for REM sleep. REM periods lengthen with each succeeding cycle of the sleep stages, of which there are usually four or five a night, lasting about 90 minutes each. By the fourth or fifth 90-minute cycle, REM may take up about 25% of the sleep time.

With age, the amount of stage 4 sleep (deep sleep) decreases by 25% to 30%. Since patterns and needs are variable, none are assumed to be abnormal.

When naps are taken in the mornings, REM sleep is found to predominate; when naps occur in the late afternoon, deep sleep is more prevalent. This pattern differs for night workers.

Sleep latency. *Sleep latency* is the term used for the time that passes between the intent to sleep (as when the light is turned out) and falling asleep, normally about 15 to 30 minutes; *REM latency* is the term used for the time from onset of sleep to the first REM, normally 70 to 80 minutes.

Problems and Disorders of Sleep

Table 53–1 shows the common disorders of sleep, their incidence, and their etiology.

Assessment

A. **LISTENING TO THE COMPLAINT**
The nurse listens carefully to the report of the sleep complaint and elicits the client's habits surrounding sleep as well as the onset of the sleep difficulty.

B. **EXPLORING THE ONSET**
Once the onset of insomnia has been identified, the nurse explores with the client the events immediately prior to the onset of the sleep difficulty. The precipitating event may be obvious, such as a major loss, or there may be an impending stressful event. Or the precipitating event may be more subtle, such as the dawn of realization. Exploration with the client can elicit the meaning of events and thoughts and can assist the client to work through the changes that these events require of the client.

C. **ASSESSING PERSISTENT PROBLEMS**
Some sleep problems require more specialized assessment and treatment techniques. The initial exploration of the complaint may disclose a persistent, recalcitrant insomnia, unresponsive to ordinary measures and requiring a more sophisticated and comprehensive evaluation and treatment:
1. The client should be evaluated for the use of substances such as hypnotic drugs, alcohol, and nicotine.

Table 53–1
PROBLEMS AND DISORDERS OF SLEEP, INCIDENCE, AND ETIOLOGY

Problem/Manifestation	Incidence	Etiology
Insomnia Initial—difficulty falling asleep (DFA) Middle—awakening during night (ADN) Terminal—early morning awakening (EMA) During the day—sleepiness, lethargy, irritability Acute, transient—related to a specific situation Chronic—persisting over time Objective—different sleep pattern shows on polysomnograph Subjective—no difference in sleep pattern on polysomnograph	Every night, one of every three persons has some sleep difficulty. Problems increase with age. Women have more problems with sleep than men. One of every two persons has some serious sleep problem at some time.	Has been attributed to pressures of modern society, natural human evolution, intrapsychic structure Insomniacs have been shown to have some neuroticism on the MMPI. Probably a combination of biology and environment of each individual
Hypersomnia Excessive daytime sleepiness, often with a pattern of sleeping more than the average person	No reliable statistics	Narcolepsy is related in over half of cases. Abuse of stimulants or hypnotics often occurs. Accompanies pregnancy and weight gain
Narcolepsy Sleep attacks—recurrent paroxysms of uncontrollable sleep lasting minutes or hours; inability to move body may occur Cataplexy—sudden transient loss of muscle tone in the extremities or trunk; may occur while fully awake and be followed by sleep Hypnogogic hallucinations—terrifying dreams at the beginning or end of a sleep attack	200,000 Americans have narcolepsy.	May be a genetic predisposition, since it has been found to run in families; tension induces REM sleep or stage 4 sleep without inducing the preceding three stages of normal sleep
Nocturnal Apnea Periods of loud snoring and then periods of no breathing occur. The quality of sleep may be severely impaired. Daytime sleepiness and lack of energy occur often, as well as hypersomnia. Deaths have been attributed to the condition (sudden infant death may be such a condition).	1 million Americans, mostly men, have nocturnal apnea.	Upper airway apnea may accompany enlarged tonsils, thick palate, or unusual jaw structure. Central apneas are cessations of breathing due to a defect of the respiratory center.

Table 53–1
(continued)

Problem/Manifestation	Incidence	Etiology
The Parasomnias Occur either singly or together		
Somnambulism—sleep walking	Common in children 5–12 years old; 15% of all children sleepwalk once; 1%–6% do so fairly often. Most eventually stop, but several million continue to sleepwalk as adults.	Occurs during stage 4 sleep; has been attributed to biophysiological predisposition, internal and external stress
Sleep terror disorder—the person screams, cries, or gasps, has a rapid pulse, rapid breathing, dilated pupils, sweating, and piloerection, is aroused with difficulty, and does not recall the experience later.	0.1%–4% of children at some time have the disorder.[1]	There is no consistently associated psychopathology in children with this disorder. In contrast, adults with the disorder do show evidence of other mental disorders, such as generalized anixiety disorder.[1]
Nightmares—bad dreams, which usually awaken the person and can be recalled	Occur commonly in children	Is related to anxiety common to the stage of development; in adults, they appear related to stress; occur also when hypnotics are discontinued
Enuresis—bed wetting while asleep	At age 5—7% of boys, 3% of girls At age 10—5% of boys, 2% of girls At age 18—1% of boys, almost nonexistent in girls[1]	May be related to biophysiological predisposition, internal or external stress
Dyssomnia Disordered sleep/wake cycle due to changes in shift work or jet lag	Occurs when person changes shift work from days to nights or travels across time zones	Caused by a disturbance in wave patterns within the various stages of sleep
Other Sleep Disorders Nocturnal myoclonus—brief clonic movements of which the sleeper is unaware, occurring in one or both legs	Unknown	Is related to tension
Restless leg syndrome—legs feel uncomfortable, as though they must be moved constantly	Unknown	Is related to tension
Bruxism—tooth grinding	Unknown	Is related to tension

2. A thorough medical examination is essential for ruling out the many possible somatic underpinnings of sleep disorder.

3. A psychological assessment will help to identify whether the sleep disorder is interrelated with depression, high anxiety, manic–depressive disorder, or other psychiatric problems.

4. A referral to a sleep disorder clinic may be required to learn what the sleep wave pattern reveals of the problem. (There are over 25 sleep clinics in the United States alone.)

5. Clients may need to be counseled to obtain these assessments, by providing information and support through their decision making.

6. The evaluations may indicate the need for special treatment, including medication of established efficacy and safety, psychotherapy, or behavior therapy.

The client may need information about the treatment approach recommended and would profit by the opportunity to discuss the options available.

Sleep Hygiene

Sleep hygiene procedures are used both for assessing and counseling a client toward improving sleep habits. Many cases of sleep disorder, especially the insomnias, have been relieved by improving sleep habits or using relaxation techniques. Following an exploration of the client's sleep routines, all or part of the information in Table 53–2 can be used by the nurse in teaching sleep hygiene.

Nursing Interventions—Counseling Specific to the Types of Sleep Disorder

When sleep hygiene does not provide relief, the nurse may use specific counseling techniques or refer the client to experts in these techniques. Chart 53–1 shows sleep disorders, nursing interventions, and the theoretical rationale for each.

Table 53–2
ELEMENTS OF SLEEP HYGIENE

Elements	Explanation
The Environment	
1. The bed	Person determines preference for firmness of mattress, texture of sheets, hardness of pillow, and weight of covers. These are then kept consistent when the client is in the hospital, if possible.
2. Noise	Noise is kept to a minimum through the use of earplugs, or by masking noise with nonengaging music, an air conditioner, fan, or white noise machine.
3. Room temperature	Optimum temperature is 60°–65°F (16°–18°C). Comfort can be controlled by adjusting room temperature or bedding.
4. Light	Sleep and night are usually associated. Light can be reduced with drapes, blinds, or eye coverings (blindfolds).
5. Physical security	Locks on windows and doors are checked before retiring to reduce anxiety about safety. In the hospital, clients may need verbal reassurance that they are in a safe place.
The Person	
1. Sleep clothing	Personal preference is followed at home or in the hospital.
2. Sleep time	Adherence to an established sleep wake cycle is desirable. In the hospital, clients are permitted to follow their usual cycle if possible.
3. Physical exercise	Physical exercise during the day increases deep sleep (stage 4 sleep). Strenuous physical exercise should not occur later than 2–3 hours prior to bedtime. Instead, relaxation should occur prior to sleep.
4. Mental activity	Mental activity and all tension-producing activities are stimulating and ought not to be scheduled for late at night.
5. Bedtime snack	Warm milk and a light snack are desirable. Most protein foods contain L-tryptophan which is necessary for the production of serotonin, believed to induce and maintain sleep. One gram of L-tryptophan (available in health food stores) reduces sleep latency and prolongs length of sleep.
6. Caffeine	Coffee and other snacks and beverages containing caffeine diminish delta sleep and increase the number of nighttime awakenings. Caffeine effects peak in 2–4 hours and

---

Table 53–2
(continued)

Elements	Explanation
	usually are gone in 8 hours, but can linger for 24 hours. Monosodium glutamate (MSG) affects some people in the same way.
7. Smoking	Heavy smokers have less REM sleep and stage 4 sleep. Light smoking does not alter sleep, but light smokers who stop smoking altogether take less time falling asleep and awaken less during the night.
8. Alcoholic beverages	A nightcap at bedtime reduces the time it takes to fall asleep but is disruptive to the normal sleep wave pattern. Fluctuations between stages are erratic, and there is reduced delta and REM sleep. Heavy drinking in the evening will induce rapid falling asleep but the person awakens a few hours later with the sensation of being ''wide awake'' for some time. A glass of wine at bedtime for geriatric clients has been shown to reduce the consumption of nighttime medication.[8]
9. Relaxing activities	Taking a warm bath, reading a pleasant book, and listening to peaceful music may induce sleep. Some persons find meditation or prayer relaxing before sleep.
10. In-bed preparation	Watching television, reading an exciting book, or participating in unsatisfying sexual activity may delay sleep. Instead, relaxing music, pleasant reading or conversation, and satisfying sex are helpful.

Chart 53–1
SLEEP DISORDERS, NURSING INTERVENTIONS, AND THEORETICAL RATIONALE

Sleep Disorder	Nursing Intervention	Theoretical Rationale
Insomnia (initial)	Advise clients to 1. Go to bed only when sleepy, rather than trying to get sleepy in bed 2. Get up if unable to sleep or when anxiety occurs about not sleeping 3. Go to another room and occupy themselves with something relaxing until sleepy	1–3. Tossing and turning in bed sets up a perceived connection between sleeplessness and the bed. This chain can reinforce sleeplessness the next night.
	4. Take a sedative–hypnotic only when insomnia occurs, not over a prolonged period or prophylactically	4. Hypnotics have a lessening effect over time and never improve the quality of sleep. Some are addictive.
Insomnia (middle or terminal)	Advise clients to 1. Follow sleep hygiene measures 2. Seek psychotherapy	1. Many clients are unaware of these. 2. Daytime stress underlies insomnia. When this stress is alleviated, insomnia will recede.
Narcolepsy	1. Explain the illness to the client and family. 2. Advise several 10-minute naps throughout the day. 3. Stress caution about activities such as driving and swimming alone.	1. Family members may be angry at the client and may not realize the hazards involved. 2. This minimizes sleep attacks and encourages regular sleep habits. 3. These are life-threatening if a sleep attack occurs.

(continued)

Chart 53–1
(continued)

Sleep Disorder	Nursing Intervention	Theoretical Rationale
	4. Discuss medications that may have been prescribed. Methylphenidate (Ritalin) is used to prevent sleep attacks. Antidepressants are helpful for a time, but effect decreases after a few months.	4. Education may ensure that client follows medication regimen.
	5. Refer client to American Narcoleptic Association, 1139 Bush Street, San Carlos, CA 94070; telephone (415) 591-7979.	5. This association can provide further education and support.
Nocturnal apnea	1. Educate client and sleeping partner about disorder.	1. Reduces anxiety
	2. Encourage client to have a medical workup and support client and family through decision for surgery if it is recommended.	2. Disorder could arise from a structural problem in the airway or in the respiratory center of the brain.
	3. Recommend gadgets (such as hard balls sewn into pajamas) which prevent client from turning onto the back.	3. Some apneas occur only when persons sleep on their backs.
The parasomnias	Advise client to	
	1. Sleep on the ground floor	1. Reduces stairway accidents
	2. Remove from the home objects that are dangerous to stumble over or walk into	2. Reduces accidents
	3. Lock windows and doors at night and give keys to another family member	3. Increases safety
	4. Acquire deep muscle relaxation before sleep through: Progressive relaxation exercises Biofeedback Hypnosis	4. Relaxation leads to more delta sleep.
	5. Seek psychotherapy	5. This may be used to explore and resolve problems of living that may account for the disturbance.
	6. Educate client about the medications frequently prescribed, including Diazepam (Valium) Flurazepam (Dalmane) Imipramine (Tofranil)	6. Education may ensure that the client follows medication regimen.
Dysomnia	1. Inform clients about natural sleep/wake cycles and the nature of the disruption that occurs when they change from day to night shifts or travel through different time zones.	1. Clients may be able to adjust schedules or take measures to minimize problems and hazards.
	2. Assure clients of the body's capacity to re-establish rhythmicities	2. Reduces anxiety

Specialized Treatments for Sleep Disorders, Especially Insomnia

A. **ENHANCING RELAXATION**

  1. Biofeedback—Signals to the client of their wave patterns, including their EMG, EEG, or other, may be employed. Clients learn to affect their own wave patterns.
  2. Progressive relaxation—Included in this group of treatments are tension release relaxation training, nontension release relaxation training,[2] muscle relaxation training for cancer patients,[3] muscle relaxation training for hemophiliacs,[9] and many others.

B. CONDITIONING

Within this group are the systematic desensitizations and classical conditioning. Habits may be restructured by stimulus control. The advice to clients to associate the bed only with sleep is an example of this. Self-punishment for nocturnal awakenings would be another example.

C. BEHAVIORAL SELF-MANAGEMENT

The strategies of this method attempt to modify a number of daytime and nighttime variables based on individual behavioral analysis and to maintain improvement by learning problem solving and self-management skills. Clients are helped to gain a greater sense of control over factors related to poor and good sleep. The method includes providing information about sleep, learning from others who have similar problems, and addressing attitudes about sleep.

D. PARADOXICAL INTENTION

This treatment is based on the theory that trying hard to go to sleep only increases anxiety and prolongs sleeplessness, whereas trying to stay awake changes the rules and frees the person for sleepiness and sleep. A typical instruction to the client would be to remain awake as long as possible and to report back, in fullest detail possible, all the thoughts that occurred during sleep latency.

E. IMPLOSIVE TREATMENT

Imagery and fantasy are used to get people to confront what they fear.

F. CHRONOTHERAPY

The body's sleep clock is reset in a clinical sleep laboratory. The technique is based on the finding that the "natural" day for people is somewhat longer than 24 hours, more like 25 hours. The theory follows that some people do not adjust well to the environmentally imposed 24-hour cycle. Their bodies tend to stay wakeful and out of "sync" with the sun and with most of their fellow human beings. Instead of trying to get these persons to get to sleep earlier, they are asked to extend their wake time further into the night, until their bedtime moves through the night and day, eventually reaching late evening once again. Through this experience the clock is reset. The technique has been highly successful when the "setting" was done in the isolation of a sleep laboratory. However, the problem returns over time. Those who are relieved of the problem for a time may be quite willing to undergo a repetition of the treatment.

G. ACUPUNCTURE

There are reports of success in individual cases.[10]

H. HYPNOSIS

There are reports of successes by this method.[5]

Substance Use in Relation to Sleep Disorders   **Alcohol.** Alcohol is commonly used by insomniacs. In studies of animals and normal humans, its hypnotic effects are manifest primarily by putting the subject to sleep quickly rather than improving the quality of sleep overall.[7] The immediate effect of alcohol is a decrease in REM sleep and an increase in slow wave sleep. Alcohol's effect is short lived, since it is metabolized at the rate of 10 to 20 mg% per hour. Chronic alcoholics have persistent EEG changes, including increased REM sleep and number of arousals, changes in sleep stages, and decreased slow wave sleep. Discontinuing the use of alcohol is often accompanied by decreased total sleep and, after a few nights, a large increase in REM, known as REM rebound. Patients in delirium tremens may experience as much as 90% of their total sleep time in REM sleep. During the period immediately following the discontinuance of alcohol (or other hypnotics), the client may complain of tiredness and nightmares. The nurse can explain this occurrence and reassure the client that the sleep patterns will re-establish themselves.

Hypnotic drugs. A host of drugs have been developed to produce sleep.[6] The use of these pharmaceutical hypnotics continues to be extensive, despite the fact that extended use becomes counterproductive.

Hypnotics reduce sleep latency. The ''ideal'' hypnotic drug would not only reduce sleep latency but would enhance the quality of sleep throughout the sleeping period without side effects and without the development of dependency. There is no ideal hypnotic drug. See Table 53–3 for a list of sedative–hypnotics, their doses, and half-lives.

Medication for narcoleptics and cataplectics. Specific medications known to be useful to persons who are narcoleptic are
   Maxinol
   D-amphetamine
   Imipramine
   Amphetamines
Those used for clients who are cataplectic are
   Fluoxamine, 25–200 mg daily
   Clomipramine, 25–200 mg daily

Antidepressants. The antidepressants (for example, Tofranil) are known to depress REM sleep; they are, in some cases, effective in improving sleep for anxious or depressive persons. They have been used effectively in the treatment of eneuretic children.

Correlates of Insomnia   The nurse ought to be aware that sleep difficulties often occur along with other conditions, either as the precursor, companion, or result of the condition. Among these conditions, most notable are
1. Anxiety
2. Depression
3. Psychiatric disorders, especially manic–depressive disorder, obsessive–compulsive symptomatology, epilepsy
4. Disorders of organic systems, such as
   a. Heart disease
   b. Ulcers
   c. Hypertension
   d. Hyperthyroidism
5. Malignancies
6. Blood dyscrasias

Evaluation   The nurse listens carefully and explores behavior much as in the initial assessment, to identify change since interventions began. The nurse elicits details of the previous nights' sleep, for example, preparation for sleep, onset, awakenings, duration, and client's degree of satisfaction with sleep.

Table 53–3
THE SEDATIVE–HYPNOTICS, DOSES, AND HALF-LIVES

Generic Name	Trade Name	Hypnotic Dose	Sedative Dose (Total Daily Dose)	Half-life (hr)
Barbiturates				
Secobarbital	Seconal	100–200 mg	90–200 mg	19–34
Pentobarbital	Nembutal	100–200 mg	60–80 mg	15–48
Amobarbital	Amytal	100–200 mg	60–150 mg	8–42
Butabarbital	Butisol	100–200 mg	20–200 mg	34–42
Phenobarbital	Luminal and others	100–200 mg	30–90 mg	24–140
Thiopental	Pentothal	Used for anesthesia		
Methohexital	Brevital	Used for anesthesia for ECT only		
Nonbarbiturates				
Benzodiazepines				
Flurazepam	Dalmane	15–30 mg		24–100
Nitrazepam	Mogadon	5–10 mg	Not available in US	18–34
Chlordiazepoxide	Librium and others	25 mg	15–80 mg	6–30
Diazepam	Valium	10 mg	6–40 mg	20–90
Oxazepam	Serax	10–30 mg	30–60 mg	3–21
Clorazepate	Tranxene and others		15–60 mg	40–200
Prazepam	Verstran	10–20 mg	20–60 mg	24–200
Lorazepam	Ativan	2–4 mg	2–6 mg	10–20
Nonbenzodiazepines				
Propanediols				
Meprobamate	Equanil Miltown and others	800 mg	0.4–1.2 gm	10
Tybamate	Solacen Tybatran		500–1,500 mg	
Quinazolines				
Methaqualone	Quaalude Parest Optimil Sopor and others	150–300 mg	250–300 mg	10–42
Acetylinic alcohols				
Ethchlorvynol	Placidyl	0.5–1 gm	200–600 mg	10–25
Piperidinedione derivatives				
Glutethimide	Doriden	250–500 mg	125–750 mg	5–22
Methyprylon	Noludar	200–400 mg	150–400 mg	
Chloral derivatives				
Chloral hydrate	Noctec Somnos and others	0.5–2 gm		
Chloral betaine	Beta-Chlor	870 mg–1 gm		
Triclofos	Triclos	750 mg–1.5 gm		
Monoureides				
Paraldehyde	Paral	3–8 gm		

(From Harris E: Sedative–hypnotic drugs. Am J Nurs 81:1329, 1981. Reprinted with permission.)

If current sleep patterns remain less than satisfactory, the evaluation includes further inquiry into the client's experience since the last session, including after-thoughts regarding the initial assessment and recommendations and any problems or obstacles encountered in attempting to follow the prescription. Problems and obstacles are explored, not as a supervisory parent might, but as a therapist participating in an exploration through which clients better understand themselves and direct change.

References

1. American Psychiatric Association, Diagnostic and Statistical Manual of Mental Disorders, 3rd ed. Washington, DC, American Psychiatric Association, 1980
2. Borkovec TD et al.: Relaxation treatment of insomnia. J Behav Anal 12:37, 1979
3. Cannici JP: Treatment of insomnia in cancer patients using muscle relaxation training. (Ph.D. dissertation, North Texas State University, 1979) Ann Arbor, MI, University Microfilms No. 8012878, 1979
4. Carrera R, Elenewski J: Implosive therapy as a treatment for insomnia. J Clin Psychol 16:729, 1980
5. Erickson M, Rossi E: Hypnotherapy: An Exploratory Casebook. New York, Irvington, 1979
6. Harris E: Sedative–hypnotic drugs. Am J Nurs 81:1329, 1981
7. Mendelson WB: The Use and Misuse of Sleeping Pills. New York, Plenum Press, 1980
8. Mishara BL, Kastenbaum R: Wine in the treatment of long term geriatric patients in mental institutions. J Am Geriat Soc 22:88, 1974
9. Varni JW: Behavioral treatment of disease related chronic insomnia in a hemophiliac. J Behav Ther Exp Psychiatr 11:143, 1980
10. Weal E: Acupuncture—a culturally relevant treatment method for select Chinese-American mental health problems—Ancient needles for modern ills. Innovations 6:14, 1979

Bibliography

Coates TJ, Thoreson CE: How to Sleep Better; a Drug Free Program for Overcoming Insomnia. Englewood Cliffs, NJ, Prentice-Hall, 1979

Dement WC: Some Must Watch While Some Must Sleep. San Francisco, WA Freeman, 1974

Demi L: The nightmare of sleep problems. J Nurs Care 13:8, 1980

Doyle NC: Breathing disorders during sleep. Am Lung Assoc Bull 66:8, 1980

Goldberg P, Kaufman D: Natural Sleep. New York, Bantam Books, 1978

Hayter J: The rhythm of sleep. Am J Nurs 80:457, 1980

Kellerman H: Sleep Disorders—Insomnia and Narcolepsy. New York, Brunner-Mazel, 1981

Kleitman N: Sleep and Wakefulness, 2nd ed. Chicago, University of Chicago Press, 1963

Martin I: Twitch and between. Nurs Times 74:953, 1978

Maxmen JS: A Good Night's Sleep. New York, WW Norton, 1981

Navin HL, Wilson JA: Caffeine consumption and sleep disturbance in acutely ill psychiatric inpatients. J Psychiatr Nurs 18:37, 1980

Oswald I: No peace for the worried—Sleep disorders and their management. Nurs Mirror 150:34, 1980

Relinger H et al: Treatment of insomnia by paradoxical intention: A time series analysis. Behav Ther 9:955, 1978

Sanis HV, Capobianco S eds: Biological Rhythms and Aging. St. Petersburg, FL, Eckerd College Gerontology Center, 1977

Turner RM, Ascher LM: Controlled comparison of progressive relaxation, stimulus control, and paradoxical intention therapies for insomnia. J Consult Clin Psychol 47:500, 1979

Walsheben J: Sleep disorders. Am J Nurs 82:936, 1982

Zelechowski GP: Helping your patient sleep: Planning instead of pills. Nurs 77, 7:62, 1977

54

The Client
Who Has Been Battered

Terry Morton

Types of Abuse The client who has been battered has been abused. Abuse takes many forms, as is shown in Table 54–1. Battering is physical abuse, and battering between adult couples is referred to as spouse abuse, whether the couple is legally married or not. Battering may range from mild physical abuse to lethal abuse.

Levels of Battering[4]

1. Throwing objects at spouse
2. Pushing, shoving, grabbing spouse
3. Slapping or hitting spouse with open hand
4. Hitting with fist, kicking, biting spouse
5. Hitting spouse with an object or attempting to do so
6. Repeated hitting or beating up
7. Torturing spouse or threatening spouse with a lethal object
8. Using a lethal object or strangling spouse

Generally, men resort to levels 2, 3, 6, 7, and 8 when battering their partners, whereas women batter their spouse at levels 1, 4, and 5.[1] Men who batter their spouses do so an average of 3.8 times a year; women who batter their partners do so at an average of 4.6 times a year.[5] It is estimated that 1.8 million women are battered per year.[5] As yet, no reliable estimates are available on the number of men who are battered each year.[5]

Battering Characteristics Like rape, battering is not always reported; therefore, only statistical estimates are available. However, generalizations from clinical cases can be made regarding characteristics of the battering itself, the batterer, and the spouse who is battered. These are as follows[3]:

1. Occurs across socioeconomic groups
2. Occurs across religious denominations
3. Occurs across races
4. Occurs within many cultures
5. Occurs within the family
6. Occurs most frequently during the hours of 8 and 11:30 PM.
7. Occurs most frequently on weekends
8. Occurs most frequently in the kitchen
9. Increases during pregnancy
10. Children may be battered by the spouse or the battered client.

Characteristics of the batterer and the battered person appear in Table 54–2.

Identifying the Battered Person **Clinical Observation.** Battered persons generally seek help from hospital emergency rooms, psychiatric emergency services, and obstetrical–gynecological clinics.[2] They may report having been physically abused, but more likely they will attribute the

Table 54–1
TYPES OF ABUSE AND EXAMPLES

Type of Abuse	Example
1. Physical	Spouse hits partner
2. Psychological	Spouse verbally degrades partner
3. Economical	Spouse earning the income controls the money and gives no money to partner
4. Social	Spouse yells at and embarrasses partner in front of others
5. Sexual	Spouse forces partner into unwanted sexual activity

Table 54–2

CHARACTERISTICS OF BATTERER AND BATTERED PERSON

Batterer	Battered Person
1. Dependent, possessive, jealous	1. Dependent, passive, submissive
2. Low self-esteem	2. Low self-esteem
3. External locus of control	3. External locus of control
4. Uses alcohol, drugs, violence when under stress	4. Uses alcohol, drugs, somatic complaints, and suicidal behavior when under stress
5. Depressed	5. Depressed
6. Anxious	6. Anxious
7. Guilty	7. Guilty
8. Omnipotent	8. Helpless
9. Contrite and remorseful	9. Omnipotent
10. Blames others for own actions	10. Accepts responsibility for another's actions
11. Uses sex to establish dominance	11. Uses sex to establish intimacy
12. Believes in traditional male, female roles	12. Believes in traditional male, female roles

battering injuries to "accidents," for example, a fall down a flight of stairs or running head first into a door. Therefore, it is most important to be able to identify the battered person. The following are clues to battering[1]:

1. Multiple injuries, such as abrasions, contusions, dislocations, lacerations, bites (*not* sprains and strains)
2. Injuries on head, face, neck, chest, abdomen and back (*not* hips or extremities)

The battered client also presents symptoms associated with trauma that leave no evidence, such as headaches, backaches, and symptoms associated with the stress of living in a violent atmosphere, such as[1]

1. Sleep disorders
2. Anxiety
3. Menstrual complaints
4. Vague abdominal pain
5. Dyspareunia
6. General malaise

The nurse should also be aware of characteristic presenting problems that are associated with battering, such as[1]

1. Suicidal ideations or gestures
2. Alcohol abuse
3. Drug abuse
4. Rape (by spouse)
5. Abortions

Medical history. If the client presents injuries and symptoms of stress, the nurse then examines the medical history for the following additional clues to battering:

1. Clusters of complaints for which the client repeatedly sought treatment. These complaints include
   a. Multiple injuries
   b. Multiple psychiatric problems
   c. Multiple medical problems

2. Self-abusive behavior over time such as
   a. Alcohol abuse
   b. Drug abuse
   c. Suicidal gestures

Battering history. After the nurse identifies the battered person (whether the client identifies self as this or not) a history is taken. This is done as follows:
1. Ask the battered person how the injury occurred or what the reason is for the presenting symptom.
2. Ask if there have been similar injuries or symptoms in the past.
3. Ask if there have been any other injuries in the past.
4. Encourage the client to describe the symptoms in detail
   a. When the symptoms began
   b. Where the client was when the symptoms began
   c. What the client was doing when the symptoms began
   d. What the symptom felt like when it began
   e. What the symptom feels like at present
5. Ask the client directly if she or he is battered

If the client denies being battered and yet there remains evidence that this is a possibility, record this and flag the chart. Perhaps the next time the client will admit to being battered.

Crisis Counseling   When the client admits to being battered, multiple treatment options are offered. The first is crisis counseling, which requires that nurses
   1. Be aware of their own thoughts, values, and feelings regarding violence in the family.
   2. Refrain from being judgmental:
      a. If the nurse criticizes the batterer, the client may only come to the batterer's defense.
      b. If the nurse tells the client to leave the batterer, this may only channel the client's energies into resisting such change.
   3. Help the client identify the consequences of the battering. Help the client connect the vague symptoms and self-abusive behavior to the battering and to realize that these symptoms and the behavior are the client's reactions to the battering.
   4. Determine together the level of the battering and thereby its seriousness. Decide
      a. What will happen if the client returns home
      b. What will happen if the client does not return home
   5. Assist the client to identify a support system.
   6. Inform the client of available resources.
   7. Develop together a plan of action incorporating
      a. The client's support system
      b. Available resources
   8. Implement the plan.
   9. Follow-up
      a. Supportive contact may need to be more frequent than once a day during the first week.
      b. During the first week, wean the client from your supportive counseling to the appropriate resources.
  10. Consider the crisis counseling a success if
      a. The client is identified as being battered.

b. The client is aware of the consequence of the battering.

c. The client is aware of the available resources.

Concrete Services   **A. EMERGENCY HOUSING**

1. Shelters for battered clients—the nurse should know
   a. How to contact the shelter
   b. The shelter's admission requirements, for example
      - Are battered men accepted?
      - Can the battered client bring dependent children?
      - Is there a monetary charge?
      - Are battered clients with alcohol or drug abuse problems accepted?
   c. The procedure for referring the client to the shelter
2. If the client is inappropriate for the shelter or no shelter exists, other avenues for emergency housing are considered, such as
   a. Admitting the client to a hospital bed until social service can find appropriate housing
   b. Arranging for the client to stay in a boarding house, hotel, or church facility in the community
   c. Admitting the client to a psychiatric inpatient unit for further evaluation if the client is suicidal or elicits behavior associated with a psychiatric state
   d. Exploring the possibility of the client staying with family or friends. The disadvantage to this is that there is a high probability that the batterer may locate the client and further battering could occur.

B. EMERGENCY MONEY

1. The nurse investigates the possibility of the client receiving financial assistance from family or friends.
2. Under Title XX of the 1974 Social Security Amendment Act, a battered *woman* is entitled to emergency monies. This is a federally funded program that is usually implemented through county welfare. These monies cover:
   a. One month's rent and utility costs
   b. Security deposit on the dwelling
   c. Food for one month
   d. Emergency clothing
   e. Emergency furniture

C. LEGAL COUNSELING

The nurse

1. Refers the client to legal aid or a lawyer who handles domestic violence cases for
   a. An injunction, which is a short-term order by the court requiring the batterer to do or not to do something. This is a civil matter heard in a civil court. An injunction is a temporary order implemented before a full hearing is conducted.
   b. A legal restraint, which is an order of longer duration implemented after a full hearing has been conducted
   c. Advice regarding support payments for the client and any dependent children involved
   d. Advice regarding bringing suit against the batterer for damage
2. Refers the battered client to the police precinct to file a complaint

a. This is a criminal matter, which will be heard in municipal court.

b. If the judge finds the batterer guilty as charged, the batterer can be reprimanded, referred to counseling, fined, or jailed.

3. May see that pictures are taken of the battered client's injuries to be used as evidence

D. **VOCATIONAL COUNSELING**

The nurse

1. Compiles a list of programs that are available for women who are displaced homemakers or in need of vocational counseling, or

2. Compiles a list of programs available to men needing vocational skills, vocational testing, or counseling.

3. Encourages the client, with assistance, to contact one of these services

Psychotherapy A. **THERAPIST'S QUALIFICATIONS**

1. Master's degree in psychiatric nursing

2. Certified or eligible for certification

B. **INDIVIDUAL PSYCHOTHERAPY**

1. *Dynamics*—Battered clients are often very anxious and are frequently depressed. One of the reasons is that they have learned through conditioning that no matter how they interact with the spouse, they cannot prevent the battering, nor can they identify which responses result in battering. The unexpressed anger they feel is often turned inward, producing depression.

Psychoanalytic theories of battered persons include the possibility that the client is reenacting earlier childhood experiences or reacting to deep unconscious guilt and low self-esteem.

2. *Goal*—Help clients to recognize

a. Their feelings about the battering

b. Their options regarding the battering

c. Their feelings about themselves and their partners

3. *Method*—Encourage the client to talk freely about anything he or she chooses. Try to identify patterns in the client's approach to life; for example, does the client tend to react passively to any problem, or to avoid open expression of anger? Help the client see the connection between this pattern and the battering behavior.

C. **COUPLE'S THERAPY**

1. *Rationale*—The interaction between the battered client and the spouse is repetitive. There are phases through which the couple progresses time and time again. These are shown in Chart 54–1.

2. *Goal*—Decrease the frequency and intensity of the battering by interrupting the cyclic nature of the couple's interactions.

3. *Methods*

a. Gather a detailed history of how the battering occurred.

• What are the stressors in the family that increase tension?

• What are the couple's individual coping mechanisms?

b. Encourage the couple to identify patterns in their interactions.

c. Teach the phases of the battering cycle.

d. Help the partners identify the phases of their own cycle.

e. Help the couple learn new ways to decrease tension without battering.

Chart 54–1
PHASES OF SPOUSE ABUSE*

Tension-Building Phase

1. Stressors of daily living occur.
2. Disagreements between the couple occur.
   a. The battered client does not assert herself and rationalizes that if this were done the spouse would get angry and might resort to battering.
   b. Client withdraws in an attempt to prevent expressing any anger verbally or nonverbally.
   c. Spouse senses the client's anger and experiences the increasing emotional distance between the two of them.
   d. Spouse becomes possessive, jealous, and fearful the client will leave.
   e. Spouse rationalizes the client's nonassertiveness as acceptance and permission to vent his tensions on the client.
3. Tension insidiously increases.
   a. Minor abusive incidents occur.
   b. Client does not assert that the abuse is not acceptable for fear more severe abuse would follow.
   c. Spouse once again rationalizes the nonassertiveness as acceptance of the abusive behavior.
4. As the tension increases, they try to reduce the tension through their individual coping mechanisms.
   a. Spouse may try to reduce the tension with alcohol or drugs, which only decreases his inhibitions, usually leading to further abusive episodes.
   b. Client may attempt to reduce the tension by somatizing, which only further perpetuates the "poor, helpless me" image.

Tension-Releasing Phase

1. Spouse releases the tension for *both of them* in an acute battering incident.
   a. Spouse is out of control and blind with rage. Spouse will not remember his behavior during the battering.
   b. Client is out of control. The battering cannot be stopped nor the degree of destructiveness controlled. Client depersonalizes during the battering and is able to remember in detail what occurred.
2. Immediately after the battering
   a. Both are in shock.
   b. There is usually a 24–hour delay before the client seeks help.
   c. Spouse begins to rationalize why he battered in an attempt to justify his loss of control.

Calm Phase

1. Spouse becomes contrite and remorseful, begs forgiveness, and makes promises. Spouse tells client that he cannot live without the client.
2. Client forgives and believes the promises. Client begins to feel less helpless and more omnipotent that spouse needs her.
3. Spouse interprets client's remaining as an act of love and acceptance of not only the spouse but also of his behavior.
4. Soon the calm will once again remit as the tension begins to build.

*The feminine pronoun is used for the client and the masculine pronoun for the spouse, since this is most often the case.

---

f. Teach assertiveness.

g. Help the couple learn positive coping skills.

h. Strengthen the support system for the couple and each individual.

Evaluation Because work with battered clients is highly charged and can be demanding and frustrating, a channel for ventilating concerns and obtaining support is recommended. These include case review with peers and supervision or consultation.

   The best objective evaluation of success in this work is cessation of the battering. Other signs of improvement are

1. Increased self-esteem
2. Decreased alcohol and drug abuse
3. Decreased physical symptoms
4. Increased satisfaction in relationships

References 1. Fliteruft A: Battered Women: An Emergency Room Epidemiology With a Description of a Clinical Syndrome and Critique of Present Therapeutics. M.D. thesis, Yale University, 1977
2. Harris L: Survey of Spousal Violence Against Women. Frankfort, Kentucky, Kentucky Commission of Women, 1979

3. Martin D: Battered Wives. New York, Gulf and Western, 1977
4. Straus M: Spouse abuse. Victimology Int J 2:444, 1978
5. United States Commission on Civil Rights: Battered Women: Issues of Public Policy. Washington, DC, 1978
6. Walker L: The Battered Woman. New York, Harper & Row, 1979

Bibliography

Gemmell FB: A family approach to the battered woman. J Psychosoc Nurs 20:22, 1982
Giles–Sims J: Wife Battering: A Systems Theory Approach. New York, Guilford Press, 1983
Jansen M, Myers–Abell J: Assertive training for the battered woman: A pilot program. Soc Work 26:164, 1981
Roy M: Battered Woman. New York, Van Nostrand, 1977

55

The Client Who Has Been Raped

Theresa S. Foley

Definition Rape is a crime of *violence* in which one person assaults another person both physically and psychologically. According to *legal* criteria, three essential elements must be present to define an act as rape[13]:
1. The use of force, threat, intimidation, or duress
2. Vaginal penetration, however slight
3. Lack of consent of the victim

Some states are changing their laws to include acts of oral and anal sodomy without a person's consent and to permit a wife to charge her husband with rape. It is important for nurses who counsel victims to be aware of the statutes on rape in their state of practice. This chapter focuses on the adult female victim of rape.*

Description The elements that describe a rape situation are as follows:

A. **STYLE OF ATTACK**

Two main styles of attack are reported by victims[5]:
1. *Blitz rape*—An unexpected surprise attack "out of the blue," in which victim and offender lack prior interaction
2. *Confidence rape*—Victim and offender have prior interaction, and the offender obtains forced sexual relations under false pretenses by using deceit, betrayal, or violence.

B. **TYPE OF NONCONSENT**

Three types of nonconsent are reported by victims[5]:
1. Rape—Sex without consent
2. Accessory-to-sex—Inability to consent due to the victim's stage of personality development or cognitive capacity. Examples of such vulnerable victims are the mentally retarded or mentally ill.
3. Sex-stress situation—Sex was initially consented to and something drastically went wrong; usually the male exploits the female's initial friendliness, or communication is misinterpreted, as in the "date rape."

C. **MOTIVES OF RAPIST**

Three motives for rape are reported by rapists[5,16]:
1. *Power rape (55%–65%)*—Is characterized by unresolved life issues over power and mastery. The offender captures and forces the victim to experience what he despises about himself, that is, being weak, helpless, and submissive. The power rapist tends to have negative self-esteem with pervasive feelings of worthlessness, vulnerability, inadequacy, and a history of poor relationships with women (mother, wife, girlfriend).
2. *Anger rape (35%–40%)*—Is characterized by more physical brutality and intimidation than is necessary to subdue the victim for sexual relations. *Temporary* relief is felt by the offender from the discharge of rage, hatred, and contempt toward the victim, and he repeats the act of rape in search of relief.
3. *Sadistic rape (55%)*—Is characterized by eroticization of aggression in which sexual and aggressive needs are fused into a single psychological experience. The offender requires violence to experience sexual excitation and misperceives the victim's anguish as sexual excitation rather than refusal of his "amorous" advances, even when she is fighting for her life. The intent of the sadistic rapist

*The author recognizes that males are victims of rape; however, to facilitate writing style, victims are referred to in this text as female or women.

is to inflict pain and torment, not sexual gratification. The act may involve bizarre ritualistic behavior or torture as the rapist makes a desperate attempt to gain a sense of omnipotence.

Assessment   Competent and sensitive assessment of rape victims requires
1. Knowledge of rape myths and facts
2. An understanding of victims at risk and offender characteristics
3. Awareness of one's personal responses to rape

Knowledge of rape myths and facts. Common rape myths that focus on the victim and corresponding facts are shown in Table 55–1.

Table 55–1
RAPE MYTHS AND RAPE FACTS

Rape Myths	*Rape Facts*
1. Rape is provoked by the victim, either consciously or by default.	1. Eighty percent of rapes are planned in advance by rapists, and the victim is threatened with death or injury if she resists. No person's dress or behavior is license for violence.
2. Only young, beautiful women are raped, particularly if they are "promiscuous" or have "bad" reputations.	2. Rapists choose victims without regard for beauty, age, race, or socioeconomic class. Victims range in age from 3 months to 93 years.
3. If women stay at home, they will not be raped.	3. Half of all rapes occur in a private residence; one third to one half of all rapes occur in the victim's home. Women are raped by their husbands, ex-husbands, boyfriends, lovers, friends, and neighbors.
4. Women who avoid strangers will avoid being raped.	4. Over half of *reported* rapes are by strangers; the majority of adults report rape by strangers, whereas the majority of children and adolescents report rape by persons known to them. Victims who know the rapist often do not report for fear that others will not believe them.
5. No woman can be raped against her will.	5. A majority of victims are threatened with death if they resist. Eighty percent of rapists carry a weapon or threaten death, 30% manhandle victims, 20% use verbal threats, and 15% use no force (usually with child victims); percentages reflect use of more than one mode of force.
6. Rape occurs only in large cities.	6. Rape occurs everywhere. Reported rapes in urban areas are increasing. People in rural communities often believe rape myths and do not report rapes.
7. Most rapes involve black men and white women.	7. Rape is predominantly *intraracial*. Three percent of rapes involve interracial assaults.
8. Rape is an impulsive act to achieve sexual gratification.	8. Rapists report a lack of sexual gratification from rape and describe their motives as power, anger and sadism aimed at humiliating or degrading the victim.
9. Rapists are abnormal perverts or mentally deranged.	9. Rapists exhibit poor impulse control and a greater tendency toward expressing violence; otherwise they do not differ from the "normal" man.

(continued)

Table 55–1
(continued)

Rape Myths	Rape Facts
10. It is easy to prosecute rapists, thus failure to prosecute implies that the victim is guilty.	10. Only 3% of *reported* rapes result in convictions; when multiplied by estimates of unreported rapes, the rate is 0.3%. Rapists report 13 offenses for every convicted offense.
11. Women frequently cry rape for revenge.	11. The false report rate for rape is the same as for other felonies (2%).
12. Rape is a minor crime affecting only a few women.	12. 1980 FBI Crime Index figures record 76,000 rapes; estimates of unreported rapes raises the figure to 760,000 (10:1) or 7,600,000 (20:1). Chances of a woman being raped in her lifetime are 1:15, some cities estimate figures as high as 1:3. Chances of a person being sexually abused before the age of 18 are 1:4. A rape is reported every 7 minutes in the United States.
13. Rape is predominantly a hot-weather crime.	13. Research reports a higher incidence of *reported* rape in summer months and warmer weather areas. Rape occurs year round.
14. Elderly women are not bothered by rape because they have already had sex.	14. Rape of elderly women is more brutal and violent than rape of younger victims.
15. Psychiatrically ill women are raped more often than women without prior psychiatric histories.	15. Victims with psychiatric histories are not raped more frequently but do have a more severe response to being raped.
16. Homosexual rapes differ from heterosexual rapes.	16. Motives for homosexual rape are the same as for heterosexual rape; only the available object (person) differs, and more brutality may occur as the offender subdues a resisting victim.
17. Gang rape is harmless activity by young boys "sowing wild oats."	17. Gang rapes occur for hours and are brutal as each offender attempts to outdo the "performance" of his predecessor in demonstrating masculinity and "adequacy." Alcohol and drug abuse, which lower inhibitions toward violence, is frequently associated with gang rapes.
18. Victims of repeat rape are unlike first-time victims.	18. Repeat rape reflects greater victim vulnerability. Victims of repeat rape tend to be newly relocated or transient, have a higher incidence of seeking help for emotional problems, and come from lower socioeconomic classes; otherwise repeat rape victims are similar to first-time victims.

(Adapted from Foley TS: Counseling the victim of rape. In Stuart GW, Sundeen SJ (eds): Principles and Practice of Psychiatric Nursing, 2nd ed. St Louis, © 1983, CV Mosby, p. 840. Printed with permission [Modified from Keller E, Remus S: Statistics on sexual assault. Minnesota Program for Victims of Sexual Assault, 430 Metro Square Building, St Paul, MN, 55101; Travis MN: The most common myths concerning rape—and the facts. *Brainerd Daily Dispatch*, May 15, 1976; and the collected publications of AW Burgess and LL Holmstrom])

Victims at risk and offender characteristics. *All* people face the possibility of rape; however, some people are more at risk than others, based on *reported* statistics. These include black, single females between the ages of 13 and 24 with low socioeconomic status. It is important that nurses realize that reported victim high-risk figures are relative, that is, infants, children, and the elderly are victims of rape, just as offenders are also young adolescents or middle aged men who are perceived as "respectable" citizens.

Awareness of personal responses to rape. Nurses providing care to rape victims find that they experience strong responses to the violent crime. These responses follow a pattern of phases, each of which is interrelated to subsequent and foregoing phases. Four phases have been identified.[13]

1. Conflict over who is to blame, the victim or the offender
2. Anxiety over the threat of this happening to the nurse
3. Anger toward the rapist, society, and the victim for allowing this to happen
4. Action to resolve feelings, for example, learning more about rape

Factors Influencing Victim Response

Developmental level. The victim's developmental level and life stage affects response patterns to rape. To plan interventions, it is important for the nurse to assess the interaction of the victim's developmental level with the crisis of a rape experience. Table 55–2 presents common victim responses to rape according to developmental stages.[5,13]

Table 55–2
DEVELOPMENTAL LEVEL AND REACTION TO RAPE

Developmental Level	Reaction to Rape
Infancy (birth–3 years) and preschool	1. Trust in adults shaken 2. Assertion of autonomy disrupted 3. Parental rage at offender is seen as directed to self
Childhood (4–7 years)	1. Increased focus on genitals 2. Concern over genital damage 3. Preoccupation with ''wrong'' acts 4. Stifled initiative 5. Regression
Latency (7 years–puberty)	1. Industry temporarily disrupted 2. Sex and aggression confused 3. Increased awareness of sex 4. Tension dissipated by anxious laughter 5. Misperception of rape as a sexual act 6. Academic difficulties 7. School attendance disrupted
Adolescence (puberty–18 years)	1. Increased concern over identity 2. Independence threatened; help seen as regression to dependence 3. Desire to resolve rape independently 4. Concern over pregnancy and venereal disease 5. Focus on here-and-now events versus long-term reorganization 6. Confusion about normal sexual behavior 7. Hesitancy in reporting owing to feared reactions of parents, police and peers 8. Idealism, blaming society for rape 9. Disrupted school/work attendance 10. Academic difficulties
Young adult (18–24 years)	1. Disrupted parenting and work 2. Change of job and residence 3. Inability to verbalize needs and responses

(continued)

Table 55–2
(continued)

Developmental Level	Reaction to Rape
	4. Spontaneity in discussing concerns of pregnancy and venereal disease
	5. Anxiety over premarital sex, if victim is single
	6. Threatened sense of intimacy
	7. Confusion of intimacy and sexuality
	8. Concern over husband's or boyfriend's reaction
	9. Concern about independence and ability to take care of oneself
	10. Concern over body integrity, intactness
	11. Concern over credibility, life-style, morality, and character
Adulthood (25–45 years)	1. Concern over ability to carry out responsibilities (*e.g.*, parenting, job)
	2. Concern over how rape will affect family
	3. Concern over how rape will affect life-style
	4. Concern over community reaction
	5. Concern over how to tell others of rape
	6. Concern over pregnancy and venereal disease
Older adult (45+ years)	1. Concern over societal processes and future generations, quality of life
	2. Fear of death
	3. Concern over family's reaction
	4. Secrecy to "protect" others and self
	5. Concern over physical safety
	6. Tendency to view rape as sexual act
	7. Concern over reputation and respectability
	8. Threatened independence
	9. Increased feelings of helplessness
	10. Often severe physical trauma

(Data from Assault Crisis Center, The Adolescent Sexual Assault Victim, Ann Arbor, MI, 1981; Burgess AW, Holmstrom L: Rape: Victim of Crisis. Bowie, MD, Robert J Brady, 1974; Fletcher P: Criminal victimization of elderly women: A look at sexual assault. April 28, 1977, Rape Crisis Center of Syracuse, Inc; Notman MT, Nadelson CC: The rape victim: Psychodynamic considerations. Am J Psychiatry 133:408, 1976)

Offender type. Victims respond differently to rape, depending on their personalities, the type of offender, and the motive for the rape.[16] The differing responses of victims guide nursing interventions. The post-rape response to an encounter with a sadistic rapist, in which the victim's efforts to relate meaningfully to the assailant were futile and only served to increase his rage, will be very different from that observed in the victim of an assault in which the rapist focused on humiliating and degrading the victim (power rape) and the victim attempted to gain her freedom by reassuring the assailant about his sexual adequacy ("You're loving me better than any man ever has"). This desperate attempt to obtain release may later become a source of guilt, anger, and self-blame. The nurse plans interventions based on the victim's account of the experience and an assessment of the victim's response to the type of rapist. The nurse can reduce the victim's sense of stress by validating the victim's belief that she did whatever was necessary to survive the assault.

Phases of Victim Response Victims respond to rape as a stressful, life-threatening event with symptoms characteristic of a post-traumatic stress disorder.[13] Two phases of response to rape have been identified: an acute reaction and a longer-term reorganization process,[5] which can be understood in terms of stress-adaptation theory.[13] See Chart 55–1 for the acute reaction and Chart 55–2 for the reorganization reaction. Chart 55–3 shows a maladaptive stress reaction.

Chart 55–1
ACUTE STRESS REACTION FOLLOWING RAPE[5,13,29]

Impact reactions
    Denial
    Shock
    Disbelief
Styles of emotional response
    Expressed style: verbal, crying, angry
    Controlled style: calm, composed, "all's under control"
Emotional reactions
    Anxiety, from mild to panic
    Fear for one's life
    Guilt, self-blame
    Embarrassment
    Humiliation
    Anger
    Desire for revenge
    Secrecy about the rape
Somatic reactions
    Physical trauma
    Skeletal muscle tension
    Gastrointestinal irritability
    Genitourinary disturbances

Cognitive reactions
    Recurrent recollection of the rape
    Dreams and nightmares of the rape
    Evaluation of failure to escape
    Assessment of participation or complicity in the act
    Decision to seek or refuse medical care and counseling
Crisis requests
    Medical attention
    Police intervention
    Psychological intervention
Counseling requests
    Confirmation of concern
    Ventilation
    Clarification
    Advice
    Overt refusal of help

Chart 55–2
REORGANIZATION STRESS REACTIONS FOLLOWING RAPE[5,13,29]

Changes in life-style
    Moving residence
    Changing telephone number
    Fear of going out alone
    Reduced functioning gradually improving at work, school, and home
Emotional reactions
    Denial and suppression of anxieties and fears
    Lack of interest in talking about the rape
    Return to pursuits at work, home, or school
    Refusal of counseling and reporting of adaptation
    Emergence of inner sense of depression and need to talk about anger at the rapist, homicidal rage toward rapist (may be acted out), resentment ("Why me?"), relationship with offender

Resolution of doubts about responsibility for rape
    Concern over long-term impact of rape on disrupted relationships with men or family and disrupted satisfaction in sexual relationships
Phobias or avoidance behaviors
    Fear of being indoors or outdoors
    Fear of being alone
    Fear of crowds
    Fear of people walking behind one
    Fear of sexual relations
    Fears specific to assailant's characteristics
    Global fear of everyone
Dreams and nightmares (two types)
    Dreams similar to actual rape
    Violent and murderous dreams

Chart 55–3
MALADAPTIVE STRESS REACTIONS FOLLOWING RAPE[5,14,29]

Silent rape syndrome
    Failure to disclose the rape to anyone
    Feelings and reactions unresolved
    Increased psychologic distress
    Prior history of incest or rape undisclosed and unresolved

Compounded reaction
    Prior psychiatric history
    Psychotic behavior stemming from social/physical difficulties
    Depression
    Suicidal behavior
    Psychosomatic disorder
    Acting-out behaviors
        Alcohol/drug abuse
        Sexual promiscuity

The victim often experiences a period in which she wishes to forget about the rape but later returns to thoughts of the assault to settle the event as part of her history, and to settle depressed feelings that were temporarily put aside. There is no universal adaptation response to rape: victims raped by the same man demonstrate unique and individualized trauma responses to the assault. Maladaptive responses are observed when the victim fails to disclose the rape to anyone and carries the psychological burden alone like a "pressure cooker" with no outlet. A woman who decides not to disclose a rape may seek help for another problem, for example, somatic reactions. Maladaptive responses are also seen when the victim has a prior psychiatric history, including psychosocial limitations, depressive or suicidal behavior, and acting-out behaviors, which reflect a devaluation of self. An understanding of developmental issues helps nurses explore with victims their particular needs and the consequences of decisions being considered.

Planning   Planning of nursing care requires that the client be encouraged to make self-care decisions and to be involved in the treatment program. The intent of collaborative planning is to help victims regain mastery over their lives as soon as possible, because the experience of rape divests one of self-control. Nurses employ skills of creative or active listening throughout all phases of the planning process.[15]

During the acute reaction, phase 1, the nurse helps the rape victim get in touch with feelings about the rape experience and work through seven issues that confront victims at this time[29]:

1. Police contacts and legal matters, including reporting and prosecuting
2. Notification of family and friends
3. Medical attention, including rape examination and follow-up care
4. Emotional responses
5. Current practical concerns, including safety, transportation, absence from work/school
6. Clarification of factual information
7. Psychiatric consultation, if necessary

During the process of planning, nurses assess the phase of response that victims report and intervene accordingly. For example, in the acute phase of stress reactions to rape, nurses plan crisis intervention approaches to assist victims and in longer-term reorganization stress reactions, nurses plan counseling approaches based on a synthesis of models of care. During the long-term reorganization process, nurses remain available and supportive to victims for follow-up counseling and medical care. Victims resolve a rape experience at their own pace; thus planning nursing care is partially determined by what the victim is experiencing.[13,15] The nurse encourages

1. *Self-exploration*—In which the presenting problem and all its ramifications are explored
2. *Understanding*—By which victims make sense out of the rape experience by exploring feelings about themselves and the assailant
3. *Action*—Directed at correcting an identified problem, for example, prosecuting an assailant, cognitive restructuring of self-blame, or re-establishing task performance.

Intervention　The type of intervention nurses use depends on an assessment of the victim's physical and psychological status, the victim's response to the rape and phase of resolution, the setting in which the victim is seen for care, and the nurse's theoretical perspective. Four models of care are described here[2,5,8,12,13,19,22,24,25]:

Medical model. The medical model focuses on illness and disease and starts with an assumption that altered or pathologic conditions can be cured. Goals of the medical model include relief from pain and somatic treatment of diseased states. Nurses implement a medical model of care when assisting physicians or nurse practitioners in the conduct of a rape examination, including treatment of and follow-up care for venereal disease and pregnancy. It is important that nurses know the protocol for a rape examination, as evidence collected corroborates a victim's accusation of rape in a court trial. If evidence of a rape is not properly collected, the professional has contributed to the loss of a conviction of the rapist in court.[7] A general outline of the medical examination of the rape victim is presented in Chart 55–4.[11]

　　Nursing care in this early stage focuses on the client's needs and rights in relation to the following areas[11,13]:

1. Informing rape victims of their rights
2. Giving rape victims priority in emergency treatment when possible
3. Providing privacy in a waiting room while awaiting treatment or interviews
4. Respecting the victim's right to confidentiality
5. Obtaining the victim's consent for and explaining all procedures
6. Assigning a primary nurse to provide nursing care
7. Maintaining a nonjudgmental attitude toward the victim
8. Using empathetic listening skills to foster psychological healing
9. Providing for victim's comfort throughout the rape examination
10. Explaining the reasons for any delays in treatment
11. Offering the assistance of an advocate from a rape crisis center
12. Offering anticipatory guidance to avert alarm about responses to rape
13. Acting as a liaison with health team members and the public
14. After victim consent, facilitating notification of family, friends, and police
15. Ensuring a ''chain of evidence'' for contents of rape examination
16. Scheduling follow-up care for medical and counseling needs

　　If the client is extremely upset, the nurse may assess the client's mental status (see Chap. 1) and her suicide potential (see Chap. 3); in rare cases, hospitalization may be necessary.

Social network model. In order to resolve a crisis state, the victim must adequately balance three factors:

1. Realistic perception of the event (which is not common because many victims believe rape myths and blame themselves for the assault)

Chart 55–4
MEDICAL EXAMINATION OF THE RAPE VICTIM

History

A medical history should be obtained and a statement taken about time and place of the event, relationship to the assailant, if any, nature of suspected physical and sexual acts, time lapse between assault and current examination, victim's physical state, and whether there have been any physical changes since the assault (*e.g.,* if victim bathed, douched, showered, urinated, or defecated, changed clothes, used or removed a tampon, treated wound, etc, prior to examination)

Examination, Treatment, and Follow-up Care

Equipment Recommended for Evidentiary Material
1. Fresh-sealed package of microscopic slides with frosted ends
2. Eyedropper bottle with 0.9% saline
3. Six to twelve packages of sterile cotton swabs
4. Nine to twelve test tubes with stoppers
5. Urine container
6. Sterile, new comb
7. Sterile scissors
8. Nail scraper—plastic or orangewood
9. Envelopes
10. Package of gummed labels
11. Glass-cutting pencil
12. Sterile gauze and envelope for saliva sample

Complete Physical and Gynecologic Examination
1. Evaluate vital signs, general appearance, and mental status.
2. Identify and measure cuts, bruises, and scratches; record and photograph (only black and white admissible in court).
3. Take fingernail scrapings, particularly if nails are broken or victim scratched the assailant.
4. Examine for extragenital sexual trauma to mouth, breasts, neck, and other body parts. Take swabs and smears from mouth, throat, or anus in the case of sodomy to check for semen presence.
5. Do a "baseline" check for venereal disease (VD) and gonorrhea, followed 6 weeks later with another set of tests. Sometimes massive doses of penicillin are given to help prevent VD infection. The victim should understand what is being given and may refuse any medication.
6. Discuss with the victim her birth control practices, use of oral contraceptives and IUDs, and belief system surrounding abortion. A discussion of possible types of post-coital contraception wtih a full explanation of possible effects is indicated (diethylstilbestrol [DES] has been shown to cause nausea and vomiting, and cancer in daughters born to women who have taken it during pregnancy).
7. Discuss with the victim the sexual functioning of the rapist (impotence, retarded ejaculation, premature ejaculation, masturbation).
8. Pregnancy testing and information on abortion, location of free clinics, women's health services, and crisis and counseling centers in the community should be provided.
9. Pelvic examination should include the following:
   a. Observation for matted or free hair
   b. Combings of pubic and head hair to find any traces of assailant's hair and collection of pubic and head hairs from victim for reference
   c. Description of vulvar trauma, redness, lacerations, and bruises and photography in black and white
   d. Examination of condition of hymen
   e. Determination of parity
   f. Determination of date of last menstrual period
   g. Determination of date and time of last voluntary coitus
   h. Determination of condition of anus and rectum
   i. Vaginal examination with lubricated, water-moistened speculum
   j. Specimen of victim's blood for matching
   k. Examination of adnexa for hematoma
   l. Swabs and smears from vagina, vulva, rectum, and thighs to check for presence of semen
10. Clothing should be checked for tears, blood, semen, and stains. Victim's clothing should be preserved, marked, photographed, and collected in a paper bag (never plastic).

Chart 55–4
(continued)

Evidentiary Material
Evidentiary material should be gathered and held for release to the police. It should not be released without consent of the patient or guardian, except by subpoena or court order. Specimens should be gathered and handled as follows:
1. Take swab from the vaginal pool and from any suspicious area about the vulva and protect in dry test tube. These can be examined by a hospital or police laboratory for the following:
   a. Acid phosphatase test
   b. Blood group antigen of semen test
   c. Precipitin test against sperm and blood
2. Examine wet sample from fornix immediately for motile sperm. This examination should be performed only by an experienced person who understands the limitations of examining sperm material.
3. Take separate smears from vulva.
4. Culture for *Neisseria* in appropriate medium such as Thayer-Martin.
5. Comb pubic and head hair for free hairs; pull (do not cut) a minimum of 25 of victim's pubic and head hairs.
6. Take fingernail scrapings.
7. Chain of evidence: laboratory specimens should be gathered by a physician in presence of a witness and personally handed to a technician or pathologist. Slides and containers should be clearly labeled with patient's name. Victim should be advised that turning bloody, torn, or stained clothing over to police may help their investigation and prosecution of case (if she chooses to prosecute). It is critical that a chain of evidence be established identifying all persons responsible for handling or keeping evidentiary material.

Follow-up Care
Patient should be examined for lacerations, contusions, and other wounds. Retesting and examining for pregnancy, VD, and gonorrhea should be completed. Counseling to assess and prevent long-term psychological effects should be provided or made available.

Medical Records

Medical record should contain complete documentation of history, examination, and treatment provided. It should describe physician's findings and what was done. It should state what evidentiary materials were given and to whom. Only medical conclusions, opinions, and diagnosis should be in medical record. Above all, it must be legible, and preferably typed, to avert case dismissal in court proceedings. Medical personnel and record may be subpoenaed. Misinterpretations can be avoided if all data are exact and detailed. Negative findings are as important as positive ones and may assist in protection of all concerned parties.

(Foley TS: Counseling the victim of rape. In Stuart G, Sundeen S [eds]: Principles and Practice of Psychiatric Nursing. St Louis, CV Mosby, 1979. Reprinted with permission [Adapted from The Hospital Association of Pennsylvania and the Pennsylvania Medical Society: Guidelines for treatment of suspected victims of sexual assault. Penn Med 79:73, June, 1976; Bragonier R, Nadelson CC: Caring for the rape victim. In Interact: New perspectives for the clinical management of sexual problems. Chicago, 1977, GD Searle & Co; and the collected publications of AW Burgess and LL Holmstrom])

2. Adequate coping mechanisms
3. Support systems

Social network theory focuses primarily on the third balancing factor: support systems. A social network is "that group of persons who maintain an ongoing significance in each other's lives by fulfilling specific human needs."[1] The focus of the social network model of care is on the way in which the individual functions within a social system, for example, with peers, family, school or work systems, and the community. Theory posits that social forces determine the norms for behavior, including the fostering or sanctioning of deviant behavior. Hence, social network theory contributes to an understanding of the relationship between social variables and victim response patterns, of factors motivating men to rape, and society's attribution of fault to the victim.

Treatment focuses on having clients connect with helpful individuals or groups and by reorganizing the social system itself. Nurses encourage a victim to activate *multiple* support systems in resolving a rape experience. Specifically, medical and legal systems provide assistance to victims in crises, as well as primary and secondary support networks. Chart 55–5 presents interviewing guidelines that nurses use with rape victims in crisis.

Chart 55–5
INTERVIEWING GUIDELINES WITH RAPE VICTIMS IN CRISIS

Date _____ Time _____

General Information

Introduction: Hello. This is _____
from _____ .
  How can I help you?
Name of victim/caller _____
Phone number calling from _____
Address or general area _____
  Location/neighborhood of assault _____
  Why in the area _____
When did assault occur (date, time)? _____
Are you in a safe place? _____
Are you hurt? _____
How are you feeling now? _____
Time between assault and call to crisis line _____

Demographic Data

Age of victim _____
Race and sex of victim _____
Marital status _____
Description of assailant:
  Who did it? _____
  Age _____
  Race and sex _____
  Acquainted with victim _____
    Describe relationship:

Crisis Status

Perception of the event _____
Response to the event _____
Situational supports _____
Coping mechanisms _____

Type of Assault

_____ Rape
_____ Attempted rape
_____ Involuntary deviate sexual intercourse
_____ Indecent assault
_____ Sexual assault of a minor
_____ Other degrading acts
    Describe:
_____ Use of weapon
    Type:
_____ Struggle by victim
    feelings now about that
_____ Threats (describe)
    Verbal _____
    Physical _____

Services Requested and Questions to Consider

1. Medical intervention (hospital): Has the victim had a medical examination? Encourage going to the emergency room for treatment of injuries and collection of evidence pending decision to prosecute.
   a. **If not examined:** If she does not want to go to the hospital, does she know about the importance of testing for VD, GC, pregnancy now and later? Is she injured other than the sexual assault? What supportive network is available to her? Does she want/need an advocate to accompany her to a shelter/care facility? Give her information about the local hospital procedure and what to expect, her rights.

   b. **If examined:** How did she get to the hospital? What did she expect would be done for her at the hospital? Were tests for VD, GC, pregnancy done? Did she change clothes or clean up before going to the hospital? Was medical evidence collected (what, where)? Was she treated for lacerations, abrasions, bruises? Is she on any medications or DES? Specify these. Does she know their side effects and risks involved? Is she having any medical problems? Was follow-up care discussed/planned? How does she feel she was treated by the health professionals? What is her reaction to this experience? Did she decide to obtain help or did someone else pressure her to seek help?

Chart 55–5
(continued)

c. **Abuse:** Is there evidence of physical abuse to a child or elderly person or battered wife syndrome? Describe the data. Has the evidence been reported to the police, hospital, and/or Child Welfare?

2. Shelter and transportation intervention: Does she need emergency transportation?

From _____ to _____ Date _____
Time _____
Does she need emergency shelter? _____
Contributing factors _____
Length of time requested _____
Accompanied (children) or alone _____
Economic/financial concerns (describe) _____

3. Police and legal intervention: Has she reported to the police?

a. **If not reported:** Does she want to report? Does she want the report kept anonymous? Does she want to press charges? Does she want to talk about the pros and cons of not reporting/reporting? What feelings/factors are contributing to a no-report decision? Does she know about victim compensation–restitution (that she can be compensated for unpaid medical expenses if she reports the crime within 72 hours)?

b. **If reported:** Does she understand the legal procedure and what to expect at the preliminary hearing, pretrial, trial? Is she aware of the possibility of a trial postponement and of a not-guilty verdict? To whom did she report (which police station and name of officer taking the report)? Was a report taken? Was she encouraged or discouraged from prosecuting? What is happening with the police follow-up at this time? Is she aware of the procedures necessary to identify the assailant? Has the assailant been picked up by the police? Is the assailant in jail, out on bond? Is she being harrassed or threatened by him or others? Describe. Does she have any intent to retaliate against the assailant? Name of officer arresting the assailant and police station(s) he is assigned to? Who is the district attorney? How does she feel the police treated her? What is her reaction to the experience of reporting?

4. Psychological intervention

a. **The victim:** How did she feel at the time of the assault? And now? Does she feel the rape was her fault? Does she believe in the myths? Which ones and their impact on her as noted by _____. Does she perceive anyone as able to assist her? Did she go or not go to the police/hospital as a result of outside pressure/advice? Is she ambivalent regarding what to do? Describe. Is she seeking others' opinions? (Whose? What content? What action taken?) Was she or the assailant affected by the use of alcohol and/or drugs? (What ingested? When? Amount? By which party? Feelings about this?) Is she unable to verbalize her needs? Is she psychotic? Mentally retarded? History of social difficulties? History of physical difficulties? Hospitalized or under a physician's care now or previously? Mentally status is (describe). What is the most painful part to recall/discuss? Has she been raped before? Is this her first sexual experience? What is her usual sexual style? What does this sexual assault mean to her? How did she react to sexual acts demanded (feelings, behaviors [*e.g.,* compliance, resistance])?

b. **Family and friends:** Who are her friends, relatives? Where do they live? Quality and frequency of contacts? Persons most and least in touch with? Does she have a therapist, minister? Does she attend any women's groups, any rap sessions? Does she want to talk with other victims of rape? Can she rely on her support systems if she wants to talk about the rape? Will they listen? How will she feel if they don't or reject her? How is her church community a support system for her? Has she decided to talk about the incident? (Discuss pros/cons of doing so and with whom—she is the best judge of her situation.) Who knows about the assault? Describe their response. Do family/friends want to talk with a counselor, or does she want a counselor to talk with them? Is the family responding with (1) caring for the victim's welfare, empathy, support, anger directed at the assailant, ability to give to the victim or (2) blaming the victim, caring for their own welfare (*e.g.,* what others will think), recriminations, anger directed at the victim, blaming themselves?

5. Narrative summary

Services requested _____ Medical
_____ Police/legal
_____ Shelter
_____ Transportation
_____ Counseling (specify type)
_____ Other

Nursing diagnosis _____
Plans _____
Contacts made (e.g., police, hospital, name of person/agency)
Referrals made or suggested _____
Follow-up indicated and type _____
Self-evaluation
Describe feelings about the call, personal reactions, influence of biases/myths. List additional information/training that would help improve services. Delineate learning needs.

(From Foley TS: Counseling the Victim of Rape. In Stuart G, and Sundeen S (eds): Principles and Practice of Psychiatric Nursing. St Louis, CV Mosby Co., 1983, pp 447–449. Reprinted with permission. [Adapted from Pittsburgh Action Against Rape: Crisis call form, 211 S Oakland Ave, Pittsburgh, PA 15213; Burgess AW, Holmstrom LL: Crisis and counseling requests of rape victims. Nurs Res 23:198, 1974])

The victim is encouraged to use primary and secondary social networks for supports during the period of vulnerability post-rape. Primary social networks are comprised of persons whom *the victim* identifies as most meaningful or relevant, for example, a peer may be more meaningful than a parent. Secondary social networks are comprised of persons the victim identifies as less meaningful or relevant, for example, employers, police officers, and health care providers. The *victim* decides who to contact. Disclosing a rape to family and significant others often means that victims work through fears of disapproval, rejection, and scorn from those persons most important in their lives. It also means telling someone loved about an event the victim would rather spare them from knowing. Sometimes victims feel unable to tell family members and will seek out counselors in rape crisis centers or community mental health centers for support. The nurse helps a victim weigh the "pros" and "cons" of any decision and abides by the *victim's decision,* even if it is one the nurse does not agree with, because the philosophy of self-care is essential in resolving a rape experience.

Treatment that implements a social network model also focuses on reorganizing social systems, including the family and society. Focusing on social systems includes interventions directed toward realigning the family system to be supportive to the victim and opening the system to communicate effectively with its members and other systems. Stress reactions by the victim's social network often require nursing intervention.[5,6,13,18,28] Some of these include

1. Shock, disbelief, dismay, and helplessness
2. Blaming or finding a scapegoat
3. Overprotecting or infantilizing the victim
4. Keeping the rape a secret, resulting in psychologic disease
5. Reacting to rape as a sexually motivated act
6. Insisting on sexual relations and re-establishing sexual relations
7. Viewing the victim as their "damaged property"
8. Thoughts about or acts of violent retribution
9. "If only" reactions
10. Disrupted relationships (separation, divorce)
11. Coping with the victim's phobic behavior and nightmares

The victim is encouraged to seek out significant others to talk to about the rape. Talking about the rape helps the victim settle the crisis experience, reduces the sense of emotional isolation, helps weigh the "pros" and "cons" of suggestions, thereby enhancing problem-solving abilities, and may lead to the use of further available support systems.

Reorganizing social systems also includes continuing education. Professional nurses teach other nurses about the nature of rape and the nursing care of victims, and educate the public and youth of society with a view toward prevention. Large systems issues are addressed in an effort to influence major social change in systems, for example, revising the rape laws and the ways in which victims are treated by health care providers and the judicial system, educating police officers, developing rape examination protocols for hospitals, dissipating poverty as a stimulus toward violent behavior, helping to prosecute rapists, and making policy recommendations for improving institutional response to rape victims. The overall goal of the social network model is to maintain or establish adequate supportive systems for rape victims and to prevent rape.

Psychological model. Crisis intervention and individual insight therapy are provided as a part of this model (see Chap. 21 and 25). Cognitive therapy may also be employed.

Cognitive therapy. In cognitive therapy the nurse uses cognitive restructuring techniques to help the client resolve psychodynamic conflicts by focusing on victims' distorted views of themselves and their world. Attention is drawn to common errors in thinking, which include arbitrary inferences, selective abstraction, overgeneralization, magnification and minimization, personalization, and absolutistic, dichotomous thinking.[3] A person's thought processes or cognitions include both verbal and visual events although the person is not always aware of these cognitions. Cognitions are believed to be based on assumptions or attitudes derived from previous interpersonal experience.[3] For example, if a victim tends to place moral values on her experiences she may be dominated by the assumption: "If the rapist does not get a guilty verdict I am a bad person." The victim would then believe that significant others were also making value judgments about her worth. Thus, when *assessing* a rape victim's distressing thought processes, it is important for nurses to begin by identifying what seem to be the victim's faulty assumptions.

Identifying and correcting faulty cognitions is achieved through the use of a "Daily Record of Dysfunctional Thoughts" which involves five steps: situation, emotion, automatic thoughts, rational response, and outcome[3] (see Chart 55–6).

Chart 55–6
DAILY RECORD OF DYSFUNCTIONAL THOUGHTS

	Situation	Emotion(s)	Automatic Thought(s)	Rational Response	Outcome
	Describe:				
	1. Actual event leading to unpleasant emotion, or	1. Specify sad/ anxious/angry, and so forth.	1. Write automatic thought(s) that preceded emotion(s).	1. Write rational response to automatic thought(s).	1. Re-rate belief in automatic thought(s), 0–100%.
	2. Stream of thoughts, daydream, or recollection, leading to unpleasant emotion	2. Rate degree of emotion, 1–100.	2. Rate belief in automatic thought(s), 0–100%.	2. Rate belief in rational response, 0–100%.	2. Specify and rate subsequent emotions, 0–100.
Date 2-14-80	On the bus going to work, I see several passengers that look like the rapist. I suddenly realize this is the bus the rapist usually takes to work.	Fear = 80	1. I might run into (the rapist). I don't want to face him until absolutely necessary. He might try to rape me again. 2. 80%	1. Running into him would help prepare me for confrontation at the trial, give me a chance to say stuff to him that has been on my mind. He can't persuade me to go with him again. He isn't allowed to come near me, so I don't need to be frightened. If he bugs me I'll notify the police. 2. 80%	1. 10% 2. Fear = 20

EXPLANATION: When you experience an unpleasant emotion, note the situation that seemed to stimulate the emotion. (If the emotion occurred while you were thinking, daydreaming, and so forth, please note this.) Then note the automatic thought associated with the emotion. Record the degree to which you believe this thought: 0% = not at all; 100% = completely. In rating degree of emotion: 1 = a trace; 100 = the most intense possible. (From Beck AT, Ruch AJ, Shaw BF, Emerg GD: Cognitive Therapy of Depression. New York, Guilford Press, 1979. Copyright © 1978 by Aaron T. Beck, M.D. Further information about this scale and/or permission to use the scale may be obtained from: Center for Cognitive Therapy, Rm 602, 133 S 36th St, Philadelphia, PA 19104)

The victim is instructed to record a *situation* in which unpleasant emotions arise along with the automatic thoughts and emotions that occur in that situation. The victim is asked to rate the extent to which she believes the automatic thoughts on a percentage scale ranging from 0 (not at all) to 100% (completely) and to rate the extent to which she believes in the emotion on a numerical scale ranging from 1 (a trace) to 100 (the most intense possible). This initial step teaches the rape victim to identify faulty automatic cognitions and emotions, and their relationship to specific situations. After the victim has mastered self-monitoring of affect and is able to label emotions correctly, recognizing their relationship to specific cognitions and situations, she is ready to begin refuting nonproductive cognitions (step 2). In the second step of the cognitive exercise, the victim is instructed to write a "rational" response to automatic nonproductive thoughts previously listed. The extent to which the victim believes in the rational response is indicated on a percentage scale of 0 (not at all) to 100% (completely). Then belief in the automatic thoughts are re-rated using the same percentage scale (0–100%). Emotions are specified after the victim gives a rational response full consideration, and are then re-rated.[3]

Behavioral model. A variety of behavioral strategies are used in treating rape victims. Two well-known behavioral strategies are[5,13,27]

1. *In vivo* desensitization—The rape victim gradually faces a real life stimulus that is feared, such as work setting where she was raped.
2. Systematic desensitization—The victim is gradually exposed to a hierarchy of imaginary stimuli that are feared.

Desensitization strategies help victims regain mastery over feared behaviors such as socializing at parties, re-establishing sexual relations, and seeing the rapist on the street or in the courtroom.[5,13,27] Keeping a diary is another behavioral strategy used to help victims record all of the rape events, thereby reducing their fears about loss of memory and assisting them with control over recall at the time of the trial, which can be 6 to 12 months postrape. Rape victims experiencing homicidal rage toward the rapist following a "not-guilty" verdict are instructed to write out their fantasies of what they would like to do to the rapist, thereby mobilizing anger to prevent depression. Another therapeutic behavioral intervention is to instruct the victim to draw pictures of the rapist and his cohorts on paper bags, place these on an air-inflated punching bag, and punch the symbolic figure to release rage through action behaviors. The value of exercise, swimming, walking, jogging, tennis, and so forth is stressed as a measure to reduce increased psychological tension. The following measures have been found to be therapeutically effective in treating depression[3,14]:

1. *Weekly activated schedules* in which a report is recorded of activities during the week
2. *Mastery and pleasure schedules,* in which activities are graded daily for a sense of mastery and pleasure
3. *Graded task assignments,* in which tasks are assigned on a graded, sequential basis
   Talking is a behavior, and thus talking out troubling thoughts and feelings is viewed as a behavioral intervention. Talking about the painful parts of the rape helps to desensitize the victim to the memory of the assault and helps her depersonalize the event. The goal of behavioral interventions is to assist the rape victim to return to pre-rape or higher levels of functioning by modifying problematic behaviors and, in some cases, learning new coping behaviors.

Evaluation Treatment of the rape victim is considered successful when there is a return to the pre-rape level or a higher level of functioning. To date, most counseling programs lack internal and external evaluation although a few researchers are beginning to study comparable treatment approaches in rape victim care.[14,20] After 10 years of descriptive data on rape victim response, professionals can begin to evaluate treatment effectiveness, epidemiologic variables identifying victim vulnerability to both rape and difficulty in resolving a rape experience. Further, variables characterizing treatment refusers (victims who do not feel the need for intervention by professionals and whose symptoms remit without treatment) can be further explicated. Comparisons can be made between rape victims' responses and responses to other crimes, for example, burglary and assault. In essence, the understanding of rape victim response has developed to a point of readiness for experimental studies testing the effectiveness of differing treatment interventions. Nurses are encouraged to respond to this challenge.

References

1. Adams B: Intervention theory and the social network. Sociometry 30:64, 1967
2. Aguilera D, Messick J: Crisis Intervention: Theory and Methodology. St Louis, CV Mosby, 1978
3. Beck A et al: Cognitive Therapy of Depression. New York, The Guilford Press, 1979
4. Brownmiller S: Against Our Will: Men, Women and Rape. New York, Simon & Schuster, 1975
5. Burgess AW, Holmstrom LL: Rape: Victims of Crisis. Bowie, MD, Robert J Brady, 1974
6. Burgess AW, Holmstrom LL: Rape: Sexual disruption and recovery. Am J Orthopsychiatry 4:648, 1979
7. Burgess AW, Laszlo AT: Courtroom use of hospital records in sexual assault cases. Am J Nurs 77:64, 1977
8. Burgess A, Lazare A: The social context of mental illness. In Burgess A, Lazare A (eds): Psychiatric Nursing in the Hospital and the Community. Englewood Cliffs, NJ, Prentice-Hall, 1976
9. Ellis A: Humanistic Psychology. New York, McGraw-Hill, 1973
10. Ellis A, Harper R: A New Guide to Rational Living. North Hollywood, CA, Wilshire, 1975
11. Foley T: Counseling the victim of rape. In Stuart G, Sundeen S (eds): Principles and Practice of Psychiatric Nursing, St Louis, CV Mosby, 1983
12. Foley T, MacDonald C: Models of Treatment. Lecture notes, University of Pittsburgh School of Nursing, 1975–1976
13. Foley T, Davies M: Rape: Nursing Care of Victims, St Louis, CV Mosby, 1983
14. Frank E, Turner S: The rape victim: Her response and treatment. NIMH study #RO 1 MH 29692, Western Psychiatric Institute and Clinic (3881 O'Hara St, Pittsburgh, PA, 15213)
15. Gazda G et al: Human Relations Development: A Manual for Educators. Boston, Allyn and Bacon, 1977
16. Groth AN, Birnbaum HJ: Men Who Rape: The Psychology of the Offender. New York, Plenum Press, 1979
17. Holmstrom LL, Burgess AW: The Victim of Rape: Institutional Reactions. New York, John Wiley & Sons, 1978
18. Holmstrom LL, Burgess AW: Rape: The husband's and boyfriend's initial reactions. Fam Coordinator 71:321, 1979
19. Kalkman M: Models of psychiatric treatment. In Kalkman M, Davies A: New Dimensions in Mental Health–Psychiatric Nursing. New York, McGraw-Hill, 1974
20. Kilpatrick D, Veronen L: Treatment of fear and anxiety in victims of rape. NIMH study #RO 1 MH 29602, Medical University of South Carolina, Charleston, SC, 29401
21. Kliman A: Crisis: Psychological First Aid for Recovery and Growth. New York, Holt, Rinehart & Winston, 1978
22. Lazare A: Hidden conceptual models in clinical psychiatry. New Engl J Med 188:345, 1973
23. Ledray L, Chaignot MJ: Services to sexual assault victims in Hennepin County. Special Issue 131, 1980
24. Leighton A: Conceptual perspectives. In Kaplan B, Wilson R, Leighton A: Further Explorations in Social Psychiatry. New York, Basic Books, 1976
25. Matheney R, Topalis M: Psychiatric Nursing. St Louis, CV Mosby, 1974
26. May R: The Meaning of Anxiety. New York, Ronald Press, 1950
27. Rimm D, Masters J: Behavior Therapy: Techniques and Empirical Findings. New York, Academic Press, 1974
28. Silverman D: Sharing the crisis of rape: Counseling the mates and families of victims. Am J Orthopsychiatry 48:166, 1978
29. Sutherland S, Scherl D: Patterns of response among victims of rape. Am J Orthopsychiatry 40:503, 1970
30. Thio A: Deviant Behavior. Boston, Houghton Mifflin, 1978
31. Webster's New Collegiate Dictionary. Springfield, MA, G and C Merriam, 1977

Part V

Psychiatric

Nursing

Procedures

56

Admission
to the Hospital

Kathleen Rekasis

OVERVIEW

Criteria for Admission
Intake
Nursing Intervention
Nursing Assessment

Criteria for Admission   The Joint Commission of Accreditation of Hospitals (JCAH) Section 16:5 states

Acceptance of a patient for treatment shall be based on an intake procedure that results in the following conclusions:[1]

1. the treatment required by the patient is appropriate to the intensity and restrictions of care provided by the facility or program component; and/or
2. the treatment required can be appropriately provided by the facility or program component; and
3. the alternatives for less intensive and restrictive treatment are not available.

Chart 56–1

NURSING ACTIONS AND RATIONALE JUST BEFORE ADMISSION

Nursing Action	Rationale
1. Clients are told that they are being admitted to the hospital.	1. To give clients information from which to make a decision to admit themselves voluntarily
2. Clients, if capable, are involved in the decision to admit themselves.	2. To enhance compliance with the decision
3. The family or significant others, if available, are involved.	3. To gather information and to provide support to clients
4. The nature and goals of the treatment program are provided.	4. To enhance compliance with the treatment program
5. Clients and family are told the hours during which services are available.	5. Same as #1
6. Clients and family are told the cost to them, if any.	6. Same as #1
7. Clients are told their rights and responsibilities.	7. To help prevent misunderstandings that might block treatment

---

Chart 56–2

NURSING ACTIONS AND RATIONALE DURING ADMISSION PROCEDURE

Nursing Action	Rationale
1. The nurse is responsible for admitting clients to the unit and meets them in the admitting office.	1. To provide clients with a positive attitude toward hospital staff and a feeling of support from the nurse
2. The nurse explains the admitting process to clients and makes sure that they are aware of their rights.	2. To decrease clients' anxiety and afford proper legal protection
3. The admitting nurse accompanies clients and families to the nursing unit and completes the nursing history, assessment, and plan.	3. To provide the client and family with a positive feeling toward the unit, and to gather necessary data
4. Clients' belongings are listed and checked for dangerous articles and medication.	4. To promote a safe and secure environment for all clients
5. Valuables clients may not keep are sent home with the family or sent to the hospital vault for safekeeping.	5. To prevent loss to clients due to their confusion or poor judgment
6. Clients and families are shown around the unit. This includes introductions to staff, explanations of routine procedures, and provision of a copy of the client handbook.	6. To foster a feeling of safety and security
7. The nurse stays with clients until they feel comfortable in the new environment.	7. To help create a feeling of safety
8. The physician is notified, if necessary, to obtain admitting orders.	8. So that treatment can begin
9. Other departments of the hospital that may be providing services to clients are notified of their admission.	9. Same as #8

Intake   Although intake in many cases is done by a private physician before the client comes to the hospital, clients who arrive without an admission reservation or private physician may require intake on the spot.

A qualified person as defined by the state mental health code, who in many cases can be a psychiatric nurse, must screen the client, using the above criteria, prior to admission. The nurse gathers the data for the assessment on the appropriate hospital forms.

Included are

1. Identifying data (name, address, age, and so on)
2. Complaint (reason the client is seeking help)
3. Nursing assessment of behavior relative to the complaint
4. Plan to
   a. Recommend admission (see Chap. 72 for types of admission)
   b. Recommend alternative treatment

If the client is to be admitted, the nurse carries out the actions shown in Chart 56–1.

Nursing Intervention   Chart 56–2 outlines nursing interventions during the admission procedure, and the theoretical rationale for each.

Nursing Assessment   A complete nursing assessment* is done within the first 24 hours after the admission. The objectives are

1. To collect data regarding the clients' illness, background, and social, developmental, and emotional responses
2. To assess the data in order to help establish a multidisciplinary treatment plan, and a nursing care plan
3. To involve clients in planning and individualizing the treatment plan and nursing care plan
4. To evaluate the effectiveness of treatment over time

Reference   1. Joint Commission on Accreditation of Hospitals: Consolidated Standards Manual for Child, Adolescent, and Adult Psychiatric, Alcoholism, and Drug Abuse Facilities, 1981

Bibliography   McFarland GK, Apostoles FE: The nursing history in a psychiatric setting: Adaptations to a variety of nursing care patterns and patient populations. J Psychiatr Nurs 13:12, 1975

*See Chapter 1 for the nursing assessment.

57

Rapid Tranquilization

Rachel Parios

OVERVIEW

Purpose
Considerations
Risks
Nursing Intervention

Rapid tranquilization is a pharmacological intervention used to rapidly diminish severe symptoms accompanying acute psychosis. Antipsychotic chemotherapy is preferable; it may be used in conjunction with physical management of psychiatric clients when their psychotic behavior could cause harm to themselves or others.

This method of chemical administration is in oral concentrate or intramuscular dosages prescribed every 15 minutes, ½ hour, 1 hour, or 2 hours. The physician's order may be for a limited number of doses or may cover a 24-hour period on an "as needed" basis. Careful observation and assessment of the client are required by the nursing and medical staff.

Chart 57–1
NURSING INTERVENTIONS AND RATIONALE WITH RAPID TRANQUILIZATION

Nursing Intervention	*Rationale*
1. Obtain a physician's order including 　a. Name of medication 　b. Dosage 　c. Method—oral concentrate or intramuscular 　d. Administration schedule 2. Prepare medication as prescribed.	1–2. Antipsychotic medication diminishes psychotic symptoms
3. Tell client name of medication and its effects. 4. Remain at client's side for reassurance and observation.	3–4. Reduces client's anxiety
5. Assess effects of medication: 　a. Monitor blood pressure and pulse	a. Alpha-adrenergic blockade of peripheral vascular system lowers blood pressure and causes postural hypotension
b. Monitor symptom reduction	b. Antipsychotic medication diminishes psychotic symptoms
c. Monitor anticholinergic effects of medication	c. Antipsychotic medication having higher dosage, lower potency, for example, chlorpromazine hydrochloride (Thorazine), thioridazine (Mellaril), or chlorprothixene (Taractin), with higher anticholinergic action lowers blood pressure, is more sedating, and tends to produce fewer extrapyramidal side effects. Antipsychotic medication having lower dosage and higher potency, for example haloperidol (Haldol), perphenazine (Trilafon), thiothixene hydrochloride (Navane), and fluphenazine hydrochloride (Prolixin) with lower anticholinergic action, is less hypotensive and less sedating and causes more extrapyramidal side effects.
6. Monitor extrapyramidal side effects, observing for any signs and symptoms of the following: 　a. Dystonia—prolonged, persistent, firm, tonic contractions of muscle groups of the head, neck and jaw including torticollis, spasms of lips, tongue, face, or throat, oculogyric crisis, opisthotonos 　b. Dyskinesia—clonic, uncoordinated, involuntary contraction and relaxation of muscle groups 　c. Akathesia—involuntary motor restlessness of lower extremities 　d. Akinesia—rigidity, cogwheeling, stiffness, and slowness of involuntary movements	6. These side effects cause clients much distress and discomfort. Unless attended to they can become permanent.
7. Obtain physician's order for and medicate with antiparkinsonian medication, for example, benztropine mesylate (Cogentin), trihexyphenidyl hydrochloride (Artane), and biperiden (Akineton)	7. Rapidly relieves the pseudo-Parkinsonian, extrapyramidal side effects of antipsychotic medication
8. Tranquilize client until symptoms of psychosis diminish and client is tranquil.	8. Assures necessary drug concentration level in brain and reduction of psychotic symptoms.

Purpose	Antipsychotic medication is used to rapidly tranquilize clients exhibiting acute psychotic symptomatology and is implemented to rapidly accomplish the following: 1. Diminish severely aggressive, assaultive, violent behavior, agitation, delusions, hallucinations, and disordered thinking present in acute psychosis 2. Provide adequate dosage of medication to achieve necessary drug concentration in the brain (Very high ranges are necessary in some individuals.) 3. Reduce the client's experience of psychic pain 4. Assess the client's drug tolerance, thus establishing a maximal daily dose and determining the client's sensitivity toward undesirable side effects
Considerations*	1. Client's history of drug response 2. Family history of drug response 3. Wide range of drug effectiveness 4. Benefit-risk ratio (When client is in psychotic crisis, intravenous medication may be given as initial dose.)
Risks*	1. Antiadrenergic effects 2. Alpha-adrenergic blockade of the peripheral vascular system 3. Electrocardiographic changes[1] 4. Anticholinergic or atropinelike effects 5. Co-administration of antipsychotic and antiparkinsonian medication 6. Overdosage 7. Drug interactions 8. Altered laboratory values
Nursing Interventions	Chart 57–1 shows the nursing interventions and rationale associated with providing rapid tranquilization.
Reference	1. Bernstein JG (ed): Clinical Psychopharmacology. Massachusetts, PSG Publishing, 1978
Bibliography	The Psychiatrist's Compendium of Drug Therapy. New York, Biomedical Information Corporation, 1982–1983

*See Part VI, Psychopharmacology and Psychiatric Nursing.

58

Administration
of Medications

Cynthia M. Taylor

Role of Medication in Psychiatric Treatment   The role of medication in the treatment plan for a psychiatric client depends on the orientation of the practitioner. Practitioners who have a strong biological orientation use medication to treat the client's behavior, whereas other practitioners may use medication to offer some degree of symptom relief while employing psychotherapy to resolve the underlying problem.

Nursing Responsibilities   The nursing responsibilities in administering medication follow the nursing process.

A. **ASSESSMENT**

The nurse makes a complete assessment of the client's drug history at the time of admission or later as part of a medication work-up. Areas to be assessed include the client's

1. Prior and current experiences with prescription and nonprescription drugs
2. Reactions to various medications taken previously
3. Attitudes about medication

B. **PLANNING**

Before the client is started on medication, the nurse begins teaching the client and family about

1. The purpose of the medication
2. Possible side effects
3. The client's responsibilities while taking the medication

If the decision is made to have the client self-administer the medication, more detailed instruction is necessary (see Chap. 63).

C. **IMPLEMENTATION**

1. Generally speaking, in inpatient settings, the nurse administers the medication. Prior to the administration of a drug the nurse must have a thorough knowledge of the drug's absorption, destruction, biotransformation, and excretion. The nurse must also be aware of the therapeutic range, dosage schedule, and effects of the drug, including contraindications.
2. The nurse must be technically skilled in administering drugs orally and intramuscularly. It is rarely necessary to administer drugs intravenously or subcutaneously in a psychiatric setting.
3. If the client refuses to take the prescribed medication, the nurse has additional responsibilities. In most states, the client has the right to refuse medication. The nurse must be familiar with the state's mental health code as it relates to giving clients medication against their will in an emergency situation. When a client refuses medication, the nurse always documents this in the medical record and notifies the physician.

D. **EVALUATION**

The nurse evaluates the client's response to the medication, including behavior, symptom reduction, side effects, tolerance, and attitude about taking the medication. This evaluation is an important part of the nurse's responsibility because many times several types of medication are tried before the right medication is found.

Procedure*   1. Physician's orders for medication are filled in the pharmacy department and sent to each nursing unit by the pharmacist.

*This procedure assumes the use of a unit dose system.

CHICAGO LAKESHORE HOSPITAL

MEDICATION ADMINISTRATION RECORD

Enter Here
IN PENCIL
Number of
Forms in Use

| 1 |

NAME *John Doe*

DIAGNOSES: *Major Affective Disorder*

CASE NO. *111-333-555*

ALLERGIC TO: *Tetracycline*   DIET: *General*
(Record in Red)

ROOM NO. *400 B.*

DATES GIVEN

OR DATE INITIALS	STOP DATE	MEDICATION-DOSAGE-FREQUENCY-RT OF ADM.	HR	5/1	5/2	5/3	5/4	5/5	5/6	5/7	5/8	5/9	5/10	5/11	5/12	5/13	5/14
5/1/81	5/22	Thorazine 50 mg PO BID	9 A	ct	ct	ct	ct	ct									
			5 P	JS	JS	JS	JS	JS									
5/1/81	5/29	Cogentin 2 mg PO 9 AM	9 A	ct	ct	ct	ct	ct									
5/1/81	—	Prolixin Enthamate 25 mg	11 AM	ct	←												
		1 cc IM q̄ wks.					Give next dose 5-15-81										

Single Orders

OR DATE INITIALS	MEDICATION-DOSAGE-FREQUENCY-RT. OF ADM.	TO BE GIVEN DATE	TIME	NURSE INITIAL	OR DATE INITIALS	MEDICATION-DOSAGE-RT. OF ADM.	TO BE GIVEN DATE	TIME
5/5/81	Thorazine 50 mg IM STAT	5/5/81	9 PM	JS				

AGE *32*   DOCTOR *Weiss*   DATE/TIME ADMITTED *5-1-81   5 AM*

NAME *John Doe*

FIG. 58–1   Medication record. (Reprinted with the permission of Chicago Lakeshore Hospital, Chicago, IL)

ct	*Cynthia M. Taylor*	R.N.	*J.S.*	*Jane Schultz*	R.N.			
Initials	Full Signature	Title	Initials	Full Signature	Title			

RN Medications

OR DATE INITIALS	STOP DATE	MEDICATION-DOSAGE-FREQUENCY RT. OF ADM.	DOSES GIVEN																	
5-1-81	*5-22-81*	*A.S.A. gr. X PRN*	DATE	5/2																
		for headache	TIME	3p																
		q̄ 4 hours.	INIT	*ct*																
			DATE																	
			TIME																	
			INIT																	
			DATE																	
			TIME																	
			INIT																	
			DATE																	
			TIME																	
			INIT																	
			DATE																	
			TIME																	
			INIT																	
			DATE																	
			TIME																	
			INIT																	

FIG. 58–1 *(continued)*

2. To ensure an accurate record, the night nurse goes through the medex and checks each medication sheet against the physician's orders. On units with primary nursing, the primary nurse checks the medex for accuracy daily.
3. The nurse who recopies current orders on new medication sheets initials the upper right corner of the new sheet.
4. Before the medication orders go to the pharmacy, the medication nurse goes through the client's charts to check for any new medication orders.
5. Each bin in the medication cart designates the client's name and room number.
6. At the time designated for passing medication, the nurse wheels the cart to the predetermined area for dispensing medication and the clients come to receive their medications.
7. The nurse makes sure the medication label on the container corresponds with the medex for each client prior to dispensing the medication.
8. Medication is placed in appropriate medication cups and given to the client.
9. Before administering medication, the nurse identifies each client by checking the name band and asking the client's name.
10. The nurse makes certain that the client receives and takes the medication at the time it is given. The client is not allowed to carry off the medication to take later, nor is the medication left at the bedside.
11. If the client refuses to take medication, the nurse indicates this on the chart with the reason and informs the physician. In some settings, the medication is returned to the pharmacy, and in others, unused medication is destroyed.
12. The nurse indicates medications administered at other times (for example, prn) in the chart.
13. After medication is administered, the nurse initials and signs the client's medication sheet before administering medication to the next client.
14. When the medication delivery process has been completed, the medication cart is locked and placed in the appropriate storage area.

Figure 58–1 is an example of a typical medication record.

Bibliography

Cain R, Cain N: A compendium of psychiatric drugs. In Backer B et al (eds): Psychiatric/Mental Health Nursing. New York, Van Nostrand Reinhold, 1978

Falconer M: The Drug, The Nurse, The Patient. Philadelphia, WB Saunders, 1978

Hollister L: The Clinical Use of Psychotherapeutic Drugs. Springfield, IL, Charles C Thomas, 1973

Rodman M, Smith D: Pharmacology and Drug Therapy in Nursing. Philadelphia, JB Lippincott, 1979

Shader R: Manual of Psychiatric Therapeutics. Boston, Little, Brown & Co, 1975

59

Electroconvulsive _____

Treatment _____

Rachel Parios / *Cynthia M. Taylor*

OVERVIEW

Description
Mode of Action
Purpose
Indications
Contraindications
Risk Factors
Side Effects
Measurement
Procedure

Electroconvulsive therapy (ECT) was introduced in 1933 as a treatment to "cure" psychosis by inducing convulsions. Although it has undergone modifications, ECT remains a useful treatment for a limited number of psychiatric conditions. However, it has come under severe criticism from consumer groups. Many of these criticisms have been directed at the use of outdated techniques or poor client selection.

Knowledge of the actions, indications, and contraindications of ECT is essential for establishing guidelines for the effective use of this treatment. The administration of ECT can take place in an inpatient or outpatient treatment area where the client is monitored before and after treatment by a physician, a nurse, and an anesthetist. Clinicians vary in the frequency with which they give treatments: from two to three times weekly, every day, or twice a day. As a general rule, the briefer the client's illness and the more acute the onset, the fewer the number of treatments over time.

Description In ECT, Atropine gr $\frac{1}{150}$ im is administered $\frac{1}{2}$ hour before treatment, and a grand mal seizure is induced by passing an electric current (200–1600 milliamperes) through the temporal lobes of the brain and into the hypothalamus after the client has been anesthetized intravenously. A short-acting barbiturate, methohexital sodium (Brevital Sodium), 5 ml to 10 ml (10 mg/1 ml), and a short-acting muscle relaxant, suxamethonium chloride (Anectine chloride), 0.3 ml to 5 ml (20 mg/1 ml), are given intravenously. The physician regulates the ECT machine to produce the voltage (90–170 V) of alternating current across the electrodes for 0.1 to 1 second's duration. The tonic phase of muscle contraction lasts approximately 10 seconds, and the clonic phase of movements lasts approximately 30 to 40 seconds. With the use of succinylcholine chloride, the modified convulsion is so attenuated that there is only a mild grimace or blepharospasm when the current is applied. There is a slow plantar flexion (reverse Babinski) during the tonic phase, and there are tiny movements of the toes (fasciculations) during the clonic phase. The muscular contraction during the grand mal seizure still allows the effect of the treatment to occur but greatly reduces the posttreatment complication formerly seen with unmodified ECT. Electroconvulsive therapy can be administered bilaterally or unilaterally; the latter method is believed to reduce memory loss and confusion. Unilateral ECT is done on the person's nondominant side (if the client is righthanded, electrodes are placed on the *right* side).

Mode of Action Changes in behavior from ECT result from certain correlates rather than from a simple cause-and-effect relationship. When the electrical current from ECT is transmitted through the temporal lobe of the brain, it passes down into the diencephalon, increasing activity of central neurotransmitters and releasing hypothalamic peptides, which relieve the primary depressive syndrome and foster change in behavior.[1] Chemicals are stimulated and discharged into the brain, autonomic nervous system, body musculature, and endocrine glands, with the following correlates[1]:

1. Molecular activity increases the turnover and synthesis rates of serotonin.
2. Polypeptides from the hypothalamus alter neuroendocrine activity believed to disrupt thalamocortical pathways.
3. Biochemically there is alteration of the cerebrovascular system, with increased choline and cholinesterase blood levels.
4. Electrocardiogram (EEG) wave pattern is altered, demonstrating
   a. Neuron activity on the nondominant side
   b. Persistence of these chemicals in the brain, which alters cerebral biochemistry
   c. Slow wave activity resulting from deep central cerebral structural change
5. With the EEG changes noted on the nondominant side, psychological testing also demonstrates evidence of this change.

Purpose   ECT is used to rapidly relieve the following symptoms in acute psychosis[1]:
1. Catatonia
2. Stupor
3. Suicidal attempts and thoughts
4. Uncontrollable excitement and exhaustion
5. Anorexia
6. Insomnia
7. Delusions (guilt, worthlessness, somatic)
8. Diurnal mood swings
9. Weight loss
10. Inability to concentrate
11. Inhibition of motor activity

Indications   A. SELECTED DIAGNOSES
ECT is chosen as a psychiatric treatment modality for clients with the following diagnoses:
1. Major affective disorder
2. Psychotic depression
3. Unipolar–bipolar depression
4. Involutional depression
5. Depression (geriatric, postpartum)
6. Mania
7. Catatonia
8. Schizophrenia that is unresponsive to other therapies

B. SELECTION OF THERAPY
ECT is preferred when[1]:
1. Previous episodes of the same illness have been unresponsive to drug therapy
2. The client has a history of drug idiosyncrasies
3. Illness occurs in the first trimester of pregnancy and drugs are contraindicated
4. The client's illness progresses so rapidly and severely that there is no time for drug trial

Contraindications   Electroconvulsive therapy is contraindicated for clients diagnosed as follows[1]:
1. Reactive depression (neurotic, personal)
2. Psychoneurosis (hysteria, hypochondriasis, anxiety state)
3. Schizophrenia (paranoid, hebephrenic, simple)
4. Drug dependence
5. Personality disorder

Risk Factors   The following are considered high risk factors for ECT, and caution is indicated in applying ECT in their presence[1]:
1. Pregnancy
2. Fractures or history of recent fractures
3. Organic brain syndrome
4. Brain tumors
5. Advanced coronary or myocardial disease
6. Cardiac arrhythmias
7. Acute and chronic endocarditis
8. Hypertension–hypotension
9. Aortic aneurysms
10. Thrombophlebitis

Chart 59–1

PRETREATMENT PROCEDURE FOR ADMINISTERING ELECTROCONVULSIVE THERAPY

Nursing Intervention	*Rationale*
Monitor Medical Screening	
1. Check client's record for history of cardiovascular or neurologic illnesses.	1. Anesthesia and seizure provide potential risks for clients with these illnesses.
2. Check client's record to be sure physical examination included the following and that all are within normal limits:	2. Reduces possibility of posttreatment complications
a. Cardiovascular—EKG, pulse, blood pressure, temperature, respirations	a. To prevent cardiovascular complications
b. CBC and blood chemistries	b. Same as a
c. Chest, spine x-rays	c. To prevent orthopedic complications
d. Brain or CT scan when there are signs of neurologic problems or organicity, or history of aneurism	d. To prevent neurologic complications
e. Urinalysis	e. To rule out infections or other complications
f. Funduscopic eye examination when there is a history of glaucoma	f. To rule out presence of glaucoma
g. Dental examination	g. To make sure there are no loose teeth, which could dislodge and block airway
h. Memory test	h. To establish baseline data for post-ECT memory loss
i. Suxamethonium sensitivity (Pseudocholinesterase) blood level	i. To prevent allergic reaction
3. Bring any abnormal findings to the attention of the physician.	3. Client must be medically cleared to prevent complications
Monitor Consent	
1. Remind physician to obtain signature for consent. (Client or family may sign in some states.) Nurse acts as witness.	1. If client and family are sensitively informed of ECT, the potential benefits, hazards, and aftereffects, they are better able to make an informed decision about using it.
2. Assure that consent includes	2. Ensures informed consent
a. Name of client	
b. Name of psychiatrist	
c. Explanation of treatment, how it is administered	
d. The number of expected treatments	
e. The risks involved, including possible confusion and temporary recent memory loss, which will disappear	
f. The possibility of the client or family discontinuing treatments at any time	
g. Date	
h. Client, guardian, or family member's signature	
Monitor Client and Family's Psychological Condition	
1. Help client and family to understand anything that is still confusing about the treatment.	1. Reduces anxiety
2. Show client the treatment area prior to treatment, when possible.	2. Reduces anxiety
3. Have other clients who have responded to ECT talk with the client, when possible.	3. Reduces anxiety

   11. Narrow-angle glaucoma

   12. Ocular hypertension with atropine

   13. Liver disease

   14. Low cholinesterase activity

   15. Barbiturate or suxamethonium chloride toxicity

(Text continues on page 512)

Chart 59–2

PROCEDURE FOR ADMINISTERING ELECTROCONVULSIVE THERAPY

Nursing Intervention	*Rationale*
1. Ensure that the client receives nothing by mouth after midnight.	1. Reduces possibility of vomiting or aspiration of contents of stomach
2. Take vital signs.	2. Alerts staff to cardiovascular problems
3. Administer atropine grains, 1/150 IM, about 1/2 hour to 1 hour before treatment.	3. Prevents cardiac arrhythmias produced by vagal stimulation; decreases salivary secretion and potential for aspiration during seizure
4. Reassure client about treatment.	4. Reduces anxiety
5. Have client void and defecate prior to treatment.	5. Prevents voiding or defecation during seizure
6. Have client dress in loose clothing.	6. Prevents bodily constriction during seizure
7. Make sure physician, anesthesia, and staff are present for ECT.	7. Increases client safety
8. Make sure all equipment is in the treatment room, including medication for anesthesia, muscle relaxant, CPR cart, endotracheal tubes, and oxygen.	8. Expedites safe treatment
9. Assist client onto stretcher.	9. Reassures client
10. Have client remove any dentures or partial dentures.	10. Prevents damage to dentures and mouth
11. Provide patent airway.	11. Prevents mouth injuries; eases artificial ventilation with oxygen; reduces possibility of brain anoxia
12. Prepare client as follows: *For bilateral ECT*—Prepare anterior portion of client's temples with alcohol swab and conductive jelly. *For unilateral ECT*—Prepare anterior portion of client's nondominant temple (if right handed, right temple) and posterior scalp at any location 2 inches from anterior temple with alcohol swab and conductive jelly. Apply 1–1½-inch round flat metal electrodes to head band, and apply conductive jelly to electrodes.	12. Use of alcohol cleanses skin and aids friction. Use of conductive jelly aids in current conduction and prevention of burns to client's temples or scalp.

13. *For Monitored ECT* (occlusion of vessel)
  a. Assist physician or anesthesiologist with butterfly needle for IV injection of Brevital and Anectine.
	13.
	  a. Allows needle to remain in vein, keeping vein open during ECT, facilitating rapid IV therapy during emergency, if necessary

b. Assist with administration of O₂ pre and post treatment.	b. Client awakens and becomes alert more rapidly after the treatment
c. When physician or anesthesiologist has injected all but 1 ml of Brevital, inflate blood pressure cuff, which has been placed on arm opposite to one with IV. (Blood pressure cuff is inflated to 10 mm above client's previous systolic B/P and maintained.) Physician injects Anectine and last 1 ml of Brevital.	c. Occludes circulation in one extremity, preventing paralytic effects of Anectine in that extremity, and fosters observation of client's seizure Forces Anectine through butterfly tubing into client
d. Wait with physician and anesthesiologist until small muscular fasciculations around neck, face, toes and fingers have ceased.	d. Differentiates Anectine fasciculations from motor activity of seizure
e. When client is anesthetized, and has stopped fasciculating (about 45–60 seconds after injection of intravenous medication), apply electrodes, making sure hands are on rubber, not metal portion.	e. Assures total effect of Brevital and Anectine have been reached
f. Have physician give treatment.	f. Current and electrodes are monitored simultaneously.
g. Observe client's extremity, gently protecting same while timing duration of seizure (at least 23 seconds), both tonic and clonic phases.	g. Determines that client has had a seizure

Chart 59–2
(continued)

Nursing Intervention	Rationale
h. At the same time *gently* protect shoulders and upper and lower extremities.	h. Client may not be paralyzed by Anectine and have more visible motor reaction to seizure. Prevents fractures and dislocations of joints
14. When seizure is finished, anesthetist will give oxygen.	14. Helps client awaken
15. Take blood pressure. It will be elevated just after treatment and will then return to normal level.	15. Helps determine that client is physically stabilized
16. Awaken client by calling name. Reassure client.	16. Client will be confused. Reassurance reduces anxiety.
17. Help client down from stretcher when awake and aware of surroundings.	17. Client will be confused. Reassurance reduces anxiety.
18. Serve client breakfast. Offer reassurance and information about time and place. "Your treatment is over. You are in the hospital. Your memory will come back."	18. Helps client resume daily routine; reduces anxiety

---

CONSENT TO ELECTROCONVULSIVE THERAPY

1) I AUTHORIZE Dr. _____, and/or a qualified physician under his/her direction to administer electroconvulsive therapy (also known as electroshock treatment) and preliminary anesthesia with hypnotic or sedative drugs supplemented by a drug that induces muscular relaxation to _____ and to continue such treatment at such intervals as he/she and the physician may deem advisable.

2) The purpose of the treatment is to attempt to relieve, reduce, and remove the existing symptoms. The effect and nature of this therapy and possible alternative methods of treatment have been explained. I understand that electroconvulsive therapy, like medical and surgical procedures, involves an element of calculated risk despite precautions. I have discussed this with the above-mentioned doctor and have been duly advised of the implications and risks involved in this form of therapy.

3) The number varies from case to case; up to 12 treatments may be required during this hospital stay in order for this form of therapy to be effective. Should additional treatments be necessary, a psychiatric consultation will be sought.

4) Frequently, a period of amnesia may occur during and following the course of electroconvulsive therapy.

5) No guarantee or assurance has been given by anyone as to the results that may be obtained.

6) I understand that I may withdraw this consent at any time.

DATE:_____   SIGNED:_____
                                                                Client, Guardian, or Family Member

                                                WITNESS:_____
                                                                Primary Nurse

                                                WITNESS:_____
                                                                Attending Psychiatrist

FIG. 59–1 Example of a consent form for electroconvulsive therapy (ECT). (Reprinted with the permission of Chicago Lakeshore Hospital, Chicago, IL)

16. Porphyria (familial metabolic disorder)
17. Paget's disease (bone overgrowth of spine)
18. Advanced osteoporosis
Note: ECT is NEVER given when the client has signs of intracranial pressure.

Side Effects A. **DYSMNESIA**

     B. **CONFUSION**
     This varies from no confusion with first treatment to confusion lasting for several hours. With an increased number of treatments, more severe confusion may be seen.

     C. **MEMORY LOSS**
     Recent memory disturbance often occurs but is time limited. With an increased number of treatments, memory loss goes farther back, and there is a more global memory disturbance. It is sometimes unclear whether the memory disturbance or difficulty with concentration is the result of ECT or the original illness.

Measurement It is possible to measure the client's vital signs, EEG, EKG, and the length of the convulsions during treatment by the use of specialized equipment, for example, the MECTA machine. In the absence of such equipment, the nurse is responsible for taking vital signs. Observation of the client's seizure (monitoring) is done by the nurse in the following way: The vessels in one arm are occluded by a blood pressure cuff so that this arm, which does not receive the muscle relaxant, can be observed, and the exact length and strength of the seizure can be observed and measured.

Procedure Chart 59–1 shows the pretreatment procedure for ECT. The procedure for administering ECT is presented in Chart 59–2. Nursing interventions and rationale are indicated in both charts. An example of a consent form for ECT is shown in Figure 59–1.

Reference 1. Fink M: Convulsive Therapy, Theory and Practice. New York, Raven Press, 1979

Bibliography Mulaik JS: Nurses' questions about electroconvulsive therapy. J Psychiatr Nurs 19:15, 1979
Thomas SP: Uses and abuses of electric convulsive shock therapy. J Psychiatr Nurs 16:17, 1978

60

Administration
of Cold Wet Pack

Cynthia M. Taylor

OVERVIEW

Indications for Use
Application of Cold Wet Pack
  Equipment and Personnel
  Preparatory Steps
  Procedure

Hydrotherapy is defined as the treatment of a disease by the use of water in any form. The cold wet pack (CWP) is a form of hydrotherapy used to treat severely agitated clients.

The procedure renders the client totally immobilized in a CWP. The sheets are initially cold. (Cold sheets are very important because the client can easily become overheated.) The initial contraction of the subcutaneous vessels when they come in contact with the cold wet sheet is followed by dilation of the vessels, which floods the body surface with blood and creates the feeling of warmth and relaxation.[1]

Several factors are involved in the effect produced by the CWP. Clients often cite the external control of impulses as reassuring. Another factor is the concrete expression of care taking, as evidenced by the bodily contact with the nursing staff who are wrapping the client in the sheets. Dependency gratification is inherent in the procedure.[3]

Indications for Use

CWPs are typically used for clients who exhibit combative, impulsive, or severe acting-out behavior and are not responding to medication (or cannot take psychotrophic medication), or when the medication has not yet taken effect.[3]

CWP has also been seen as symbolic of the regressed state of infancy, and positive results are attributed to the nurturing effect.[2] The difference between total immobilization in a CWP and localized restraints has been pointed out. Total immobilization is seen as inducing passive relaxation and acceptance, while being tied up locally (such as with full leather restraints) leaves the client free to struggle and actually provokes a struggle.[3]

Application of Cold Wet Pack*

A. **EQUIPMENT AND PERSONNEL**
Pack bed with bars on each side of frame and waterproof mattress (Fig. 60–1)
Suction machine
6 Sheets for pack bundle
1 Sheet to cover pack bed mattress
1 Cotton bath blanket
1 Waterproof pillow and regular pillow case
1 Regular blanket to cover client when sheet envelopment is completed
Watch with a second hand
Pen and paper
Liquid beverage cup with drinking straw
A minimum of 4 staff members, 2 on each side of pack bed

B. **PREPARATORY STEPS**
1. Obtain written physician's order to employ the CWP for a period of 1 to 3 hours. If client is sleeping in the pack, an order may be obtained to extend the time to its limit of three hours. See state mental health code, since times vary from state to state.
2. Prepare client by explaining treatment. *The pack is never presented as a threat or form of punishment.*
3. Fold safety sheets, body sheets, and arm and leg sheets as shown in Figure 60–2.
4. Fill deep sink or bathtub with cold water. Ice may be added if water is tepid.

---

*This procedure was developed by the Nursing Department, The New York Hospital–Cornell Medical Center, Westchester Division, Department of Psychiatry. Illustrations adapted from drawings by Dennis Thornton. Reprinted with permission.

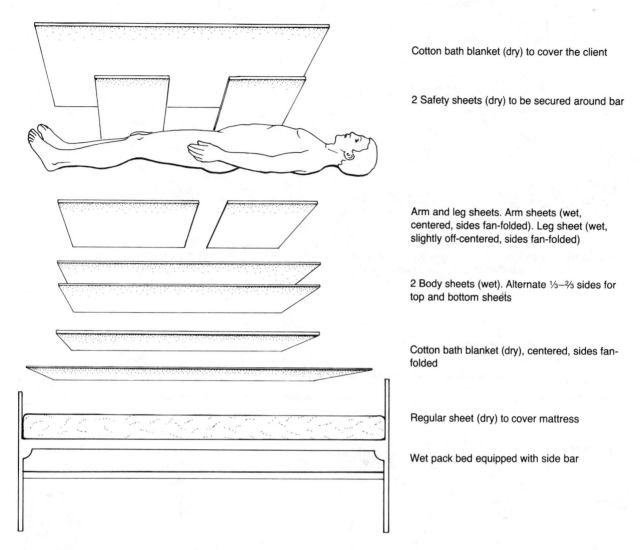

Cotton bath blanket (dry) to cover the client

2 Safety sheets (dry) to be secured around bar

Arm and leg sheets. Arm sheets (wet, centered, sides fan-folded). Leg sheet (wet, slightly off-centered, sides fan-folded)

2 Body sheets (wet). Alternate ⅓–⅔ sides for top and bottom sheets

Cotton bath blanket (dry), centered, sides fan-folded

Regular sheet (dry) to cover mattress

Wet pack bed equipped with side bar

FIG. 60–1 Schematic of equipment for cold wet pack procedure. (Nursing Department, The New York Hospital, Cornell Medical Center, Westchester Division, Department of Psychiatry. Illustrations for cold wet pack procedure based on drawings by Dennis Thornton. Reprinted with permission)

5. Set aside cotton bath blanket, regular bed blanket, two safety sheets, cover sheet, pillow, and pillow case from CWP bundle. Keep these dry.

6. Immerse remaining four sheets (two body and arm and leg sheets) in water. Allow them to saturate thoroughly through their folds; soak approximately 15 minutes. Cold water must be used because the combination of body heat and warm, wet sheets would become uncomfortably warm after about ½ hour. Warm water may be used to soak sheets when wet packing is for a shorter duration, for example, for tube feeding.

7. Bring pack bed to location where client will be packed; cover bed with cover sheet, which was set aside. Miter corners.

8. Bring suction machine to bedside. Since the client will be immobilized and restrained, a suction machine must be on hand in case of aspiration.

9. Place dry cotton bath blanket (removed earlier from bundle) across bed widthwise; fold top edge over about 6 inches at neck height. Fan-fold sides; smooth

(*Text continues on page 518*)

A. *SAFETY SHEETS*

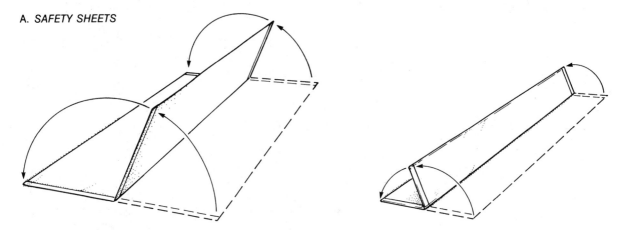

Each safety sheet will be folded in quarters lengthwise. To do so, fold sheet in half by bringing the nonhemmed edges together. Then fold in half again by bringing new edges together.

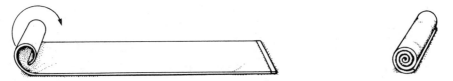

Take one open end and roll compactly to the other end, producing a single roll. Repeat entire procedure for second sheet.

B. *BODY SHEETS*

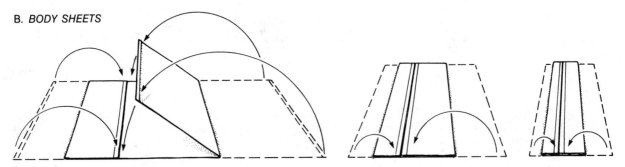

Open regular sheet completely on a flat surface. Bring each hemmed edge together so that one section is twice as wide as the other (*i.e.*, ⅓ and ⅔ sections). Smooth out wrinkles. Take new ends and fold in half to hem line again. Do this twice on each side. Smooth out wrinkles.

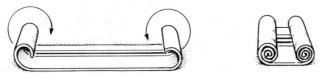

Roll the open edges of the sheet compactly toward the center on each side, giving it a scroll-like effect when completed. Repeat entire procedure for second body sheet.

FIG. 60–2 Methods for folding sheets. (*A*) Safety sheets. (*B*) Body sheets. (*C*) Arm and leg sheets. (*D*) Alternate method of folding arm and leg sheets.

C. ARM AND LEG SHEETS

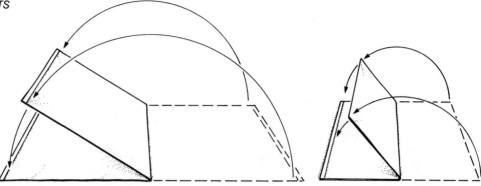

Arm and leg sheets will be folded in quarters widthwise. To do so, fold sheet in half widthwise by bringing hemmed edges together. Then fold in half again by bringing new edges together.

Turn sheet sideways. Take open edges and roll compactly toward center, producing a scroll-like effect when completed. Repeat entire procedure for second sheet.

D. ALTERNATE METHOD OF FOLDING ARM AND LEG SHEETS

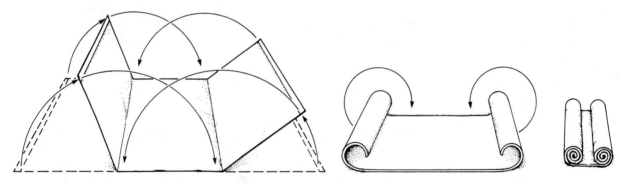

For most individuals, folding the arm and leg sheets in quarters widthwise will be adequate. However, clients who are taller and/or have long arms and/or legs may require that the width of the sheet be increased. Increasing the length of the sheet is to prevent body surfaces from touching. If you determine that a longer width is necessary follow the method described below. *Note:* Folding the sheet in thirds widthwise will increase the width of the sheet approximately 9 inches.

With the sheet on a flat surface, bring one hemmed edge toward the center of the sheet approximately ⅓ the length of the sheet. Take the opposite hemmed edge and fold similarly so that this third overlaps the already folded portion.

Turn sheet sideways. Take open edges and roll compactly toward center, producing a scroll-like effect when completed.

It is possible that you may want a combination of these two methods (*e.g.,* arm sheet folded in thirds and leg sheet folded in quarters). If so, follow the instructions for folding and then fold one of the two scrolls in half in order to distinguish one from the other.

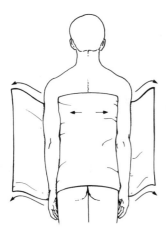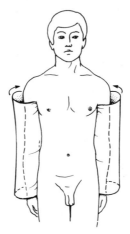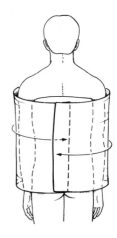

(A) Place client on top of prepared sheets. Adjust arm sheet if necessary (*i.e.,* so that top of sheet is even with axilla).

(B) Lift one arm and draw sheet up close to body, and then wrap around outside of arm. Roll client to opposite side so that end of sheet can be wrapped smoothly across the back.

(C) Repeat for other arm so that ends of sheet overlap smoothly across client's back.

FIG. 60–3 Procedure for wrapping arms. Arm sheet is placed on bed (atop body sheets) so that the top of the sheet will be even with the client's axilla and will be of equal length on both sides. Fan-fold sides. Proceed as shown above.

out wrinkles in center. Wring out four wet sheets and bring them to pack bed. Length of sheet should be equal to client's body length; fold top edge of sheet accordingly. Avoid dry, abrasive areas on sheets by having them thoroughly saturated.

10. Center one wet body sheet on bed, unrolling it lengthwise like a scroll. Place upper edge even with top edge of the blanket, unfolding sheet so that one fan-folded side remains wider than the other (*i.e.,* 1/3 and 2/3 proportions); smooth out center.

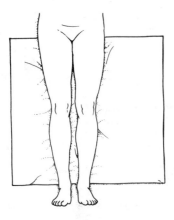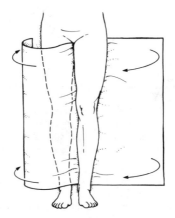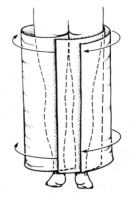

(A) With client lying on his back, adjust sheet so that top of sheet is even with client's crotch and bottom is even with the ankles. Do not cover feet during the procedure.

(B) Lift right leg and draw sheet out from under same leg. Bring 1/3 side up between client's legs and over top of the right leg. Wrap excess sheet behind same leg.

(C) Bring 2/3 side over outside of left leg and wrap across top of both legs. Wrap excess sheet around back of both legs so that the two ends overlap behind client's legs.

FIG. 60–4 Procedure for wrapping legs. Place folded leg sheet on bed so that sheet is divided into 1/3 and 2/3 sections, with the 1/3 side under client's right leg. Fan-fold sides of sheet. Proceed as shown above.

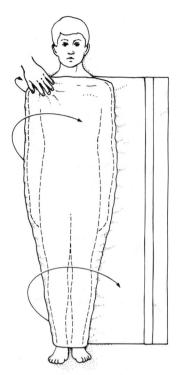 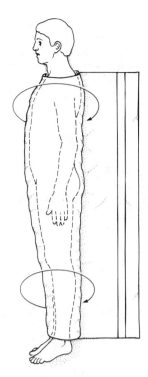 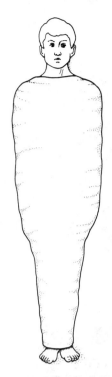

(A) Having wrapped arms and legs, bring the top end of the ⅓ side of the body sheet up over top of client's shoulder and down toward body. Hold edge of sheet in position on shoulder. Grasp end of sheet with other hand and bring remainder of sheet up at an angle across chest, thereby making a mitered corner at the shoulder. Simultaneously pull remainder of body sheet across torso and legs.

(B) Roll client toward you (*i.e.*, onto shoulder just wrapped) and smoothly wrap remainder of sheet across back and legs.

(C) Bring other side (⅔ side) of body sheet across body, mitering shoulder pocket as just described. Continue to wrap, turning client as necessary until client is enveloped in entire sheet. Remember to smooth out sheets as much as possible when wrapping client. Repeat this procedure for second body sheet and finally with pack blanket. Secure safety sheets.

FIG. 60–5 Procedure for wrapping body sheets.

11. Place second wet body sheet on top of the first, again centering it, but place the wider (2/3) fan-folded side on top of the narrower (1/3) fan-folded side of the first sheet. Smooth out wrinkles. At this point, the two body sheets should alternate (1/3) and (2/3) sides from bottom to top sheets.
12. Center wet arm sheet and unfold on bed, top edge approximately even with client's axilla. Fan-fold edges; smooth out center.
13. Unfold wet leg sheet, placing it in a position to cover client's knees. Leave one side slightly longer than the other, fan-fold edges, and smooth out center. During the procedure, prevent any two body surfaces from rubbing together, especially bony protuberances.

C. PROCEDURE
1. Having explained procedure to client, suggesting toileting, assist with undressing as needed and cover client with a robe or sheet. Clients wear underpants only. Bring client back to pack bed. Avoid exposing the client unnecessarily. Ask client to lie flat on back, on sheets. Explain that the initial

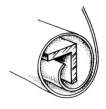

(A) Pull sheet down from bed, bringing sheet around outside of securing bar. Wrap about 12″ of the sheet under and around the bar so that the sheet is tucked under itself. Holding this end of the sheet in place, pull remainder across client's body.

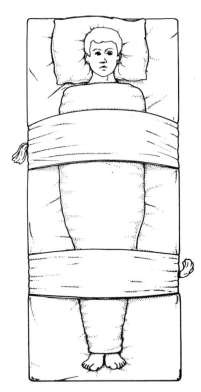

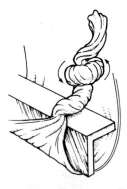

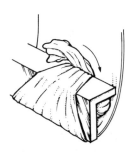

(B) With end of sheet taut across client's body, guide sheet under the inside of the securing bar and pull up toward you. Keeping sheet taut around bar, twist sheet until a large knot is formed. Shove knot over and under the top of the bar so that the knot is wedged under the upper lip of the bar.

(C) Repeat procedure for second safety sheet. However, alternate the side on which the knot is formed. Place pillow under client's head. Make sure that suction machine and drinking fluid are readily available. Cover client with extra blanket, leaving feet uncovered.

FIG. 60–6 Securing safety sheets. One safety sheet is secured across the client's chest, the other across the knees.

contact with the cold sheets will be uncomfortable. Reassure client that warmth will ensue.

2. Assemble two staff members on either side of the bed to prevent client from being rolled too near the edge.

3. Wrap arms (Fig. 60–3). With client on his/her back and arms flat at sides, bring one side of arm sheet under arm and back around arm, ending smoothly across his back. Do the same with the other side. Client's arms and hands should be in a comfortable position. Work rapidly to avoid chilling the client.

4. Wrap legs (Fig. 60–4). Bring shorter side of leg sheet up between client's knees, wrapping the excess around back of knees.

5. Wrap body sheets (Fig. 60–5). Having completed wrapping of arms and legs, bring corner of narrower (1/3) side of body sheet up over top of client's shoulder and down toward body. Hold in position with other hand and bring remainder of sheet up at an angle across body, thereby making a mitered corner at the shoulder. Roll client toward you and smoothly wrap remainder of sheet across back. Avoid wrinkles under body by putting folds of excess sheet under natural curves of body, that is, under curves of buttocks.

6. Bring other side (2/3) of sheet across body, mitering shoulder pocket as in step #5; continue to wrap, turning client as necessary until enveloped in entire sheet.

7. Repeat steps #5 and #6 with second body sheet and finally with pack bath blanket.

8. Secure safety sheets (Fig. 60–6). Attach one safety sheet, previously removed from CWP bundle and kept dry, to bar on bed at one side near client's chest.

    a. Secure safety sheet to bar by looping edge toward you and tucking about 12″ of sheet under itself around bar tightly.

    b. Draw rest of safety sheet across chest, fastening it firmly to bar on opposite side of bed by twisting end several times, drawing twisted end under bar toward you, and tucking it back against itself around bar. Leave a short piece hanging loose to facilitate quick release, if necessary.

9. Attach second safety sheet to bar alongside client's knees as in step #8-a. Draw it securely across his knees and attach it to bar on opposite side of bed, anchoring it as in step #8-b.

10. Place pillow under client's head and cover client with a light blanket or sheet. While clients are in pack, they must be on constant observation, fluids must be offered, and temporal pulses taken and recorded every 15 minutes.

11. When the client has completed the prescribed amount of time in pack, the pack must be removed promptly. If client is to be repacked, a second CWP bundle is prepared.

12. Clients may experience the sensation of having to void while in the cold wet pack. The CWP is not removed, and the client is told that it is acceptable to void while in the pack.

13. Document on chart the use of CWP, reason for its use, time involved, and results.

References

1. Bailey H: Nursing Mental Diseases. New York, MacMillan, 1920
2. Feinsilver DB: Transitional relatedness and the containment in the treatment of a chronic schizophrenic patient. Int Rev Psychoanal 7:309, 1980
3. Kilgalen R: Hydrotherapy—Is it all washed up? J Psychiatr Nurs 10:3, 1972

61

Use of Seclusion and Restraints

Mary Ann Zillman

OVERVIEW   *Verbal Intervention*
Use of Seclusion
Use of Leather Restraints

In psychiatric–mental health nursing, the behavior of aggressive clients is usually detrimental to self-preservation or protection. The aggressive behavior is generally directed outward toward the physical environment or toward others, but may be directed toward the self. The management of aggressive clients is intended to prevent injury to clients themselves, to other clients, and to staff, and to prevent the destruction of property.

Verbal Intervention   Nursing intervention in the management of aggressive clients must begin as soon as the nurse notes that clients are acting in an aggressive manner or that their anxiety is increasing and an aggressive act is likely to occur. Nursing intervention begins with the least restrictive form of action, which is verbal intervention. Nursing interventions may progress to more restrictive forms of interventions depending on the success of earlier actions (see Fig. 61–1). Verbal intervention is described in Chart 61–1.

(Text continues on page 527)

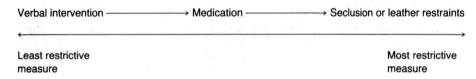

Verbal intervention ⟶ Medication ⟶ Seclusion or leather restraints

Least restrictive measure   Most restrictive measure

FIG. 61-1   Interventions with aggressive clients.

Chart 61–1
VERBAL INTERVENTION WITH AGGRESSIVE CLIENTS

Nursing Intervention	*Rationale*
1. If possible, identify issues leading to aggressive behavior.	1. To reassure clients that the nurse is concerned about these issues
2. When aggressive behavior begins, approach clients as if you expect them to be in control of their behavior.	2. To expect clients to be in control increases the possibility that they will take control of their behavior
3. Maintain eye contact with clients.	3. To assure clients that they have your undivided attention, concern, and support
4. Approach clients in a calm, direct manner; do not be aggressive yourself.	4. To reduce client's own sense of lack of control
5. Give clients a choice of controlling themselves or having staff help to control them. Indicate preference that clients control themselves.	5. To increase clients' safety and security
6. Reassure clients that their concerns will be discussed after they regain control.	6. To reinforce the expectation that they act in a responsible, controlled manner
7. If clients calm down with verbal interaction, escort them to a place of minimal stimulation.	7. To decrease anxiety in a less stimulating environment
8. Spend time with clients to explore issues and alternative behaviors.	8. To provide support, reassure, and give positive reinforcement for positive behavior
9. If clients do not respond to verbal intervention, medication may be offered as an alternative intervention, if ordered and appropriate.	9. To continue to use least restrictive interventions

Chart 61–2
NURSING INTERVENTIONS AND RATIONALE IN THE USE OF SECLUSION

Nursing Intervention	*Rationale*

Policy

1. Upon determination that the use of a seclusion room is necessary, the written order of a physician or, in an emergency, the order of the charge nurse is obtained. If the charge nurse orders the use of quiet room, an order from the attending physician is obtained within a reasonable period of time and countersigned by the physician on duty.

2. All orders for the use of seclusion room must be in compliance with state laws.

3. The charge nurse documents the justification for the use of seclusion room to include the following:
   a. Events leading up to the need for seclusion
   b. Alternative intervention used
   c. Purpose for which the seclusion is being used
   d. Length of time the seclusion room is being used
   e. Clinical justification for length of time

4. A qualified person (registered nurse, licensed practical nurse, or nursing asistant) is assigned to observe clients at least every 15 minutes or more often, if necessary.

5. All appropriate administrative personnel, including the medical director, are informed of action taken.

1. To ensure compliance with local laws and provide adequate clinical justification for use of seclusion

2. To protect the client

3. To ensure adequate documentation and to provide continuity of communication and nursing care

4. To reassure clients of staff concern and to ensure their safety

5. To maintain communication

Procedure

1. Before the client is placed in the seclusion room, the procedure and purpose of the seclusion room is explained to him/her.

2. The client is escorted to the quiet room in a manner that does not cause undue physical discomfort, harm, or pain.

3. The charge nurse is present when the client is placed in the quiet room.

4. A qualified person checks the client every 15 minutes and supervises mealtimes, use of washroom, and smoking (see Fig. 61–2).

5. Use of bathroom is offered at least every 2 hours.

6. All food served in the seclusion room is served on plastic dishes.

7. The seclusion room is free of all articles that clients might use to cause harm to themselves or others.

8. In case of fire, the seclusion room door should automatically open when alarm is sounded.

9. Only the physician, nurses, and primary therapist are allowed to enter the seclusion room.

10. Nursing documentation includes
   a. Precipitating factors and client behavior prior to use of the seclusion room
   b. Alternative interventions that were tried
   c. Time the physician or charge nurse was notified and time the client was seen for purpose of ordering use of the seclusion room
   d. Name of nurse who accompanied client to seclusion room
   e. Name of qualified person who supervised and checked client

1. To reassure the client and provide support; to decrease anxiety

2. To ensure the client's safety

3. To give direction to staff involved

4. To ensure safety, provide support, reassure, and afford the opportunity for clients to express their concerns

5. To provide for basic needs
6. To prevent clients from harming themselves

7. To ensure client's safety

8. To ensure client's safety

9. To decrease stimulation and to provide continuity of interpersonal relationships

10. To provide continuity of care through adequate documentation

Chart 61–2
(continued)

Nursing Intervention	Rationale

    f. Client's response to the seclusion room
    g. Time removed from the seclusion room
11. The physician, medical director, and all appropriate administrative personnel are notified.
12. The nurse approaches the client and provides an opportunity to talk.

11. To provide closure to the incident

12. Clients coming out of seclusion may need to talk about their feelings.

CLIENT'S NAME: _____

Date & Time	Purpose	Ordered By

DATE: _____   **15 MINUTE CHECK**

	Time	By:	Time	By:	Time	By:	Time	By:
1	12:00		12:15		12:30		12:45	
2	1:00 AM		1:15		1:30		1:45	
3	2:00		2:15		2:30		2:45	
4	3:00		3:15		3:30		3:45	
5	4:00		4:15		4:30		4:45	
6	5:00		5:15		5:30		5:45	
7	6:00		6:15		6:30		6:45	
8	7:00		7:15		7:30		7:45	
9	8:00		8:15		8:30		8:45	
10	9:00		9:15		9:30		9:45	
11	10:00		10:15		10:30		10:45	
12	11:00		11:15		11:30		11:45	
13	12:00		12:15		12:30		12:45	
14	1:00 PM		1:15		1:30		1:45	
15	2:00		2:15		2:30		2:45	
16	3:00		3:15		3:30		3:45	
17	4:00		4:15		4:30		4:45	
18	5:00		5:15		5:30		5:45	
19	6:00		6:15		6:30		6:45	
20	7:00		7:15		7:30		7:45	
21	8:00		8:15		8:30		8:45	
22	9:00		9:15		9:30		9:45	
23	10:00		10:15		10:30		10:45	
24	11:00		11:15		11:30		11:45	

R.N. Signature _____   Initial _____

FIG. 61–2   Seclusion and restraint check form. (Reprinted with the permission of Chicago Lakeshore Hospital, Chicago, IL)

Chart 61–3

NURSING INTERVENTIONS AND RATIONALE IN THE USE OF LEATHER RESTRAINTS

Nursing Intervention	*Rationale*
Policy	
1. Restraints are applied only after less restrictive measures have failed.	1. To control clients who cannot provide their own controls on the unit or in the seclusion room
2. Restraints are used only upon the written order of a physician or registered nurse in an emergency situation after he or she has observed and examined clients.	2. To ensure compliance with state laws and provide adequate clinical justification for use of leather restraints
3. All orders for restraints must include: a. Events leading up to the need for restraints b. Purpose for which such restraints are employed c. Length of time restraints are to be employed d. Clinical justification for such length of time	3. To ensure adequate documentation and to provide continuity of communication and nursing care
4. Other than the attending physician, state mental health code laws will determine who must be notified and length of time allowed.	4. To be in compliance with laws
Procedure	
1. An adequate number of trained staff is available.	1. To prevent injury to clients or staff
2. The minimum amount of restraints are used to control clients.	2. To ensure client's safety
3. An explanation of the reason for the use of restraints is given to clients.	3. To reassure clients that the staff is in control
4. If time allows, restraints are set up on bed in advance. However, restraints are never left unattended at the bedside.	4. To ensure orderly application of restraints To ensure safety
5. Leather restraints are applied to all four extremities in a manner that will control clients but will not cause undue physical discomfort.	5. To control clients and to prevent injury to clients or staff
6. All of the above are done under the supervision of the charge nurse.	6. To provide supervision to staff
7. A qualified staff person checks clients every 15 minutes (see Fig. 61–2).	7. To reassure clients of staff concerns and to prevent isolation
8. Relief is provided from restraints at least every 2 hours, including: a. Active range of motion by allowing client to be up limited period or b. If unsafe to release clients from restraints, then passive range of motion exercises are performed on each extremity every 2 hours.	8. To maintain muscle tone
9. Bathroom facilities are offered every two hours.	9. To provide for basic needs
10. Circulation and skin condition are checked as frequently as necessary.	10. To maintain good circulation and prevent skin breakdown
11. Fluids and nutrition are offered.	11. To meet basic needs
12. Registered nurse documentation includes a. Events leading up to necessity for restraints b. Documentation of less restrictive measures attempted (including use of medication) c. Documentation that a registered nurse was present when client was placed in restraints d. Individual who ordered the use of restraints, and whether client was examined prior to being placed in restraints e. Time restraints were applied f. Summation of client's response to restraints and relief periods	12. To provide continuity of care through adequate documentation

Chart 61–3
(continued)

Nursing Intervention	Rationale
g. Time client was removed from restraints and client's behavior	
When client is removed from restraints	
13. Those individuals required by law are notified.	13. To comply with state laws
14. The attending physician is notified.	14. To inform the physician and plan future care
15. In case of fire, clients are released from restraints immediately.	15. To ensure client's safety
16. The nurse approaches the client and provides an opportunity to talk.	16. Clients just out of restraints may need to talk about their feelings.

Use of Seclusion   If verbal intervention and medication do not work, the next measure of intervention is more restrictive. State mental health codes will determine whether the use of seclusion or the use of restraints is possible.

The use of the seclusion room is intended to provide external controls for aggressive clients to protect them from harming themselves, causing harm to others, or destroying property. In no event shall seclusion be used

1. To punish or discipline clients
2. At the convenience of the staff
3. As a mechanism to produce regression

Use of the seclusion room means placing clients alone in a room that they cannot leave. In the event that clients initiate the request for the use of the seclusion room, the same policies and procedures will apply. Chart 61–2 shows nursing interventions and theoretical rationale when using seclusion.

Use of Leather Restraints   The same principles that govern the use of the seclusion room govern the use of leather restraints.

Chart 61–3 shows the policy and procedure associated with the use of leather restraints.

Bibliography   DiFabio S: Nurses' reactions to restraining patients. Am J Nurs 81:973, 1981

62

Suicide
Precautions

Mary Ann Zillman

OVERVIEW   *Description*
                 Nursing Intervention

Chart 62–1
NURSING INTERVENTION AND THEORETICAL RATIONALE WITH SUICIDE PRECAUTIONS

Nursing Intervention	Theoretical Rationale
1. After evaluation and assessment, suicide precautions may be instituted either by the physician or the registered nurse (consult local state laws regarding who can institute suicide precautions). If suicide precautions are implemented by the nurse, the attending physician is notified for the appropriate order.	1. To prevent clients from harming themselves
2. The client is assigned a primary nurse who meets with the client daily and who supervises care of the client	2. To provide a person with whom the client can discuss self-destructive and other feelings
3. Clients are told why they are on suicide precautions, and the procedure is explained to them.	3. To reassure clients and to decrease anxiety
4. Clients' belongings and person are searched for dangerous items. Examples of such items are razor blades, cords, belts, drugs, and glass objects.	4. To remove articles that can be used harmfully
5. If the client is on level 1 (constant awareness precautions), 15-minute checks are made of the client's behavior and documented. If the client is on level 2 (constant observation), nurses are assigned to stay with the client on a one-to-one basis, and are rotated hourly.	5. To decrease isolation of clients and to provide continuous observation
6. The order for suicide precautions is communicated to all members of the staff. Order is noted on cardex and front of chart.	6. To ensure continuity of suicide precautions
7. All off-unit privileges are discontinued, or clients are accompanied by staff on a one-to-one ratio.	7. To prevent elopement
8. The administration of medication is monitored and given in liquid form if necessary.	8. To prevent saving of medication
9. Daily assessment of continued need for suicide precautions is made by the physician and nursing staff, including the client's primary nurse.	9. To determine whether the precaution is still necessary
10. Documentation on a daily basis includes: a. The reason for instituting precautions, including behavioral observations and the clients' verbalizations indicating suicidal ideas b. Client responses to the precautions c. Evaluation of the continued need for precautions d. Discontinuance of precautions and reason	10. To provide accurate and daily clinical justification for suicide precautions and their discontinuance

Description   Suicide precautions are instituted to protect clients from their own self-destructive behavior. The decision to place clients on suicide precautions may be based on behavioral assessments or clients' overt spoken wishes to harm themselves. A behavioral assessment might include information on disturbances in sleep or eating patterns, lack of interest in personal appearance, and so on. Verbalizations may include statements such as "I can't go on anymore," "What's the use? Nobody cares about me," or "I want to kill myself." See Chapter 3 for suicide assessment and Chapter 43 for counseling the suicidal client.

Nursing Intervention   Chart 62–1 shows the procedure for suicide precautions, including nursing intervention and rationale. Figure 61–2 shows a form for recording fifteen-minute checks for the client on suicide precautions.

Bibliography
Floyd GJ: Nursing management of the suicidal patient. J Psychiatr Nurs 13:23, 1975
Leonard CV: Treating the suicidal patient: A communication approach. J Psychiatr Nurs 13:19, 1975
Vollen KH, Watson CG: Suicide in relation to time of day and day of week. Am J Nurs 75:263, 1975
Wekstein L: Handbook of Suicidology: Principles, Problems, Practice. New York, Brunner-Mazel, 1979

63

Elopement

Precautions

Mary Ann Zillman

OVERVIEW   *Description*
              Nursing Intervention

Description   Elopement precautions may be instituted when clients who are harmful to self and others attempt to leave the hospital without proper authorization. These clients may be adults who are confined to the hospital against their will or adolescents who have been admitted by their parents. The decision to place clients on elopement precautions is individualized, based on sound clinical judgment and in accordance with state mental health codes.

Nursing Intervention   Chart 63–1 shows nursing interventions and theoretical rationale aimed at preventing elopement. In the event that the hospital security and the precautions presented in Chart 63–1 fail to prevent clients from leaving the hospital, the actions in Chart 63–2 may be instituted according to local state laws.

Chart 63–1
NURSING INTERVENTIONS AND RATIONALE TO PREVENT ELOPEMENT

Nursing Intervention	*Rationale*
1. Elopement precautions are instituted by the physician or registered nurse after assessment and evaluation of escape risk. If elopement precautions are implemented by the nurse, the physician is notified to give the appropriate order.	1. To prevent clients from leaving the hospital
2. Clients are told why they are on escape precautions, and the procedure is explained to clients.	2. To reassure clients that they will be taken care of, to give knowledge to decrease anxiety, and to provide support
3. The client is assigned a primary nurse who meets with the client daily and supervises care of the client.	3. To provide a person with whom the client can discuss thoughts and feelings
4. Clients are moved to a room near the nursing station.	4. To ensure better observation
5. The order for elopement precautions is communicated to all members of the staff.	5. To ensure continuity of elopement precautions
6. All off-unit privileges are discontinued, or clients are accompanied by staff in a 1:1 ratio.	6. To prevent elopement
7. A staff member is assigned to check location and activity of clients every 15 minutes or more often, as necessary. Fifteen-minute checks are made and documented in the chart (see Fig. 61–2).	7. To know status of clients at all times
8. Daily assessment of continued need for elopement precautions is made by the physician and nursing staff, including the primary nurse.	8. To assess need for continuation of precautions

9. Documentation on daily basis includes
  a. Rationale for instituting precautions, including behavioral and verbal assessment
  b. Clients' responses to precautions
  c. Evaluation of continued need for precautions
  d. When precautions are discontinued and reason
	9. To provide daily and accurate clinical justification for elopement precautions

---

Chart 63–2
NURSING INTERVENTION AND THEORETICAL RATIONALE WHEN THE CLIENT HAS ELOPED

Nursing Intervention	*Rationale*
1. Upon discovery that a client is missing, an internal communication system is activated that alerts all personnel.	1. To communicate to all staff that a client is missing
2. If the identity of the client is not known, a head count of all clients is made.	2. To identify the missing client
3. The identity of the client, including physical description and how the client was dressed, is communicated to all staff, and a search of the premises is conducted.	3. To return the client to the unit

(continued)

Chart 63–2
(continued)

Nursing Intervention	Rationale
4. The charge nurse notifies the nursing supervisor, medical director, and appropriate administrative personnel.	4. To keep all responsible personnel informed
5. At the direction of the attending physician, the charge nurse notifies the client's family	5. To make the family aware of client's status and elicit their help in returning the client to the hospital
6. If a client is seen leaving the building, state mental health laws will determine who can pursue the client.	6. To be in compliance with laws
7. If law permits, the police may be notified of the client's elopement.	7. To assist in returning the client to the hospital
8. If the client is found and returned to hospital, a search of the client is conducted in accordance with hospital policy.	8. To prevent illicit or dangerous items from being brought onto the unit
9. On return of the client, the charge nurse notifies the attending physician, nursing supervisor, medical director, appropriate administrative personnel, family, and police.	9. To keep all responsible personnel informed
10. If the client has not returned in a reasonable period of time, the charge nurse contacts the physician for further orders. The physician may then discharge the client.	10. To determine future course of action. If the physician has heard from the client or family and believes the client to be safe, a discharge order may be given.
11. If the client is discharged, all responsible personnel are notified.	11. To keep all personnel informed
12. The client's belongings and valuables are collected and stored for safekeeping until pick-up.	12. To ensure that the client receives all his/her belongings

Bibliography   Almeida E, Chapman AH: The Interpersonal Basis of Psychiatric Nursing. New York, GP Putnam & Sons, 1972

Haber J et al (eds): Comprehensive Psychiatric Nursing. New York, McGraw-Hill, 1982

64

Record

Keeping

Kathleen Rekasis

OVERVIEW

The Medical Record
General Principles for Recording Data
Components of the Problem-Oriented Record
Progress Notes
SOAP Progress Notes

The Medical Record The client's medical record is a confidential report to be used for communication, accountability, and coordination of care. Various methods are used to organize the data that make up the client record. The record format being discussed here is the problem-oriented system.[1]

General Principles for Recording Data

1. The client's record is a legal document and, as such, must be handled with confidentiality.
2. It is important to state facts and observations, not inferences.
3. The use of slang, abbreviations, or coded language is avoided.
4. Language, including use of appropriate vocabulary, is understandable to the intended audience.
5. Entries are dated and signed.
6. Data are recorded as soon as possible to prevent distortion of facts.

Components of the Problem-Oriented Record The basic components of the problem-oriented record are the data base, the complete problem list, initial plans, and progress notes (see Chap. 3 for the first three components).

Progress Notes Progress notes provide a concise record of the client's response to the treatment plan and a way to communicate assessment and plans for care. Entries may include physiologic responses, psychosocial responses, progress relevant to the treatment plan, and any unique or unusual occurrences relevant to the client or treatment.

The SOAP format (Subjective, Objective, Assessment, Plan) is here discussed as a framework for recording the progress note. The SOAP note includes subjective and objective observations of the problem, the problem, the problem assessment, and the nursing plan of action regarding the problem. All the SOAP components are not necessary for each entry, but each entry follows this sequence. Considering each component in greater detail, the documentation is as follows:

Chart 64–1
SAMPLE PROGRESS NOTE

Mrs. Hill, 36 years old, is a housewife and mother with two preschool children, who was widowed 6 months prior to admission. Precipitating the admission, her first to a psychiatric unit, was information from her sister and a neighbor, who report that during the past 3 months she has become increasingly negligent in the care of herself, her children, and her home. The admitting nurse made the following note:

S. The client presents herself with a sad expression, speaking in short sentences and low tones. Her clothing is wrinkled and too large for her weight, which is 20 pounds less than that on her driver's license. Client has no somatic complaints but complains of loss of appetite and difficulty sleeping. There is poor recollection of recent events. She states that her husband is "away."

O. Pulse 72 and regular, blood pressure 90/60, weight 106. Poor eye contact, low voice, poor hygiene, poor skin turgor, pale color.

A. Client has loss of self-worth, evidenced by lack of interest in self-care, possible malnutrition, anorexia: insomnia is present. Because this is the first hospitalization and follows the death of her spouse, it probably is episodic.

P. 1. Help with daily hygiene and instruct about rules as to dress in milieu.
2. Provide nutritional diet, perhaps fortified with vitamins and high calorie beverages.
3. Encourage exercise and socialization during the day.
4. Provide quiet, dark room for sleep and possibly a temporary sleeping aid.
5. Provide daily one-to-one session with primary nurse. Confront client with reality of spouse's death by asking her to talk about it.

SOAP Progress Notes S—Subjective

      a. Primary source—Information about the client's perception of problem(s), treatment, or general response

      b. Secondary source—Information from spouse, parents, friend, and so forth about their perceptions of the problem, treatment, or response.

O—Objective

      a. Clinical observations made by the nurse

         1. Measurable signs and symptoms including mental status (see Chap. 1)

         2. Behavioral observations

      b. Laboratory data specific to the problem

A—Assessment

      a. What is happening to the client and why? A nursing explanation for S and O data

         1. Draws from S and O data

         2. May reflect progress of the client

         3. Should reflect a rationale for the nursing action plan to follow

P—Plan

      a. Follows from the assessment rationale

      b. Explains what is to be done, by whom, and when

      An example of a progress note is provided in Chart 64–1.

Reference

1. Grant RL, Maletzky BN: Application of the Weed system to psychiatric records. Psychiatry in Med 3:119, 1972

Bibliography

Siegel C, Fischer S: Psychiatric Records in Mental Health Care. New York, Brunner-Mazel, 1981

Simonton MJ: The open medical record: An educational tool. J Psychiatr Nurs 15:25, 1977

65

Teaching
Self-Medication

Nancy Sargent

OVERVIEW   *The Medication Group*
Goals for Self-Administration
Criteria for Selection of Clients Who May Benefit from Self-Administration
Procedure

One of the major reasons for relapse in psychotic clients is failure to continue to take medications after discharge.[2] For this reason, clients are often taught in the hospital to take their own medications. In addition, they learn important information about their medications.

The Medication Group Clients meet weekly in a medication group as soon as they are able to understand and learn about their medications. They begin by viewing five slide–tape programs,[1] 6 to 10 minutes in length, on the following topics:
1. Medication and You
2. Lithium
3. Tricyclic Antidepressants
4. Neuroleptics
5. Anti-anxiety Medications

The medication group meets for 60 minutes and is led by a professional nurse and, if possible, a clinical pharmacist. Clients are told upon entering the group what medications they are taking, the dosage, and how often to take them. In the course of the group sessions clients learn[2]
1. The reason for the medications
2. The importance of taking it as prescribed
3. The length of time it takes for symptoms to return if medication is stopped
4. The side effects of the medications and how to treat them
5. Why and how medications may be changed
6. Where prescriptions can be filled
7. How much medications cost
8. How to ask for generic medication
9. How to keep track of when medications were taken
10. How to handle questions about medications from employers, co-workers, and friends
11. The effect of alcohol ingested with medications
12. What foods to avoid with certain medications
13. How long medications will be needed

The client may remain in the medication group throughout the hospital stay, but is ready to begin learning to self-administer medications when it is demonstrated that the client knows[3]
1. Name of medication and benefits
2. Dose
3. Time of day for each medication
4. Side effects
5. How to open bottle with safety cap
6. Why the previous points are important to know

Goals for Self-Administration
1. Sustain independence in those clients who were adequately managing their own medications before admission.
2. Prepare clients who will be responsible for their own medications after discharge.
3. Offer support to those clients who are ambivalent or fearful about chemotherapy.
4. Encourage independence and responsibility in those clients who are passive and dependent.
5. Help establish healthy norms in clients who have abused medications in the past.
6. Offer support to clients who were or are currently noncompliant with medication schedules.

Criteria for Selection of Clients Who May Benefit from Self-Administration

High priority clients are those
1. Who have any of the problems listed above in 3, 4, 5, and 6 *and*
2. Whose dosage schedule is reasonably well-adjusted

Clients who are not ready for the program are those who
1. Are severely psychotic
2. Are actively suicidal
3. Are severely depressed and nonfunctional
4. Have moderate to severe organic brain syndrome
5. Are taking medications that are in the process of being adjusted

Procedure
1. Talk with the client to gain cooperation.
2. Record goals and approaches in the nursing care plan.
3. Schedule times of medication preparation to avoid conflict with regularly scheduled medication administration for the remaining clients.
4. Record decisions on the "Special Instructions for Medications" section of the med cardex and sign name.
   Examples:
   a. Client will prepare and administer valium only. M. Jones, R.N.
   b. Client will prepare and administer all of her own medications at 9 AM and 1 PM. The nurse will give medications on 3–11 shift. B. White, R.N.
   c. Client will prepare and administer all of her own medications at all times. S. Green, R.N.
   d. Client will prepare and administer all of her own medications *only when I am on duty*. F. Nightingale, R.N.
5. Using principles of teaching–learning, question the client about names, dosage, and times of medications.
6. Guide the client by using a procedure similar to the general procedure, working from the cardex.
7. Ensure that the client takes all scheduled medications.
8. Chart the medication as usual. The client will have no responsibility for documentation.
9. Chart in the nursing notes the client's response.

References

1. Batey SR: Drug information for patients. Hosp Community Psychiatry 31:685, 1980
2. Batey SR, Ledbetter JE: Medication education for patients in a partial hospitalization program. J Psychosoc Nurs 20:7, 1982
3. Franclemont J, Sclafani M: Self-medication program for the emotionally ill. J Psychiatr Nurs 16:15, 1978

Bibliography

Lane DE: Self-medication of psychiatric patients. J Psychosoc Nurs 19:27, 1981
Larkin AR: What's a medication group? J Psychosoc Nurs 20:35, 1982

66

Discharge

Planning

Linda St. Germain

Discharge planning is an essential part of clients' treatment; therefore, clients are included in the planning. Discharge planning begins at the time of admission or shortly thereafter. It involves the collaborative efforts of clients, families, significant others, and health professionals.

Objective

The objective of discharge planning is to ensure that continued support and assistance are available and accessible to clients and their families after discharge to improve or maintain the current health status of clients.

The Discharge-Planning Process

In some settings, the nurse assumes the responsibility for discharge planning and coordinates the recommendations of other disciplines involved, such as social service; medicine; physical, occupational, and recreational therapies; and dietary, as well as the wishes of the clients and significant others.

Assessment of Clients and Families

A. OBJECTIVE DATA
   1. Demographic information
   2. Medical history
   3. Nursing history
   4. Psychosocial/financial history
   5. Current status
      a. Diagnosis
      b. Behavioral manifestations, level of functioning

B. SUBJECTIVE DATA
   1. What do clients perceive as their needs and problems?
   2. Whom do the clients perceive as part of their support system?
   3. What are the clients' and families' expectations of the health care system, presently the hospital?
   4. What are the clients' plans for discharge? What are their goals?

Plan

A multidisciplinary conference is held. This conference is a forum in which the clients' needs and problems are shared and discussed among the representatives from the different disciplines. Goals are identified and a plan for discharge is formulated, target dates are set.

Interventions

The suggested plan and goals are shared with the client and significant others. The plan is negotiable, and the client's involvement from the start increases follow-through with the plan.

   The nurse contacts appropriate community services available and accessible to the client with the authorization of the client. Examples of services to be contacted by the nurse or the client are
   1. Outpatient psychotherapy resources, that is, mental health clinics, or private practitioners such as psychiatric nurses, social workers, psychologists, and psychiatrists
   2. Day-treatment programs
   3. Nursing homes
   4. Chemical dependency rehabilitation programs
   5. Sheltered workshops
   6. Half-way houses
   7. Residential hotels or boarding homes

Documentation

1. The Joint Commission of Accreditation of Hospitals (JCAH) Standard IV of Nursing Services states "the plan of care must be documented and should reflect current standards of nursing practice, including patient discharge planning."[1]
2. Doumentation reflects the ongoing progression of the discharge planning such as
   a. Summaries of multidisciplinary conferences, dates, members present
   b. Interactions with the client regarding the plans
   c. Community services contacted, appointments and interviews scheduled, and outcomes of contacts

Discharge Forms

1. Referral forms are completed when appropriate in transfer of the clients to other facilities.
   a. Written communications between hospital and outside agencies are made.
   b. Referral forms are similar to the discharge summaries written in the medical record. They include summaries of clients' progress, based on assessment of needs and problems and treatment provided, as well as recommendations to ensure continuity of care.
2. Discharge Summaries
   a. Written summaries that reflect clients' responses to treatment provided are placed in the medical records.
   b. Provisions made for posthospitalization follow-up care include
      • Teaching that has been provided to clients and significant others
      • Referrals and reasons for referrals

Evaluation

Members of the various disciplines meet to discuss the discharge-planning process, including their own effectiveness and efficiency. This includes an ongoing assessment and evaluation of community services' strengths and weaknesses.

Reference

1. Joint Commission on Accreditation of Hospitals: Accreditation Manual for Hospitals. Chicago, JCAH, 1980

Part VI

Psychopharmacology and Psychiatric Nursing

67

General Nursing Roles in Psychopharmacology

Linda S. Beeber

OVERVIEW   *Introduction*
General Nursing Roles in Caring for Clients Receiving Psychotropic Medications

Introduction   No medical treatment of the psychiatric client has had a greater impact on psychiatric nursing than the psychotropic medications introduced in the mid-1950s. Chemical alteration of clients' psychiatric symptoms has decreased the role of nursing in controlling behavior through mechanical means and increased the role of nursing in therapeutic interpersonal contacts with the client. The nurse's fear of the client's unpredictable behavior may be lessened when the client is treated with medication. The nurse's sense of hope (as well as the client's) may be bolstered by rapid remission of symptoms. Unfortunately, the nurse may become dependent on the use of medication and bypass interpersonal means of reducing the client's symptoms. Failure to offer correct interpersonal interventions when the client is anxious, frightened, resistant, or highly symptomatic may force the use of a traumatic medication route, or lead to greater dosage of medication than necessary. The nurse may feel anxious and resort to medication for the client when interpersonal interaction with the client is the correct response. The nurse may withhold medication out of misunderstanding of or reactivity to its uses and cause the client to suffer needlessly. Identification of the uses of medication and the nursing roles and actions related to psychotropic medication will help reduce reactivity and overmedication or undermedication by the nurse.

The following sections present the dependent, collaborative, and independent roles of nursing care of the psychiatric client who is receiving psychotropic medication, and integrates the roles into the nursing process. Since medication therapy changes according to the acute or stable nature of the client's symptoms, the body of information about each medication group is organized into chronologic phases of treatment and nursing care. Since the client may attach significance to the nurse's *action* of giving medication, nurses must be sensitive to the interpersonal significance of their actions to the client. The nurse may be seen as feeding, nurturing, punishing, withholding, poisoning, curing, and having other significant intentions. Excellent technique in communicating with the client will allow these dynamic factors to be explored.

Chart 67–1

GENERAL NURSING ROLES IN PSYCHOTROPIC MEDICATION THERAPY

Functional Nursing Roles	*Sample Nursing Interventions*
A. *Dependent Role* 1. Dispensing medication (see Chap. 58)	• Assuring that the amount, time, and so forth, are within acceptable limits • Documenting that medication was given
B. *Collaborative Role* 1. Choosing optimal medication for the client's symptoms	• Observing behaviors helped by medication • Validating observations • Providing a comprehensive assessment, including medication, sexual, social life-style history, functional strengths, factors affecting receptiveness to medication
2. Deciding dosage, frequency, route, dosage adjustment (prn), reduction, and conclusion criteria	• Expert observing for changes or stabilization in behaviors helped by medication • Validating observations • Providing information about effect of interpersonal interventions • Acting on the client's behalf to ascertain that the least injurious route is chosen

Chart 67–1
(continued)

Functional Nursing Roles	Sample Nursing Interventions
3. Gaining and maintaining client's acceptance of medication therapy	• Securing agreement between physician and nurse as to shared teaching responsibilities • Establishing therapeutic relationship and alliance • Diagnosing client's resistance to medication • Intervening when resistance to medication exists • Securing informed consent to medication therapy
C. *Independent Role* 1. Providing anticipatory/ongoing counseling about medication	• Assessing client's operative defenses • Introducing information appropriate to the client's defenses and capacity to integrate data • Providing support • Encouraging the client to assume the role of active learner and collaborator
2. Postmedication monitoring of physiologic baselines	• Identifying critical physiologic behavioral criteria for each medication group • Identifying premedication baselines • Monitoring present physiologic status using client-derived baselines • Documenting physiologic state
3. Recognizing adverse effects of medication and intervening appropriately	• Observing for signs of adverse reactions • Validating through use of critical client-derived baselines • Withholding medication • Notifying physician; requesting medical evaluation • Supporting and monitoring the client • Providing additional prescribed treatments for adverse effects • Collaborating with physician to alter dosage or conclude medication therapy
4. Preventing complications arising from therapy *Sample nursing diagnoses:* Exacerbation of physiologic instability; iatrogenic problem (for example, tardive dyskinesia, dependence); misuse of medication (for example, overdose); multiple medication interaction	• Assessing all variables potentially affecting medication therapy: a. Laboratory data and physical assessment b. Medication and other concurrent therapies c. Psychologic variables, for example, suicide potential • Detecting complications early • Counseling the client about complications • Withholding medication when indicated • Collaborating with physician to alter dosage or conclude medication therapy
5. Maintaining optimal health level	• Providing health maintenance and improvement • Treating side effects
6. Preparing client to self-administer medications at highest level of independence possible (see Chap. 65)	• Assessing the client's present and potential capacity for self-administration of medications • Providing supervised learning experiences • Providing support • Assisting the client to mobilize available supports when indicated
7. Reducing symptoms through interpersonal alterations	• Assessing the client's operative interpersonal skills • Intervening to promote greater use and mastery of existing skills • Encouraging the client to use interpersonal means in addition to medication • Encouraging the client to use interpersonal means in lieu of medication

The goal of nursing must never be forgotten. Although nurses are involved in furthering the client's treatment with psychotropic medication, nursing assessment and intervention must be directed toward diagnosing and treating the client's response to dysfunction and treatment, preventing complications of dysfunction and treatment, and promoting or maintaining optimal degrees of wellness and progression along the human developmental continuum. These functions are stressed heavily throughout the following sections.

General Nursing Roles in Caring for Clients Receiving Psychotropic Medications

When nurses collaborate with physicians regarding psychotropic medication, the nurse makes use of extended contact with clients to influence type, dosage, and route of medication. The quality of the nurse's interpersonal interventions can determine the quantity of medication administered and the duration of treatment. The provision of qualitative information about a client's progress and regression influences all dimensions of medication therapy. Failure to correctly diagnose and resolve clients' resistance to medication therapy leads to failure of the therapeutic alliance and the loss of the client's cooperation in medication therapy. Chart 67–1 shows general nursing roles in psychotropic medication therapy.

Bibliography Refer to Selected Bibliography following Chapter 71 at the end of this unit.

68

Antipsychotic Medications

Linda S. Beeber

OVERVIEW

Description
Use
Chemical Groups
Method of Action
Symptoms Helped by Antipsychotic Medications
General Medical Treatment Guidelines
Side Effects and Adverse Effects
Antiparkinsonian Medications
Nursing Care

Description   Antipsychotic medication is the general term referring to the groups of medications used to treat symptoms of psychosis. Psychosis is a state in which a person's ability to recognize reality, to communicate, and to relate to others is severely impaired.[3]

These drugs are often called major tranquilizers, neuroleptics, or phenothiazines. These terms are sometimes used imprecisely. Tranquilization is a side effect; these medications exert a direct effect upon psychosis, so that a withdrawn client may be more *active* after medication.

Use   Antipsychotic medication is commonly used for the following:
1. Treatment of acute schizophrenic disorders
2. Treatment of paranoid disorders
3. Treatment of psychotic disorders of the brief or atypical form
4. Management of acute mania before lithium is begun
5. Combined treatment of psychotic depression with antidepressants

Use is questioned in the following groups because of long-term side effects[1]:
1. Anxiety disorders
2. Organic mental disorders
3. Schizophrenic disorders not responsive to medication
4. Chronic schizophrenic disorders

See Table 68–1 for commonly used antipsychotic medications ranked according to potency.

These medications reduce psychotic symptoms but are not curative. When receiving adequate doses, 95% of acute schizophrenic clients (by diagnosis) will show *some* improvement within 6 to 8 weeks, and 50% will show *moderate to marked* improvement. Therapeutic effects may be evident within 2 days to 2 weeks.[1] Maintenance on antipsychotic medication reduces the relapse rate but does not improve social adjustment.[1]

Chemical Groups   Five chemically different groups exist. They are the
1. Phenothiazines
2. Butyrophenones
3. Thioxanthenes
4. Oxoindoles
5. Dibenzoxazepines

Table 68–1
COMMONLY USED ANTIPSYCHOTIC MEDICATIONS RANKED ACCORDING TO POTENCY[2]

	Medication
Most Potent	1. Fluphenazine (Prolixin D, E)
	2. Fluphenazine (Prolixin)
	3. Haloperidol (Haldol)
	4. Thiothixene (Navane)
to	5. Trifluoperazine (Stelazine)
	6. Perphenazine (Trilafon)
	7. Molindone (Moban)
	8. Loxapine (Loxitane)
Least Potent	9. Thioridazine (Mellaril)
	10. Chlorpromazine (Thorazine)

Note: High potency does not mean "more effective" but that a lower quantity of medication will produce therapeutic effects.

No group has proven to be either superior in antipsychotic effect or more specific for the treatment of certain symptoms or syndromes.[1] Potency varies among the groups and medications within groups. Individuals may show a varied response among groups, and side effects vary among groups. Familiarity with one frequently used medication from *each chemical group* is sufficient to meet most medical and nursing clinicians' needs. It is not efficacious to use more than one antipsychotic preparation at a time. Clients who do not respond or who develop side effects in response to one chemical group should be moved to a different group.

Table 68–2 shows the classification of antipsychotic medications according to chemical group.

Method of Action   It is postulated that antipsychotic drugs block the neurotransmitter dopamine at the postsynaptic neurons throughout the brain, and specifically in the mesolimbic system and the basal ganglia, which exert control over behavior and muscular contractions.

Table 68–2
CLASSIFICATION OF ANTIPSYCHOTIC MEDICATIONS ACCORDING TO CHEMICAL GROUP

| Chemical Group | Trade Name | Oral Dose Range | How Supplied | | | | Comments and Drug-Specific Considerations |
			Tabs	Liq	Inj	Other	
I. Phenothiazines							
Aliphatic							
Chlorpromazine	Thorazine Chlor-PZ Cromedazine Promachel Promapar Sonazine	50–1200 mg/day	x	x	x	Suppositories	Aliphatic phenothiazines— higher sedation, hypotension; lower extrapyramidal symptoms; IM form is low potency—therapeutic dose requires multiple injections of large volume; abscesses and erosion into sciatic nerve complications
Triflupromazine	Vesprin	30–150 mg/day	x	x	x		More potent than chlorpromazine
Promazine	Sparine	100–2400 mg/day	x	x	x		See note under chlorpromazine
Piperazine							
Trifluoperazine	Stelazine	5–40 mg/day	x	x	x		Piperazine phenothiazines— lower sedation, hypotension; higher EPS
Perphenazine	Trilafon	12–64 mg/day	x	x	x		Used in combination with amitryptyline as Etrafon, Triavil; generic drugs given separately preferable to fixed-dosage trade combinations, which allow less flexibility in altering dosage
Fluphenazine	Prolixin Permitil	2–20 mg/day	x	x	x	*Long-acting preparations:* Prolixin Enanthate,	Short-acting form can be used to assess client's tolerance in preparation for depot injection. *Always use PO test trial before administering*

(continued)

Table 68–2
(continued)

Chemical Group	Trade Name	Oral Dose Range	Tabs	Liq	Inj	Other	Comments and Drug-Specific Considerations
						dose 12.5–100 mg (IM)— duration 10 days–2 weeks; Prolixin Decanoate, dose 12.5–100 mg (IM)— duration 3 to 4 weeks	*depot injection* to assess allergic/idiosyncratic reactions. Maintenance goal with long-acting forms is *lowest dose* at *longest interval* to prevent relapse.
Acetophenazine	Tindal	40–120 mg/day	x	no	no		
Carphenazine	Proketazine	25–400 mg/day	x	x	no		
Butaperazine	Repoise	50–100 mg/day	x	no	no		
Piperidines							
Thioridazine	Mellaril	50–800 mg/day	x	x	no		Piperidine phenothiazines lowest extrapyramidal symptoms of phenothiazine group; data shows high incidence of orthostatic hypotension, cardiac effects, ejaculatory inhibition; caution in use with elderly; unsafe in high doses; caution in use with suicidal patients
Piperacetazine	Quide	40–160 mg/day	x	no	x		
Mesoridazine	Serentil	150–400 mg/day	x	x	x		
II. Butyrophenones							
Haloperidol	Haldol	2–100 mg/day	x	x	x		Extrapyramidal symptoms more common than with phenothiazines
Droperidol	Inapsine	none	no	no	x		
III. Thioxanthenes							
Thiothixene	Navane	5–60 mg/day	x	x	x		More potent of the two common thioxanthenes
Chlorprothixene	Taractan	75–600 mg/day	x	x	x		Potency similar to that of phenothiazine Side effects similar to those of phenothiazine
IV. Oxoindoles							
Molindone	Moban Endo Lidone	15–225 mg/day	x	no	no		Clinically similar to phenothiazines
V. Dibenzoxazipines							
Loxapine	Loxitane Daxolin	15–100 mg/day	x	no	no		

Choosing one or two *target symptoms* of psychosis to observe consistently is helpful in assessing the effectiveness of medication. Agreement on the target symptom(s) is reached by the physician and the nurse. Supporting staff are trained to recognize shifts in target symptoms. Choosing an anxiety-provoking target symptom (violence, disrobing) will decrease objectivity. Target symptoms likely to respond to drugs include *agitation, hallucinations, sleep disturbance,* and *anxiety.*[1,2]

Other symptoms of schizophrenic psychosis that may be helped (though to a lesser degree) by antipsychotic drugs include

A. **DISORDERED THOUGHT**
1. Delusions
2. Combativeness (secondary to suspicion, fear, misperception, autistic commands)
3. Associative looseness
4. Flight of ideas
5. Ideas of influence (one's thoughts, feelings, actions are being imposed by an external force)
6. Thought broadcasting (one's thoughts are escaping aloud from one's head)

B. **WITHDRAWAL** (secondary to catastrophic anxiety)
1. Apathy
2. Waxy flexibility, posturing
3. Disrupted socialization
4. Self-neglect

A. **DOSAGE MUST BE INDIVIDUALIZED**

Agitated			Withdrawn
More psychotic	High	Low	Slower clearance rate
Young	dose ↔	dose	Dehydrated
Heavy			Elderly
Male			Low weight
			Female

B. **ACUTE TREATMENT PHASE GUIDELINES AND TREATMENT OPTIONS**
    (First 48–72 hours)
1. Test dose is administered before treatment begins.
    1. 25 mg–50 mg PO/25 mg IM, chlorpromazine or equivalent (see Table 68–1)
    b. Observe for orthostatic hypotension and other side effects for 2 hours.
2. Dosage can be increased gradually until symptoms subside or side effects develop. Reaching adequate dosage is important. The most common cause of treatment failure is inadequate dose of antipsychotic medication. (Noncompliance contributes to inadequate dosage.)
3. Medication should be given in divided doses.
4. *Treatment of side effects*
    a. Extrapyramidal side effects: Individuals vary in vulnerability to side effects. Since multiple medications complicate clinical observations, antiparkinsonian medications are generally not given until extrapyramidal side effects develop.
        Note: Antiparkinsonian medications do not prevent extrapyramidal side effects. Antiparkinsonian medications can worsen anticholinergic side effects of antipsychotics.
    b. *Dose reduction* may be as effective in eliminating side effects as antiparkinsonian medication.

5. *Special aspects of acute treatment*—Rapid tranquilization, psychotolysis (see Chap. 57)
   a. Large IM dose every 30–60 minutes until improvement is observed or side effects appear.
   b. Observe for orthostatic hypotension.
   c. *Long-term adverse effects of high dose treatment have not yet been documented.*

C. **STABILIZATION—MAINTENANCE PHASE**
   (Subsequent to 72 hours)
   1. Long half-life of these medications allows one or two doses during 24-hour period.
   2. Single dose at bedtime reduces orthostatic hypotension and subjective discomfort of sedative and anticholinergic side effects and is easier for client to remember.
   3. Medication cannot be judged ineffective until at least 6 weeks at adequate doses. If it is judged ineffective, a different *group* of antipsychotic medications should be chosen.
   4. Preparation for self-medication is begun as soon as possible.
   5. Dosage can be reduced when symptoms have subsided. Goal is reduction to the lowest dose that will prevent relapse. Suggested protocol to reach maintenance level is to reduce dose by 25% of acute treatment dose every 1 to 3 months. Maintenance goal is 25% to 30% of acute treatment dose.[1]

D. **CONCLUSION PHASE**
   1. Clients continuing medication according to standard postpsychosis treatment guidelines are less likely to relapse than clients on placebo.[1]
   2. Guidelines for discontinuing medication[1]
      a. First episode—6 months' maintenance
      b. Second episode—1 year's maintenance
      c. Three or more episodes—consider indefinite maintenance
   3. Risk of tardive dyskinesia necessitates periodic consideration of discontinuation of drug therapy. No sufficient data are available to identify a group of schizophrenic clients who can manage in the community without medication. Chronic clients over 60 years old and clients with a poor prognosis may not benefit sufficiently from medication to warrant exposure to tardive dyskinesia. Clients who struggle to comply may be tried on long-acting phenothiazines.

E. **SPECIAL CONSIDERATIONS**[2]
   1. Pregnant and lactating women
      a. Antipsychotic medications *do* cross the placenta. Newborns of mothers treated with antipsychotic medications have shown transitory neurologic side effects. Infants of mothers treated with antipsychotic medications *do not* show a higher incidence of birth defects, perinatal mortality, or developmental disruptions than infants of nontreated mothers.
      b. Antipsychotic medications are secreted in breast milk. The concentration passed in breast milk is not judged to be harmful to the infant.
   2. Elderly persons
      a. At risk for side effects
         1) Cardiovascular problems may be aggravated. Orthostatic hypotension can aggravate central nervous system (CNS) confusion owing to poor circulation. Low blood pressure can lead to falls resulting in fractures of the hip.

2) Extrapyramidal side effects are increased, as is tardive dyskinesia, especially in women.
3) Anticholinergic side effects may aggravate glaucoma, gait unsteadiness, and dysuria in men with benign prostatic hypertrophy.
4) Allergic reactions are more common in the elderly, including adverse reactions (agranulocytosis, monocytosis, cholestatic jaundice).

b. At risk for drug–drug interactions and toxic overdose
1) The elderly are more likely to be treated concurrently with other medications.
2) The elderly are less reliable in remembering dosage and may live in settings with poor supervision and where overmedication to achieve behavioral control is likely.

c. The physiologic aging process increases blood triglycerides and decreases hepatic enzyme production.
1) Lipid soluble antipsychotic medications will remain in higher concentrations in blood.
2) Antipsychotic medications will break down more slowly.

3. Children
a. Child is dependent upon adult for administration of medication.
1) Strongly positive or negative parental attitudes may lead to overdosage or underdosage. Parental expectations for cure of both parent and child may be idealistic and magical.
2) The child may perceive medication with fear or sense of loss of control, as punishment, or as love.

b. Physiologic differences in the child
1) Neurologic immaturity may produce paradoxical responses.
2) Generally, *higher doses are tolerated* by children than adults, making weight and age unreliable guidelines for determining dosage.

c. Side effects
1) Are likely to be expressed in an action rather than verbal mode
2) Are reduced, in general, in the child
3) On long-term growth and development are incompletely known and must be weighed in the fact of clinical symptoms. Some evidence suggests that sedating antipsychotic medications (for example, aliphatics, piperidine, phenothiazines) decrease learning in psychotic and retarded children.

Side Effects and Adverse Effects　　　"Neuroleptic" refers to the capacity of these medications to produce CNS side effects that mimic extrapyramidal disease (Parkinson's). These medications carry serious acute and permanent side effects and should be used cautiously. Chart 68–1 shows

---

Chart 68–1
SIDE EFFECTS OF ANTIPSYCHOTIC MEDICATIONS AND NURSING INTERVENTIONS

Side Effect	*Nursing Intervention*
A. Autonomic Nervous System Side Effects	
1) *Symptoms due to Interference with Acetylcholine (Anticholinergic)*	
Dry mouth	1. Examine periodically for fungal infection.
	2. Encourage use of mouthwash or sugarless gum and lozenges.

(continued)

Chart 68–1
(continued)

Side Effect	Nursing Intervention
Blurred vision	1. Examine periodically for insidious development of retinitis pigmentosa, corneal deposits (see Chart 68–2). 2. Reassure client of transient nature of side effect. 3. Suggest magnifying lens or "dime-store" glasses to help reading.
Constipation	1. Provide adequate hydration, dietary bulk. 2. Provide stool softener, laxative. 3. Establish regular routines for eating and toileting.
Urinary hesitance/retention	1. Record intake and output to establish urinary retention. 2. Seek reduction of dose, intervene in any underlying problems. 3. Observe for symptoms of infection or obstruction—*withhold medication pending medical evaluation.*
Paralytic ileus	1. Observe for signs of abdominal distention. 2. *Withhold medication pending medical evaluation.*

2) *Symptoms due to Interference with Epinephrine (Antiadrenergic)*

Orthostatic hypotension	1. Secure BP baselines; check BP against control before administering medication; elderly are at high risk; *greater than 5 mm fall upon standing—withhold medication pending medical evaluation;* check BP ½ hour after medication. 2. Teach client to rise slowly and dangle legs before standing; if client too disoriented to carry this out reliably, provide supervision upon rising, especially at sleep periods. 3. Provide elastic stockings and isometric exercises while supine.
Inhibition of ejaculation	1. Encourage relationship in which client can discuss sexual concerns. 2. Listen for covert cues that client is concerned about difficulty ejaculating (in a setting where staff is mixed by gender, male staff needs to be alert for cues, since client may approach another male with this concern). 3. Reassure client of cause; pursue with physician reducing dose or changing medication.

B. Extrapyramidal Effects

(Action of medication on extrapyramidal tracts of central nervous system)

1) *Dystonias*—Severe, often rapidly developing contractions of muscles of tongue, jaw, neck (producing torticollis), extraocular muscles; combined torticollis and extraocular spasm results in *oculogyric crisis,* in which eyes look upward, head is turned to one side. Dystonias are a sometimes painful and always frightening experience for clients. Many clients incorporate the symptoms into other altered sensations that accompany psychosis. To have a nurse distinguish a sensation as a reversible side effect and offer reassurance and rapid treatment is a significant trust-building experience for the client. Since these side effects occur early in treatment, the nursing intervention will be critical in the client's acceptance of treatment.	1. Secure prn dose of antiparkinsonian medication when client is begun on antipsychotic medication. Time spent securing medication orders when side effect appears can be agonizing to the client. 2. Observe client closely during acute treatment; follow up any communications concerning altered body by close examination; check tendons for "cogwheel" jerkiness. 3. Teach client to recognize onset of dystonic symptoms. 4. Respond to symptoms of dystonia immediately by remaining or having a staff member remain with client, administer antiparkinsonian drug, continue to remain with client, offering reassurance until side effect has abated. 5. Pursue dose reduction and/or antiparkinsonian drug regimen for 2–4 weeks maximum.

Chart 68–1
(continued)

Side Effect	Nursing Intervention
2) *Pseudoparkinsonian Syndrome*—Extrapyramidal side effects mimicking Parkinson's disease, including mask-like face, shuffling gait, rigidity with flexion of arms, outward-rotating tremor of hands	1. Speed is not necessary in intervention, but client will need reassurance that the side effect is reversible. 2. Administer antiparkinsonian medication.
3) *Akinesia*—Lethargy, subjective sense of fatigue, muscle weakness often mistaken for withdrawal and apathy	1. Speed is not necessary in intervention, but client will need reassurance that the side effect is reversible. 2. Administer antiparkinsonian medication. 3. Do not allow antipsychotic drug to be increased without vigorous differentiation of symptoms of relapse from this side effect.
4) *Akathisia*—Restless, "walking in place," inability to rest, shifting weight from foot to foot, rocking—symptoms of this side effect are mistaken for anxiety and autistic behavior. Client can be taught to distinguish this from agitation by recognizing the unrelenting nature of the restlessness. Agitation will be more episodic.	1. Speed is not necessary in intervention, but client will need reassurance that the side effect is reversible. 2. Administer antiparkinsonian medication. 3. Do not allow antipsychotic drug to be increased without vigorous differentiation of symptoms of relapse from this side effect.
5) *Tardive Dyskinesia*	See adverse effects, Chart 68–2
C. Endocrine Disruptions 1) Menstrual irregularities, including amenorrhea and false-positive pregnancy test	1. Assess client's behavior. If client is sexually active, pregnancy must be considered. Undereating and anxiety may also account for these symptoms. 2. Investigate and reassure client. Consider dose reduction or switch to different group.
2) Breast enlargement, lactation	1. Assess the meaning to client. (May provoke pregnancy fantasies, fears of changing gender.) 2. Offer reassurance and explanation; consider drug change.
3) Weight gain	1. Assessment dimensions; weight baseline 2. Provide reduction diet.
4) Glycosuria; hyperglycemia	1. Assess for history of diabetes in client and family, and other symptoms of diabetes. (Presence may go unnoticed except in diabetic clients and clients undergoing diagnostic tests.)
D. Skin—Photosensitivity, Pigment Deposits	1. Protect from sun, ultraviolet light sources (use true *sunscreen*, not suntan preparation). 2. Observe skin carefully, especially in dark-skinned persons.

the side effects of antipsychotic medications and appropriate nursing interventions; Chart 68–2 shows the adverse effects of antipsychotic medications and nursing interventions.

Antiparkinsonian Medications These medications are of major use in clients receiving antipsychotics because they are helpful in treating extrapyramidal side effects. Early recognition of extrapyramidal side effects will allow enough time to give the antiparkinsonian medication orally. In an acute, massive dystonic reaction (such as oculogyric crisis) injectable forms may be given.

Side effects of these medications are dry mouth, blurred vision, constipation, urinary hesitance and retention, nausea, and vomiting. Table 68–3 shows the common antiparkinsonian medications, and Table 68–4 the adverse effects of these medications.

(Text continues on page 567)

Chart 68–2
ADVERSE EFFECTS OF ANTIPSYCHOTIC MEDICATIONS AND NURSING INTERVENTIONS

Adverse Effect	Nursing Interventions
A. Lowering of Seizure Threshold	1. Secure seizure history. 2. Observe closely, especially when dosage is increased. 3. Carefully monitor clients with known seizure disorder who may need increased seizure-control medication.
B. Hypersensitivity Reactions 1) Blood dyscrasias (agranulocytosis, monocytosis)	1. Distinguish through careful physical assessment—elevated temperature, sore throat, itching, bruising and nosebleeds. CBC not always reliable confirmation. 2. Withhold medication until medical evaluation. 3. Note that elderly, debilitated women are at high risk; symptoms appear between 4–12 weeks.
2) Cholestatic jaundice	1. Assess for yellowing of sclera, skin; discoloration of urine and feces. 2. Withhold medication until medical evaluation.
3) Dermatitis	1. Withhold medication until medical evaluation. 2. Treat symptoms.
C. Cardiac Arrhythmias Including sudden death in asymptomatic clients (rare)	1. Assess for change in cardiac baselines.
D. Tardive Dyskinesia Potentially irreversible disorder of involuntary muscular movements of insidious onset; may appear when antipsychotic dosages are being reduced or discontinued; represent injury to basal ganglion areas. Symptoms are worsened by administering antiparkinson drugs. Tardive dyskinesia symptoms may increase clients' perception of self as bizarre and uncontrollable, as well as alienate others around them.	1. Assess for changes in gait, facial and extremity movements; risk factors—elderly, female, extended treatment with or high doses of antipsychotic drugs Administer Abnormal Involuntary Movement Scale (AIMS) to high risk or suspected clients.* 2. Do not withhold medication (symptoms will worsen). 3. Immediately contact physician for medical evaluation. If tardive dyskinesia is confirmed, client should either be informed of the symptom and removed from antipsychotic medications or be informed of the symptom and implications, and give informed consent for treatment to continue. Written consent is required in at least one state and may become standard for practice.
E. Ocular Changes Deposits in lens, conjunctiva, cornea may produce star-shaped opacities; retinitis pigmentosa can produce vision impairment.	1. Assess for symptoms (onset generally not as early as anticholinergic blurriness). 2. Seek ophthalmological evaluation.

*AIMS may be obtained by writing to Chief, Schizophrenic Disorders Section, Pharmacologic and Somatic Treatments Research Branch, National Institute of Mental Health, Rockville, Maryland 20857.

Table 68–3
ANTIPARKINSONIAN MEDICATIONS

Generic Name	Trade Name	Daily Dosage Range	Tablet	Liquid	Injectable
Benztropine mesylate	Cogentin	0.5 mg–6 mg	X	no	X
Biperiden	Akineton	2 mg–8 mg	X	no	X
Procyclidine	Kemadrin	10 mg–20 mg	X	no	no
Trihexyphenidyl	Artane	6 mg–10 mg	X	X	no
Diphenhydramine	Benadryl	75 mg–150 mg	X	X	X

Table 68–4
ADVERSE EFFECTS OF ANTIPARKINSONIAN MEDICATIONS

Adverse Effect	Comments
Aggravation of narrow-angle glaucoma	Hyperpyrexia, heat stroke due to interference with sweating; watch for in elderly clients while on outings
Psychosis characterized by *visual* hallucinations, illusions due to toxic levels of these drugs Aggravation of tardive dyskinesia	Watch for in rapid tranquilization, when client is receiving multiple doses of antiparkinsonian medications

---

Chart 68–3
NURSING CARE OF CLIENTS RECEIVING ANTIPSYCHOTIC MEDICATIONS

Phase of Treatment	Assessment and Formulation Dimensions	Nursing Interventions	Criteria for Evaluating Response to Nursing Intervention
Diagnostic/ Preparatory Phase *Collaborative Role* Collaborating in choice of optimal medication for client's symptoms	1. Symptoms of psychosis must be differentiated from symptoms of organic brain syndrome, alcohol withdrawal, organic diseases, drug abuse and drug–drug toxicities, severe anxiety, and transient panic states.	1.1. Observe for recurring behaviors.	a. Validation by more than one observer of specific behaviors occurring in many different settings b. Validation by client
		1.2. Observe for recurring behaviors in interpersonal settings (predictably higher anxiety). *Suggestions*—One-to-one relationships with nurse and colleagues; group settings/therapy; group settings/social, religious, family interactions	a. Validation by more than one observer of specific behaviors occurring with a rise in anxiety b. Validation by client
		1.3. Observe client when not involved in interpersonal settings; look for times throughout the 24-hour day when symptoms appear. *Suggestions*—Early morning, upon awakening, look for more confusion; evening, approaching darkness, look for more loss of boundaries, fear	a. Validation by more than one observer of specific behaviors occurring with a rise in anxiety b. Validation by client
		1.4. Carefully document content, form, rhythms of symptoms; behavioral predictors	a. Themes and predictable stressors will arise; behavior will take on greater meaning.

(continued)

Chart 68–3
(continued)

Phase of Treatment	Assessment and Formulation Dimensions	Nursing Interventions	Criteria for Evaluating Response to Nursing Intervention
		of rising anxiety and validated predictable times of stress in the client's day are especially valuable (environmental change—new personnel, new clients, visitors).	
	2. Historical dimensions of importance for client's receptivity to medication: Relationship with parents and siblings; relationships with peers, especially during adolescence (includes pleasure drug taking, sexual pursuits), self-care skills (includes cooking, health care, money management, purchasing); these predict ultimate level of self-medication. Occupational, esthetic, religious pursuits, including hobbies, creative releases (long-term medication must not interfere with these if functional) Previous experience with nurses' administering medication	2.1. Document relevant information. 2.2. Elicit client's feelings about areas relating directly to medication. 2.3. Encourage client to contribute to decision to medicate and choice of medication based on subjective experiencing of symptoms. 2.4. Reach agreement with prescribing physician as to target symptoms to observe for effect of medication.	a. One or two target symptoms will be documented.
Collaborating in decisions about dosage, frequency, route, dosage adjustment (prn)	1. Psychosis is a disrupting experience in which linkages between experience and meaning are lost. Provision of an environment with structure, routine, predictability, acceptance, and kindness is essential for recovery. The quality of the physical and emotional setting will determine the *amount* and *route* choice for medication. These supportive factors can be constructed in the home and community as long as the client/significant others are not in danger and the client/family is able to carry out adequate care.	1.1. Provide an optimal environment; provide or assist others to provide Limit setting Reality provision Positive interpersonal presence(s) Diversion and suggestion Reduction of stimuli when overstimulated Scheduling	a. Reduction in anxiety and, in turn, symptoms or psychosis
	2. Wherever nursing is involved directly with the client, the skill of the interpersonal nursing interventions will determine the amount and route of the medication.	2.1. Establish a therapeutic relationship including consistency, positive contact, compassion, decoding and interpretation, role/purpose definition, intuitive responses to expressed needs.	a. Recognition of nurse b. Neutral/"seeking-out" behaviors toward nurse c. Reduction of anxiety as demonstrated by reduced symptoms in the presence of the nurse.

Chart 68–3
(continued)

Phase of Treatment	Assessment and Formulation Dimensions	Nursing Interventions	Criteria for Evaluating Response to Nursing Intervention
	3. Communicating accurate changing data about the client is essential to decision making by the physician.	3.1. Document and communicate responses to interpersonal interventions by the nurse. 3.2. Observe target symptoms; communicate exacerbation/stabilization to physician.	
	4. Acting as an advocate to assure client's optimal safety and choice of treatment maintains dignity and fosters growth. Long periods of time spent with the client allow the nurse to offer medication when the client is less resistant and hence may accept oral form. Treatment of acute extrapyramidal symptoms should begin as quickly as possible after recognition to prevent worsening of discomfort to the client. Encouraging the client to ask for additional medication may strengthen his/her sense of control in the treatment process.	4.1. Be certain that client receives least injurious route possible. 4.2. Maintain flexible route to encourage choice of less injurious route. 4.3. Secure (PO) option if injection is being used in order to allow client to choose less injurious route when amenable. 4.4. Secure prn antiparkinsonian medication for acute extrapyramidal side effects. 4.5. Secure prn doses of medication in order to respond to client's need for extra medication.	a. Medication regimen will be client-centered, more than one route is allowed, and provision for emergency treatment of side effects exists.
Gaining client's acceptance of medication therapy	1. Agreement should be reached between nurse and physician concerning mutual assessment of information relevant to the client's understanding and acceptance of medication therapy	1.1. Write a teaching plan outlining information to be given to client, by whom; outline content to be reinforced by all persons working with client.	
	2. Developing trust in nurse is foundation of accepting medication. Preparation for medication therapy can be beginning of therapeutic relationship as medication can be viewed as "giving."	2.1. Establish therapeutic relationship (See I.a, Intervention 2.1).	
	3. Resistance to medication is expected and may give cues as to client's conflicts and operative strengths. Resistance during psychosis usually takes form of active and passive refusal due to fear, suspicion, loss of boundaries, confusion, or ambivalence.	3.1. Convey a complete but brief explanation of medication choice and procedure. 3.2. Encourage client to participate in preliminary decision-making. 3.3. Present unified, nonambivalent decision to client. 3.4. Apprise client of when treatment is to begin. 3.5. Encourage open sharing of resistant feelings; empathize.	a. Resistance will be expressed verbally. b. Client will begin to collaborate.

(continued)

Chart 68–3
(continued)

Phase of Treatment	Assessment and Formulation Dimensions	Nursing Interventions	Criteria for Evaluating Response to Nursing Intervention
		3.6. Respond correctly to source of resistance to convey understanding.	
Independent Role Establishing control values for critical physiologic and behavioral criteria	1. Review of side effects of antipsychotic medication—cardiovascular, neuromuscular, central nervous system, endocrine, renal, and hepatic systems may sustain adverse reactions.	1.1. Review laboratory data according to established guidelines. Suggestions—Blood and hepatic function studies, electrocardiogram	a. Data will fall within normal range.
	2. Review client's physical health, age, gender, seizure, and drug history.	2.1. Establish documented baselines by observing and documenting a. Blood pressure (orthostatic regimen)—Lying, standing, morning, evening	a. Blood Pressure—5-mm fall upon standing indicates significant orthostatic hypotension (see Chart 68–1, Side Effects of Antipsychotic Medications, for further indications).
		b. Pulse—Quality, rate, apical may be necessary	b. Pulse—Significant arrhythmias, apical/radial deficit should be reported and confirmed through EKG/physical examination.
		c. Weight	c. Weight—Document (see section 2.1–3 for indications if client is over/underweight).
		d. Sleep record	d. Sleep—Document sleep–wakefulness, quality, presence-absence of dreams CNS functioning upon awakening.
		e. Tongue and facial movements f. Walking gait g. Resting behavior—Absence/presence of abnormal involuntary movements in e, f, and g should be noted	e–g. Describe any abnormal movements in narrative form, noting factors that increase/decrease movements, absence of movement in sleep.
		h. Eyesight—Abnormalities should be noted.	h. Eyesight—Note accommodation difficulties, glaucoma, other vision disturbances, corrective devices.
		i. Intake/output if history of urinary retention 2.2 Establish and document absence/presence of a. Medication ingestion b. Pregnancy c. Seizure disorder	i. Urinary—Note any hesitance, symptoms of residual urine.
	3. Measure consistently and accurately over several days to 1 week to establish normal range; when rapid treatment		

Chart 68–3
(continued)

Phase of Treatment	Assessment and Formulation Dimensions	Nursing Interventions	Criteria for Evaluating Response to Nursing Intervention
	is required, secure as many measurements before treatment as possible. 4. Look for effects of anxiety and daily biorhythms on readings.		
Establishing optimal health level prior to medication therapy	1. Psychosis is characterized by self-neglect. The patient may show evidence of poor nutrition, hydration, skin integrity, and exercise, and may be similarly uninterested in improving these conditions.	1.1. Assess operative level of self-caring. 1.2. Establish plan to remedy deficient areas. 1.3. Intervene at level to which client has regressed.	a. Deficient areas will begin to show signs of improvement. b. Client will respond by decrease in anxiety.
	2. Food and drink are potent means with which to establish contact with psychotic clients. In the obese individual, be certain that caloric reduction does not result in oral deprivation or power struggles. Offering low-calorie foods in abundance will help.	2.1. Offer high-calorie foods at frequent intervals if client is underweight. 2.2. Offer low-calorie foods at frequent intervals if client is overweight. 2.3. Offer low-sugar fluids frequently.	a. Weight gain in underweight clients will begin. b. Weight reduction in obese clients will begin. c. Symptoms of dehydration will subside. d. Signs of hydration will continue.
	3. Prepare for the development of side effects.	3.1. Have order for prn antiparkinsonian medications.	

Prevention of complications arising from therapy	1. Some adverse effects of the medication are rare, in itself a complication, since many nurses do not see these reactions enough to recognize the onset. Regular comprehensive physical assessment is best preventative intervention. Begin this prior to medication therapy. Psychotic clients generally do not resist vital sign measurement if it is routine and explained carefully.	1.1. Plan for physical assessment on regular basis including
		  a. Review of baselines
		  b. Skin turgor, color, rashes
		  c. Review reports by client of physical discomforts
		  d. Menstrual, sexual activities of women
		  e. Sexual activities of men
			a. Documentation of comprehensive health state prior to therapy will be available.

Acute Treatment Phase
  Collaborative Role
    Validating choice of medication for client's symptoms
	1. Reliability among nursing observers is helped by clearly delineating behavioral form of target symptoms. If this is delegated to nursing support persons, establish that staff can distinguish the symptom from other symptoms and can reliably observe the target symptom without infusing the	1.1. Clearly outline target behaviors in nursing care plan.
		1.2. Use two validators when making observations.
		1.3. If observations *consistently* differ from established target symptoms, or if target symptoms worsen markedly, institute new planning with physician.
			a. During first 72 hours of treatment, documented observations will assume a consistent form; patterns to the symptoms will emerge.

(continued)

Chart 68–3
(continued)

Phase of Treatment	Assessment and Formulation Dimensions	Nursing Interventions	Criteria for Evaluating Response to Nursing Intervention
	observation with subjectivity. Failure to distinguish between agitation/increased activity, combativeness/assertiveness, aggression/fear is common because of anxiety provoked in observers.		
Collaborating in dosage adjustment	1. Since these drugs are long acting, dosage schedules do not need to be strictly followed even in acute treatment phase. This frees the nurse to use "windows" of receptivity with the client. *Consistency is the enemy of ambivalence.* Frequent approaches to the client with statements indicating that the nurse is aligning with the receptive feelings of the client. "This medicine will help *you* control (symptoms)." Capitalize on distractibility and short attention span by withdrawing from power struggles and returning again after an interval. Search for areas where client can have control over medication.	1.1 Offer medication at frequent intervals by trusted nurse (preferably with established relationship). 1.2. Do not engage in power struggles but withdraw and return later. 1.3. Allow client decisions as tolerated about medication	a. Client will accept medication with increasing frequency. b. Client will indicate capability to make decisions.
	2. Nurse's feelings influence client's receptivity. When possible, avoid giving medications when feeling angry, punitive, or frightened. If not possible, identify your own feeling to client and differentiate the medication from the feeling.	2.1. Continually self-examine feelings about medicating and controlling clients, reactions to perceived helplessness when clients suffer, and fears of physical or psychological harm.	a. Nurse's anxiety will decrease upon identifying feelings; behaviors will be task and client centered, not reactive.
	3. Additional medication (prn) is best given in anticipation of anxiety rather than to control outbursts. In acute treatment phase, prn medications are useful in controlling situational rises in anxiety. If a prn medication begins to be used at a predictable time each day, substitute an anticipatory standing dose increasing reliability of delivery to the client. Because of the long-acting nature of the drugs, consistent acceptance of the medication by the client is	3.1. Establish medication schedule in anticipation of high/low stress times. 3.2. Specify nonchemical interventions to be used before medication is offered. 3.3. Establish clear criteria for additional medication. (Criteria should be within legal guidelines for the setting.)	

Chart 68–3
(continued)

Phase of Treatment	Assessment and Formulation Dimensions	Nursing Interventions	Criteria for Evaluating Response to Nursing Intervention
	more useful than episodic control.		
	4. Skilled, anticipatory interventions by the nurse will reduce traumatic medicating (IM) and unnecessarily high dosages. Client will quickly become a collaborator.	4.1. Establish protocol by which several successive attempts at oral medication must be attempted before parenteral medication is given. 4.2. Establish safe procedure for administering additional medication.	a. Medication will be administered with no injury to client.
Gaining and maintaining client's acceptance of medication therapy	1. Continue to offer information according to what client can integrate.	1.1. Update teaching plan. 1.2. Assess client's operative defenses; support defenses.	
Independent Role			
Monitoring critical physiologic and behavioral criteria	1. Encourage client to report bodily sensations to nurse; client can begin to distinguish important body stimuli from nonimportant or symptomatic stimuli.	1.1. Continue observations; compare measurements to developing baseline data. 1.2. Establish criteria for withholding medications and requesting medical evaluation. 1.3. Withhold medications according to established criteria; notify physician.	
Maintaining Optimal Health Level	1. Side effects reduce optimal health level and must be remedied. Dystonias require immediate intervention. Other side effects will require collaborative decisions about dosage reduction, ongoing antiparkinsonian medications, conclusion of treatment.	1.1. Continue to remedy deficient areas. 1.2. Begin to give functions to client and reinforce attempts to care for self. 1.3. Diagnose early onset of dystonia. 1.4. Remain with client; administer antiparkinsonian medication. 1.5. Observe; collaborate with physician. 1.6. Diagnose side effects. 1.7. Provide measures according to Chart 68–1.	a. Level of wellness will be maintained or show improvement. b. Side effects will diminish. c. Anxiety and discomfort of client will diminish. d. Client will remain allied with therapy.
Recognition–intervention into adverse effects	1. Adverse effects require immediate cessation of the drug in most cases, medical evaluation, and institution of supportive therapies. Tardive dyskinesia is an exception.	1.1. Compare observations to developing baseline movement data. 1.2. Carry out AIMS evaluation every week (tardive dyskinesia).	a. Client will avoid complications and injury. b. Client will remain allied with therapy.

(continued)

Chart 68–3
(continued)

Phase of Treatment	Assessment and Formulation Dimensions	Nursing Interventions	Criteria for Evaluating Response to Nursing Intervention
	The nurse makes use of extended time and unusual settings with clients to observe for early signs of tardive dyskinesia. The nurse might observe tongue movements while a client cleans her dentures, or vermicular movements of her toes during a bath.		
Maintenance and Conclusion Phase *Collaborative Role*			
Collaborating on decisions about reduction and conclusion criteria	1. During this phase of treatment, the nurse and client work more closely on interpersonal concerns of the client. The accuracy of the nurse's interpersonal interventions has increased, as has the client's acceptance of the interventions. Despite greater intimacy and confrontation of real problems, the client requires less medication to control symptoms.	1.1. Observe against reduction and conclusion criteria and communicate observations. 1.2. Involve client as a full collaborator; allow maximal input into decisions. 1.3. Reduce dosage to once a day at bedtime.	
Collaborating to reduce medication	1. If the client has been hospitalized transition from hospital to community occurs at this point and may cause relapse or exacerbation of old symptoms. Medication may need to be increased, although thorough preparation and careful management of the therapeutic relationship can prevent this. The client may be terminating relationships with hospital nurses and establishing relationships with a community nurse.	1.1. Continue to support client and help connect symptoms to phenomena in the relationship. 1.2. If termination is occurring, encourage client to learn new strategies of coping with symptoms. Clients may need validation that they are not relapsing.	
Collaborating to conclude medication therapy	1. Conclusion of medication therapy should be accomplished by clients' having a felt sense of mastery over their symptoms using conscious means in interpersonal situations.	1.1. Help client practice conscious coping strategies such as relaxation techniques, exercise, interpersonal distance or contact, music, and creative hobbies.	a. Client controls symptoms or is asymptomatic without increasing medication.

Chart 68–3
(continued)

Phase of Treatment	Assessment and Formulation Dimensions	Nursing Interventions	Criteria for Evaluating Response to Nursing Intervention
Collaborating to teach client self-medication at most independent level possible	1. Assessment of client's resistance or alliance with medication therapy, available supports, suicide potential will determine level of self-medication possible. Client should always be in charge of medicating even if this means using slow-acting injectable forms. Placing members of the family "in charge" of medicating adds validation to their role as the "asymptomatic ones" and may sabotage client's medication therapy.	1.1. Collaborate on teaching plan, which should include identification of drug, symptoms helped by drug, dose schedule, general pharmacologic information, side effects, adverse effects, drug–drug/food interactions. 1.2. Carry out plan with practice demonstrations.	a. Client will state basic knowledge taught in plan. b. Client will medicate self under supervision over specified time.
Independent Functions Baseline monitoring Optimal health maintenance includes side effects Prevention of complications of adverse effects	1. Throughout these phases of therapy, information used by the nurse should pass to the client such that he/she is able to recognize the onset of complications. This teaching can be generalized to include aspects of health maintenance and normal physiology never learned by the client. Schizophrenic clients, in particular, having experienced disrupted interpersonal relationships, often have never learned basic information about body processes, including sexuality. This teaching leads to other areas where the client has distortions or absences of information.	1–3.1. Introduce information according to client's capacity to integrate information. 1–3.2. Look for cues that client wants to explore related areas; encourage exploration.	

Nursing Care Chart 68–3 shows the nursing care of clients receiving antipsychotic medications, considering the phase of treatment, assessment, interventions, and criteria for evaluating response to intervention.

References
1. Kessler K et al: Clinical use of antipsychotics. Am J Psychiatr 138:202, 1981
2. Shader R: Manual of Psychiatric Therapeutics. Boston, Little, Brown, & Co, 1975
3. Wilson H, Kneisel C: Psychiatric Nursing. Menlo Park, Addison-Wesley, 1979

Bibliography Refer to Selected Bibliography following Chapter 71 at the end of this unit.

69 _____

Antidepressant _____
Medications _____

_____

Linda S. Beeber

OVERVIEW   *Introduction*
Types
Method of Action
Medical Treatment Guidelines
Side Effects and Adverse Effects of the Tricyclics and Tetracyclics
Side Effects and Adverse Effects of MAO-Inhibitors
Nursing Care

Introduction	Affective disorders involve a disturbance in mood. Feeling tone may be perpetually sad and melancholic, as in depression, or elated and euphoric, as in bipolar disorder, mania. Medications used for treating affective disorders include tricyclic and tetracyclic antidepressants and monoamine oxidase (MAO)-inhibitors. These medications are not stimulants but exert a direct effect on the disturbed affect. Antidepressants are not effective in all disorders in which depression exists. Work among the medico-psychiatric community progresses toward greater distinction among affective disturbances and clearer identification of which disorders are helped by antidepressants (see Chap. 42). At present, several groups of affective disorders seem to be treatable by antidepressants:

A. **ENDOGENOUS (ENDOGENOMORPHIC) DEPRESSION**

This depression occurs seemingly without a relationship to life events. There is slowing of thought and speech, loss of energy, severely depressed mood, agitation, and *vegetative signs,* including inability to experience satisfaction, early-morning awakening, anorexia, constipation, and sleep disturbances. This disorder can be differentiated from grief reactions (response to a major loss), reactive depression (response to a blow to self-esteem), and characterological depression (inherent part of the personality).

B. **AGITATED INVOLUTIONAL DEPRESSIVE SYNDROMES**

This depression can be seen as a subgroup of endogenous depression and includes agitation, delusions, and profound guilt. These clients are generally over 45 years of age.[1]

Clients diagnosed with either of these forms of depression seem to respond to tricyclic antidepressants. Additional affective disorders are presently being studied that do not fit into the categories mentioned. Some clients with these "atypical" depressions are responsive to MAO-inhibitors.

Types	Efficacy of the tricyclic and tetracyclic antidepressants seems affected by idiosyncratic responses of the client. Clients on identical doses of tricyclic antidepressants will show markedly different blood levels. Clients who do not respond to imipramine will often respond to amitriptyline and vice versa. Measurements of metabolites of biogenic amines in urine (urinary MHPG) and cerebrospinal fluid (5-HIAA) point toward the potential for predicting which clients will respond to specific antidepressant medications.[2]

MAO-inhibitors are potent drugs with the potential to interact with many drugs and foods. Clients who are treated with MAO-inhibitors must be reliably able to manage complex diet and medication restrictions. Both groups are highly toxic in excess. Danger of successful overdose in the depressed client must always be evaluated.

Table 69–1 shows the tricyclic and tetracyclic antidepressants, and Table 69–2 shows the MAO-inhibitors.

Method of Action	It is postulated that reduced levels of norepinephrine (NE) and serotonin (5-HT) are present in depressions that respond to tricyclic and tetracyclic antidepressants and MAO-inhibitors. Both groups increase the NE and serotonin 5-HT available to the synaptic receptors in the central nervous system. Tricyclic antidepressants block the re-uptake of NE and 5-HT into the storage vesicles after release (about 85% available biogenic amines); MAO-inhibitors block the action of monoamine oxidase in breaking down excess NE and 5-HT at the presynaptic neuron (about 15% available amine).

Table 69–1
TRICYCLIC AND TETRACYCLIC ANTIDEPRESSANTS*

Chemical Group	Trade Name	Starting Dosage (mg/day)—Maximum Daily Dosage (mg/day)
Tricyclic Antidepressants		
Imipramine	Tofranil	75 mg–300 mg
	Presamine	
	SK-Pramine	
	Janimine	
	Imavate	
Trimipramine	Surmontil	
Amitriptyline	Elavil	75 mg–300 mg
	Endep	
	Amitril	
	Amitid	
Desipramine	Pertofrane	75 mg–300 mg
	Norpramin	
Nortriptyline	Aventyl	40 mg–100 mg
	Pamelor	
Protriptyline	Vivactil	30 mg–60 mg
Doxepin	Sinequan	75 mg–300 mg
	Adapin	
Tetracyclic Antidepressant		
Maprotilene	Lidiomil	75 mg–300 mg

*Major use—Unipolar depression of major proportions, but not all unipolar depressions respond to antidepressant therapy. More discrete criteria are being developed.

Medical Treatment Guidelines[1]

A. **DOSAGE**

1. Individual clients vary in absorption of tricyclic and tetracyclic antidepressant and MAO-inhibitors. The relationship of blood level to therapeutic effect is not known at present. There is probably a "therapeutic window" in some of the tri/tetracyclic antidepressants, that is, a specific dosage range where therapeutic activity occurs.

2. Dosage is begun at low level and increased over a number of days to reach a therapeutic level. Body weight can be used to determine dosage (3.5 mg/kg/day).

Table 69–2
MAO-INHIBITORS*

Generic Name	Trade Name	Dosage Range/Day
Isocarboxazid	Marplan	10 mg–60 mg
Phenelzine Sulfate	Nardil	15 mg–90 mg
Tranylcypromine sulfate	Parnate	10 mg–60 mg

*Major use—Formerly for hospitalized clients with severe endogenous depressions who have not responded to tricyclic or tetracyclic antidepressants. Presently being tried with "atypical" depressions, a depression characterized by pananxiety, phobias, hypochondriasis, and dysphoria.

3. It is recommended that upper ranges of dosage be administered in a controlled environment.
4. Elderly clients tolerate these drugs less well. The dose used is 1 mg/kg of body weight.
5. *Acute Treatment Phase*
   a. Test dose—25 mg
   b. Observe for orthostatic hypotension.
   c. If there are no untoward effects, increase by 25 mg/day to 150 mg/day.
   d. Divided doses reduce cardiac and hypotensive side effects.
   e. Use twice daily dose schedule with loaded bedtime dose.
   f. Response will not be immediate and is often very gradual.
   g. If no improvement occurs in 2 weeks, increase to 300 mg/day without evidence of adverse effects.
   h. Full response may take 4 to 6 weeks.
   i. Watch for suicide attempts.
6. *Stabilization–Maintenance Phase*
   a. Remission of symptoms should be complete in responding client.
   b. Dosage can be lowered to one-half the therapeutic dose.
   c. Dosage should be lowered *gradually*.
   d. Continue to watch for suicide attempts.
7. *Conclusion Criteria*
   If client is asymptomatic for 6 months
   a. Decrease dosage by 25 mg every 7 to 14 days.
   b. Watch for recurrence of depression.
   c. If depression is recurrent, maintenance may be longer.

B. **SPECIAL CONSIDERATIONS**
1. Suicide is always a threat with depressed persons. Danger of attempts is very high when depression lifts and psychic energy returns but suicidal impulses are present. Overdose with tricyclic or tetracyclic antidepressants is common.
2. Elderly persons or children
   a. See section on Antipsychotics
   b. *Benign prostatic hypertrophy* may contraindicate use in susceptible clients.

Side Effects and Adverse Effects of the Tricyclics and Tetracyclics

A. **SIDE EFFECTS**
Tricyclics and tetracyclic antidepressants have side effects similar to those of antipsychotic medications. These include
1. Dry mouth
2. Blurred vision
3. Constipation
4. Urinary hesitance/retention
5. Orthostatic hypotension
6. Excessive perspiration

B. **ADVERSE EFFECTS**
1. Exacerbation of psychosis
2. Cardiac arrhythmias (A/V block)

Side Effects and Adverse Effects of MAO-Inhibitors

A. **SIDE EFFECTS**
1. Orthostatic hypotension
2. Blurred vision
3. Dry mouth
4. Constipation
5. Urinary hesitance/retention

(Text continues on page 579)

Chart 69–1

ADVERSE EFFECTS OF MAO-INHIBITORS AND NURSING INTERVENTIONS

Adverse Effect	Nursing Intervention
1. *Cardiac Complications* of orthostatic hypotension Contraindicated in clients with congestive heart failure	1. Monitor cardiac baselines. 2. Withhold medication; request medical evaluation.

2. *Drug–Drug Interactions*
Potentiates:
   Anticholinergics
   Antiparkinsonians
   Barbiturates and hypnotics
   Chloral hydrate
   Cocaine
   Curare
   Dopamine
   Insulin (oral)
   Meperidine and other narcotics (hypotension increased)
   Analgesics
   Antianxiety agents
   Sympathomimetics—may cause extreme hypertension
   Thiazide diuretics—may cause hypotension
   Antihypertensives
   Antihistamines
   Anesthetics
   Alcohol
   Bee stings
	1. Provide continual comprehensive physical assessment, particularly when other conditions requiring treatment arise.
	2. Provide extensive teaching to help client avoid dangerous interactions. *WARN CLIENT OF DRUGSTORE COLD REMEDIES* containing ephedrine (sympathomimetic) combinations.

3. *Jaundice* (rare)	1. Assess for cause.

4. *Hypertensive Crisis*
Monoamine oxidase is essential in metabolism of tyramine; MAO-inhibitor prevents breakdown of ingested tyramine leading to pressor effect of tyramine.
Tyramine-containing foods
Cheese (aged)
Whiskey
Beer
Cream
Chocolate
Canned figs
Coffee
Licorice
Pickled herring
Chicken livers
Soy sauce
Pickles
Sauerkraut
Smoked salmon
Snails
Raisins
Wine (chianti, sherry)
Live yeast, yeast extracts
   (Bovril, Marmite, yogurt)
Fava beans (broad beans)
	1. Provide extensive teaching, warning clients to avoid tyramine-containing foods and food combinations and menu items of "unknown" ingredients. Diet must be maintained 2 weeks postdiscontinuation of MAO-inhibitors.
	2. If acute hypertensive crisis occurs
	  a. Seek immediate medical intervention.
	  b. Secure BP, vital signs.
	  c. Medical treatment will include
	    1) Phentolamine (Regitine) 5 mg (IV)
	      or
	    2) Chlorpromazine (Thorazine) 50 mg–100 mg (IM)
	    to reduce blood pressure.

Chart 69–2

NURSING CARE OF CLIENTS RECEIVING ANTIDEPRESSANT MEDICATIONS
(Tri- and Tetracyclic Antidepressants and MAO-Inhibitors)

Phase of Treatment	Assessment and Formulation Dimensions	Nursing Interventions	Criteria for Evaluating Response to Nursing Intervention

Diagnostic/ Preparatory Phase
 	
Collaborative Role
Collaborating on choice of optimal medication for client
	1. Symptoms of depression presented by the client must be organized and compared to symptom clusters most helped by antidepressants. Vegetative signs are significant because of their connection with so-called endogenous depression. Presence of psychosis may necessitate addition of antipsychotic medication. A life adjustment indicative of schizophrenia may be reason to withhold or give antidepressant cautiously so as not to provoke psychosis.	1.1. Observe for recurring behaviors over time in various settings.
		1.2. Observe for recurring behaviors in interpersonal situations.
		1.3. Observe throughout 24-hour clock for rhythm to symptoms, for example
		   Early morning awakening
		   Lightening of depression toward afternoon or evening
			a. All observations will be validated by other observers.
			b. Observations will be validated by the client.

	2. History is significant with respect to presence or absence of mania in client or family, presence or absence of response to treatment with antidepressant and suicidal capabilities.	2.1. Establish a nurse–client relationship. 2.2. Assess client's symptoms and ways of responding to symptoms (coping behaviors), suicidal capabilities and intent, absence or presence of significant event prior to depression. 2.3. Encourage client to contribute to decision to take medications.	a. Client will indicate nurse is a significant person. b. Symptoms will begin to be documented. Form and theme will emerge. Suicidal intent, plan or absence of plan, method availability or unavailability will be documented. c. Client will contribute to decision.
	3. Symptoms expected to respond to medication should be documented, since a lag period of 2–6 weeks may elapse, and criteria will be forgotten.	3.1. Establish target behaviors probably responsive to medication.	a. Target behaviors will be documented.
Collaborating on decisions about dosage and frequency	1. Decisions about dosage tend to be made according to physiologic response of the client to antidepressants, and this will be determined by remission of symptoms and development of untoward side effects. Endogenous depression includes symptoms of slowed thought processes,	1.1. Provide an optimal environment; provide or assist others to provide safety from self-destructive acts; provide reduced decision-making graduated responsibilities; provide graduated *successes;* prevent isolation and withdrawal; provide other areas of expression,	a. Client will experience reduced suicidal intent. b. Client will experience moderate relief of anxiety once dependency needs are addressed. c. Client will engage in therapeutic relationship.

(continued)

Chart 69–2
(continued)

Phase of Treatment	Assessment and Formulation Dimensions	Nursing Interventions	Criteria for Evaluating Response to Nursing Intervention
	loss of energy, inability to experience pleasure, agitation, sleep disturbance, hopelessness, helplessness, worthlessness, and guilt. Provision of an environment with support and socialization opportunities, distraction from rumination, progressive opportunities to succeed in tasks, and opportunities to engage in supportive therapeutic relationships is necessary. Protection from self-harm and careful monitoring of response to antidepressants are two essential factors.	especially nonverbal (clay, movement, and exercise). 1.2. Establish a therapeutic relationship including low reactivity by nurse to extreme mood, criticism, demanding behavior; clear, concise communications; encouragement of expression of feeling; acceptance of hostility; firm, nonparticipation in guilt-inducing behaviors. 1.3. Document response to interpersonal interventions. 1.4. Provide expert observation of depressive symptoms.	
Gaining client's acceptance of medication therapy	1. Agreement should be reached between physician and nurse concerning mutual assessment information relevant to the client's understanding and acceptance of medication therapy.	1.1. Write teaching plan outlining information to be given to the client and by whom; outline content to be reinforced by all persons working with client.	a. Client will participate in medication therapy.
	2. Clients who are depressed are often *too* ready to accept medication since it meets oral dependency needs and allows conceptualization of the client's difficulties in a concrete, cause-and-effect manner. This may not be antitherapeutic since vigorous investigation of problems during the acute stage may undermine functional areas and promote regression. Such intervention may be best done during recovery. Overacceptance of medication can pose a nursing problem by undermining nurses' confidence in their interpersonal interventions through the client's overconfidence in the medication and hostility toward the nurses' approaches.	2.1. Allow overdependence on medication, as it may increase confidence. 2.2. Continue therapeutic interventions.	

Chart 69–2
(continued)

Phase of Treatment	Assessment and Formulation Dimensions	Nursing Interventions	Criteria for Evaluating Response to Nursing Intervention

Independent Role
 Establishing control values for critical physiologic and behavioral criteria
	1. Side effects of antidepressants involve cardiovascular, central nervous system, and hepatic systems.	1.1. Obtain laboratory data—CBC, EKG, liver function tests.
		 1.2. Obtain baselines
		   a. BP—orthostatic reassurement
		   b. Pulse—apical/radial
		   c. Weight
		   d. Sleep
		   e. Eyesight
		   f. Intake/output
		   g. Bowel record
		   h. Presence/absence of
		     (1) Pregnancy
		     (2) Seizure disorder
		     (3) Tyramine in diet
			a. See criteria for baselines 1.2 under Antipsychotics, Independent Role (1).

	2. Dietary and drug ingestion is critical. Age, cardiovascular, genitourinary, bowel difficulties are significant.	2.1. Assess present or recent medication intake according to Chart 69–1. Document and report to physician.	a. Documentation of complete dietary and medication history will be present before medication is begun.
	3. Suicide potential is a critical element. Most suicides occur as depression lifts, allowing psychic energy to return but before suicidal ideation has resolved. Antidepressants may chemically re-energize the client as well as provide means (through overdose and dietary intake) of self-harm. The following list of behaviors associated with levels of depression should be scrutinized because depressed persons are often less aware of improvement than are their immediate observers:	3.1. Choose critical behaviors (may be target symptoms) to observe for *any shift*. Clearly spell out behaviors to nursing support persons prior to starting antidepressant medications.	a. Critical behaviors to watch for improvement will be documented.

Mild Depression	Moderate Depression	Severe Depression
1. Sadness; weepiness	1. Gloom and pessimism	1. Intense despair and desolation. At first glance, seems flat or blunted.
2. Transitory anxiety	2. Overt pervasive anxiety	2. Anxiety may be bound into delusions and thus not as freely communicated.
3. Transitory irritability	3. Indirect but pervasive hostility	3. Hostility less outward directed

(continued)

Chart 69–2
(continued)

	Mild Depression	Moderate Depression	Severe Depression
	4. Loss of energy and involvement in interests, but not narrowed	4. Narrowed thoughts and interests; indecisiveness	4. No interests; no decision-making activity
	5. Preoccupation with death, loss, and morbid themes	5. Ruminations and obsessive thoughts	5. Delusions; intense self-persecutory ruminations
	6. Transitory sleep, GI disturbances	6. Vegetative signs	6. Severe vegetative signs
	7. Overeating or undereating with transitory weight change	7. Disordered eating patterns; weight change	7. Disorganized eating patterns; tardive weight change
	8. Transitory somatic complaints	8. Frequent somatic complaints and altered perceptions of body	8. Detachment from body; self-neglect
	9. Sarcasm, put-downs; jabs	9. Depreciation of self or others	9. Augmented depreciation
	10. *Lower suicidal risk*	10. *Active suicidal risk*	10. *Lower suicidal risk*

Phase of Treatment	Assessment and Formulation Dimensions	Nursing Interventions	Criteria for Evaluating Response to Nursing Intervention
	The nurse must closely observe the client on antidepressant medication. Some signs of improvement can easily be mistaken for worsening depression, for example, increasing free-floating anxiety, outward hostility, increased complaints of somatic troubles. To mistake this transition could be lethal for the suicidal client.		
Establishing optimal health level prior to medication therapy	1. Severe depression involves slowed metabolic processes. Neglect may occur, not because of disturbed boundaries or intense anxiety, as in psychosis, but because small tasks seem insurmountable to the depressed person. Delusions of internal decay, often expressed as a fear of contaminating others, may partially express anxiety and hostility toward the nurse who attempts to keep the client in good health. Persistence helps.	1.1. Assess operative levels of self-caring. 1.2. Establish a plan to remedy deficient areas. 1.3. Intervene at the level to which the client has regressed.	a. Deficient areas will begin to show improvement. b. Level of health will be maintained.
	2. Food and drink are also potent means of contact to the depressed person—but contrary to the "hunger" of the psychotic client, the depressed client will use the nurse's nurturant contacts as	2.1. Hydrate. 2.2. Maintain hydration. 2.3. Facilitate weight gain or reduction as needed.	a. Signs of hydration will appear. b. Weight will change in desired direction.

Chart 69–2
(continued)

Phase of Treatment	Assessment and Formulation Dimensions	Nursing Interventions	Criteria for Evaluating Response to Nursing Intervention
	a focus to express hostility and dependency (medication will also be a focus for these feelings).		
Prevention of complications arising from therapy	1. Ongoing physical assessment will identify adverse effects and complications.	1.1. Plan for ongoing physical assessment.	a. Documentation of physical health state will be available.
Acute Treatment Phase *Collaborative Role* Validating choice of medication for client's symptoms	1. See Chart 68–3 for full discussion. 2. Reliability among nursing observers must be established.	2.1. Validate observations. 2.2. Notify physician if there is consistent deviation from established target symptoms or shift in target symptoms.	a. Pattern and consistency of client's target symptoms will develop.
Collaborating in dosage adjustment	1. Factors in dosage adjustment are rate of absorption by the individual and development of side effects. Tolerance of the medication will allow increase to therapeutic range.	1.1. Observe for therapeutic effects on target symptoms. 1.2. Observe for presence of side effects/adverse effects.	a. Client will reach therapeutic range safely.
Gaining and maintaining client's acceptance of medication therapy	1. The depressed client may express resistance to medication by being noncommittal, overtly compliant but hostile through criticism of the medication (and those who give it), or passive–aggressive (forgetting, overzealously reporting side effects). *Occasionally, the very prompt, compliant, nonquestioning client may be hoarding uningested tablets in preparation for a suicide attempt.* Often, overly compliant depressed persons fear loss of caring by significant helpers if they question the medication.	1.1. Observe and diagnose resistances to medication. 1.2. Allow expressions of hostility without retaliation. 1.3. Confront directly any suspicious behaviors indicative of hoarding medication. 1.4. Diagnose resistance and intervene.	a. Client will express resistance openly.
Independent Role Monitoring critical	1. See Chart 68–3 for full discussion.		

(continued)

Chart 69–2
(continued)

Phase of Treatment	Assessment and Formulation Dimensions	Nursing Interventions	Criteria for Evaluating Response to Nursing Intervention
physiologic and behavioral criteria			
Maintaining optimal health level	1. Early side effects will be orthostatic hypotension and sedation. Injuries from orthostatic hypotension are more frequent than from cardiac complications.	1.1. Promptly intervene in side effects.	a. Level of wellness will be maintained or improve.
Recognition/ intervention into adverse effects	1. Early adverse effects will be cardiovascular.	1.1. Monitor cardiovascular baselines closely.	
Maintenance Conclusion Phase *Collaborative Role* Collaborating to establish reduction and conclusion criteria	1. See 1, 2, 3, Chart 68–3		
Collaborating to reduce medication dosage	1. See 1, 2, 3, as above		
Collaborating to conclude medication therapy	1. See 1, 2, 3, as above		
Collaborating to teach client self-medication at most independent level possible	1. Assessment of suicidal intent is essential before clients can be taught to medicate themselves. Preferably, clients will have begun to develop interpersonal solutions to the problems presented to them.	1.1. Provide continual comprehensive assessment of suicide potential. 1.2. Provide continual assessment of client's present life and stressors. 1.3. Dispense only medication necessary for short trials of self-medication. 1.4 Supply Medic-Alert bracelet for clients taking MAO-inhibitors.	a. Client will begin to use a wider repertoire of skills to cope with daily stresses.

Phase of Treatment	Assessment and Formulation Dimensions	Nursing Interventions	Criteria for Evaluating Response to Nursing Intervention
Independent Functions Baseline monitoring. Optimal health maintenance Prevention of suicide	1. Suicide can occur at this point when dosage is within therapeutic ranges.	1. *WATCH CLOSELY FOR SUICIDAL CUES!*	

Chart 69–2
(continued)

B. **CENTRAL NERVOUS SYSTEM SIDE EFFECTS**
These may require dose reductions:
1. Jittery hyperexcitement
2. Excessive activity
3. Confusion

C. **ADVERSE EFFECTS**
The adverse effects of MAO-inhibitors and corresponding nursing interventions are shown in Chart 69–1.

Nursing Care   Chart 69–2 shows the nursing care of clients receiving anti-depressant medications.

References   1. Shader R: Manual of Psychiatric Therapeutics. Boston, Little, Brown, & Co, 1975
2. Stern S et al: Toward a rational pharmacotherapy of depression. Am J Psychiatr 137:547, 1980

Bibliography   Refer to Selected Bibliography following Chapter 55.

70

Lithium Therapy for Bipolar Disorder

Linda S. Beeber

Introduction   Whereas the tricyclic and tetracyclic antidepressants and the MAO-inhibitor medications are given for *major depressions,* lithium is given for control of *bipolar disorder,* more commonly understood as mania or manic depression. Although lithium is extremely effective in the treatment of mania, differentiating clients who will respond to lithium is difficult. Clients exhibiting mania appear for treatment infrequently in comparison to clients exhibiting depression. Symptoms of mania include euphoria, irritability, hyperactivity, pressured speech, flight of ideas, grandiosity, intrusiveness, joviality, and joking.[3] The "manic triad" isolates three critical symptoms: dysphoric mood, motor hyperactivity, and pressured speech.[4] Observed at a single point in time, mania is difficult to distinguish from acute schizophrenia. Clear cyclic mood shifts and a familial history of affective disorders and alcoholism but not schizophrenia are helpful diagnostic cues.

Method of Action   The source of the therapeutic effect of lithium is unclear. The lithium ion may alter abnormalities in the transport of sodium and potassium ions through nerve cell walls. This action may favorably affect the balance between norepinephrine and serotonin in the parts of the central nervous system involved in emotional responses.[2] The competition of the lithium ion in ionic exchange at the cellular level produces a reciprocal relationship between sodium and lithium:

$$\uparrow Na - \downarrow Li$$
$$\downarrow Na - \uparrow Li$$

The latter direction is extremely important to nursing because the implication of sodium depletion is potential lithium toxicity. Any condition altering fluid and electrolyte balance in the client taking lithium *must* be assessed carefully by the nurse. Any condition interfering with elimination of lithium from the body (for example renal disease) must likewise be considered.

Use   The major use of lithium is the treatment of manic episodes and prophylaxis of recurrent episodes.

Available Lithium Salts   Available lithium salts by trade name are
1. Eskalith
2. Lithane
3. Lithonate
4. Lithobid (slow-release spansule)
5. Lithonate-S (syrup)

Dosage
1. For acute manic episodes—600 mg–900 mg tid
2. For maintenance—300 mg tid
3. Dosage must be individualized

Medical Treatment Guidelines   A. **SELECTION OF CLIENTS**
1. Careful determination that the client is appropriate for treatment with lithium, including the determination whether treatment is to be only for the acute symptoms or as a maintenance treatment, client alliance with treatment, reliability, and support system are important considerations for maintenance.
2. Consideration of physiologic status, including cardiac disease, organic brain disease, and sodium restrictions.

B. DOSAGE

Treatment can be divided into two phases:

1. Stabilization of the acute manic episode (5–10 days)
   a. Lithium is administered orally, approximately 1–3 grams in divided doses over 24 hours; by 5 or 6 days a steady state between intake and elimination should be reached.
   b. Blood levels should be determined every 3 to 4 days; blood samples should be drawn 12 hours after the last intake of lithium; 0.8–1.5 mEq/L is acceptable.
   c. The client should be watched for signs of toxicity (Table 70–1) *A blood level of 2.0 mEq/L is unacceptable and lithium must be stopped immediately.*
   d. If violence is a problem, an antipsychotic drug may be added to the medication regimen and gradually discontinued as the lithium takes effect.[3]
2. Maintenance
   a. When the manic symptoms remit, the high dose of lithium should be reduced until a stable blood level is reached.
   b. During maintenance, lithium intake should equal lithium excretion; measurements of renal lithium clearance is critical, since lithium is excreted primarily by the kidneys. One fifth of the creatinine clearance can be used as a measure of renal clearance.
   c. Blood level lithium should measure between 0.6 and 1.2 mEq/L.
   d. Prophylactic treatment of indeterminate duration may be decided upon after maintenance is achieved.

Side Effects and Toxic Effects

Therapeutic plasma levels of lithium are quite close to toxic plasma levels of lithium. The nurse observing the client treated with lithium must rely on clinical signs of toxicity. Continuing to administer lithium while waiting for a plasma lithium level may be dangerous for the client. Changes in central nervous system functions are the most discrete signs of developing toxicity.

At any appearance of toxic effects, the nurse must withhold lithium and seek medical evaluation. Toxicity should be ruled out and documented before administering more lithium.

Table 70–1
ROUTINE SIDE EFFECTS AND TOXIC SYMPTOMS OF LITHIUM CARBONATE

Routine Side Effects	*Toxic Symptoms*
1. Mild gastrointestinal disturbance—anorexia, mild and *transient* diarrhea, vomiting, nausea	1. Marked and persistent gastrointestinal disturbance
2. Thirst, polyuria	2. Marked and persistent thirst and polyuria
3. Persistent fine hand tremor	3. Persistent coarse hand tremor
4. CNS symptoms—fatigue, drowsiness	4. CNS Symptoms—somnolence, ataxia, slurred speech, confusion, slowed thought, metallic taste
5. Blood pressure, pulse, electrocardiogram within normal limits	5. Hypotension, irregular pulse, electrocardiogram changes
	6. Other symptoms of progressive toxicity—hyperactive deep tendon reflexes, muscle twitching, choreoathetoid movements, epileptiform seizures, coma

Chronic side effects of lithium are

1. Diabetes insipidus-like syndrome
2. Elevated blood sugar
3. Thyroid disturbances
4. Elevated white blood cell count

Table 70–1 shows routine side effects and toxic symptoms of lithium carbonate.

Nursing Care The nursing process and roles throughout the phases of medication therapy will proceed in a fashion similar to the preceding chapters on antipsychotic and antidepressant medications. Refer to these chapters for general care-planning approaches.

Preparatory Phase of Treatment

A. **COLLABORATIVE ROLE**
  1. Choice of medication—Make observations to discriminate between mania and schizoaffective schizophrenia, organic diseases, and toxic states.
  2. Dose adjustment—If the client is subject to gastrointestinal disturbances, arrange dosage times to coincide with meals. Choose spansules because gastrointestinal disturbances generally occur with peaks in absorption, and spansules give more even release.
  3. Help the client accept the medication.
    a. Interpersonal interventions do not have an impact on medication dosage, since this is fixed by renal clearance rate; interventions do produce a climate for the client to become a collaborator. Suggested interpersonal interventions:
      • Provision of one consistent, accepting person
      • Clear, concise communication with minimal demands for decisions
      • Acceptance of dependency needs (expressed in defiance and power struggles)
      • Limits (consistent, fair, nonpunitive)
      • A noncluttered environment with as much space as possible and room for large-muscle activities
      • Interpersonal neutrality to mood extremes (euphoria, hostility)
    b. Document which interpersonal interventions work.
    c. Teach client critical information in a concise manner.

B. **INDEPENDENT ROLE**
  1. Physiologic baselines
    a. Check physiologic status, including complete blood count, thyroid function, organic brain disease workup, renal assessment, pregnancy test.
    b. Nursing assessment baselines. Check
      • Blood pressure
      • Pulse
      • Weight
      • Intake/output/urine specific gravity
      • Edema (ankle, tibial)
      • Speech, thought, level of consciousness (CNS status)
  2. Establish optimal health level.
    a. The acutely manic client will exhibit poor health maintenance as a manifestation of poor self-esteem, distractibility, and grandiosity.
    b. Physiologic supports are necessary. Frequent small offerings of *fluids* are especially important. Offer foods in an on-the-run fashion. Offer a diversity of foods to produce adequate sodium intake.

c. Since lithium is a suspected teratogen, absence of pregnancy must be established.

Acute Treatment Phase

A. **COLLABORATIVE ROLE**
1. Choice of medication(s); report improvement in symptoms; seek conclusion of concurrent antipsychotic medication.
2. Help client to accept medication—continue to introduce small amounts of information to client according to ability to concentrate.

B. **INDEPENDENT ROLE**
1. Assess client's physiologic response to treatment:
   - Monitor baselines, withhold lithium if critical symptoms of toxicity appear or adverse response occurs.
2. Provide early recognition of complications:
   - Observe for conditions altering fluid and electrolytes.
   - Observe for conditions altering dietary sodium intake.
3. Provide maintenance of optimal health level:
   - Provide solutions for discomfort caused by side effects.
   - As symptoms subside, introduce health improvement measures.

Maintenance/Conclusion Phase

A. **COLLABORATIVE ROLE**
Dosage
1. Continue to participate in dose reduction until stabilization is reached.
2. Help client to accept medication in spite of low self-esteem, resistance to losing euphoric symptoms, and denial of difficulties.

B. **INDEPENDENT ROLE**
1. Physiologic baselines/recognition of adverse effects—Teach clients to monitor one or two critical systems themselves. Teach someone in their immediate support network to help clients obtain treatment if they are showing signs of toxicity (especially CNS signs). Help client secure a Medic-Alert tag/bracelet. Refer client to outpatient department or community health nurse. Set up regular schedule for plasma lithium monitoring.
2. Maintenance of optimal health level—Provide nutritional counseling to maintain sodium in diet at 3.0–6.0 grams sodium per day.

References

1. Kessler K et al: Clinical use of antipsychotics. Am J Psychiatry 138:202, 1981
2. Rodman M, Smith D: Pharmacology and Drug Therapy in Nursing. Philadelphia, JB Lippincott, 1979
3. Shader R: Manual of Psychiatric Therapeutics. Boston, Little, Brown, & Co, 1975
4. Wilson H, Kneisel C: Psychiatric Nursing. Menlo Park, CA, Addison-Wesley, 1979

Bibliography

Refer to Selected Bibliography following Chapter 71 at the end of this unit.

71

Antianxiety Medications

Linda S. Beeber

OVERVIEW   *Introduction*
Use
Types
Nursing Care

Introduction   Anxiety arises as a signal that a threat is presenting itself and mobilizes one to cope with the threat. Some sources of anxiety are clear (e.g., situations of evaluation or physical alteration), while other sources of anxiety are unclear to the person. Anxiety is discussed in detail in Chapter 41.

Confusion about medical approaches to anxiety is reflected in the degree of disagreement about proper use of antianxiety medications. When the cause of the anxiety is known, it is best treated by removing the source of the anxiety.[1] Chart 71–1 shows some sources of anxiety and related medical or nursing interventions.

Treatment of anxiety is designed to lessen learned avoidance responses and to diminish anticipatory responses to external or imagined danger. Optimal health is achieved when this lessening of learned responses permits insight into the cause and direct activity related to removing the cause. Anxiety drives psychotherapy. To treat anxiety before the person has identified the source often removes motivation for examination of the cause in psychotherapy.

Use   Antianxiety medications should never be used in lieu of good nursing care. Short staffing, fatigue, or perceived helplessness on the nurse's part can sometimes lead to use of an antianxiety medication when skilled nursing care is more appropriate. Antianxiety medications are used in the following situations:
1. To reduce severe and moderate anxiety to mild to moderate levels appropriate for an investigative approach to the source of the anxiety
2. To reduce short-term anxiety when this anxiety may complicate the outcome of a medical procedure, for example, preoperative anxiety
3. To treat alcohol withdrawal
4. To potentiate seizure-control medication
5. To relieve muscle spasms
6. To provide short-term sleep induction (30 days)

Antianxiety agents should always be used in a time-limited regimen.

Types   Common antianxiety drugs are shown in Table 71–1 according to chemical group. Their major use is the time-limited treatment of anxiety.

NURSING CARE   A. COLLABORATIVE ROLE
1. Choice of medication—The nurse's expert observations are critical in determining the source of anxiety.

Preparatory Phase
2. Dose and route
   a. Use oral dose, particularly in situations where immediate action is desired (preoperatively) as intramuscular doses of benzodiazepines are *poorly* absorbed.

Chart 71–1
SOURCES OF ANXIETY AND MEDICAL OR NURSING INTERVENTIONS

Source of Anxiety	Medical/Nursing Intervention
Preoperative anxiety	Assessment of client's defenses Education and support of client
Anxiety in depression	Treatment of depression with antidepressants
Anxiety in psychosis	Treatment of psychosis with antipsychotics
Anxiety after major disaster	Crisis intervention counseling
Anxiety in medical conditions	Treatment of underlying medical condition

---

Table 71–1
ANTIANXIETY AGENTS ORGANIZED BY CHEMICAL GROUP

Chemical Group	Generic Name	Trade Name	Daily Dose Range	Tablet	Liquid	Injectable
Propanediols	Meprobamate	Equanil	1.2 gm–1.6 gm	x	no	no
		Miltown	1.2 gm–1.6 gm	x	no	no
		SK-Bamate	1.2 gm–1.6 gm	x	x	no
		Tybamate	1.2 gm–1.6 gm	x	no	no
Benzodiazepines	Chlordiazepoxide	Librium	15 mg–100 mg	x	no	no
	Diazepam	Valium	6 mg–50 mg	x	no	x
	Oxazepam	Serax	30 mg–120 mg	x	no	no
	Chlorazepate	Tranzene	11.25 mg–60 mg	x	no	no
		Azene				
Antihistamines	Hydroxyzine	Atarax	30 mg–200 mg	x	x	x
		Vistaril	30 mg–200 mg	x	x	x

      b. Seek time-limited treatment.
  3. Gaining client's acceptance—The nurse may be in a position to help the client redefine the problem and begin investigation into the source of anxiety. The goal should be to help the client build confidence in interpersonal solutions. Psychological dependence on antianxiety medications is discouraged.

B. **INDEPENDENT ROLE**
  1. Establish baselines:
    a. Gait (ataxia is a minor side effect)
    b. Sleep record
    c. Absence of pregnancy (teratogenic potential)

Acute Treatment Phase C. **INDEPENDENT ROLE**
  1. Monitor baselines; watch sleep curve for changes.
  2. Prevent complications arising from therapy:
    a. Observe closely for other sources of anxiety and symptoms associated with the source, for example, depression or suicidal cues.
    b. Watch for dependence on medication.
    c. Observe for alcohol abuse (antianxiety medication may potentiate alcohol).
  3. Provide interpersonal interventions to replace medication:
    a. Develop a relationship with the client and work on causes of anxiety.
    b. Investigate new ways of handling anxiety, for example, talking about it, exercise, and so forth.
    c. Explore new measures to induce sleep (see Chap. 53).
    d. Insist that treatment have a definite end.

Reference 1. Shader R: Manual of Psychiatric Therapeutics. Boston, Little, Brown, & Co, 1975

Selected Bibliography Appleton WS: Third Psychoactive drug usage guide. Dis Nerv System 37:39, 1976
Aslam M et al: Drugs in psychiatry. Nurs Times 75:1539, 1979
Bachinsky M: How psychotropic drugs can go astray. RN 41:50, 1978
Doller JC: Tardive dyskinesia and changing concepts of antipsychotic drug use: A nursing perspective. J Psychiatr Nurs 15:23, 1977

JOURNALS

General Psychotropic Medications

Doughty B: Understanding neurotransmitters and related drugs. Can Nurse 72:38, 1976

Dwyer M et al: Effect of hospitalization on weight of psychiatric patients. J Adv Nurs 3:433, 1978

Flynn W: Psychotropic drugs and informed consent. Hosp Community Psychiatry 30:51, 1979

Hecht A: Improving medication compliance by teaching outpatients. Nurs Forum 13:112, 1979

Newton M et al: How you can improve the effectiveness of psychotropic drug therapy. Nursing 78, 8:46, 1978

Pilette W: What is an adequate trial of psychotropic medication? Perspect Psychiatr Care 15:170, 1977

Ramsey A et al: Individual drug supply in a psychogeriatric ward: An evaluation of the system. Nurs Times 73:537, 1977

Rappolt R: N.A.G.D. regimen for the coma of drug-related overdose. Ann Emer Med 9:357, 1980

Raynes N: Factors affecting the prescribing of psychotropic drugs. Psychological Med 4:671, 1979

Sayle D: Drugs used in the treatment of mental disorder. Nurs Mirror 142:61, 1976

Sclafani M: Medication classes for the emotionally ill. J Psychiatr Nurs 15:13, 1977

Smith M: Appeals used in advertisements for psychotropic drugs. Am J Public Health 67:171, 1977

Thorner N: Nurses violate their patients' rights. J Psychiatr Nurs 14:7, 1976

Watts R: The psychological interrelationships between depression, drugs, and sexuality. Nurs Forum 17:168, 1978

Weiner J: Psychotropic drugs therapy: Knowledge of health care practitioners. Am J Hosp Pharm 33:237, 1976

Weinstein M: Progress and problems: Antipsychotics, antidepressants, antianxiety. Hosp Formulary 13:118, 1978

Psychotropic Medications with Specialized Populations

Ananth J: Side effects in the neonate from psychotropic agents excreted through breast feeding. Am J Psychiatry 135:801, 1978

Bachinsky M: Geriatric medications: How psychotropic drugs can go astray. RN 41:50, 1978

Blau S: A guide to the use of psychiatropic medications in children and adolescents. J Clin Psychiatry 39:766, 1978

Burgess H: When the patient on lithium is pregnant. Am J Nurs 79:1989, 1979

Fitzgerald C: Physiological changes affecting psychotropic drug handling in the aged. J Gerontol Nurs 6:207, 1980

Rosenbaum J: Widows and widowers and their medication use: Nursing implication. J Psychiatr Nurs 19:17, 1981

Slone, D et al: Antenatal exposure to the phenothiazines in relation to congenital malformations, perinatal mortality rate, birth weight, and intelligence quotient scores. Am J Obstet Gynecol 125:486, 1977

Werry J: Principles of use of psychotropic drugs in children. Drugs 79, 18:392, 1979

Antipsychotic Medications

Berezowsky J: Nursing the acutely psychotic patient. Can Nurse 73:30, 1977

Cohen M et al: A single bedtime dose self-medication system. 30:30, 1979

Daller J: Tardive dyskinesia and changing concepts of antipsychotic drug use. J Psychiatr Nurs 15:23, 1977

Donlon P et al: Overview: Efficacy and safety of the rapid neuroleptization method with injectable haloperidol. Am J Psychiatry 136:273, 1979

Hansell N: Services for schizophrenics: A lifelong approach to treatment. Hosp Community Psychiatry 29:105, 1978

Hitchens EA: Helping psychiatric outpatients accept drug therapy. Am J Nurs 77:464, 1977

Kessler K et al: Clinical use of antipsychotics. Am J Psychiatry 138:202, 1981

Kurucz J et al: Dose reduction and discontinuation of antipsychotic medications. Hosp Community Psychiatry 31:117, 1980

McAfee H: Tardive dyskinesia. Am J Nurs 78:395, 1978

Opler L: Tardive dyskinesia and institutional practice: Current issues and guidelines. Hosp Community Psychiatry 31:239, 1980

Pyke J: Nutrition and the chronic schizophrenic. Can Nurse 75:40, 1979

Ray WA et al: A study of antipsychotic use in nursing homes: Epidemiologic evidence suggests misuse. Am J Public Health, 70:485, 1980

Rodman M: Controlling acute and chronic schizophrenia. RN 41:75, 1978

Antidepressants and Lithium Carbonate

Callahan M: Tricyclic antidepressant overdose. JACEP 8:413, 1979

Cooper P: The tricyclic antidepressants. Midwife Health Visitor Community Nurse, 16:339, 1980

Goldstein B: Drug therapy for the depressed patient. Hosp Formulary 12:855, 1977

Stern S et al: Toward a rational pharmacotherapy of depression. Am J Psychiatry 137:545, 1980

Antianxiety Medications

Edmiston S: The medicine everybody loves. Family Health 10:24, 1978

Fritz G: Use of minor tranquilizers in a C.H.M.C.. Hosp Community Psychiatry 30:540, 1979

Greenspan K: The consequences of stress: The medical and social implications of prescribing tranquilizers. Occupational Health Nursing, 27:49, 1979

Lader M: Tranquilizers: Panacea or plague. Nurs Mirror, 148:16, 1979

Schiele B: Chemotherapy for anxiety: The place of the minor tranquilizers. Hosp Formulary, 11:423, 1976

BOOKS

Bernstein JG: Handbook of Drug Therapy in Psychiatry. Littleton, MA, John Wright, 1983

Cain R, Cain N: A compendium of psychiatric drugs. In Psychiatric/Mental Health Nursing, Backer B et al (eds): New York, D. Van Nostrand, 1978

Falconer M: The Drug, The Nurse, The Patient. Philadelphia, WB Saunders, 1978

Haber J et al (eds): Comprehensive Psychiatric Nursing. New York, McGraw-Hill, 1978

Hollister I: Clinical Use of Psychotherapeutic Drugs. Springfield, IL, Charles C Thomas, 1973

Part VII

Special Issues in Psychiatric Nursing

72

Legal Issues in Psychiatric Nursing

Marie E. Snyder

Introduction

Psychiatric–mental health nurses today must be aware of the legal ramifications of treatment. The state's interest in both the organization and delivery of mental health services, and in the mentally ill themselves, particularly those clients who demonstrate a potential for harming others, has sparked years of litigation. Mental health care has been more carefully examined by the courts than any other aspect of the health care system, partly because of the legal issues raised by involuntary civil commitment.

Types of Admissions to Inpatient Psychiatric Facilities

A. **VOLUNTARY**
Clients must be mentally ill, in need of inpatient care, and able and willing to consent to treatment. Clients must be released upon their own request.

B. **CONDITIONAL VOLUNTARY**
Clients have the same status as voluntary clients but may be detained only for a reasonable period of time (2–3 days) if they request release.

C. **EMERGENCY INVOLUNTARY**
Clients who are mentally ill and need inpatient care, that is, who are a danger to themselves or others but who refuse to consent to treatment, may be hospitalized on an involuntary basis for a period of time for evaluation and emergency care (7–10 days).

D. **INVOLUNTARY (CIVIL COMMITMENT)**
Clients are mentally ill and need inpatient care but refuse to consent. Upon hearing by the courts, clients may be hospitalized for treatment if they are thought to pose an immediate threat of serious harm to themselves or others.

Civil Commitment

A. **JUSTIFICATION**
1. *Parens patriae power*—The state has the responsibility to care for those unable to care for themselves.
2. *Police power*—Granted by Federal Constitution: The state has the responsibility for the health and welfare of its citizens, including responsibility to protect citizens from potential harm resulting from action or inaction of others.

B. **RIGHTS OF CLIENTS REGARDING POTENTIAL COMMITMENT**
1. An effective and timely notice to the client of the commitment proceedings and reason for them[4]
2. Detention no longer than 2 weeks without a full hearing on the necessity of commitment[4]
3. Representation by counsel[4]
4. That they not be committed without adequate proof of dangerousness.[4] The proof must be greater than a preponderance of the evidence and a "clear unequivocal and convincing" evidence is constitutionally adequate.[1]
5. That persons accused of a crime not be held in an inpatient psychiatric hospital in indefinite status as incompetent to stand trial[2]

C. **CIVIL COMMITMENT OF MINORS**
In the absence of evidence of clear-cut abuse of process by parents, or evidence that admitting psychiatrists acted in bad faith, children may be committed. Review of parents' request for commitment by a neutral and independent physician is

required. No distinction is made between children living with parents and children who are juvenile wards of the state. Ages 14 to 16 are the usual upper limit to those considered children.

Patients' Rights

A. **GENERAL RIGHTS**
1. Right to adequate treatment and that confinement for treatment not to generate into punishment[15]
2. Criteria for treatment[9]
   a. Humane psychological and physical environment
   b. Qualified staff personnel in sufficient numbers
   c. Individualized treatment plans
3. Right to release
   Nondangerous civilly committed persons must be provided an opportunity for treatment beyond custodial care or they have a right to be released.[6]
4. Right to aftercare
   Every client must have an individualized post-hospitalization plan. Hospital must adopt a functional approach to discharge planning, with emphasis on linkage with community mental health and social service agencies.[1]

B. **SPECIFIC RIGHTS OF INSTITUTIONALIZED CLIENTS**
   These are generally established by state statute and regulation. Typically, they include:
1. Right to stationery and postage in reasonable amounts
2. Right to have letters forwarded unopened
3. Right to be visited by personal physician, attorney, and clergyman
4. Right to be visited by other persons unless a representative of the facility writes a statement, consistent with treatment goals, of the reasons for denial on the treatment record
5. Right to keep and use personal possessions, including clothing, unless there is a written statement, consistent with treatment goals, of reasons for denial
6. Right to keep and be allowed to spend a reasonable sum of money for small purchases
7. Right to have access to individual storage space for private use
8. Right to reasonable access to the telephone to make and receive confidential calls
9. Right not to be deprived of civil rights by virtue of admission or commitment to a facility (*e.g.*, to marry, to hold or convey property, to vote in local, state, or federal elections)
10. Right to education
11. Right to notice of recommendation that guardian or conservator is indicated
12. Right to challenge retention at a facility

C. **LEAST RESTRICTIVE ALTERNATIVE**
   Some states have enacted statutes that require treatment of mentally ill clients in the least restrictive alternative. These statutes are based on the principle that the state may have a legitimate reason for wanting to treat a person, but treatment must be provided in the least restrictive manner and one that can provide sufficient care for the client's needs. There is no federal mandate for treatment in the Least Restrictive Alternative.[7]

Competence, Conservatorship and Guardianship

There is a popular misconception that a civilly committed client is assumed incompetent. Actually, the law presumes every adult to be competent even if committed to a mental health facility. State probate courts have jurisdiction to make the finding of incompetence and to appoint a guardian or conservator. Competence to take care of self or property does not require faultless decision-making but does require the ability to understand the consequences of actions and decisions.[3] If the client is found incompetent, the state may appoint a

Conservator—Confers authority only over property or estate of the client, or

Guardian—Confers authority over both person and property of the client

Informed Consent

Civilly committed clients are presumed competent to give informed consent or, conversely, to refuse treatment unless there is a judicial determination that the client is incapable of making treatment decisions. Informed consent should include the following:

1. A fair explanation of the procedures to be followed, together with their purposes, including identification of any procedure that is experimental
2. A description of any attendant discomforts and risks reasonably expected
3. A description of any benefits reasonably to be expected
4. An offer to answer any inquiries concerning the procedure
5. Instruction that the client is free to withhold or withdraw consent and to discontinue participation at any time
6. A disclosure of any appropriate alternative procedures that may be advantageous for the client
7. A reasonable description of any controlled substances and any other drugs to be used, and their anticipated effects, side effects, and interactions

Right to Refuse Treatment

1. Without a client's informed consent, facilities may not use involuntary seclusion, mechanical restraint, or forced psychotropic medication, except in an emergency situation to protect the safety of the client or others, and when delay could result in significant deterioration of the client's mental health. In an emergency, a qualified physician must find that the possibility of side effects is less serious than the need to prevent violence and that there are no less restrictive alternatives.[5]
2. Lobotomy or shock treatment may *not* be performed without the consent of the client or the client's legal guardian.
3. A guardian may consent to forced medication or other treatment in nonemergency situations.

Access to Records/ Confidentiality/ Privilege

A. CONFIDENTIALITY

It is the responsibility of the facility and the professional to keep all information, records, and correspondence confidential and to allow access to them only under specifically defined circumstances.

B. ACCESS

Mental health records are private and not open to public inspection except:

1. Upon a judicial order compelling discharge
2. To an attorney or other health care provider if requested by the client, or
3. To be used to enable the client to receive third-party reimbursement for services

C. **PRIVILEGE**
   1. Specifically refers to the relationship of a particular professional to a client and provides the client with protection against the release of any information obtained through the relationship
   2. Each state defines which professionals are privileged and whether privilege is absolute.
   3. Communication with nurses in client–therapist relationships generally is not privileged.
   4. Privilege is generally granted to communication with psychiatrists, licensed psychologists, clergymen, and attorneys, except:
      a. To place or retain the client in a hospital
      b. Under court examination, when the client has been informed that the examination would not be privileged
      c. When the client cites mental or emotional condition as a claim or defense in any court proceeding (except a child custody case)
      d. In a child custody case in which mental condition bears significantly on the client's suitability to provide care

Duty of Therapist to Warn Third Parties

A duty to warn third parties exists when a therapist determines, or pursuant to the standards of the profession *should* determine, that the client presents a serious physical danger to another person. "The protection of privilege ends where public peril begins."[8]

Malpractice

TORT LAW

Civil liability for nursing practice falls into the area of tort law. A *tort* is an action brought by a person on the basis of harm done to him by another. Torts may be intentional, as in defamation, or may be unintentional, as in negligence.

NEGLIGENCE

Negligence is an unintentional tort that involves harm resulting from the failure of a person to conduct himself in a reasonable and prudent manner. *Malpractice* refers to the negligent acts of persons with specialized professional education and experience. Performing an act of malpractice necessarily constitutes negligence, but not all negligence constitutes malpractice.

NURSING MALPRACTICE

The major aspects of nursing malpractice may be outlined as follows:

A. **DEFINITION**
   Nursing malpractice is an act or failure to act by a nurse that causes harm to a client.

B. **ELEMENTS**
   To prove nursing malpractice, a client plaintiff must be able to show each of the following:
   1. The defendant nurse owed the client a duty of care.
   2. The defendant nurse breached the duty of care.
   3. The breach was the direct or proximate cause of harm to the client.
   4. The client was really harmed or damaged.

C. **DUTY OF CARE**
   1. The nurse–client relationship is a legal relationship arising whenever a nurse renders nursing care to another person.
   2. How or by whom the nurse's services are engaged is of no significance; the act of providing nursing care creates the relationship.

D. **STANDARD OF CARE**
   1. Standard of care is a relative one, determined by the circumstances
   2. Nurse's qualifications, education, and experience are considered in determining breach of standard of care
   3. The legal yardstick is whether a nurse acted the same as a nurse similarly educated and experienced would have acted in similar circumstances
   4. Standard of care may be established by:
      a. Professional standards of practice
      b. Testimony of nurse expert witnesses

Standard of Care for Clinical Specialists

When nurses have acquired the necessary education and the experience to act as clinical specialists in a specialized field of nursing (e.g., psychiatric–mental health nursing), they are held to a higher standard of care than the nurse generalist, but only while performing services in the specialty.

Rules of Personal Liability

The principles of personal liability may be summarized as follows:
1. Nurses who are negligent are always personally liable for their own malpractice, even though another party also may be sued and held liable.
2. Supervisors may be held liable for the acts of someone they supervise if they are either negligent in making an assignment clearly beyond the latter's capabilities, or do not provide adequate supervision of a nurse who, because of inexperience, requires close supervision in carrying out a specific function.
3. The doctrine of *respondeat superior* holds employers legally liable for the negligent acts of employees that arise out of and in the course of the employment. The legal basis of *respondeat superior* is employer–employee relationships, employers being held responsible for the acts of those whom they have a right to supervise or control.

Nurse Practice Acts

A. **PRINCIPLES RELATING TO LEGAL REGULATION OF NURSING PRACTICE**
   1. The primary purpose of a licensing law for the regulation of the practice of nursing is to protect the public health and welfare by establishing legal qualifications for the practice of nursing.
   2. Nursing Practice Acts usually provide for the legal regulation of nursing without reference to a specialized area of practice.
   3. Two general models of statutory construction have dealt with expanded nurse practice, including psychotherapy.
      a. *Authorization states* have redefined nursing through the use of language authorizing nurses to perform additional acts beyond the standardized definition in the statute itself. (This is sometimes called "expanded definition.")
      b. *Administrative states* have redefined nursing by allowing nurses to perform such additional tasks as may be authorized by appropriate regulatory state agencies (usually the state board of nursing or the state board of medicine, alone or in conjunction with one another). This is sometimes called "regulatory definition."

B. AMERICAN NURSES' ASSOCIATION (ANA) MODEL NURSE PRACTICE ACT OF 1976: DEFINITION OF NURSING

The *practice of nursing* means the performance, for compensation, of professional services requiring substantial specialized knowledge of the biological, physical, behavioral, psychological, and sociological sciences and of nursing theory as the basis for assessment, diagnosis, planning, intervention, and evaluation in the promotion and maintenance of health; the casefinding and management of illness, injury, or infirmity; the restoration of optimum function; or the achievement of a dignified death. Nursing practice includes but is not limited to administration, teaching, counseling, supervision, delegation, and evaluation of practice and execution of the medical regimen, including the administration of medications and treatments prescribed by any person that state law authorizes to prescribe. Each registered nurse is directly accountable and responsible to the consumer for the quality of nursing care rendered.

The *practice of practical nursing* means the performance, for compensation, of technical services requiring basic knowledge of the biological, physical, behavioral, psychological, and sociological sciences and of nursing procedures. These services are performed under the supervision of a registered nurse and make use of standardized procedures leading to predictable outcomes in the observation and care of the ill, injured, and infirm; in the maintenance of health; in action to safeguard life and health; and in the administration of medications and treatments prescribed by any person that state law authorizes to prescribe.

TABLE OF CASES

1. *Goodwin* v. *Shapiro.* 545 F. Supp. 826, 1982
2. *Jackson* v. *Indiana.* 406 U.S. 715, 1972
3. *Lane* v. *Candura.* 385 N.E. 2nd 1024, 1979
4. *Lessard* v. *Schmidt.* 349 F. Supp. 1078, Wis. 1972
5. *Mills, et al* v. *Rogers, et al.* 50 V.S.L.W, 4676, June 18, 1982
6. *O'Connor* v. *Donaldson.* 422 U.S. 563, 1975
7. *Pennhurst* v. *Halderman.* 19 U.S.L.W. 4363, U.S. April 20, 1981
8. *Tarasoff* v. *Regents of the University of California.* 592 P. 2d 553, 1974
9. *Wyatt* v. *Stickney.* 325 F. Supp. 78L. M.D. Ala 1971; on submission of proposed standards by defendants. 334 F. Supp. 1341; enforced 344 F. Support 373, 1972, affirmed in part, remanded on the other grounds sub nom. *Wyatt* v. *Aderhold.* 503 F. 2nd 1305 (5th Cir.) 1974

Bibliography

American Nurses' Association: Standards of Psychiatric-Mental Health Nursing Practice. Kansas City, MO, 1982

American Nurses' Association: The Nursing Practice Act: Suggested State Legislation. Kansas City, MO, 1981

Annas GJ: The Rights of Hospital Patients: A.C.L.U. Handbook. New York, Avon Books, 1975

Annas GJ, Glantz LH, Katz BF: The Rights of Doctors, Nurses and Allied Health Professionals: A.C.L.U. Handbook. New York, Avon Books, 1981

Bernzweig EP: The Nurse's Liability for Malpractice: A Programmed Course, 2nd ed. New York, McGraw–Hill, 1969

Cazalas MW: Nursing and the Law. Germantown, MD, Aspen Systems Corporation, 1978

Cole, Mills v. Rogers, Advisor: Notes from Mental Health Legal Advisors' Committee. 3(5):3, 1982

Creighton H: Law Every Nurse Should Know, 4th ed. Philadelphia, WB Saunders, 1981

Cushing M: A judgment of standards. Am J Nurs 81:797, 1981

Ennis B, Seigel L: The Rights of Mental Patients: A.C.L.U. Handbook. New York, Avon Books, 1973

Hall VC: Summary of statutory provisions governing legal scope of nursing practice in various states. In Bliss A, Cohen E (eds): The New Health Professionals. Germantown, MD, Aspen Systems Corporation, 1977

Hofling CK: Law and Ethics in the Practice of Psychiatry. New York, Brunner–Mazel, 1981

Laben JK, MacLean CP: Legal aspects of psychiatric–mental health nursing. In Burgess AW (ed): Psychiatric Nursing in the Hospital and the Community. Englewood Cliffs, NJ, Prentice–Hall, 1980

Mental Disability Law Reporter: U.S. Supreme Court declines to decide right to refuse treatment issue. 6(4):221, 1982

Roth LH: Mental health commitment: The state of the debate, 1980. Hosp Community Psychiatry 31:385, 1980

Saphire RB: The civilly committed public mental patient and the right to aftercare. Florida State University Law Review, 4:229, 1976

Schell–King M, Finneran MR: The role of forensic psychiatry and the insanity defense. Perspect Psychiatr Care 20:55, 1982

Shindul JA, Snyder ME: Legal restraints on restraint. Am J Nurs 81:393, 1981

Stone A: Mental Health and the Law: A System in Transition. Bethesda, MD, National Institute of Mental Health, 1975

Thorner N: Nurses violate their patients' rights. J Psychosoc Nurs 14:7, Jan 1976

Trandel–Korenchuk and Trandel–Korenchuk: How state laws recognize advanced nursing practice. Nurs Outlook, 78:713, 1978

73

Women's Issues
in Psychiatric Nursing

Cynthia M. Taylor

Introduction   More than 50% of the clients receiving psychiatric services are women. Although the number of male nurses is increasing dramatically, psychiatric nursing remains a female-dominated profession. Hence, in psychiatric nursing the most common client–therapist dyad is female–female.

Because of the high percentage of women as clients and as therapists, it is important to understand the gender-rate bias that can affect the treatment of female clients. It is also important to consider female development and implications for treatment and psychopathology influenced by gender.

Female Development   Our understanding of female development affects our therapeutic interventions with women in treatment. Today, studies abound concerning new theories of female development. A number of these current studies are critical of the traditional Freudian concept of women. However, an examination of the concepts of female development of Sigmund Freud and Karen Horney, and the conflict between the two, will be a helpful backdrop for subsequent theories and their implications for treatment.

Freud   Basically, Freud's theory of the development of feminine identity is based on penis envy. Female development begins when a girl realizes that she does not have a penis. Before this realization, a girl's sexual development is very similiar to that of a boy. Freud believed that it is by repressing her masculine, active, clitoral sexuality that the girl acquires feminity. This theory is developed further by Freud in his differentiation of the transfer of sexual arousal from the clitoris to the vagina.

Freud also asserted that femininity is achieved when the girl blames mother for her defect (lack of penis) and turns to her father for fulfillment of her wish to gain a penis. This wish for a penis is replaced very shortly by the wish for a baby. The girl then becomes jealous of the mother, and the father is her love object.

As a result of penis envy, Freud found several limitations in a woman's psychic development. Some of these limitations were

1. Women have less stringent moral development (because they do not have castration fear).
2. Normal jealous tendencies become excessive.
3. Women are more vain.
4. Women have excessive claims to privileges.

Freud saw girls as having three paths to follow in feminine development:

1. Developing masculine characteristics (maybe to the extent of homosexuality) as a reaction formation
2. Developing sexual inhibitions or becoming neurotic
3. Accepting their condition (lack of penis) and becoming feminine

Even though Freud thought that the third path was positive, he believed women's lives to be fraught with difficulties.[6]

Horney   Horney's theory of female development brought a major break from Freudian theory. Though Horney recognized penis envy in girls, she viewed it in a different light than did Freud. She identified two types of penis envy, primary and secondary.

Horney saw primary penis envy occurring in the pre-Oedipal years and having the following sources:

1. The desire to urinate as a man does.
2. The boy's greater freedom to exhibit himself and have his sexual curiosity satisfied.
3. Because a boy held his penis to urinate, he appeared to have greater permission to masturbate.

Horney saw primary penis envy arising from the restriction of the wish to gratify the impulses arising in the pregenital period. She believed further that because of these restricted impulses the girl does suffer developmental complications but not pathologic consequences. Horney did not see these complications as debilitating or producing intense feelings of inferiority.

Horney saw secondary penis envy occurring in relation to the Oedipal complex. She believed that the girl is disappointed in her expectation of her father's love for her. She wishes to have children with him. When her love and wishes are not reciprocated, the girl represses her womanly feelings towards her father. This repression renews earlier feelings of penis envy. According to Horney, it is at this point that penis envy has pathologic consequences.[6]

Horney believed that if little girls were made aware of their specific female sexuality, they would not have to repress masculine sexuality to achieve femininity. She believed very strongly in the importance of sociocultural influences on feminine development. Some of Horney's observations of women in this culture were

1. Overvaluation of love
2. Excessive dependency on external sources of gratification
3. Devaluation of a woman's mature years
4. Women placing more emphasis on developing their love life than their personalities

Horney led the way for a number of theorists who continued to emphasize the importance of social and cultural attitudes toward women on female development. Several general statements can be made from the study of feminine psychology that have strong implications for our interventions with women clients. Relative to men these statements include the following:

1. Women have a vulnerable sense of self-esteem.
2. Women continue to have a great need for approval from others, and their behavior tends to be guided by a fear of rejection or fear of loss of love.
3. Women perceive the world in interpersonal terms. They regard themselves with esteem insofar as they are esteemed by those they love.
4. For many women, feminine sexual identity depends on success in heterosexual affiliations.[1]

Psychopathology: Influences by Gender

A recent study of the use of psychiatric services related to gender found more women than men seeking services. This finding occurred in every data source studied. These sources included first admissions to psychiatric hospitals, psychiatric admissions to general hospitals, psychiatric care in outpatient clinics, psychiatric care in private practice, and psychiatric disorders among the general practice of physicians.[4] A recently published study on antidepressants revealed the statistics from a consumer-owned cooperative that fills prescriptions for 98% of its 280,000 members living in Seattle, Washington. Table 73–1 shows the frequency of tricyclic antidepressant prescriptions for outpatient use, related to age and sex.[7]

Table 73–1
NUMBER OF CLIENTS TREATED WITH TRICYCLIC ANTIDEPRESSANT DRUGS: DISTRIBUTION BY AGE AND SEX[7]

	Age (years)			Total No. of Clients
	20–34	35–49	50–70	
Male	472	520	765	1757 (26%)
Female	1672	1538	1862	5072 (74%)
Total	2144 (31%)	2058 (30%)	2627 (39%)	6829

Psychopathology Found More Often in Women Than in Men

Depression   Statistics show that women are more prone to depression than men in every age group studied.[9] Evidence for the preponderance of women with depression can be found in the following sources:

1. *Diagnostic studies*—A 2:1 sex ratio is fairly consistent for women over men with the diagnosis of depression (treated depressive patients). When a specific subtype is given, ratios are lower for manic-depressive clients and higher for neurotic clients.

2. *Community surveys of persons not under treatment*—These surveys involve a random sample drawn from a total community and provide information on many persons who have had the disorder but have not received treatment. Women predominate in all studies and over all periods of time.

3. *Suicide studies*—Suicide attempters tend to be young women whereas suicide completers are older men. Rates of suicide attempters are an indirect index of depression, since many suicide attempters are depressed.

   Explanations put forth about why women suffer depression more often than men include:

1. *Differences in help-seeking behavior*[9]—Researchers have looked at the possibilities that women perceive, acknowledge, report, and seek help for symptoms differently than men, and that these factors account for the sex-ratio findings. However, all available evidence shows that women *do not* experience or report more stressful life events. Men and women do not appear to evaluate standard lists of life stress events as having different impacts on their lives. Women do appear to experience more depressive symptoms, though health-care–seeking behavior does not account for the higher rate for females.

   An interesting hypothesis regarding men and alcoholism is that men use alcohol to self-medicate for symptoms of depression. It cannot be ruled out that a substantial number of depressed men may be diagnosed as alcoholics or drug abusers.

2. *Biological explanations*[9]—There is reasonable evidence that a genetic factor is responsible for higher rates of depression among women. Studies show that persons who have a family history of depression are more at risk for depression. This risk is even greater if the person has a depressed twin.

   The patterns of the relationships between female depression and hormones are inconsistent; however, there seems to be good evidence that:

   a. Premenstrual tension and the use of oral contraceptives have a small effect.

   b. The postpartum period predisposes women to depression.

   c. Menopause does not increase rates of depression.

3. Psychosocial explanations[8]—Several hypotheses exist regarding the disadvantaged social status of women and how it may contribute to clinical depression in women. The first emphasizes low social status and the legal and economic discrimination against women. It is believed that these inequities lead to legal and economic helplessness, dependency on others, low self-esteem, low aspiration, and eventually to clinical depression.

   The second hypothesis emphasizes women's internalization of role expectations, leading to learned helplessness. It is believed that traditional feminine values are redefined as a variant of the learned helplessness that is characteristic of depression. Young girls learn to be helpless during their socialization and believe that this behavior is normal and expected.

Probably the most convincing evidence that social role plays a part in the higher rates of depression among women is the data on marital status and depression. Being married has a protective effect for males and a detrimental effect for females. Women with young children living at home have the highest rates of depression. Data indicating that unmarried women have lower rates of mental illness than unmarried men, but that married women have higher rates than married men are cited as evidence that the conflicts generated by the traditional female role play a large part in female depression.

Hysterical Personality

It is obvious in all psychiatric settings that the diagnosis of hysteria is very commonly given to females and very rarely given to males. Hysterics are generally described as demanding, dependent, overdramatic, scatterbrained, and sexy but frigid. These characteristics are thought to result from the consistent use of repression and denial as defenses.

Freud initially believed that women were more likely to exhibit hysterical features because they tend to repress rather than resolve conflicts of the Oedipal period. In later years, Freud believed that women may be more frightened of the loss of love than castration. This later belief is more consistent with interpersonal interpretations of hysterical personalities.

Studies focusing on sociocultural explanations note that the hysterical personality is an exaggeration of the female stereotype and suggest that girls are "trained" to become hysterics. Women have a tendency to be more dependent on the reactions of others, which is a key attribute of the hysterical personality.

For most women, a hysterical personality mode does not signify the existence of psychopathology, especially since the hysterical traits are highly congruent with the female stereotype. Nevertheless, this personality style often is associated with the development of serious psychiatric problems. It has been shown that under stressful circumstances *agoraphobia* (anxiety hysteria) and conversion reactions may develop, but more often in women than men.[3]

Anorexia Nervosa[2,3]

In the last 15 to 20 years, cases of anorexia nervosa have been occurring at a rapidly increasing rate. It tends to affect young and healthy girls who have been raised in privileged environments. It does occur in boys usually still in puberty, but at less than one tenth of the incidence in girls and young women.

It is a commonly held view today that anorexia is a rejection of femininity. Most anorectic women suffer from amenorrhea and interruption of the menstrual cycle. The anorectic client has very low self-esteem, a distorted body image, a striving to be perfect, a sense of inadequacy, and an inability to have satisfying relationships with men, all characteristics believed to be socialized in women in our culture.

Treatment

In reconstructive psychotherapy, individual, group, or family, with women who present symptoms that seem to be exaggerated forms of socialized sex-role stereotypes, nurses must keep several things in mind. First, the goal of therapy is the same with these women as with any client. That is, the nurse helps the client to uncover the unconscious meaning of the symptoms that she presents. Once this is done, the woman is in a position to choose what *she* truly wants, based on a thorough understanding of herself.

Second, though it may be tempting to "straighten out" the client regarding the ways in which she is living out sex-role stereotypes, the nurse must be careful to avoid turning the psychotherapy into "political activity." At the same time, it is appropriate to introduce the client to ways of viewing her life that may have escaped her because of strict traditional female upbringing. For example:

Client: "I'd love to continue therapy but my husband just doesn't earn enough money to pay for it."

Nurse: "Have you thought about getting a job to pay for it yourself?"

Client: (indignant) "Of course not! I have children who need me at home when they return from school!"

Nurse: "You want to protect them from coming home to an empty house?"

Client: "Yes, like my mother was there for me."

Nurse: "Is a part of you protecting *you* from going out into the world?"

APA Guidelines for Therapy with Women

The American Psychological Association (APA) has described the characteristics that therapists should have when working with women. These are presented in Chart 73–1.

Chart 73–1
APA GUIDELINES FOR THERAPY WITH WOMEN*

1. Counselors/therapists are knowledgeable about women, particularly with regard to biological, psychological, and social issues that have impact on women in general or on particular groups of women in our society.
2. Counselors/therapists are aware that the assumptions and precepts of theories relevant to their practice may apply differently to men and women. Counselors/therapists are aware of those theories and models that proscribe or limit the potential of women clients, as well as those that may have particular usefulness for women clients.
3. After formal training, counselors/therapists continue to explore and learn of issues related to women, including special problems of female subgroups, throughout their professional careers.
4. Counselors/therapists recognize and are aware of all forms of oppression and how these interact with sexism.
5. Counselors/therapists are knowledgeable and aware of verbal and nonverbal process variables (particularly with regard to power in the relationship) when these affect women in counseling/therapy, so that the counselor/therapist-client interactions are not affected adversely. The need for shared responsibility between clients and counselors/therapists is acknowledged and implemented.
6. Counselors/therapists have the capability of using skills that are particularly facilitative to women in general and to particular subgroups of women.
7. Counselors/therapists ascribe no preconceived limitations on the direction or nature of potential changes or goals in counseling/therapy for women.
8. Counselors/therapists are sensitive to circumstances in which it is more desirable for a woman client to be seen by a female or male counselor/therapist.
9. Counselors/therapists use nonsexist language in counseling/therapy, supervision, teaching, and journal publications.
10. Counselors/therapists do not engage in sexual activity with their women clients under any circumstances.
11. Counselors/therapists are aware of and review continually their own values and biases and the effect of these on their women clients. Counselors/therapists understand the effect of sex-role socialization upon their own development and functioning, and the consequent values and attitudes they hold for themselves and others. They recognize that behavior and roles need not be sex-based.
12. Counselors/therapists are aware of how their personal functioning may influence their effectiveness in counseling/therapy with women clients. They monitor their functioning through consultation, supervision, or therapy so that it does not adversely affect their work with women clients.
13. Counselors/therapists support the elimination of sex bias with institutions and individuals.

*Copyright (c) 1978 by the American Psychological Association. Reprinted with permission from the author and publisher.

References

1. Bardwick J: Psychological conflict and the reproductive system. In Walker E (ed): Feminine Personality and Conflict. Belmont, CA, Brooks/Cole, 1970
2. Boskind-Lodahl M: Cinderella's Stepsisters: A Feminist Perspective on Anorexia Nervosa and Bulimia. In Howell E, Bayes M (eds): Women and Mental Health. New York Basic Books, 1981
3. Chambless D, Goldstein A: In Brodsky A, Hare-Mustin R (eds): Women and Psychotherapy. New York, Guilford Press, 1980
4. Grove W: Mental illness and psychiatric treatment among women. Psychol Women Quart 4:345, 1980
5. Guidelines for Therapy with Women. American Psychological Association, Washington, DC
6. Howell E: Women: From Freud to the Present. In Howell E, Bayes M (eds): Women and Mental Health. New York, Basic Books, 1981
7. Jirk H et al: Tricyclic antidepressants and convulsions. J Clin Psychopharmacol 3:183, 1983
8. Weissman M: Depression. In Brodsky A, Hare-Mustin R (eds): Women and Psychotherapy. New York, Guilford Press, 1980
9. Weissman M, Klerman G: Sex Differences and the Epidemiology of Depression. In Howell E, Bayes M (eds): Women and Mental Health. New York, Basic Books, 1981

Bibliography

Bruch H: Eating Disorders. New York, Basic Books, 1973

Chesler P: Women and Madness. New York, Doubleday, 1973

Franks V, Burtle V: Women in Therapy. New York, Brunner/Mazel, 1974

Horney K: Feminine Psychology. New York, WW Norton & Co, 1973

Miller J: Toward a New Psychology of Women. Boston, Beacon Books, 1976

Muff J (ed): Socialization, Sexism, and Stereotyping: Women's Issues in Nursing. St. Louis, CV Mosby, 1982

Scarf M: Unfinished Business. New York, Doubleday, 1980

Thompson CM: On Women. New York, New American Library, 1971

Williams J: Psychology of Women. New York, WW Norton, 1977

74

Cultural Issues

in Psychiatric Nursing

Kem Betty Louie

Introduction

Ethnic background is one factor that determines the way that people experience their environment, helping to provide goals, expectations, values, and attitudes, as well as a sense of security. The meaning of behavior varies according to the norms and rules of each culture and subculture.

Cultural groups vary in the incidence and symptoms of mental illness. Though there are basic symptoms of neurosis and psychosis that appear the same in all cultures, variations in the symptoms show the influence of culture.

Studies have shown that the content and choice of sense organs in expressing hallucinations vary from culture to culture. For example, auditory hallucinations are observed more frequently in Western countries, whereas in non-Western countries the people tend to exhibit more visual, olfactory, and tactile hallucinations.[1]

It is postulated that in non-Western cultures, visual and other senses are more culturally emphasized as a means of communication and contact with the social environment than these senses are in Western societies. With this borne in mind, the determination of mental illness should be based on mental state and not social behavior. Behaviors that are ambiguous or unfamiliar to the nurse may not be necessarily indicative of a psychiatric disorder.

If health planning and treatment are to be effective, consideration of the client's cultural beliefs, attitudes, values, and goals must be assessed. Although clients come from a specific culture or subculture, individual variations exist and therefore nurses are cautioned against stereotyping clients or families.

Cultural Sensitivity

Cultural sensitivity refers to nurses' ability to be aware of and to respect the client's values and life-style even when these differ from the nurses' own. Before nurses can transmit an open and nonjudgmental attitude toward ethnic clients, they must understand and develop insight into their own cultural belief systems. Otherwise, they are apt unwittingly to transmit negative feelings, attitudes, and values to the client, causing further anxiety and discomfort.

Considerations in Conducting an Assessment

A guide to a cultural assessment is presented in Chart 74–1. These items serve only as a guide and should be incorporated in a nursing history.[3]

A. **PSYCHOLOGICAL TESTS**

Psychological tests should be interpreted flexibly, keeping in mind the following:
1. The norms of the test: What is the normal range of scores for this client, taking into consideration the age, sex, culture, and diagnosis? The standard norms of this test may not be applicable to this client.
2. The client's view of the test-taking situation: Does the client view this situation as a threat, a challenge, or a humiliating situation?
3. The client's responses to the specific items or answers: Does the client understand clearly what is being asked? Ethnic clients may answer the questions literally or give responses in which they think the interviewer is interested.

B. **INTERVIEWING**

When interviewing the ethnic client, nurses should bear in mind the following:
1. Clients may expect an initial period of polite exchange of "small talk" before getting down to business. Direct questioning about their problems immediately may be considered offensive and rude.

Chart 74–1
GUIDE TO CULTURAL ASSESSEMENT

	Example
Ethnicity	
Identify the following: specific cultural group and subgroup, degree of identification with group, citizenship or immigrant status, and length of time in this country	Chinese, a student in this country for 3 years, states she is Buddhist
Identify the language: 1. Language usually spoken in public and at home (include dialect) 2. Fluency in English 3. Degree of confort in giving information (disclosure) 4. Nonverbal communcation (gestures, posture, eye movements)	Speaks "broken" English in public and Toy Shan Chinese at home. Client is hesitant to give information regarding her illness. Answers questions literally. Speaks in a low voice and does not maintain eye contact with interviewer.
Family Constellation Identify the: 1. Type of family structure, matriarchal or patriarchal 2. Memers in the family/household, gender, and sibling rank	States that her father is head of the household. There are five members in her family, her husband, mother-in-law, son and daughter. Client is the oldest of three children.
Diet and Nutritional Preferences Identify the following: 1. Ethnic food preferences 2. Food taboos 3. Any special food preparations	Enjoys oriental foods, will not eat cold or raw foods
Health and Illness Beliefs • How does the client perceive this hospital admission? • What is believed to be the cause of the illness? • How is this condition usually treated in this group?	Has difficulty expressing her emotions. States she is tired all the time and is unable to sleep. She is not doing well in her studies. She has taken herbal medicines and has not found them effective. She believes that there is an imbalance in her body.

2. Communication barriers can occur because of cultural differences in the connotative and denotative meaning of words and phrases. For example, a client may say to you, "The devil is behind these walls." The denotative or common meaning of devil is a demon or evil spirit. The connotative meanings of a devil may include a wicked or cruel person, an unhappy person, or, in black subculture, a select group of people or a woman.[6]

3. Display of emotions and expressions of emotions may be different in various cultures. For example, what may be called "hysteria" in one ethnic group is a genuine, appropriate expression of love in another.

4. Time orientations, including tempo or speed of conversation, vary among cultural groups. Interrupting clients before they have finished a thought may be considered insulting in many cultures.

5. Nonverbal facial and body gestures and expressions, as well as social distance, are culturally interpreted. The nurse's own verbal and nonverbal expression may influence the responses in the interview.

6. Content within the assessment form biased toward middle class values and beliefs can cause misunderstanding or hostility.

7. Developing rapport and trust may be difficult. For example, mistrust or reserved behavior may be the typical response within black or Asian cultures when talking with strangers and need not indicate hostility.

8. Information from secondary sources such as family, friends, and others may be collected to understand the total situation.

C. **USE OF TRANSLATORS**

The need for translators or interpreters is fairly common for non-English–speaking clients. Interpreters may be professionals, local volunteers, relatives, or friends. There are several ways of communicating effectively with clients through an interpreter.[2]

1. Explain the reason for the interview and the type of questions to the interpreter. This information will assist the interpreter in eliciting general or literal responses, essay or short answers from the client.
2. Introduce the interpreter to the client and family. If possible, allow some time for them to become acquainted.
3. Speak directly to the client and allow the interpreter to translate. Do not interrupt the interpreter or client when either is speaking.
4. After the interview, spend some time with the interpreter to share information about the nonverbal communication and ease of obtaining information from the client.
5. Whenever possible, arrange for clients to speak to the same interpreter each time they are interviewed.

D. **MENTAL STATUS ASSESSMENT**

Among the information obtained from the mental health assessment, four areas are particularly culturally sensitive:

1. *Affect or emotional state:* For example, certain Asian clients respond automatically in a passive and quiet manner. Other groups may respond with hostility and aggression.
2. *General intellectual level:* Client's intelligence is often judged by their ability to use factual information in a comprehensive manner. This is difficult to assess if the client has had little or no education.
3. *Reasoning and judgment:* The values of many cultural groups are different from white middle class values. Differences in reasoning and judgment may be merely differences in values. For example, an Asian client may attempt suicide to "save face" in the family.
4. *Abstract thinking:* The content and terms must be within the client's cultural understanding. The client's response to proverbs such as "A rolling stone gathers no moss", may not be indicative of the client's ability to think abstractly, but rather of unfamiliarity with the proverb.

Nursing Intervention

To deliver relevant care to clients, consider strategies tailored to ethnic clients in general and to specific groups. See Chart 74–2 for overall nursing intervention and rationale, and Table 74–1 for specific information about three ethnic groups. Subgroups and individual groups will exist within this outline. These cultural groups were chosen because they represent beliefs and values that generally are different from the larger American society.

Transference and Counter-transference

Intervention must also take place within a cultural context acknowledging cultural coping mechanisms and patterns.

Chart 74–2
NURSING INTERVENTIONS AND RATIONALE WITH ETHNIC CLIENTS

Intervention	Rationale
1. Use the client as a primary cultural informant.	1. Ethnic clients are generally aware of the differences between the dominant culture and their own cultural group.
2. Understand the perception and meaning of the identified behaviors for the client and family.	2. Culture is an important determinant in the expression of behaviors.
3. Establish therapeutic goals and plan of care within a cultural context. Develop distinct and flexible approaches to care.	3. Individualized care is a goal of nursing. A plan of care that takes into consideration the cultural aspects of clients increases their cooperation in implementing the plan.
4. Set up groups of clients with the same ethnic background to reduce situational crises and expand the range of coping patterins.	4. Clients from the same ethnic group can help each other to understand and anticipate the normal patterns and stresses of individual and community living by sharing these problems in group situations.
5. Collaborate and consult with community leaders and organizations.	5. For many cultural groups, the neighborhood is thought of as their extended family. Additional information can be sought there.

Table 74–1
CULTURAL INFORMATION AND THERAPEUTIC STRATEGIES

Values and Beliefs	Accepted Cause of Mental Illness	Traditional Solutions	Coping Patterns	Therapeutic Strategies
Blacks				
Family unity, loyalty, assertive behavior, religion, work and achievement, predominately matriarchal, extended family	Environmental hazards, oppression, racism, divine punishment, impaired relationships	Family, church, friends, root doctors	Low disclosure, hostility, open expression of pain, withdrawal	Deal with specific problems, immediate goals and needs rather than abstract matters, deal with transference and countertransference
Puerto Ricans				
Sense of dignity, respect and deference to authority figures; *machismo;* patriarchal family structure, extended family important; "voices" and "visions"	"Mal ojo" (evil eye), evil spirits and forces, punishment by God and envious others	Folk healers, spiritualists, family	Low disclosure, open expression of pain	Deal with language barrier, specific matters which are problem focused, include father and family in therapy
Asians				
Respect and deference to authority figures, maintenance of self-control, patriarchal family, social sensitivity	The individual, divine punishment, imbalance of the ying and yang	Folk healers, herbalists	Low disclosure, reserve, avoid confrontation, physical complaints are more acceptable than emotional problems	Approach problems subtly. Concrete behavior-oriented solutions are preferred; approach is formal, include family in discussion of goals and therapeutic plans

(Adapted from a grid designed by Murillo–Rhodes, I; Downstate University, New York, New York. Printed with permission)

A. **TRANSFERENCE**

It is important that nurses become aware of the possible transferences clients have toward the culturally different therapist. Feelings and attitudes such as viewing the nurse therapist as an authority figure, as oppressive, or as a racist should be explored.

B. **COUNTERTRANSFERENCE**

Nurses may be unaware of their own ethnic prejudices. They must be carefully attuned to any unusual or irrational thoughts and feelings while counseling ethnic clients. For example, three different roles of group therapists in dealing with racism have been described:[5]

1. The "democrat" believes that race is irrelevant to the client's behavior and that the therapist's responsibility is to treat human disability and suffering. Race is seen only within the context of a social issue, not an individual issue. This therapist may miss countertransference cues by avoiding the issue altogether.

2. The "white expert" believes that clients must work hard and adopt middle class values for success in life. This therapist is condescending toward clients and is minimally aware of racist behavior.

3. The "humanist" believes that clients are all alike under the skin and treats all clients as though they were the same color. Racial issues are viewed as interferences in relating to others and "effective" psychotherapy is designed to eliminate feelings of racism. This therapist runs the risk of helping clients repress or suppress angry feelings, preventing real growth.

Potential Problems

Four factors that may interfere with the therapeutic treatment of ethnic clients have been identified:[4]

A. **MISMATCHING THERAPIST AND CLIENT**

Research shows that therapist and client of similar ethnicity or social class are better able to effect therapeutic outcomes than those of differing ethnicity and social class.

B. **LACK OF CREDIBILITY OF THE THERAPIST**

Therapists who do not know the norms, beliefs, and values of the cultural group will not appear credible. The therapist must also be able to experience a variety of roles in the therapeutic relationship, such as a change agent or ombudsman.

C. **CULTURAL MISUNDERSTANDING**

The therapist may confuse a client's appropriate cultural response with a neurotic transference, as in the case of aggressive or passive behavior.

D. **CLIENT'S EXPECTATIONS VERSUS THOSE OF THE THERAPIST**

The therapy should help clients to find the most personally satisfying solution to their own problems, apart from what the therapist may see as a solution. Because goals in therapy are influenced by cultural expectations, the therapist must guard against imposing goals based on the therapist's, and not the client's, culture.

When working with the culturally different client the therapist must decide to what extent to focus on the difference and to what extent the therapist should emphasize the universal human attributes of the client. One point of view is that the therapist guides clients to change to fit into the environment or mainstream of the client's dominant culture. The more common point of view is that the therapist helps clients to adjust to the situation, with a view toward eventually changing it for the better.

References

1. A1-Issa I: Sociocultural factors in hallucinations. Int J Soc Psychiatry 167:24, 1978
2. Kohut SA: Guidelines for using interpreters. Hospital Progress 56:39, 1975
3. Mosley HJ, Clift V: The Evaluation of Cultural Dimensions on the Curriculum, Cultural Dimension in the Baccalaureate Nursing Curriculum. New York, National League for Nursing, 1977
4. Pedersen P et al: Counseling Across Cultures. Hawaii, University Press of Hawaii, 1981
5. Ruffin J: Racism as countertransference in psychotherapy groups. Perspect Psychiatr Care 11:172, 1973
6. Tubbs S, Moss S: Human Communication: An Interpersonal Perspective. New York, Random House, 1974

Bibliography

Beaton SR: The function of color blindness. Perspect Psychiatr Care 18:80, 1974

Becerra R et al: Mental Health and Hispanic Americans: Clinical Perspectives. New York, Grune & Stratton, 1982

Bevilacqua J: Voodoo: Myth or mental illness? J Psychiatr Nurs 18:17, 1980

Braxton ET: Structuring the black family for survival and growth. Perspect Psychiatr Care 14:165, 1976

Chin JL: Diagnostic considerations in working with Asian Americans. Am J Orthopsychiatr 53:100, 1983

Davis AJ: Preventive intervention: Healing in West Africa. J Psychiatr Nurs 12:20, 1974

DeGracia RT: Filipino cultural influences. Am J Nurs 79:1412, 1979

DiAngi P: Barriers to the black and white therapeutic relationship. Perspect Psychiatr Care 14:180, 1976

DiAngi P: Erickson's theory of personality development as applied to the black child. Perspect Psychiatr Care 14:184, 1976

Diaz–Duque OF: Advice from an interpreter. Am J Nurs 82:1380, 1982

Delgado M: A model for mental health education in Hispanic communities. J Psychiatr Nurs 18:16, 1980

Delgado M: Therapy Latino style: Implications for psychiatric care. Perspect Psychiatr Care 17:107, 1979

Flaskerud J: Community mental health nursing: Its unique role in the delivery of services to ethnic minorities. Perspect Psychiatr Care 20:37, 1982

Gonzales HH: The consumer movement: Implications for psychiatric care. Perspect Psychiatr Care 14:186, 1976

Grasska MA, McFarland T: Overcoming the language barrier: Problems and solutions. Am J Nurs 82:1376, 1982

Graw A: Cross-cultural Psychiatry. Boston, John Wright PSG, 1982

Hankins–McNary LD: The effects of institutional racism on the therapeutic relationship. Perspect Psychiatr Care 17:25, 1979

Harwood A (ed): Ethnicity and Medical Care. Cambridge, Harvard University Press, 1981

Henderson G (ed): Understanding and Counseling Ethnic Minorities. Springfield, Charles C Thomas, 1979

Henderson G, Primeaux M (eds): Transcultural Health Care. California, Addison–Wesley Publishing, 1981

Jaffe MC: A Hispanic male experiencing difficulty handling hostility. In Riffle K (ed): Rehabilitative Case Studies. New York, Medical Examination Publishing, 1979

Kiev A: Transcultural Psychiatry. New York, The Free Press, 1972

Krcek–Frank R: Psychosomatic problems in the people of China. J Psychiatr Nurs 18:15, 1980

Leininger M: Transcultural Health Care: Issues and Conditions. Philadelphia, FA Davis, 1976

McGoldrick M, Pearce J, Giordano J (eds): Ethnicity and Family Therapy. New York, Guilford Publications, 1982

Mei–Li L: Folk beliefs of the Chinese and implications to psychiatric nursing. J Psychiatr Nurs 14:38, 1976

Mindel D, Haberstein R (eds): Ethnic Families in America: Patterns and Variations. New York, Elsevier–Dutton, 1976

Murillo–Rohde I: Life among mainland Puerto Ricans in New York City slums. Perspect Psychiatr Care 14:174, 1976

Osborne O: Unique needs of ethnic minority clients in a multiracial society: A psychosocial perspective. In Affirmative Action: Toward Quality Nursing Care for a Multiracial Society. Kansas City, American Nurses' Association, 1976

Paramola SO: The traditional treatment of the psychiatric patient in Nigeria. J Psychiatr Nurs 17:28, 1979

Pasquali EA: East meets west: A transcultural aspect of the nurse–patient relationship. J Psychiatr Nurs 12:20, 1974

Ruffin JE: The relevance of racism to the goals of psychotherapy. Perspect Psychiatr Care 14:160, 1976

Santora D: Research studies in American Indian suicides. J Psychosoc Nurs 20:25, 1982

Schlesinger R: Cross-cultural psychiatry: The application of western Anglo-psychiatry to Asian Americans of Chinese and Japanese ethnicity. J Psychosoc Nurs 19:26, 1981

Spector R, Spector M, Zola I: Cultural Diversity in Health and Illness. New York, Appleton–Century–Crofts, 1979

Spratlen LP: A black client group in day treatment. Perspect Psychiatr Care 18:176, 1974

Sue D: Counseling the Culturally Different: Theory and Practice. New York, John Wiley & Sons, 1981

Tamez EG: Curanderismo: Folk Mexican-American health care system. J Psychiatr Nurs 16:54, 1979

Tamez EG: Families machismo and child rearing practices among Mexican Americans. J Psychosoc Nurs 19:24, 1981

Timmreck TC, Stratton LH: The health opinion survey translated into Spanish as a measure of stress for Hispanic cultures. J Psychiatr Nurs 19:9, 1981

Timmreck TC, Stratton LH: The schedule of recent events: A measure of stress due to life change events translated for the Spanish speaking. J Psychiatr Nurs 16:20, 1978

Wintrob R: Belief and Behavior: Cultural factors in the recognition and treatment of mental illness. In Foulks E, et al (eds): Current Perspectives in Psychiatry. New York, Spectrum Publishers, 1977

Appendices _____

Appendix A
ANA Standards of Psychiatric and Mental Health Nursing Practice*

INTRODUCTION

The purpose of Standards of Psychiatric and Mental Health Nursing Practice is to fulfill the profession's obligation to provide a means of improving the quality of care. The standards reflect the current state of knowledge in the field and are therefore provisional, dynamic, and subject to testing and subsequent change. Since standards represent agreed-upon levels of practice, they have been developed to characterize, to measure, and to provide guidance in achieving excellence in care.[1]

The standards presented here are a revision of the standards enunciated by the Division on Psychiatric and Mental Health Nursing Practice in 1973. They apply to any setting in which psychiatric and mental health nursing is practiced, and to both generalists and specialists in psychiatric and mental health nursing. Standards V-F (psychotherapy) and X (community health systems) apply specifically to the specialist. The standards are written within the framework of the nursing process, which includes data collection, diagnosis, planning, treatment, and evaluation.[2]

The treatment or intervention phase of the nursing process is elaborated upon in order to highlight the specific interventions or nursing care activities commonly carried out by psychiatric and mental health nurses: therapeutic interventions, health teaching, activities of daily living, somatic therapies, therapeutic environment, and psychotherapy. In addition to the standards concerned with the nursing process are standards that address professional performance, such as use of the-

ory, peer review, continuing education, interdisciplinary team collaboration, community health systems, and research. Accountability of the provider to the client, client rights, and client advocacy are implicit throughout the standards.

A rationale is provided for each standard, and criteria are developed to measure each standard. The criteria are divided into structure, process, and outcome. They are intended to provide a means by which attainment of the standard may be specifically measured. The criteria for each standard are not exhaustive.

Standards of Psychiatric and Mental Health Nursing Practice should be used in conjunction with the following ANA publications: (a) Standards of Nursing Practice, (b) Statement on Psychiatric and Mental Health Nursing Practice, (c) Nursing: A Social Policy Statement, and (d) Code for Nurses with Interpretive Statements.

PROFESSIONAL PRACTICE STANDARDS

Standard I. Theory

THE NURSE APPLIES APPROPRIATE THEORY THAT IS SCIENTIFICALLY SOUND AS A BASIS FOR DECISIONS REGARDING NURSING PRACTICE.

Rationale
Psychiatric and mental health nursing is characterized by the application of relevant theories to explain phenomena of concern to nurses, and to provide a basis for intervention and subsequent evaluation of that intervention. A primary source of knowledge for practice rests on the scholarly conceptualizations of psychiatric and

---

*From Standards of Psychiatric and Mental Health Nursing Practice, published by the American Nurses' Association, Inc. Reprinted with permission.
[1] American Nurses' Association: A Plan for Implementation of the Standards of Nursing Practice, p 4. Kansas City, MO, the Association, 1975 4
[2] Ibid

mental health nursing practice and on research findings generated from intradisciplinary and cross-disciplinary studies of human behavior. The nurse's use of selected theories provides comprehensive, balanced perceptions of clients' characteristics, diagnoses, or presenting conditions.

Structure Criteria

1. Access to resource materials on theories is provided in the practice setting.
2. Continuing education programs on theories of human behavior are available and accessible.
3. Theory-based nursing actions are recognized within the practice setting and are congruent with overall agency philosophy.

Process Criteria

The nurse—
1. Examines basic assumptions on the nature of persons
2. Corrects erroneous beliefs
3. Utilizes theory and critical thinking to
   a. Formulate generalizations, for example, opinion, speculation, and assumption
   b. Generate and test hypotheses.
4. Utilizes inferences, principles, and operational concepts
5. Applies relevant theories

Outcome Criterion

Measurable objectives and relevant interventions for clients are based on scientific theory.

Standard II. Data Collection

THE NURSE CONTINUOUSLY COLLECTS DATA THAT ARE COMPREHENSIVE, ACCURATE, AND SYSTEMATIC.

Rationale

Effective interviewing, behavioral observation, and physical and mental health assessment enable the nurse to reach sound conclusions and plan appropriate interventions with the client.

Structure Criterion

A means by which data are gathered, recorded, and retrieved is available in the practice setting.

Process Criteria

The nurse—
1. Informs the client of their mutual roles and responsibilities in the data-gathering process

2. Uses clinical judgments to determine what information is needed. Health data undergirding the nursing process for psychiatric and mental health clients are obtained through assessing the following:
   a. Biophysical, developmental, mental, and emotional status
   b. Spiritual or philosophical beliefs
   c. Family, social, cultural, and community systems
   d. Daily activities, interactions, and coping patterns
   e. Economic, environmental, and political factors affecting the client's health
   f. Personally significant support systems, as well as unutilized but available support systems
   g. Knowledge, satisfaction, and change motivation regarding current health status
   h. Strengths that can be used in reaching health goals
   i. Knowledge of pertinent legal rights
   j. Contributory data from the family, significant others, the health care team, and pertinent individuals in the community

Outcome Criteria

1. The client participates in the data-gathering process.
2. The client affirms the value of the data-gathering process. If illness precludes this capacity in the client, affirmation of the quality and ethical handling of the data is sought from the client's significant others and/or the nurse's peers.
3. The data base is synthesized and recorded in a standardized format.

Standard III. Diagnosis

THE NURSE UTILIZES NURSING DIAGNOSES AND/OR STANDARD CLASSIFICATION OF MENTAL DISORDERS TO EXPRESS CONCLUSIONS SUPPORTED BY RECORDED ASSESSMENT DATA AND CURRENT SCIENTIFIC PREMISES.

Rationale

Nursing's logical basis for providing care rests on the recognition and identification of those actual or potential health problems that are within the scope of nursing practice.

Structure Criterion

In the practice setting, opportunities are provided for validation of diagnosis by peers and for exchange of information and research findings regarding the scientific premises underlying nursing diagnosis among peers.

Process Criteria

The nurse—

1. Identifies actual or potential health problems in regard to
   a. Self-care limitations or impaired functioning whose general etiology is mental and emotional distress, deficits in the ways significant systems are functioning, and internal psychic and/or developmental issues
   b. Emotional stress or crisis components of illness, pain, self-concept changes, and life process changes
   c. Emotional problems related to daily experiences, such as anxiety, aggression, loss, loneliness, and grief
   d. Physical symptoms that occur simultaneously with altered psychic functioning, such as altered intestinal functioning and anorexia
   e. Alterations in thinking, perceiving, symbolizing, communicating, and decision-making abilities
   f. Impaired abilities to relate to others
   g. Behaviors and mental states that indicate the client is a danger to self or others or is gravely disabled
2. Analyzes available information according to accepted theoretical frameworks
3. Collects sufficient data to verify a diagnosis
4. Makes inferences regarding data from phenomena
5. Formulates a nursing diagnosis subject to revision with subsequent data

Outcome Criteria

1. Nursing diagnoses are validated with the client when validation has a therapeutic purpose and is not clearly impossible or contraindicated. If illness precludes this capacity in the client, affirmation of the nursing diagnosis is sought from the client's significant others and/or the nurse's peers.
2. Nursing diagnoses are recorded in a manner that facilitates nursing planning and research.

Standard IV. Planning

THE NURSE DEVELOPS A NURSING CARE PLAN WITH SPECIFIC GOALS AND INTERVENTIONS DELINEATING NURSING ACTIONS UNIQUE TO EACH CLIENT'S NEEDS.

Rationale

The nursing care plan is used to guide therapeutic intervention and effectively achieve the desired outcomes.

Structure Criteria

1. The practice setting is one in which the nurse has opportunities to collaborate with others in the development of nursing care plans compatible with overall treatment plans.
2. Within the practice setting, mechanisms exist for nursing care plans to be recorded, communicated to others, and revised as necessary.

Process Criteria

1. The nurse collaborates with clients, their significant others, and team members in establishing nursing care plans.
2. In the care plan, the nurse—
   a. Identifies priorities of care
   b. States realistic goals in measurable terms with an expected date of accomplishment
   c. Uses identifiable psychotherapeutic principles
   d. Indicates which client needs will be a primary responsibility of the psychiatric and mental health nurse and which will be referred to others with the appropriate expertise
   e. Stresses mutual goal setting and shared responsibility for goal attainment at the level of the client's abilities
   f. Provides guidance for the client care activities performed by others under the nurse's supervision
3. The nurse revises the care plan as goals are achieved, changed, or updated.

Outcome Criteria

1. The nursing care plan is recorded and available for review.
2. The nursing care plan shows evidence of revision and deletion of prescribed nursing actions as goals are achieved, changed, or updated.

Standard V. Intervention

THE NURSE INTERVENES AS GUIDED BY THE NURSING CARE PLAN TO IMPLEMENT NURSING ACTIONS THAT PROMOTE, MAINTAIN, OR RESTORE PHYSICAL AND MENTAL HEALTH, PREVENT ILLNESS, AND EFFECT REHABILITATION.

Rationale

Mental health is one aspect of general health and well-being. Nursing actions reflect an appreciation for the hierarchy of human needs and include interventions for all aspects of physical and mental health and illness.

Structure Criteria

1. Independent nursing interventions are promoted within the practice setting.
2. Professional staffing patterns in psychiatric and mental health care settings are determined by the documented health care needs of the population served.
3. A mechanism exists to review and revise nurse-client ratios on at least a biennial basis to assure implementation of the standards of psychiatric and mental health nursing practice.

Process Criteria

The nurse—

1. Acts to ensure that health care needs are met either by using nursing skills or by obtaining assistance from other health care providers when indicated
2. Acts as the client's advocate when necessary to facilitate the achievement of health
3. Reviews and modifies interventions based on patient progress

Outcome Criteria

1. A record of intervention is derived from the nursing care plan.
2. Interventions are validated with client and peers.
3. Peers corroborate that interventions are guided by the nursing care plan and are therapeutic.

Standard V-A. Intervention: Psychotherapeutic Interventions

THE NURSE USES PSYCHOTHERAPEUTIC INTERVENTIONS TO ASSIST CLIENTS IN REGAINING OR IMPROVING THEIR PREVIOUS COPING ABILITIES AND TO PREVENT FURTHER DISABILITY.

Rationale

Individuals with and without mental health problems often respond to health problems in a dysfunctional manner. During counseling, interviewing, crisis or emergency intervention, or daily interaction, nurses diagnose dysfunctional behaviors, engage clients in noting such behaviors, and assist the client in modifying or eliminating those behaviors.

Structure Criterion

The nurse who engages in psychotherapeutic interventions is minimally prepared as a generalist in psychiatric and mental health nursing.

Process Criteria

The nurse—

1. Identifies the client's responses to health problems
2. Reinforces those responses to health problems that are functional and helps the client modify or eliminate those that are dysfunctional
3. Employs principles of communication, interviewing techniques, problem solving, and crisis intervention when performing psychotherapeutic interventions
4. Uses knowledge of behavioral concepts such as anxiety, loss, conflict, grief, and anger to assist the client in coping, adapting, and dealing constructively with feelings
5. Demonstrates knowledge about and skill in the use of psychotherapeutic interventions specifically useful in the modification of thought, perception, affect, behavior, and motivation
6. Utilizes health team members to help evaluate the outcome of interventions and to formulate modification of psychotherapeutic techniques
7. Reinforces useful patterns and themes in the client's interactions with others
8. Uses crisis intervention to promote growth and to aid the personal and social integration of clients in developmental, situational, or suicidal crisis

Outcome Criterion

Clients state that they have been assisted in regaining or improving their previous coping abilities.

Standard V-B. Intervention: Health Teaching

THE NURSE ASSISTS CLIENTS, FAMILIES, AND GROUPS TO ACHIEVE SATISFYING AND PRODUCTIVE PATTERNS OF LIVING THROUGH HEALTH TEACHING.

Rationale

Health teaching is an essential part of the nurse's role with those who have mental health problems. Every interaction can be utilized as a teaching–learning situation. Formal and informal teaching methods can be used in working with individuals, families, groups, and the community. Emphasis is on understanding principles of mental health as well as on developing ways of coping with mental health problems. Client adherence to treatment regimens increases when health teaching is an integral part of the client's care.

Structure Criteria

1. Opportunities to use varied and appropriate teaching methodologies are available.
2. Appropriate teaching facilities and resources are provided within the practice setting.
3. Health teaching by nurses is specified in job descriptions.

Process Criteria
The nurse—
1. Identifies health education needs of clients
2. Employs principles of learning and appropriate teaching methods
3. Teaches the basic principles of physical and mental health
4. Teaches communication, interpersonal, and social skills
5. Provides opportunities for clients to learn experientially.

Outcome Criteria
1. Health teaching activities are recorded.
2. The client and/or family demonstrates acquisition of knowledge as a result of health teaching.

Standard V-C. Intervention: Activities of Daily Living

THE NURSE USES THE ACTIVITIES OF DAILY LIVING IN A GOAL-DIRECTED WAY TO FOSTER ADEQUATE SELF-CARE AND PHYSICAL AND MENTAL WELL-BEING OF CLIENTS.

Rationale
A major portion of one's daily life is spent in some form of activity related to health and well-being. An individual's developmental and intellectual levels, emotional state, and physical limitations may be reflected in these activities. Nurses are the primary professional health care providers who interact with clients on a day-to-day basis around the tasks of daily living. Therefore, the nurse has a unique opportunity to assess and intervene in these processes in order to encourage constructive changes in the client's behavior so that each child, adolescent, and adult can realize his potential for growth and health or maintain that level previously achieved.

Structure Criteria
1. A policy specifies a time frame in which an initial appraisal of self-care needs is made.
2. A method of communicating information about the client's self-care needs that assures consistency in approach is established and utilized within the practice setting.
3. Nurses are authorized to prescribe self-care activities in the practice setting.

Process Criteria
The nurse—
1. Respects and protects the client's rights
2. Encourages the client to collaborate in the development of a self-care plan

3. Sets limits in a manner that is humane and the least restrictive necessary for assuring safety of the client and others

Outcome Criteria
1. The level of the client's ability in self-care activities is recorded.
2. By the end of the acute phase, the client will—
   a. Maintain adequate food and fluid intake
   b. Maintain hygiene with minimal assistance
   c. Demonstrate the ability to maintain appropriate self-control
   d. Interact in socially appropriate manner for short periods of time
   e. Discuss reactions to the events leading up to the need for psychiatric care
   f. Participate in the evaluation of progress made toward achievement of goals formulated during the acute phase
3. By the end of the rehabilitation phase, the client will—
   a. Determine and obtain adequate sleep
   b. Assume full responsibility for personal hygiene
   c. Maintain adequate physical activity
   d. Interact in a socially appropriate manner
   e. Control impulses and demonstrate appropriate behavior
   f. Use appropriate resources for support in coping
   g. Name prescribed medication, dosage, and frequency, and be able to state a course of action to be followed if side effects are experienced, or has a parent or significant other who will do this
   h. Accurately take prescribed medication, with assistance if necessary
   i. Verbalize thoughts and feelings related to self-care, and work toward additional self-determined goals related to activities of daily living
   j. Participate in the evaluation of progress made toward achievement of goals
   k. When severely impaired, participate in the development of a plan for maintenance of self in the community with consideration of the available support system, personal life-style, cultural variables, and socioeconomic factors

Standard V-D. Intervention: Somatic Therapies

THE NURSE USES KNOWLEDGE OF SOMATIC THERAPIES AND APPLIES RELATED CLINICAL SKILLS IN WORKING WITH CLIENTS.

Rationale
Various treatment modalities may be needed by clients

during the course of illness. Pertinent clinical observations and judgments are made concerning the effect of drugs and other somatic treatments used in the therapeutic program.

Structure Criteria
1. There are policies and guidelines for provision of nursing care in somatic therapies.
2. Organizational policies regarding the client's rights for treatment or refusal of treatment are congruent with applicable laws.

Process Criteria
The nurse—
1. Utilizes knowledge of current psychopharmacology to guide nursing actions
2. Observes and interprets pertinent responses to somatic therapies in terms of the underlying principles of each therapy
3. Evaluates effectiveness of somatic therapies and recommends changes in the treatment plan as appropriate
4. Collaborates with other team members to provide for safe administration of therapies
5. Supervises the client's chemotherapeutic regimen in collaboration with the physician
6. Provides opportunities for clients and families to discuss, question, and explore their feelings and concerns about past, current, or projected use of somatic therapies
7. Reviews expected actions and side effects of somatic therapies with clients and their families
8. Uses prescribing authority for medications as congruent with the state nursing practice act

Outcome Criteria
1. Client responses to drugs and other somatic therapies are recorded.
2. The client incorporates knowledge of somatic therapies into self-care activities.

Standard V-E. Intervention: Therapeutic Environment

THE NURSE PROVIDES, STRUCTURES, AND MAINTAINS A THERAPEUTIC ENVIRONMENT IN COLLABORATION WITH THE CLIENT AND OTHER HEALTH CARE PROVIDERS.

Rationale
The nurse works with clients in a variety of environmental settings such as inpatient, residential, day care,

and home. The environment contributes in positive and negative ways to the state of health or illness of the client. When it serves the interest of the client as an inherent part of the overall nursing care plan, the setting is structured and/or altered.

Structure Criteria
1. Mechanisms exist within the practice setting that govern the establishment and maintenance of settings that are clean, safe, humane, and attractive.
2. Written policies and procedures that govern the safe use of seclusion, restraint, or aversive measures are utilized when staff institute such activity.
3. The environment is characterized by features that facilitate therapeutic gains on the part of clients.

Process Criteria
The nurse—
1. Assures that clients are adequately oriented to the milieu and are familiar with scheduled activities and rules that govern behavior and daily living
2. Observes, analyzes, interprets, and records the effects of environmental forces upon the client
3. Assesses and develops the therapeutic potential of the practice setting on behalf of clients through consideration of the physical environment, the social structure, and the culture of the setting
4. Fosters communications in the environment that are congruent with therapeutic goals
5. Collaborates with others in the development and institution of milieu activities specific to the client's physical and mental health needs
6. Articulates to the client and staff the justification for use of limit setting, restraint, or seclusion and the conditions necessary for release from restriction.
7. Participates in ongoing evaluation of the effectiveness of the therapeutic milieu
8. Assists clients living at home to achieve and maintain an environment that supports and maintains health

Outcome Criteria
1. Within 24 hours after admission to a psychiatric setting, the client has been oriented to the milieu, including scheduled activities and rules governing behavior, unless unusual client circumstances interfere with the orientation process.
2. If restrained or secluded, the client can state the reason for such action and the conditions necessary for release, unless unusual client circumstances prevail.
3. The client demonstrates an awareness of the effects of environment on his health and incorporates that knowledge into self-care.

Standard V-F. Intervention: Psychotherapy

THE NURSE UTILIZES ADVANCED CLINICAL EXPERTISE IN INDIVIDUAL, GROUP, AND FAMILY PSYCHOTHERAPY, CHILD PSYCHOTHERAPY, AND OTHER TREATMENT MODALITIES TO FUNCTION AS A PSYCHOTHERAPIST, AND RECOGNIZES PROFESSIONAL ACCOUNTABILITY FOR NURSING PRACTICE.

Rationale

Acceptance of the role of psychotherapist entails primary responsibility for the treatment of clients and entrance into a contractual agreement. This contract includes a commitment to see a client through the problem presented or to assist the client in finding other appropriate assistance. It also includes an explicit definition of the relationship, the respective role of each person in the relationship, and what can be realistically expected of each person.

Structure Criteria

1. The nurse who engages in psychotherapy shall be qualified as a psychiatric and mental health nurse specialist.
2. An agency policy specifies the educational and experiential qualifications required of the nurse who functions as a psychotherapist.
3. Job descriptions of nurses expected to function as psychotherapists and to use specific treatment modalities shall include educational and experiential qualifications.
4. Work assignment and staffing patterns provide adequate time for conducting psychotherapy when that responsibility is included in the job description.
5. A mechanism for peer review exists within the agency or is established by the nurse in solo or group practice.
6. The psychiatric and mental health nurse specialist who conducts psychotherapy in private practice maintains an ongoing, regular, formal consultative relationship with a professional colleague.
7. The psychiatric and mental health nurse specialist in private practice utilizes physician services when needed.

Process Criteria

The nurse—

1. Structures the therapeutic contract with the client in the beginning phase of the relationship, including such elements as purpose, time, place, fees, participants, confidentiality, available means of contact, and responsibilities of both client and therapist

2. Engages in interdisciplinary and intradisciplinary collaboration to achieve treatment goals
3. Engages the client in the process of determining the appropriate form of psychotherapy
4. Identifies the goals of psychotherapy
5. Uses knowledge of growth and development, psychopathology, psychosocial systems, small group and family dynamics, and knowledge of selected treatment modalities as indicated
6. Articulates a rationale for the goals chosen and interventions utilized
7. Fosters increasing personal and therapeutic responsibility on the part of the client
8. Provides for continuity of care for client in the therapist's absence
9. Determines, with the client when possible, that goals have been achieved and facilitates the termination process
10. Refers clients to other professionals when indicated
11. Respects and protects the client's legal rights
12. Avails self of appropriate opportunities to increase knowledge and skill in the therapies utilized in nursing practice
13. Obtains recognized educational preparation and ongoing supervision for types of psychotherapy utilized, for example, individual psychotherapy, group and family psychotherapy, child psychotherapy, and psychoanalysis
14. Uses clinical judgment in determining whether providing physical care (especially procedures prone to misinterpretation, for example, injections, enemas) will enhance or impair the therapist–client relationship and delegates such care as needed

Outcome Criteria

1. The client articulates the elements of the therapeutic contract.
2. The client demonstrates responsibility for the therapeutic work.
3. The client demonstrates movement toward therapeutic goals or objectives.

Standard VI. Evaluation

THE NURSE EVALUATES CLIENT RESPONSES TO NURSING ACTIONS IN ORDER TO REVISE THE DATA BASE, NURSING DIAGNOSES, AND NURSING CARE PLAN.

Rationale

Nursing care is a dynamic process that implies alterations in data, diagnoses, or plans previously made.

Structure Criteria

1. Supervision and/or consultation with psychiatric and mental health nurse specialists is available within the practice setting to enable the nurse to analyze the effectiveness of nursing actions.
2. The client or those of necessity acting in behalf of the client are asked to participate in evaluating the nursing process.

Process Criteria

The nurse—

1. Pursues validation, suggestions, and new information
2. Evaluates observations, insights, and data with colleagues
3. Documents the results of evaluation of nursing care

Outcome Criteria

1. Nursing care plans and activities are revised on the basis of an evaluation.
2. Evaluation of nursing care is recorded in a manner that promotes evaluation and refinement of psychiatric and mental health nursing theory.

PROFESSIONAL PERFORMANCE STANDARDS

Standard VII. Peer Review

THE NURSE PARTICIPATES IN PEER REVIEW AND OTHER MEANS OF EVALUATION TO ASSURE QUALITY OF NURSING CARE PROVIDED FOR CLIENTS.

Rationale

Evaluation of the quality of nursing care through examination of the clinical practice of nurses is one way to fulfill the profession's obligation to ensure that consumers are provided excellence in care. Peer review and other quality assurance procedures are utilized in this endeavor.

Structure Criteria

1. A formal mechanism for peer review is provided within the practice setting.
2. Nurses are represented on peer review and/or quality assurance teams that evaluate health care outcomes.

Process Criteria

The nurse—

1. Assumes responsibility for review and evaluation of clinical practice with peers, supervisors, and/or consultants
2. Considers recommendations for change that may arise from review

Outcome Criterion

Corrective measures are instituted as appropriate at individual, unit, or organizational level.

Standard VIII. Continuing Education

THE NURSE ASSUMES RESPONSIBILITY FOR CONTINUING EDUCATION AND PROFESSIONAL DEVELOPMENT AND CONTRIBUTES TO THE PROFESSIONAL GROWTH OF OTHERS.

Rationale

The scientific, cultural, social, and political changes characterizing our contemporary society require the nurse to be committed to the ongoing pursuit of knowledge that will enhance professional growth.

Structure Criteria

1. The governance structure of the practice setting has policies that provide for paid educational leave for continuing education of nurses.
2. The psychiatric and mental health nursing administrator, supervisor, or head nurse establishes a policy that provides for on-the-job opportunity for continuing professional development, such as professional reading time and attendance at inservice activities.

Process Criteria

The nurse—

1. Initiates independent learning activities to increase understanding and update skills
2. Participates in in-service meetings and educational programs either as an attendee or as a teacher
3. Attends conventions, institutions, workshops, symposia, and other professional meetings
4. Systematically increases understanding of theories related to psychiatric and mental health nursing
5. Assists others in identifying areas of educational needs
6. Communicates formally and informally new knowledge regarding clinical observations and interpretations with professional colleagues and others

Outcome Criteria

The nurse—

1. Meets continuing education requirements for licensure as appropriate

2. Incorporates advances in the field into practice

Standard IX. Interdisciplinary Collaboration

THE NURSE COLLABORATES WITH OTHER HEALTH CARE PROVIDERS IN ASSESSING, PLANNING, IMPLEMENTING, AND EVALUATING PROGRAMS AND OTHER MENTAL HEALTH ACTIVITIES.

Rationale
Psychiatric nursing practice requires planning and sharing with others to deliver maximum mental health services to the client and the community. Through the collaborative process, different abilities of health care providers are utilized to communicate, plan, solve problems, and evaluate services delivered.

Structure Criteria
1. The nurse administrator participates with other administrative colleagues in policy making and in overall agency and community planning for mental health services.
2. A mechanism exists for interdisciplinary collaboration.

Process Criteria
The nurse—
1. Participates in the formulation of overall goals, plans, and decisions
2. Includes the client in the collaboration of the mental health team whenever possible and appropriate
3. Recognizes, respects, accepts, and demonstrates trust in colleagues and their contributions
4. Consults with colleagues as needed and is available to be consulted by them
5. Articulates knowledge and skills so that they may be coordinated with the contributions of others working with a client or program
6. Collaborates with other disciplines in teaching, supervision, and research

Outcome Criterion
Treatment plans reflect interdisciplinary collaboration.

Standard X. Utilization of Community Health Systems

THE NURSE PARTICIPATES WITH OTHER MEMBERS OF THE COMMUNITY IN ASSESSING, PLANNING, IMPLEMENTING, AND EVALUATING MENTAL HEALTH SERVICES AND COMMUNITY SYSTEMS THAT INCLUDE THE PROMOTION OF THE BROAD CONTINUUM OF PRIMARY, SECONDARY, AND TERTIARY PREVENTION OF MENTAL ILLNESS.

Rationale
The high incidence of mental illness in our contemporary society requires increased effort to devise more effective treatment and prevention programs. Nurses must participate in programs that strengthen the existing health potential of all members of society. Such concepts as primary prevention and continuity of care are essential in planning to meet the mental health needs of the community. The nurse uses organizational, advisory, advocacy, and consultative skills to facilitate the development and implementation of mental health services.

Structure Criterion
The nurse who assesses, plans, implements, and evaluates psychiatric and mental health services in community health systems is prepared as a psychiatric and mental health nurse specialist.

Process Criteria
The nurse—
1. Uses knowledge of community and group dynamics and systems theory to understand the structure and function of the community system
2. Recognizes current social and political issues that influence the nature of mental health problems in the community
3. Encourages active consumer participation in assessing and planning programs to meet the community's mental health needs
4. Brings the community's needs to the attention of appropriate individuals and groups, including legislative bodies and regional and state planning groups
5. Plans and participates in didactic and experiential educational programs related to the community's mental health
6. Uses consultative skills to facilitate the development and implementation of mental health services
7. Interprets mental health services to others in the community.
8. Participates with other health care professionals and members of the community in the planning, implementation, and evaluation of mental health services
9. Participates in the delineation of high-risk population groups in the community and identifies gaps in community services.
10. Assesses strengths and coping capacities of individuals, families, and the community in order to

promote and increase the mental health of those individuals and groups

11. Uses knowledge of community resources to assist consumers' referral to and appropriate use of health care resources
12. Collaborates with staff at other agencies to facilitate continuity for service for individuals and families

Outcome Criteria

1. Nursing contributions to mental health services that address primary, secondary, and tertiary care are documented.
2. Comprehensive mental health services are provided in the community.
3. Nurses achieve positions of leadership on voluntary and governmental bodies within community health systems.

Standard XI. Research

THE NURSE CONTRIBUTES TO NURSING AND THE MENTAL HEALTH FIELD THROUGH INNOVATIONS IN THEORY AND PRACTICE AND PARTICIPATION IN RESEARCH.

Rationale
Each professional has responsibility for the continuing development and refinement of knowledge in the mental health field through research and experimentation with new and creative approaches to practice.

Structure Criteria

1. Formal opportunities exist for nurses to conduct and/or participate in research at appropriate educational levels.
2. Mechanisms ensure protection of human rights.

Process Criteria
The nurse—

1. Approaches nursing practice with an inquiring and open mind
2. Utilizes research findings in practice
3. Develops, implements, and evaluates research studies as appropriate to level of education
4. Uses responsible standards of research in investigative endeavors
5. Ensures that a mechanism for the protection of human subjects exists
6. Obtains expert consultation and/or supervision as required

Outcome Criterion
The nurse has published contributions to theory, practice, and research.

Appendix B
DSM-III Classification—Axes I and II Categories and Codes*

All official DSM-III codes and terms are included in ICD-9-CM. However, in order to differentiate those DSM-III categories that use the same ICD-9-CM codes, unofficial non-ICD-9-CM codes are provided in parentheses for use when greater specificity is necessary.

The long dashes indicate the need for a fifth-digit subtype or other qualifying term.

DISORDERS USUALLY FIRST EVIDENT IN INFANCY, CHILDHOOD OR ADOLESCENCE

Mental Retardation

(Code in fifth digit: 1 = with other behavioral symptoms [requiring attention or treatment and that are not part of another disorder], 0 = without other behavioral symptoms.)

317.0(x) Mild mental retardation, _____
318.0(x) Moderate mental retardation, _____
318.1(x) Severe mental retardation, _____
318.2(x) Profound mental retardation, _____
319.0(x) Unspecified mental retardation, _____

Attention Deficit Disorder

314.01 with hyperactivity
314.00 without hyperactivity
314.80 residual type

Conduct Disorder

312.00 undersocialized, aggressive
312.10 undersocialized, nonaggressive
312.23 socialized, aggressive
312.21 socialized, nonaggressive
312.90 atypical

Anxiety Disorders of Childhood or Adolescence

309.21 Separation anxiety disorder
313.21 Avoidant disorder of childhood or adolescence
313.00 Overanxious disorder

Other Disorders of Infancy, Childhood or Adolescence

313.89 Reactive attachment disorder of infancy
313.22 Schizoid disorder of childhood or adolescence
313.23 Elective mutism
313.81 Oppositional disorder
313.82 Identity disorder

Eating Disorders

307.10 Anorexia nervosa
307.51 Bulimia
307.52 Pica
307.53 Rumination disorder of infancy
307.50 Atypical eating disorder

Stereotyped Movement Disorders

307.21 Transient tic disorder
307.22 Chronic motor tic disorder
307.23 Tourette's disorder
307.20 Atypical tic disorder
307.30 Atypical stereotyped movement disorder

*From American Psychiatric Association: Diagnostic and Statistical Manual of Mental Disorders, 3rd ed. Washington, DC, A.P.A., 1980

Other Disorders with Physical Manifestations

307.00   Stuttering
307.60   Functional enuresis
307.70   Functional encopresis
307.46   Sleepwalking disorder
307.46   Sleep terror disorder (307.49)

Pervasive Developmental Disorders

Code in fifth digit: 0 = full syndrome present, 1 = residual state.

299.0x   Infantile autism, _____
299.9x   Childhood onset pervasive developmental disorder, _____
299.8x   Atypical, _____

Specific Developmental Disorders

Note: These are coded on Axis II.

315.00   Developmental reading disorder
315.10   Developmental arithmetic disorder
315.31   Developmental language disorder
315.39   Developmental articulation disorder
315.50   Mixed specific developmental disorder
315.90   Atypical specific developmental disorder

ORGANIC MENTAL DISORDERS

Section 1

Organic mental disorders whose etiology or pathophysiological process is listed below (taken from the mental disorders section of ICD-9-CM).

Dementias Arising in the Senium and Presenium

Primary Degenerative Dementia, Senile Onset
290.30   with delirium
290.20   with delusions
290.21   with depression
290.00   uncomplicated

Code in fifth digit: 1 = with delirium, 2 = with delusions, 3 = with depression, 0 = uncomplicated.

290.1x   Primary degenerative dementia, presenile onset, _____
290.4x   Multi-infarct dementia, _____

Substance-induced

Alcohol
303.00   intoxication
291.40   idiosyncratic intoxication
291.80   withdrawal
291.00   withdrawal delirium
291.30   hallucinosis
291.10   amnestic disorder

Code severity of dementia in fifth digit: 1 = mild, 2 = moderate, 3 = severe, 0 = unspecified.

291.2x   Dementia associated with alcoholism, _____

Barbiturate or Similarly Acting Sedative or Hypnotic
305.40   intoxication (327.00)
292.00   withdrawal (327.01)
292.00   withdrawal delirium (327.02)
292.83   amnestic disorder (327.04)

Opioid
305.50   intoxication (327.10)
292.00   withdrawal (327.11)

Cocaine
305.60   intoxication (327.20)

Amphetamine or Similarly Acting Sympathomimetic
305.70   intoxication (327.30)
292.81   delirium (327.32)
292.11   delusional disorder (327.35)
292.00   withdrawal (327.31)

Phencyclidine (PCP) or Similarly Acting Arylcyclohexylamine
305.90   intoxication (327.40)
292.81   delirium (327.42)
292.90   mixed organic mental disorder (327.49)

Hallucinogen
305.30   hallucinosis (327.56)
292.11   delusional disorder (327.55)
292.84   affective disorder (327.57)

Cannabis
305.20   intoxication (327.60)
292.11   delusional disorder (327.65)

Tobacco
292.00   withdrawal (327.71)

Caffeine
305.90   intoxication (327.80)

305.90   intoxication (327.90)

292.00   withdrawal (327.91)

292.81   delirium (327.92)

292.82   dementia (327.93)

292.83   amnestic disorder (327.94)

292.11   delusional disorder (327.95)

292.12   hallucinosis (327.96)

292.84   affective disorder (327.97)

292.89   personality disorder (327.98)

292.90   atypical or mixed organic mental disorder (327.99)

Section 2

Organic brain syndromes whose etiology or pathophysiological process is either noted as an additional diagnosis from outside the mental disorders section of ICD-9-CM or is unknown.

293.00   Delirium

294.10   Dementia

294.00   Amnestic syndrome

293.81   Organic delusional syndrome

293.82   Organic hallucinosis

293.83   Organic affective syndrome

310.10   Organic personality syndrome

294.80   Atypical or mixed organic brain syndrome

SUBSTANCE USE DISORDERS

Code in fifth digit: 1 = continuous, 2 = episodic, 3 = in remission, 0 = unspecified.

305.0x   Alcohol abuse, _____

303.9x   Alcohol dependence (Alcoholism), _____

305.4x   Barbiturate or similarly acting sedative or hypnotic abuse

304.1x   Barbiturate or similarly acting sedative or hypnotic dependence, _____

305.5x   Opioid abuse, _____

304.0x   Opioid dependence, _____

305.6x   Cocaine abuse, _____

305.7x   Amphetamine or similarly acting sympathomimetic abuse, _____

304.4x   Amphetamine or similarly acting sympathomimetic dependence, _____

305.9x   Phencyclidine (PCP) or similarly acting arylcyclohexylamine abuse, _____ (328.4x)

305.3x   Hallucinogen abuse, _____

305.2x   Cannabis abuse, _____

304.3x   Cannabis dependence, _____

305.1x   Tobacco dependence, _____

305.9x   Other, mixed or unspecified substance abuse, _____

304.6x   Other specified substance dependence, _____

304.9x   Unspecified substance dependence, _____

304.7x   Dependence on combination of opioid and other nonalcoholic substance, _____

304.8x   Dependence on combination of substances, excluding opioids and alcohol, _____

SCHIZOPHRENIC DISORDERS

Code in fifth digit: 1 = subchronic, 2 = chronic, 3 = subchronic with acute exacerbation, 4 = chronic with acute exacerbation, 5 = in remission, 0 = unspecified.

Schizophrenia

295.1x   disorganized, _____

295.2x   catatonic, _____

295.3x   paranoid, _____

295.9x   undifferentiated, _____

295.6x   residual, _____

PARANOID DISORDERS

297.10   Paranoia

297.30   Shared paranoid disorder

298.30   Acute paranoid disorder

297.90   Atypical paranoid disorder

PSYCHOTIC DISORDERS NOT ELSEWHERE CLASSIFIED

295.40   Schizophreniform disorder

298.80   Brief reactive psychosis

295.70   Schizoaffective disorder

298.90   Atypical psychosis

NEUROTIC DISORDERS

These are included in Affective, Anxiety, Somatoform, Dissociative, and Psychosexual Disorders. In order to facilitate the identification of the categories that in DSM-II were grouped together in the class of Neuroses, the DSM-II terms are included separately in parentheses after the corresponding categories. These DSM-II terms are included in ICD-9-CM and therefore are acceptable as alternatives to the recommended DSM-III terms that precede them.

AFFECTIVE DISORDERS

Major Affective Disorders

Code major depressive episode in fifth digit: 6 = in remission, 4 = with psychotic features (the unofficial non-ICD-9-CM fifth digit 7 may be used instead to indicate that the psychotic features are mood-incongruent), 3 = with melancholia, 2 = without melancholia, 0 = unspecified.

Code manic episode in fifth digit: 6 = in remission, 4 = with psychotic features (the unofficial non-ICD-9-CM fifth digit 7 may be used instead to indicate that the psychotic features are mood-incongruent), 2 = without psychotic features, 0 = unspecified.

Bipolar Disorder
296.6x mixed, _____
296.4x manic, _____
296.5x depressed, _____

Major Depression
296.2x single episode, _____
296.3x recurrent, _____

Other Specific Affective Disorders

301.13 Cyclothymic disorder
300.40 Dysthymic disorder (or Depressive neurosis)

Atypical Affective Disorders

296.70 Atypical bipolar disorder
296.82 Atypical depression

ANXIETY DISORDERS

Phobic Disorders (or Phobic Neuroses)
300.21 Agoraphobia with panic attacks
300.22 Agoraphobia without panic attacks
300.23 Social phobia
300.29 Simple phobia

Anxiety States (or Anxiety Neuroses)
300.01 Panic disorder
300.02 Generalized anxiety disorder
300.30 Obsessive compulsive disorder (or Obsessive compulsive neurosis)

Post-traumatic Stress Disorder
308.30 Acute
309.81 Chronic or delayed
300.00 Atypical anxiety disorder

SOMATOFORM DISORDERS

300.81 Somatization disorder
300.11 Conversion disorder (or Hysterical neurosis, conversion type)
307.80 Psychogenic pain disorder
300.70 Hypochondriasis (or Hypochondriacal neurosis)
300.70 Atypical somatoform disorder (300.71)

DISSOCIATIVE DISORDERS (OR HYSTERICAL NEUROSES, DISSOCIATIVE TYPE)

300.12 Psychogenic amnesia
300.13 Psychogenic fugue
300.14 Multiple personality
300.60 Depersonalization disorder (or Depersonalization neurosis)
300.15 Atypical dissociative disorder

PSYCHOSEXUAL DISORDERS

Gender Identity Disorders

Indicate sexual history in the fifth digit of Transsexualism code: 1 = asexual, 2 = homosexual, 3 = heterosexual, 0 = unspecified.

302.5x Transsexualism, _____
302.60 Gender identity disorder of childhood
302.85 Atypical gender identity disorder

Paraphilias

302.81 Fetishism
302.30 Transvestism
302.10 Zoophilia
302.20 Pedophilia
302.40 Exhibitionism
302.82 Voyeurism
302.83 Sexual masochism
302.84 Sexual sadism
302.90 Atypical paraphilia

Psychosexual Dysfunctions

302.71 Inhibited sexual desire
302.72 Inhibited sexual excitement
302.73 Inhibited female orgasm

302.74	Inhibited male orgasm
302.75	Premature ejaculation
302.76	Functional dysparenuia
306.51	Functional vaginismus
302.70	Atypical psychosexual dysfunction

Other Psychosexual Disorders

| 302.00 | Ego-dystonic homosexuality |
| 302.89 | Psychosexual disorder not elsewhere classified |

FACTITIOUS DISORDERS

300.16	Factitious disorder with psychological symptoms
301.51	Chronic factitious disorder with physical symptoms
300.19	Atypical factitious disorder with physical symptoms

DISORDERS OF IMPULSE CONTROL NOT ELSEWHERE CLASSIFIED

312.31	Pathological gambling
312.32	Kleptomania
312.33	Pyromania
312.34	Intermittent explosive disorder
312.35	Isolated explosive disorder
312.39	Atypical impulse control disorder

ADJUSTMENT DISORDER

309.00	with depressed mood
309.24	with anxious mood
309.28	with mixed emotional features
309.30	with disturbance of conduct
309.40	with mixed disturbance of emotions and conduct
309.23	with work (or academic) inhibition
309.83	with withdrawal
309.90	with atypical features

PSYCHOLOGICAL FACTORS AFFECTING PHYSICAL CONDITION

Specify physical condition on Axis III.

| 316.00 | Psychological factors affecting physical condition |

Personality Disorders

Note: These are coded on Axis II.

301.00	Paranoid
301.20	Schizoid
301.22	Schizotypal
301.50	Histrionic
301.81	Narcissistic
301.70	Antisocial
301.83	Borderline
301.82	Avoidant
301.60	Dependent
301.40	Compulsive
301.84	Passive–Aggressive
301.89	Atypical, mixed or other personality disorder

V CODES FOR CONDITIONS NOT ATTRIBUTABLE TO A MENTAL DISORDER THAT ARE A FOCUS OF ATTENTION OR TREATMENT

V65.20	Malingering
V62.89	Borderline intellectual functioning (V62.88)
V71.01	Adult antisocial behavior
V71.02	Childhood or adolescent antisocial behavior
V62.30	Academic problem
V62.20	Occupational problem
V62.82	Uncomplicated bereavement
V15.81	Noncompliance with medical treatment
V62.89	Phase of life problem or other life circumstance problem
V61.10	Marital problem
V61.20	Parent–child problem
V61.80	Other specified family circumstances
V62.81	Other interpersonal problem

ADDITIONAL CODES

300.90	Unspecified mental disorder (nonpsychotic)
V71.09	No diagnosis or condition on Axis I
799.90	Diagnosis or condition deferred on Axis I

| V71.09 | No diagnosis on Axis II |
| 799.90 | Diagnosis deferred on Axis II |

Glossary

abreaction The conscious memory and emotional reliving of a past painful experience

accountability Liability for one's behavior

accreditation The method by which a group or agency recognizes a program of study or an institution as meeting predetermined standards or criteria

acting in The expression of unconscious wishes, needs, conflicts, and feelings in actions rather than words, within a therapy session

acting out The expression of unconscious wishes, needs, conflicts, and feelings in actions rather than words

addiction Physical and emotional dependence on an object or activity, such as drugs, alcohol, or work

adjustment The manner by which one fits with one's peer group, family, and society, and copes with life

adolescence Period of growth and development beginning at puberty (usually 12 or 13 years) and ending at adulthood (usually 20 or 21 years)

aerophagia Excessive pathologic air swallowing

affect One's internal and external emotional tone

affective psychosis Psychosis characterized by changes in the emotional state, usually elation or depression

aggression Forceful physical or verbal behavior

agitation Severe restlessness and anxiety

agnosia Inability to recognize and grasp the meaning of sensory stimuli owing to organic brain disorder

agoraphobia Fear of going outside or of open spaces

akathisia Continuous restlessness and uncontrolled movements

akinesia Lethargy, subjective sense of fatigue, muscle weakness often mistaken for withdrawal and apathy, but actually a side effect of some antipsychotic medications

alcoholism Habituation, dependence, or addiction to alcohol, leading to poor physical or mental health, disturbed interpersonal relations, and decreased personal effectiveness

alienation A feeling of detachment

alternative family A group of people living communally to achieve common goals

Alzheimer's disease A fatal disease characterized by brain deterioration leading to loss of memory, judgment, and interest

ambivalence Simultaneous strong feelings that are the opposite of one another, for example, love and hate

amnesia Loss of short-term or long-term memory owing to organic or functional causes

amphetamines Antidepressant drugs that produce temporary elation through cortical stimulation

anaclitic Characterized by strong dependence

anaclitic depression Depression associated with loss of strong dependence like that experienced in infancy

anal character The psychoanalytic term for one who is excessively orderly, restricted, controlled, stubborn, or miserly owing to events occurring in the anal stage

anal erotism Erotic feelings arising from anal functions or activity

analgesia Absence or reduction of pain

analogic communication Communication without words

anal stage The period of growth and development between $1\frac{1}{2}$ and 3 years, when toilet training occurs

analysand A person in psychoanalytic therapy

anger A feeling of power and aggression resulting from frustration, anxiety, and helplessness

anhedonia A state characterized by a lack of pleasure

anilingus Oral stimulation of the anus

anima A Jungian term for the inner, feminine self of a man

animus A Jungian term for the inner, masculine self of a woman

anniversary reaction An emotional state that occurs on the anniversary of a traumatic event in one's past, for example, death of a parent

anorexia Lack of appetite

anorexia nervosa A disease characterized by severe loss of appetite and weight, along with other symptoms

anticipatory guidance A method of counselling whereby the person is helped to plan for possible future events before they occur

anxiety An unpleasant feeling of tension resulting from a physical or emotional threat to self

apathy Absence of emotions, interest, and activity

aphasia Inability to pronounce words, name common objects, or arrange words in sequence owing to organic brain disease

aphonia Inability to produce normal speech owing to physical or organic causes

"as if" behavior Unconsciously derived false behavior designed to cover up or compensate for unconscious thoughts, feelings, needs, or conflicts

assaultive Physically or verbally attacking

assertive behavior Behavior designed to achieve one's goals without disturbing another's self-respect

assertiveness training A form of therapy that aims to help individuals to ask for what they want without violating the rights of others, and to refuse requests without feeling guilty

attachment Interpersonal, emotional connectedness, as between a mother and infant

attachment phase The stage of infancy when the mother and infant become emotionally connected

attitude therapy A form of milieu therapy in which staff members all assume consistent, prescribed attitudes designed to be therapeutic toward clients

atypical developmental psychosis An early childhood disorder characterized by autistic behavior

aura A physical experience that signals the onset of another experience, such as hallucinations before a grand mal seizure or visual changes before a migraine headache

autism, autistic thinking Thinking that is self-gratifying without regard for reality

autistic Private, within the self without regard for reality

autoaggression Aggression directed toward oneself

autoerotism Sexuality directed toward oneself

autonomy Self-direction, independence

aversion therapy Therapy that provides unpleasant stimuli or punishment for undesirable behavior

bad trip An acute anxiety reaction following the use of psychedelic drugs

basic human needs theory Abraham Maslow's theory based on a hierarchy of physical and emotional needs

behavior modification Therapy based on Pavlovian

conditioning and designed to change behavior in a desired direction

bestiality Sexual relations between humans and animals; also called zoophilia

bipolar disorder A condition characterized by manic and depressive phases

birth defect An abnormality found in an infant at birth owing to genetic or nongenetic causes

birth trauma Otto Rank's term referring to the shock of the birth process, which leads to anxiety and neurosis

bisexual One who engages in sex with both males and females

blended family A family composed of members who originated from two separate nuclear families, as occurs when divorced people marry, each bringing children into the new family

blind spot A repressed area in one's life

blocking Involuntary stopping of a thought process owing to unconscious emotional factors

blotting paper syndrome The acting out by staff of a feeling held by a client who is unable to express it, for example, anger

blunting of affect A state characterized by an absence of emotional tone

body image The conscious and unconscious picture one holds of one's own body

bonding The process of developing emotional connectedness, as between a mother and infant

borderline personality disorder A personality disorder that lies between neurosis and psychosis and is characterized by wide fluctuations in mood, behavior, and self-image. These clients are often angry, self-destructive, and manipulative and frequently abuse drugs and alcohol

bulimia A state of increased hunger and morbid eating

burn-out A state of apathy resulting from stress; in mental health care settings, characterized by detached, automatic, dehumanized care of clients

castration Surgical removal of the ovaries in females and the testes in males

castration anxiety Literally, a fear of loss or injury of the genitals; figuratively, tension resulting when one fears the loss of any vital object or state

catalysts Group members who stimulate others to move forward

catatonia A state characterized by immobility, muscular inflexibility, and sometimes excitability

catchment area Geographic area of 75,000 to 200,000 persons served by a community mental health center

catharsis Verbalization of thoughts and feelings, usually in therapy sessions

cathexis Conscious or unconscious investment in an object or idea

cephalalgia Head pain or headache

cerea flexibilitas Condition in which the client's arm or leg remains in the position in which it was placed by another person; also called waxy flexibility

change agent One who acts for another deliberately to improve a situation

child ego state In transactional analysis theory, the aspect of the adult that is left over from childhood

childhood psychosis A state characterized by disordered thinking, affect, motility, perception, reality testing, speech, and object relations

circumstantiality Disturbed thinking process whereby a person includes many unnecessary details in verbal communication before reaching the central idea

client The term used instead of "patient" by mental health professionals desiring a less medical, more humanistic view of mental health care

clinical psychologist A doctorally prepared psychologist who provides psychotherapy, behavior modification techniques, and psychological testing

cognitive Referring to thought, comprehension, judgment, memory, and reasoning as opposed to emotional processes

cognitive therapy Therapy that concentrates on communication and problem solving

cohesiveness The result of all the forces that act on individuals to remain in a group and to feel that they belong

collective unconscious A Jungian term referring to the aspect of the unconscious common to all people; also called racial unconscious

commitment The process of hospitalizing clients for psychiatric care by legal means

communal family A group of persons living and working together to accomplish shared goals

community mental health center A community-based facility for the prevention and treatment of mental illness. Services may include inpatient, outpatient, day hospital, emergency, consultation, and educational services

community psychiatry Psychiatry that concentrates on the environmental factors in mental illness and seeks to prevent and treat clients close to home

compensation The attempt to cover up unconscious feelings, needs, or conflicts by acting in a way opposite to them

complementarity A term referring to the two-sidedness of relationships and all communication

complementary message A nonverbal message that augments a verbal message

compromise A solution to a conflict whereby both sides give up something, and both feel relatively satisfied with the outcome

compulsion A consistent urge to perform an act repetitively, in response to unacceptable unconscious wishes, needs, or feelings

compulsive ritual A series of acts carried out compulsively, in response to unacceptable unconscious wishes, needs, or feelings

concreteness Primitive thinking that employs literal meanings for ideas, as opposed to abstract meanings; also called concrete thinking

condensation The boiling down of several concepts into a single idea or symbol, as occurs in dreams

conditioning Associating specific stimuli with specific responses

confabulation The filling in of memory gaps with data that have no basis in fact, but that the teller believes to be true

confirmation Validation by one person of the other person's thoughts or ideas

conflict A clash between two equal opposing forces within oneself, between people, or groups

confrontation Communication designed to alert a person to thoughts, ideas, and concepts previously unconsidered and often threatening

connotative meaning Meaning that comes from personal experience rather than objective sources

conscious Readily accessible to an individual through thoughts and feelings

consensual validation The process of checking with another person to determine that one's thoughts and feelings are realistic

consumer A client or patient receiving mental health services

contract A mutually agreed-upon plan of action between client and mental health worker. The contract emphasizes client behavior and worker accountability

contradicting message A nonverbal message that communicates the opposite meaning of the concurrent verbal message

conversion The expression of an unconscious wish by somatic means, for example, blindness that has no physical basis

coping mechanisms Unconscious methods by which an individual defends against anxiety

coping skill A conscious method developed by a person to overcome a problem

coprolalia Obscene language or speech

coprophagia Eating feces

coprophilia The desire to defecate on a partner or to be defecated on by a partner

corrective emotional experience The reliving in a positive, therapeutic situation of a past traumatic event, such that the person grows and benefits emotionally

counterphobic Inclining toward an object or situation that a person unconsciously fears

countertransference An irrational, unrealistic response to a client by a mental health worker, based on the worker's unconscious needs, wishes, conflicts, or feelings

covert Hidden or disguised

creative arts therapist A therapist who uses dance, movement, art, and poetry to help clients express feelings, interact with others, and improve self-esteem

crisis A state of psychological disequilibrium brought on by an event that causes extreme anxiety not assuaged by the person's usual coping mechanisms

crisis counseling Brief emergency individual, group, or family therapy designed to help persons cope with a specific issue

crisis intervention Intervention designed to help an individual cope with a sudden problem issue and emerge at a level of functioning equal to or higher than the precrisis state

culture The organized set of ideas, values, and beliefs held commonly by a group

cunnilingus Oral stimulation of the female genitalia

cyclothymic behavior Alternating elation and sadness

day hospital A psychotherapeutic program for clients who attend during the day and return home at night

death instinct A Freudian term for the unconscious drive toward death.

decompensation The breakdown of a stable emotional adjustment or defensive system

defense mechanism The unconscious operations used by an individual to defend against anxiety; also called mental mechanisms, coping mechanisms, security operations

déjà vu The feeling that a current experience happened before

delirium A state of confusion and disorientation caused by an acute organic reaction

delirium tremens A psychotic state caused by withdrawal of alcohol after long and heavy use; also called DTs, alcohol withdrawal syndrome

delusion A false, fixed belief inconsistent with reality and arising from unconscious needs

dementia Loss of mental functioning with organic causes

dementia praecox An obsolete term for schizophrenia

denial An unconscious mechanism whereby disturbing thoughts, feelings, and events are kept out of conscious awareness

denotative meaning A meaning that is commonly understood by most people in a culture, as opposed to connotative meaning, which is personal to an individual

dependency Infantile reliance on others for mothering, love, assurance, affection, shelter, protection, security, warmth, and food

depersonalization A feeling of strangeness or unreality about the self, the environment, or both

depression A feeling of profound sadness, low self-esteem, and hopelessness about one's life

desensitization The gradual exposure of a client to an object or situation that was previously feared, until the client is no longer afraid

detachment Emotional unrelatedness characterized by aloofness, denial, intellectualization, and superficiality

devaluation Consistent, exaggerated criticism used as a defense against feelings of inadequacy; seen in borderline personality disorder

developmental crisis A crisis that is linked to the developmental stage of the client

developmental lag Emotional or physical development that is lower than expected considering chronological age

developmental stages The phases of growth and development from infancy to late adulthood

deviance Behavior that is markedly different from the usual behavior in a group

differentiation Healthy separateness and independence from others

digital communication Communication that is verbal and can be validated

disconfirmation Communication that invalidates another's sense of self-worth

discrimination The ability to note differences between similar objects or circumstances

disengaged families Families in which members are emotionally disconnected

disorientation The inability to identify time, place, or person

displacement The transfer of feelings about one person to another less threatening person

disqualification Communication that invalidates other communication

dissociation The removal from conscious awareness of thoughts, feelings, and actions that would cause anxiety, were they acknowledged openly

dissociative disorders Response to stress by massive

dissociation, for example, amnesia, fugue, depersonalization disorder, and multiple personality

distance In family theory, the emotional and physical space between members

double-bind communication Communication that gives two conflicting messages simultaneously, so that the receiver cannot respond adequately

Down's syndrome A congenital developmental disability characterized by mental deficiency, defective brain development, and other deformities; also called mongolism

dream analysis Used in psychoanalytic therapy to observe and understand unconscious behavior by careful exploration of the client's dreams

drive Basic motivation, urge, or instinct

drug addiction Overpowering, chronic dependency on drugs

drug dependence Drug addiction leading to the client's inability to function, need for ever-increasing doses, physical withdrawal symptoms if the drug is stopped, and psychological dependence

dynamics Emotional forces that work to produce behavior patterns or symptoms

dysarthria Inability to speak normally, owing to organic disease

dysattention Failure to pay attention to the environment

dysmenesia Inability to recall and retain information

dyspareunia Pelvic pain, emotional in origin, experienced by women during intercourse

dysphagia Painful or difficult swallowing

dystonia Severe, often rapidly developing contractions of muscles of tongue, jaw, neck, and extraocular muscles seen as a side effect with some antipsychotic medications

echolalia Continuous repetition of words said in the client's presence; usually seen in schizophrenia

echopraxia Imitation of motions made in the client's presence; usually seen in schizophrenia

ECT Treatment used most often in depression, whereby an electrical current is passed through the brain resulting in unconsciousness and a convulsion; also called electroconvulsive therapy

EEG A method of recording the electrical activity of the brain; also called electroencephalogram

ego The aspect of personality that includes intellectual, perceptual, governing, and defensive operations

egocentric Self-involved to the point of a lack of interest in others

ego-dystonic Incongruent with one's conscious wishes or values, for example, homosexuality in a client who wants to be heterosexual

ego functions Those conscious functions that help regulate one's life, such as judgment, problem solving, reality testing, and impulse control

ego ideal Standards set for oneself that eventually become a part of the superego

ego strength Ability to maintain reality and manage the forces of the id and superego

ego psychology Personality theory that is concerned with adaptation to reality, object relations, and interpersonal relations

ego syntonic Congruent with one's conscious wishes and values

Electra complex Erotic attachment of a daughter for her father

elopement Client's departure from a psychiatric inpatient unit without permission

emotional shock waves In family theory, symptoms that appear after a crisis has passed

empathy Emotional understanding of another's experience; differs from sympathy, which is subjective and contains elements of pity, agreement, and condolence

encounter group A method of group interaction popular in the 1960s and early 1970s, which emphasized confrontation, the ''here-and-now,'' and the expression of feelings; still used in drug treatment centers

enmeshed families Families characterized by power struggles, overcontrolling mothers, and a lack of open affection among members

enuresis Bed-wetting

epigenetic principle Erickson's concept that both physical and psychosocial growth are in the genetic makeup of each individual and are triggered by social expectations

epilepsy A disorder characterized by periodic motor or sensory seizures, sometimes with loss of consciousness; may be without known organic causes (idiopathic) or caused by organic lesions (symptomatic)

est A type of ''emotional training'' founded by Werner Erhard and lasting from 15 to 18 hours each day for two consecutive weekends. The trainers employ confrontation and repressive inspirational techniques to convince participants they can change their lives through willpower and determination; also called Erhard seminar training

ethics Standards of morality regulating rules of conduct

etiology Cause

euphoria An exaggerated feeling of well-being that is not congruent with objective facts. The cause may be functional or organic

exhibitionism   The practice of exposing the genitals in public for sexual self-stimulation; also used to describe behavior whereby the individual enjoys public attention

existential psychotherapy   Therapy that focuses on the client's development of a thorough exploration of past and present experiences, and designed to change the client's "mode of being in the world."

expert power   Power attained through expert skill and knowledge

extended family   The nuclear family and relatives from descent, adoption, or marriage

extinction   The removal of a behavior through lack of reinforcement

extrapyramidal syndrome   A disorder characterized by muscular rigidity, tremors, and other involuntary movements, and caused by improper use of psychotropic drugs

facilitative communication   Communication designed to initiate, carry on, and maintain satisfying relationships with others

factitious disorders   Simulations of physical or mental disorders to obtain treatment and attention

family boundaries   Informal rules about who participates in the family system and how

family ego mass   The aspect of a family characterized by a lack of personal boundaries, retarding the individual's progress toward individuation

family life chronology   The psychosocial history of a family

family life-style   Automatic methods in a family for living out their self-images

family myths   A set of unrealistic beliefs held by family members about each other and family roles

family themes   A family's ideas about its origins and history

family therapy   Therapy involving the total family, selected members, or even one member, in which focus is on family interactions

fantasy   A daydream

fear   A physical and emotional reaction to real or imagined danger

feedback   Negative or positive reinforcement conveyed through communication

fellatio   Oral stimulation of the male genitalia

fetish   An inanimate object such as an article of clothing that produces excitement and sexual pleasure

fixation   The arrest or concentration of psychic energy at a developmental stage where emotional needs have been either overgratified or undergratified

flagellantism   Masochistic or sadistic acts in which one or both partners derive sexual satisfaction from whipping or being whipped

flashbacks   Reliving of past experiences in therapy or under the influence of drugs

flatness of affect   A lack of emotional tone and instead an apathetic, unrelated feeling tone

flight of ideas   A rapid shift from one idea to another with only vague associations between the ideas. Symptom is seen in manic depressives and schizophrenics

flow chart   A method of diagramming events and their interrelationships in a system

folie à deux   A condition in which two closely related persons share the same delusions or pathologic ideas; also called shared paranoid disorder

forensic psychiatry   The branch of psychiatry concerned with legal aspects of psychiatric disorders

foreplay   Sexual stimulation preceding intercourse

formication   The tactile hallucination that insects are crawling on the body, seen in clients suffering delirium tremens

fornication   Voluntary sexual intercourse between unmarried people

free association   Uncensored verbalization by the client of whatever comes to mind

free-floating anxiety   Intense, severe, persistent anxiety

freezing   A family therapy technique whereby the client pantomimes a problem situation and then remains motionless at an important point

frigidity   The female's inability to participate in or enjoy sexual intercourse

frustration   The feeling resulting from inability to meet one's goals

fugue state   A condition in which clients suffer amnesia without knowing this and wander from their homes to unconsciously avoid a current anxiety-provoking situation

functional   Having a psychological rather than an organic cause

fusion   Enmeshment of individuals into a state of oneness

gender identity   The child's experience of being a male or female

gender role   The behaviors expected by society according to whether one is male or female

General Adaptation Syndrome (GAS)   Measurable body changes produced by stress and occurring in the stages of alarm, resistance, and exhaustion

generalization   The process of transferring learning from one situation to other similar situations

genogram   A family chart showing births, deaths, marriages, and so forth, over three generations

genuineness Spontaneous and authentic communication

Gestalt therapy Therapy that focuses on here-and-now experiences and attempts to treat the "whole person" and the interrelations of its component parts

globus hystericus A feeling of a lump in the throat with difficult swallowing, and caused by anxiety

grandiosity An exaggerated, unrealistic perception of one's wealth, power, fame, or ability

grand mal epilepsy A disorder characterized by seizures and loss of consciousness, and often preceded by an aura

grief A self-limited reaction to loss of a person, object, place, or idea

grief work The process of consciously separating from a person, object, place, or idea and reinvesting in a new person, object, and so forth

group Two or more persons interacting in such a way that they influence one another

group therapy Psychotherapy based on the examination of group interaction with a view toward understanding and eventually changing the ways clients interact with others

groupthink "Party line" thinking engaged in by members of a highly cohesive in-group in which agreement and uniformity are crucial and critical thinking is unacceptable

guilt Self-reproach

habituation Psychological dependence on drugs or alcohol

hallucination A sensory perception based on internal stimuli and lacking external reality

hallucinogen A drug producing distorted perceptions and delirium

hebephrenic schizophrenia A disorder characterized by regressive behavior, giggling, disordered thinking, shallow and inappropriate affect, frequent hypochondriacal complaints, and occasionally transient and disorganized hallucinations and delusions; also called schizophrenia, disorganized type

hedonism Consistent pursuit of pleasure and avoidance of pain

helplessness A real or imagined state in which one is at the mercy of fate or others, unable to change

here-and-now approach In therapy, a tendency to focus on what is happening in the present, as opposed to the past

hidden agenda A goal held by one or more people that is hidden from the others in a group

holistic Concerned with the whole person rather than discrete systems or parts

homosexual One who engages in sex with members of the same gender

hopelessness A feeling of extreme pessimism about the future

hostility Anger that is destructive in nature and purpose

hot line A crisis telephone answering service employing counselors, usually on a 24-hour basis

hyperactivity Increased activity, usually accompanied by emotional lability and flight of ideas

hyperkinesis Increased activity seen in some neurologic conditions, especially in children

hyperpyrexia Extremely high fever; can be an adverse effect with antiparkinsonian medications

hypnogogic state The state just before sleep when mental images occur involuntarily

hypnosis An altered state of consciousness during which one may be receptive to suggestion and direction

hypochondriasis Excessive preoccupation with one's physical health, without organic pathology

hypomania A mild state of manic behavior

hysterical personality disorder A disorder characterized by dramatic, emotionally intense, unstable behavior; also called histrionic personality disorder

id A psychoanalytic term for the unconscious aspect of personality containing primitive urges and desires, and ruled by the pleasure principle

idealization Imbuing persons or principles with exaggeratedly positive attributes

ideas of reference The false perception that events relate directly to oneself

identification The unconscious mechanism whereby one takes on characteristics of another

identity The sense of one's self based on experience, memories, perceptions, and emotions

illusion Misperception or misinterpretation of a real experience

immediacy A communication technique in which the nurse responds to interaction between the nurse and client in the here-and-now

impotence Inability of the male to achieve or to maintain an erection

impulsive behavior Unpredictable, unexpected behavior motivated by immediate needs rather than long-range goals

inadequate personality disorder a disorder in which one reacts with ineptness and social instability

inappropriate affect Emotional tone not in keeping with one's thoughts, actions, or genuine feelings

incest Sexual relations between parents and their children or between close relatives

incorporation The symbolic, unconscious taking inside of oneself a person or the person's attributes

individuation The process of becoming a separate, distinct, autonomous person

infantile autism Psychosis in a young child

informational power Power attributed to a person based on information the person is believed to have

insanity A legal term used for mental illness or psychosis

insight Understanding the connection between one's unconscious wishes and one's behavior. Intellectual insight is a cognitive connection only, whereas emotional insight is believed to produce lasting change in behavior

intellectualization The use of thinking and talking to avoid emotions and closeness

intelligence The ability to learn, remember, apply learning to new situations, think logically, and reason abstractly

intermittent explosive disorder A disorder leading to loss of control of aggression, serious assault, and destruction of property

interpersonal theory of psychiatry Harry Stack Sullivan's theory that mental illness is the result of anxiety generated in early interpersonal interaction, and that therapy consists of corrective interpersonal interactions between the therapist and client

interpretation The process by which the therapist offers an explanation of the client's behavior to the client, based on the therapist's objective observations and theory

intimacy Emotional closeness

intoxication Excessive use of a drug or alcohol, leading to maladaptive behavior

intrapsychic Within the self

introjection The unconscious taking in of either loved or hated aspects of a person, usually a parent or significant other

introjects Those aspects of a person that have been taken in as a result of interaction with a significant other

intuition Emotional knowing without thinking or talking

involuntary commitment Confinement in a psychiatric setting without personal consent

involutional psychosis Severe depression seen in clients over 45 years of age who are reacting to changes in body function and life-style

isolated explosive disorder A single episode of loss of control of aggression leading to assault in a person not thought to be schizophrenic or antisocial

isolation The dissociation of feelings from a past thought, memory, or experience

jealousy A painful feeling brought on by the notion that a person with whom one has a close, intimate relationship has an even closer relationship with a third person

judgment The capacity for appropriate, realistic behavior based on an awareness of the consequences of one's behavior

kinesics The study of body movement

kinesthesia Awareness of the movements and positions of the body

kin network A collection of nuclear families who exchange goods and services

kleptomania The failure to resist impulses to steal objects that are then given away, returned secretly, kept, or hidden

Korsakoff's disease A disorder characterized by thiamine deficiency owing to prolonged, heavy use of alcohol

la belle indifference An inappropriate lack of concern, seen in clients with conversion hysteria

labeling A method of describing and categorizing deviant behavior

labile personality disorder A disorder characterized by alternating depression and hypomania, but not sufficiently severe or prolonged as major depressive or manic episodes; also called cyclothymic disorder

language disorders Disorders involving problems learning or using language

latency The stage of growth and development between age 6 years and puberty

latent Hidden, covert

learned helplessness Presumed powerlessness brought about by the lack of reward for assertive behavior and the extinction of assertiveness

legitimate power Power brought about by the belief in a group that this person has the right to influence others

lesbian A female homosexual

lethality assessment A study of the seriousness of a client's intent to commit suicide

libido Sexual drive or motivation

life script Eric Berne's term in transactional analysis for one's unconscious life plan

lithium therapy The use of lithium salts to treat manic or hypomanic states

local adaptation syndrome (LAS) The signs of stress in a discrete part of the body

looseness of association The free flow of thoughts or ideas that appear to have little or no connection to one another

loyalty commitments Unconscious bonds between family members

loyalty conflict A pull toward loyalty to one person, which leads to disloyalty to another

LSD (lysergic acid diethylamide) A drug that can induce a psychoticlike state

magical thinking The belief that thinking something can make it happen, seen in children and psychotic clients

malingering The presentation of false or exaggerated physical or psychological symptoms to accomplish conscious goals, such as avoiding military service, obtaining drugs, obtaining financial compensation

mania A condition of extreme excitement and euphoria, with loss of reality testing

manic depressive illness A severe condition characterized by extreme mania or deep depression; also called bipolar disorder

manifest content The remembered content of a fantasy or dream as opposed to the latent content that is disguised

manipulation The influencing of another for self-gratification

MAO-inhibitor (monoamine oxidase inhibitor) A type of antidepressant that acts by inhibiting the enzyme monoamine oxidase, which oxidizes norepinephrine and serotonin

masochism Unconscious or conscious pleasure when experiencing mental or physical pain

masturbation Sexual stimulation of oneself or another manually, orally, or mechanically

maternal deprivation The absence of adequate physical and emotional care in infancy or childhood

maturational crises Crises triggered by expected developmental life changes, as opposed to situational crises, which are triggered by unexpected events

McNaughten rules A legal precedent commonly used to decide whether a person is criminally responsible for an act, based on whether the person knows right from wrong

melancholia Profound depression

mental retardation A developmental disorder characterized by subnormal intellectual functioning, learning, social adjustment, and maturation

mental status exam An assessment of the client's cognitive impairment used when the client appears disoriented or confused

metacommunication Communication about communication

metarules Rules about rules

migraine A disorder characterized by intense, recurrent, usually one-sided headaches accompanied by nausea and vomiting and thought to be caused by a combination of emotional factors, hormonal levels, and dietary intake

milieu therapy Therapy focused on positive manipulation of the client's environment

minimal brain dysfunction (MBD) A disorder characterized by impaired perception, conceptualization, language comprehension, control of attention, motor function, and impulse control

modeling Behaving in a way designed to set an example for another

multigenerational transmission In family theory, the passing on of ideas, values, and behavior patterns from generation to generation

multi-infarct dementia A disorder caused by vascular disease and characterized by progressive neurologic deterioration, with some intellectual functions left intact. There is disturbance in memory, abstract thinking, judgment, impulse control, and personality.

multiple personality A dissociative disorder in which different distinct ''personalities'' reappear from time to time in the client

mutism refusal to speak for conscious or unconscious reasons

narcissism Self-love or self-involvement seen as normal in childhood but pathologic when extended to the same degree into adulthood

narcissistic personality disorder A personality disorder characterized by a grandiose sense of importance and an exhibitionistic need for attention and admiration

narcolepsy A disorder characterized by involuntary, brief, uncontrollable episodes of sleep

narcosynthesis Interventions used by the therapist in narcotherapy

narcotherapy The use of drugs to interview a client, facilitating the client's expression of feelings

necrophilia Sexual relations with a dead body

neologism A word invented by the client, having no public, consensual meaning

neuroleptics A group of antipsychotic drugs, which produce CNS side effects that mimic extrapyramidal disease such as Parkinson's disease

neurosis A group of disorders characterized by anxiety and nonpsychotic symptoms

nihilism The delusion that the self or part of the self does not exist

nonverbal communication Communication without words, such as body language, gestures, facial expressions

norms Rules established by a group for the ways members should behave

nuclear family Parents and their children, including two generations only

nursing care plan A plan for nursing care including the client's needs, goals for care, and suggested interventions

nymphomania A disorder characterized by an insatiable need for sexual activity in women

object relations Emotional attachments with others

obsession a recurring thought, idea, or impulse that the person is unable to stop or control

obsessive-compulsive disorder A disorder characterized by recurrent obsessions or compulsions, rigidity, perfectionism, overconformity, and self-doubt

occupational therapy A type of therapy designed to help clients to express thoughts and feelings through creative activities and to learn new skills for creative expression

Oedipus complex Sexual feelings toward the parent of the opposite sex and jealousy toward the parent of the same sex, occurring in childhood, between 3 and 6 years of age, and often appearing in unconscious ways in adulthood

omega sign Furrowing between the eyebrows, occurring with depression (Ω)

omnipotence Fantasies of greatness or exaggerated importance

one-to-one relationship A client–therapist relationship formed in the process of crisis intervention or individual therapy

operational mourning A technique in family therapy whereby family members grieve the loss of family members who may have died some years ago without the emotional "working through" of the survivors

oral phase The first phase of psychosexual development in which psychic energy is invested in the mouth, sucking, and eating

orality The persistence of oral pleasure in adulthood seen in eating, smoking, drinking, and excessive dependency

organic brain syndrome (OBS) Psychotic or non-psychotic behavior caused by organic brain damage

organicity Brain damage demonstrated by errors in judgment and memory and loss of coordination

orientation Awareness of time, place, and person

orthomolecular medicine The treatment of schizophrenia with large doses of niacin (B_3); also called megavitamin therapy, niacin therapy

overcompensation A coping mechanism whereby the person experiences an "unacceptable" thought or feeling and acts exaggeratedly the opposite of the thought or feeling

overt Open to observation, not hidden

panic The experience of high anxiety

panic attacks Periods of sudden apprehension or terror, characterized by palpitations, chest pain, choking or smothering sensations, and fear of losing control or going crazy

paradoxical injunction Therapeutic technique in which clients are instructed by the therapist to do consciously what they are doing unconsciously

paralanguage Verbal communication other than words, such as sobs, laughs, moans, and voice quality; also called paralinguistics

paranoid disorder A psychotic disorder characterized by delusions of reference and persecution, and grandiosity

paranoid personality disorder A disorder characterized by suspiciousness, pathological jealousy, hypersensitivity, hypervigilance and secretiveness

paranoid schizophrenia A type of schizophrenia in which the client has a concrete and pervasive delusional system that is usually persecutory

parataxic mode Sullivan's concept describing the experience of events or objects connected on the basis of one or two similarities, yet treated as though they were the same

parent ego strength A transactional analysis term describing aspects of the personality that have been incorporated from the parents

parentification The process by which children are forced to take on the role of "parent" to their own parents or to younger siblings

passive–aggressive behavior Behavior that is seemingly passive but is motivated by unconscious anger and calls out anger and frustration in others, such as lateness, obtuseness, forgetting, "mistakes"

pastoral counseling Counseling by a clergyman usually geared to helping clients with situational or maturational crises

pathologic gambling A condition in which the person has a chronic, progressive compulsion to gamble

pavor nocturnus Night terror brought on by an anxiety dream or nightmare

pederasty Sodomy between a man and boy

pedophilia Sexual activity between an adult and child

penis envy A Freudian term that originally referred to little girls' envy of little boys' penises but later came to mean the female desire for attributes traditionally held by men

perception The process of sensation, interpretation, and comprehension of stimuli in a personal, individual way

perseveration A symptom of organic brain disease whereby the client persists in a single response or idea continually

persona A Jungian term for the external mask or facade that people present to the world

personality The deeply ingrained traits and thoughts characteristic of each individual

personality disorder Mental disorders that originate in the personality and in which there is minimal anxiety or distress, such as compulsive personality or passive–aggressive personality

personal space The area around an individual that the person prefers to have empty or free of intrusion by another

petit mal epilepsy A disorder characterized by sudden, brief lapses of consciousness, twitches, and loss of muscle tone

phallic stage The stage of growth and development between age 3 and 6 years

phallic symbols Objects that represent the penis, such as guns, knives, cigars, bananas

phantom limb The experience of feeling a limb or other body part that has been surgically removed, as if it were still present

phenothiazine derivative A substance derived from phenothiazide and used as an antipsychotic drug

phobia A persistent, irrational fear leading to a compelling desire to avoid the feared object, activity, or situation

pica Persistent eating of a nonnutritive substance, such as plaster, dirt, paint, string, hair, and cloth

placebo A pharmacologically inert substance, such as a sugar or flour pill, used for research or because of its potential psychological effect

plasticity Malleability, the ability to be formed or molded

pleasure principle The tendency to seek pleasure and avoid pain

postpartum psychosis Psychosis following childbirth and associated with schizophrenia, organic, or toxic influences

posttraumatic stress disorder A disorder arising after a traumatic event that is generally outside the range of common experience, for example, military combat, rape, earthquake, floods. Symptoms of anxiety and depression are common

poverty of content of speech Speech that is abundant but conveys little information

poverty of speech Speech that is brief and unelaborated

power The ability to influence others

precocity Unusually early appearance of intellectual or physical characteristics

preconscious Thoughts and feelings on the fringe of awareness that can be brought into awareness with concentration

pregenital The oral and anal stages of development in children

premature ejaculation Male ejaculation early in intercourse before the female partner reaches orgasm

premature grieving Survivor grief felt during the time a person is dying, characterized by emotional withdrawal from the dying person

premorbid Before the disease

prescription of the symptom A therapeutic strategy whereby the client is encouraged to increase the symptom with the hope that this will ultimately decrease it

pressure of speech Speech that is abundant, rapid, difficult to interrupt

primal scene Sexual intercourse viewed or fantasized by a child

primal therapy A type of therapy in which clients reexperience early core pain from infancy and childhood with the goal of relieving the pain and diminishing physical and psychological symptoms

primary gain The main function or use of a symptom for a client, for example, hysterical blindness that prevents the client from reading unpleasant news

primary impotence Abiding inability to obtain or maintain an erection in a man who has never done so

primary orgasmic dysfunction Abiding inability of a female to reach orgasm in a woman who has never done so

primary prevention Attempts to obviate illnesses before they occur by removing possible causes

primary process thinking Primitive thinking such as that of early development, dreams, and psychosis, in which syntaxic logic is absent

primitive idealization An archaic form of intense idealization to protect one from recognizing strong, aggressive, angry tendencies; seen in borderline personality disorders

problem-oriented records Psychiatric records that include a data base, problem list, initial plans, and progress notes

process The nonverbal aspect of interaction between two or more people, such as tone of voice, sequence of topics, and body language

prodromal   Early signs or symptoms of a disorder

projection   The attribution to others of one's own "unacceptable" thoughts and feelings

projective identification   The attribution of one's own "unacceptable" feelings (usually anger) to others who are both feared and desired such that this is the bond between the self and the other. Seen in the borderline personality disorder

projective tests   Personality tests in which relatively unstructured and ambiguous material is presented to the client, who is asked to describe it, thereby allowing the client to project certain aspects of the personality onto the material and thus reveal unconscious thoughts, feelings, wishes, and conflicts. Examples are the Rorschach (inkblot test) and the thematic apperception test (TAT).

prostitution   The provision of sex for money

prototaxic mode   Sullivan's term for the most primitive mode of thought, in which each moment is isolated from the moment before or after it

pseudomutuality   Behavior between two or more persons who appear superficially to be close and happy, but do not have a close emotional connection

pseudoparkinsonian syndrome   Extrapyramidal side effects mimicking Parkinson's disease, including masklike face, shuffling gait, rigidity with flexion of arms, outward rotating tremor of hands seen as a side effect of some antipsychotic medications

psychedelic   Drugs that affect the mind dramatically, for example, LSD

psychiatric aide   A paraprofessional trained to work with psychiatric clients

psychiatric audit   An evaluation of psychiatric care, usually done by comparing clients' charts to predetermined standards of care

psychiatric clinical nurse specialist   A nurse who has graduated from a master's program providing clinical theory and practice in psychiatric nursing, including individual, group, and family therapy

psychiatric social worker   A graduate of a 2-year master's program in social work, with specialization in psychiatry

psychiatrist   A medical doctor who has specialized in psychiatry

psychic determinism   The idea that behavior is not random or accidental, but rather is set in motion by earlier events

psychoanalysis   A treatment modality, first described by Freud, that uses an examination of the client's unconscious processes through dream analysis, fantasies, free association, and examination of the client's transference

psychoanalyst   A physician, psychologist, social worker, or psychiatric nurse who has undergone psychoanalytic training

psychodrama   A type of therapy in which clients' emotional and interactional problems are simulated or acted out dramatically under the direction of a therapist

psychodynamic theory   The idea that current behavior is understandable in light of past behavior

psychogenic   Caused by psychological factors, in the absence of organic pathology

psychological pillow   A position in which the person's head and neck are elevated as though resting on a pillow

psychological tests   Personality tests or intelligence tests usually administered and interpreted by clinical psychologists.

psychomotor agitation   Nonproductive and repetitious motor activity that is excessive and accompanied by anxiety

psychomotor retardation   Excessively slow movement and speech often seen in depressed persons

psychophysiologic disorder   A physical condition brought on by psychological factors. Examples are obesity, tension headaches, neurodermatitis, asthma, ulcer, and ulcerative colitis.

psychosexual development   Emotional and sexual growth from birth to adulthood

psychosexual disorder   Disorders of sexual functioning caused by psychological factors. Examples include transsexualism, gender identity disorder, paraphilia, fetishism, transvestism, zoophilia, pedophilia, exhibitionism, voyeurism, sexual masochism, and sexual sadism

psychosexual dysfunctions   Disorders of psychophysiologic or appetitive changes during the sexual response cycle. These include frigidity, impotence, and ego-dystonic homosexuality

psychosis   A condition of grossly impaired reality testing usually accompanied by delusions and hallucinations

psychosurgery   Surgical removal or interruption of specific areas or pathways in the brain, especially the prefrontal lobes

psychotherapy   A method of treatment based on the development of an intimate relationship between client and therapist for the purpose of exploring and modifying the client's behavior in a satisfying direction

psychotropic Affecting the mind

pyromania A condition in which there is an obsession with setting fires and watching them burn

rage Overpowering angry feelings, usually related to frustration and originating in infantile frustration

rape Forced, involuntary sexual intercourse.

rapport A conscious feeling of mutual respect, harmony, and affection between two people

rationalization An unconscious mechanism whereby a person creates a logical, socially acceptable explanation for a thought, feeling, or action considered unacceptable

reaction formation An unconscious mechanism whereby a person acts the opposite of the actual unconscious feeling experienced, in order to avoid the true feeling

reactive depression Depression occurring as a result of an actual loss

reading disorder Significant impairment in reading development not accounted for by chronologic age, mental age, or inadequate schooling; also called dyslexia

reality principle A learned ego function in which people learn to delay gratification or tension release

reality testing The ability to differentiate one's subjective thoughts and feelings from the objective thoughts and feelings of others

recall Recent memory, the process of retrieving recent memories

reciprocal inhibition The pairing of an anxiety-provoking stimulus with another stimulus of the opposite quality, but strong enough to reduce the anxiety

recreational therapist A mental health worker who provides activities designed to help clients socialize and express thoughts and feelings in a socially acceptable way

referent power Power accorded to a person because others identify with or want to be like the person

regression A return to earlier behavior, usually prompted by anxiety

remission Abatement of illness

reinforcement Reward for a behavioral response

REM sleep The part of the sleep cycle in which rapid eye movement and dreaming occurs. REM sleep is necessary to restore one mentally and emotionally, and occurs for longer periods after a stressful day.

repetition compulsion The unconscious tendency to blindly repeat earlier experience even when there is a conscious desire to stop

repression The unconscious defense of keeping ''unacceptable'' thoughts and feelings out of awareness

rescue fantasy The unrealistic narcissistic need to relieve a client of symptoms or problems

residual The stage of an illness that follows the remission of florid symptoms or the full syndrome

resistance A process whereby powerful unconscious forces prevent clients from giving up defenses and distortions

retardation of thought Excessive slowness in expressing thoughts

reversal The process by which a person acts, thinks, or feels the opposite of an instinctual wish experienced unconsciously

reward power Power attributed to a person in a position to reward others or remove negative aspects of their lives

ritual A behavior repeated for religious, cultural, or pathologic reasons

role Behavior expected of one person by others

role model One who behaves in a way designed for others to copy

role playing A technique in group or family therapy whereby members act out the behavior of others in the group or family

role reversal Exchange of usual behavior between two persons

Rorschach test (inkblot test) A projective personality test in which the person is asked to say what comes to mind when viewing each of ten inkblot cards

rum fits Major motor seizures during withdrawal from alcoholism

rumination Continual thinking about and discussion about a specific subject

rumination disorder of infancy A disorder characterized by repeated regurgitation of food, with weight loss or failure to gain expected weight, developing after a period of normal functioning

sadism Sexual pleasure and erotic gratification obtained from inflicting physical or emotional pain

satyriasis Exaggerated sexual drive in a male

scapegoat The member of a group or family who becomes the target of the group's anger, and is perceived as bad or sick by the others

schismatic family A family that has constant controversy and conflict, particularly between the parents

schizoid personality disorder A personality disorder in which there is a defect in the capacity to form social relationships, the absence of warm, tender feelings for others, and indifference to praise, criticism, and the feelings of others

schizophrenic disorders A group of psychotic disorders that is characterized by regression, thought disturbances, including delusions and hallucinations, bizarre dress and behavior, poverty of speech, abnormal motor behavior, ritualistic behavior, and withdrawal

schizophreniform disorder A schizophrenic state lasting less than 6 months

schizotypal personality disorder A personality disorder in which there are various oddities of thought, perception, speech, and behavior without the extremes found in schizophrenia

school phobia A disorder characterized by a fear of leaving major attachment figures or home; also called separation anxiety disorder

screen memory A consciously acceptable memory, which serves as a cover for another, deeper memory, which is more painful

sculpting A family therapy technique whereby one member creates a living tableau of the other family members, placing them in actual positions vis-à-vis each other, representing their relationships and interactions with one another

secondary gains The advantages clients derive from their illnesses, for example, sympathy, attention, and financial support

secondary impotence A current inability to achieve or maintain an erection in a man who has done so successfully in the past

secondary prevention The early discovery and treatment of disease

security operation Sullivan's term for defense mechanisms used to lessen or avoid anxiety

selective inattention The process of filtering out aspects of an experience under conditions of moderate or severe anxiety

self-actualization Becoming all one is capable of becoming by using all of one's potential

self-awareness Sensitivity to one's own motives, thoughts, feelings, wishes, and so forth

self-concept A person's image of the self

self-esteem A person's degree of confidence, worth, and competence

self-fulfilling prophecy A self-destructive process by which a person holds a certain distorted belief and then unconsciously goes about making that belief a reality

self-mutilation Self-disfigurement of one's own body, frequently seen in clients with borderline personality disorder

self-system Sullivan's concept of the self developed during childhood as a result of reflected appraisals of significant others

senile dementia Progressive memory impairment, apathy, and withdrawal in clients over 65 years of age

sensorium Consciousness

sensory deprivation Diminution of sensory stimuli, leading to personality changes and inner perceptual distortions

sensory overload Increased sensory stimuli leading to signs of stress

separation anxiety Tension experienced in relation to moving away from a significant person

separation anxiety disorder A disorder of childhood and adolescence characterized by stomach aches, headaches, nausea, and vomiting when there is the threat of separation from the home or parents; also called school phobia

sex therapy Treatment of sexual dysfunction by a qualified therapist

shaping A technique designed to change a client's behavior

shared paranoid disorder A disorder developing as a result of a close relationship with another person who has persecutory delusions, such that the delusions are partially shared; also called folie à deux

sibling position A person's position vis-à-vis brothers and sisters in terms of birth order

sibling rivalry Competition among brothers and sisters

sick role A position of "patient" adopted by a person to satisfy dependency needs

sign An objective manifestation of pathology, observable by others

significant other Sullivan's term for those who played an important role in development of a child's self-system; today, used to designate those who are important to a client

single-parent family A family consisting of a mother or father and offspring

situational crisis A crisis brought on by a traumatic external event

situational orgasmic dysfunction A disorder whereby a woman is able to achieve orgasm only under certain situations

skewed families Families in which one parent has a serious personality problem, which is covered over through tacit agreement so that the family appears to function without conflict

sleep terror disorder A disorder characterized by continual episodes of abrupt awakening from sleep, screaming, intense anxiety, and agitation; also called pavor nocturnus

sleepwalking disorder A disorder characterized by continual episodes of awakening from sleep and walking, followed by amnesia for the event

SOAP A method of record keeping used in problem-oriented records. The acronym is formed as follows: S for *subjective* (client's view of the problem), O for *objective* (clinical findings), A for *assessment* (analyses and syntheses of subjective and objective data), P for *plan* (proposed method of handling the client's problems).

social network One's system of social relationships that can be used as a support system in a crisis

social network therapy Therapy designed to mobilize those around the client to be helpful, or clients to help one another

social phobia A disorder in which the client has a persistent fear of situations where there may be scrutiny by others, for example, public speaking or performance, using public bathrooms, or eating in public

sociopathic personality The client who engages in chronic antisocial behavior, is unable to sustain jobs, and often abuses drugs; also called antisocial personality disorder

sociotherapy Therapy that focuses on the environment rather than intrapsychic factors

sodomy Any sex act other than face-to-face coitus between a man and woman. The legal meaning varies from state to state.

somatic delusion A false belief that the body is changing in an unusual way, for example rotting inside

somatic language Messages that are translated into physical symptoms

somatic therapy Treatment of mental illness by physical means, for example, drug therapy or electroconvulsive therapy

somatization disorders Disorders characterized by recurrent and multiple somatic complaints of several years' duration for which medical attention has been sought but which are apparently not caused by physical disorders

somatoform disorders A category of disorders, including somatization disorder and conversion disorder, in which physical symptoms occur without demonstrable organic findings

somnambulism Sleepwalking; a dissociative state in which the person walks about while sleeping

SRO (single room occupancy) A hotel or boardinghouse where deinstitutionalized clients may live

split personality See multiple personality

splitting Active separation of affects of opposite quality so that one does not contaminate the other. The client sees people or events as all good or all bad

Stanford-Binet Scale An intelligence test for children

staus A collection of rights and duties accorded to a group member by other members

stereotyped behavior Repeated speech or motor behavior, often seen in schizophrenia. Examples include echolalia and echopraxia.

stereotyped movement disorder A group of disorders involving an abnormality of gross motor movements. Examples include all tics and Tourette's disorder

stress Tension

stress-adaptation theory A framework for understanding the effect of stress on individuals

stressor A person or experience that produces tension

sublimation The conscious or unconscious channeling of "unacceptable" drives into acceptable activities

substance use disorder A group of disorders characterized by the abuse of addictive substances such as alcohol, drugs, and tobacco

substitution The unconscious replacement of an "unacceptable" wish, goal, or emotion with an acceptable one

suicide Self-inflicted death

superego The aspect of personality, known as the conscience, that includes one's ego ideals

superficiality Lightness of interpersonal contact used to protect one from intimacy or emotional closeness

supportive psychotherapy Therapy aimed at reinforcing defenses, particularly repression

support system Aspects of the environment that provide comfort or security, including people or material objects (home, place, money, job)

suppression The process by which disturbing or "unacceptable" thoughts and feelings are consciously forced out of awareness

symbiosis The close bond between infant and mother in which both appear fused. When occurring between adults, this seeming lack of boundaries is considered pathologic

symbolization The abstract process whereby one object or idea represents another, for example, a big car may represent power and prestige

symmetrical relationships Relationships in which equality is a priority

symptom An objective or subjective manifestation of pathology

symptom substitution The replacement of one symptom with another when the first is removed. Adversaries of behavior modification believe that when one symptom is removed or extinguished, another may take its place, since the underlying problem may not be solved.

syndrome A group of symptoms that occur together and that constitute a recognizable condition

synesthesia Seeing colors when a loud sound is heard

syntaxic mode Sullivan's term for the mode of experience in which past, present, and future are recognized and events are perceived in logical sequence.

system A group of people in interaction or interrelationship, where there is a boundary around them, the whole is more than the sum of its parts, and any change in one part affects the whole group

tangentiality The tendency to deviate from the central idea in a communication and to move the conversation off in another direction

tardive dyskinesia A condition occurring after years of antipsychotic drug treatment. The client has involuntary movements of the face, jaw, and tongue, lip smacking, drooling, and protrusion of the tongue

task-oriented groups Groups brought together to accomplish a task, for example, "activities of daily living" groups

TAT (thematic apperception test) A projective test in which subjects are shown a series of drawings suggesting life situations, and are asked to tell a story about each drawing

territoriality The tendency to perceive a space or function as "belonging" to one's self or one's group

tertiary prevention The elimination or reduction of the aftermath of illness; rehabilitation

therapeutic That which is thought to heal

therapeutic alliance A relationship between a client and a helping person with the goal of helping the client

therapeutic community A method of therapy whereby clients are helped to understand their interpersonal problems through continual examination of their interactions with one another and with staff. Elements are democratization, permissiveness, communalism, and reality confrontation.

therapeutic community meetings Regularly held meetings with all clients and staff in a therapeutic community

thought disorder A condition seen often in schizophrenia in which the client shows loose, bizarre, illogical, confused, or abrupt thinking

tic An involuntary, rapid movement of a related group of muscles or the involuntary production of noises or words

tobacco dependence The continual use of tobacco for at least one month with either 1) unsuccessful attempts to stop or reduce the amount of tobacco use permanently, 2) the development of tobacco withdrawal, or 3) the presence of serious physical disorder, *e.g.*, respiratory or cardiovascular disease, that the individual knows is exacerbated by tobacco use

tolerance The condition in drug or alcohol addiction when increasing amounts are needed to produce the desired effects

Tourette's disorder A disorder characterized by recurrent, involuntary, repetitive, rapid movements (tics), including multiple verbal tics resembling clicks, grunts, yelps, barks, sniffs, coughs, or words

trance A state of diminished activity and consciousness resembling sleep and seen in hypnosis, hysteria, and ecstatic religious states

tranquilizer A drug that depresses central nervous system function, calming the person without impairing the client's ability to function

transactional analysis (TA) A system of therapy introduced by Eric Berne whereby the client carefully examines modes of interaction with others

Transcendental Meditation (TM) A learned meditation technique in which the individual sits quietly with closed eyes, concentrating on a mantra with the goal of relieving tension and improving body sensations and interpersonal relations

transference The attribution to the therapist of thoughts, feelings, wishes, and needs originally felt toward the parent or significant other

transient situational disturbance A group of disorders that involve maladaptive reactions to an identifiable psychosocial stressor, that occurs within 3 months after the onset of the stressor; also called adjustment disorder

transsexual An individual who engages in sex with members of the same gender and who longs to belong to the opposite gender

transvestite An individual who dresses in clothing of the opposite gender

trauma An event producing intense anxiety

triangle An interpersonal configuration or event involving three persons

triangulation Dysfunctional communication and behavior in an interpersonal triangle, usually involving the alliance of two people against the third

tricyclics The most commonly used antidepressant drugs

unconscious Mental processes that are dissociated or out of conscious awareness

undoing A compulsive act whereby the person reverses a previous act that caused anxiety

urolangia Sexual pleasure from urinating on another or being urinated on

vaginismus Involuntary contraction of the vagina, making intercourse painful or impossible

values Internal priorities about the worth of various aspects of life

values clarification A process by which clients become aware of their values and behave accordingly

Varaguth's sign A sign of depression in which there is angulation of the inner end of the fold of skin in the upper eyelid

vertigo Dizziness associated with faintness

voluntary commitment The process whereby a client or guardian agrees in writing to enter a mental hospital

voyeur One who receives sexual pleasure from looking at others

waxy flexibility A condition seen in catatonic schizophrenia in which the client remains in a position in which he or she is placed; also called cerea flexibilitas

Wernicke-Korsakoff disease A disorder caused by thiamine deficiency associated with prolonged alcohol use. Symptoms are amnesia, confusion, and disorientation.

withdrawal Movement away from reality or from interpersonal conflict

withdrawal symptoms Physical and psychological manifestations occurring when a person stops using an addictive substance

word salad The use of words and phrases without logical connection

zoophilia Sexual relations with animals

Index

abreaction, 635
abstract thinking, cultural aspects, 611
acceptance, of dying, 367
accountability, 635
  crisis center, 47
    record keeping, 52
  in private practice, 175
accreditation, 635
  crisis center, 52
acetophenazine (Tindol), 552
acquiescent behavior, 350
acquired immune deficiency syndrome
    (AIDS), 146
acting in, 635
acting out, 201, 635
  anxiety and, 389
  in borderline personality disorder, 420
  community response to, 65
  in deinstitutionalized client, 123
  in group therapy, 216
  in individual therapy, 204
activities of daily living (ADL) groups,
    274–283
  components, 275
  conduction, 275
  evaluation, 283
  health and personal hygiene, 276
  housing, 276, 277–278
  in inpatient program, 97
  leisure time planning, 279, 281–283
  meal planning and preparation, 278–279
  money management, 279, 280–281
  nursing interventions, 275
    health and personal hygiene, 276
    housing needs, 277–278
    leisure time planning, 281
    meal planning and preparation,
      278–279
    money management, 280–281
  professional practice standards, 623
  purpose, 275
  techniques, 275
activity group therapy, for children, 252
activity therapy
  in alcoholism program, 86
  in gerontological counseling, 362
acupuncture, for sleep disorders, 463
adaptation, in group therapy, 214
adaptive regression in service of ego
    (ARISE), assessment, 12–13
adaptive stage, in individual therapy, 204
addiction, 635
adjustment, 635
adjustment disorder, DSM-III codes, 633
administrator
  adolescent therapy program, 138
  day hospital program, 105
  outpatient therapy program, 127, 128
adolescence, 635
  affective changes, 263
  changes in relationships, 263
  changes in thinking, 263
  family therapy, 268, 269
  mental disorders, DSM-III categories
    and codes, 629
  physical maturation, 263
  problems of, 264
  reaction to rape, 479

tasks of, 264
adolescent therapy, 134–142, 262–272
  activities, 140
  administrative structure, 138
  client government, 140
  client–management relationships, 140
  community assessment, 135
  community meetings, 138
  controls, 141
  daily program schedule, 141
  day program, 134–142
  impact of puberty, 263
  individual therapy, 264–268, *see also*
    individual therapy, with
    adolescent
  inpatient program, 134–142
  meetings, 138, 139
  nursing relationships, 140
  philosophy of program, 135
  physical facility, 136
  program evaluation, 142
  psychotherapy, 138
  rituals, 141
  spontaneous groups, 140
  staff qualifications and roles, 135–137
  therapeutic milieu, 137–141
  treatment modalities, 138, 140–141
adult, reaction to rape, 479–480
adult ego state, 307–313
aerophagia, 635
affect, 635
  assessment of current status in client, 10
  blunting of, 636
  cultural aspects, 611
  in depression, 394
  inappropriate, 641
  overactive client, 442
  regulation and control, assessment of, 11
affective disorders, 569
  catatonia in, 26
  DSM-III codes, 632
  depersonalization in, 23
  organic, depression in, 19
  suicide in, 399
affective psychosis, 635
affiliation, crisis center, 47–48
aftercare
  alcoholism program, 86–87
  for schizophrenics, 152
age/aging, *see also* gerontological
    counseling
  psychodynamics of, 358
  suicide potential and, 30
aggression, 635
aggressive behavior, 350
  leather restraints for, 526
  in organically brain damaged client, 439
  seclusion for, 524–525, 527
  verbal intervention, 523
aggressive stage, individual therapy, 202
agitated involutional depression syndrome,
    569
agitation, 635
agnosia, 635
agoraphobia, 605, 635
agranulocytosis, antipsychotic medications
    and, 558
akathisia, 635

antipsychotic medications and, 557
akinesia, 635
  antipsychotic medications and, 557
Akineton (biperiden), 558
alcohol abuse
  suicide potential and, 32
  withdrawal delirium, visual
    hallucinations in, 22
alcohol use
  mental disorders and, DSM-III codes,
    630
  sleep disorders and, 461, 463–464
Alcoholics Anonymous (AA), 85–86
alcoholism, 423–427
  acute alcohol intoxication, nursing
    interventions, 425
  behavior characteristics, 424–425, 427
  biological factors, 424
  definition, 635
  delirium tremens, 425
  etiology, 424
  nonproductive reactions of nurses, 427
  nursing interventions, 426
  prevention and outreach, 87–88
  psychological theories, 424
  recovery phases, 82
  social forces, 424
  treatment, *see* alcoholism program
alcoholism program, 81–88
  Alcoholics Anonymous, 85–86
  basic principles, 82
  goals, 82
  inpatient
    activities therapy, 86
    daily routine, 83
    didactic groups, 84
    discharge/aftercare groups, 86–87
    evaluation, 87
    group therapy, 84
    rules and regulations, 83
    staff meetings, 84
    structure, 82–84
    study groups, 84
    therapists in, 87
    treatment modalities, 84–87
  outpatient, 87
  prevention and outreach, 87–88
alienation, 635
aliphatic phenothiazines, 551
alternative family, 635
Alzheimer's disease, 635
ambivalence, 635
  in suicidal state, 29
amenorrhea, antipsychotic medications and,
    557
American Nurses' Association (ANA)
  Model Nurse Practice Act of 1976, 599
  Standards of Psychiatric and Mental
    Health Nursing Practice, 619–
    628
American Psychiatric Association, DSM-III
    classification, 629–633
American Psychological Association
    (APA), guidelines for therapy
    with women, 606
amitriptyline (Elavil), 570
amnesia, 635
  organic causes, 27